Multicultural Handbook of Food,
Nutrition and Dietetics

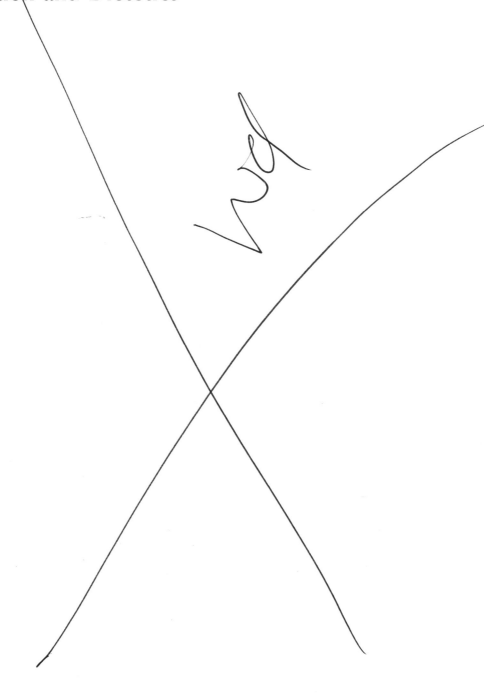

Multicultural Handbook of Food, Nutrition and Dietetics

Edited by

Aruna Thaker BSc PGDip RD

Retired Chief Dietitian

Arlene Barton MPhil BSc (Hons) RD

Lecturer in Clinical Nutrition and Dietetics
HPC Registered Dietitian, UK
University of Nottingham

WILEY-BLACKWELL

A John Wiley & Sons, Ltd., Publication

This edition first published 2012
© 2012 by Blackwell Publishing Ltd

Wiley-Blackwell is an imprint of John Wiley & Sons, formed by the merger of Wiley's global Scientific, Technical and Medical business with Blackwell Publishing.

Registered office: John Wiley & Sons, Ltd, The Atrium, Southern Gate, Chichester, West Sussex, PO19 8SQ, UK

Editorial offices: 9600 Garsington Road, Oxford, OX4 2DQ, UK
                       The Atrium, Southern Gate, Chichester, West Sussex, PO19 8SQ, UK
                       2121 State Avenue, Ames, Iowa 50014-8300, USA

For details of our global editorial offices, for customer services and for information about how to apply for permission to reuse the copyright material in this book please see our website at http://www.wiley.com/Wiley-Blackwell.

Library of Congress Cataloging-in-Publication Data
Food, nutrition, and dietetics : a multicultural handbook / edited by
Aruna Thaker, Arlene Barton
        p. ; cm.
   Includes bibliographical references and index.
   ISBN 978-1-4051-7358-2 (pbk. : alk. paper)
   I. Thaker, Aruna   II. Barton, Arlene
   [DNLM: 1. Diet–ethnology.   2. Food.   3. Cultural Characteristics.   4. Dietetics.   5. Nutritional Physiological Phenomena–ethnology.   QT 235]
   613.2–dc23
                            2011035251

A catalogue record for this book is available from the British Library.

Wiley also publishes its books in a variety of electronic formats. Some content that appears in print may not be available in electronic books.

Set in 9.5/11.5 pt Palatino by Toppan Best-set Premedia Limited
Printed and bound in Malaysia by Vivar Printing Sdn Bhd

[1   2012]

Contents

Contributors

Editors

Aruna Thaker BSc PGDip RD, Retired Chief Dietitian, Purley, Surrey. Formerly at Community Services Wandsworth, Nutrition and Dietetic Service, London

Arlene Barton BSc(Hons) MPhil RD, Lecturer in Clinical Nutrition and Dietetics, The University of Nottingham, Sutton Bonington, Loughborough, Leicestershire

Contributors

Zenab Ahmad BSc RD, Dietitian, King George Hospital, Goodmayes, Ilford, Essex

Lorraine Bailey BSc RD MSc, Nutrition Specialist, Nestlé Research Centre, Lausanne, Switzerland

Dr Suzanne Barr BSc(Hons), MSc, PhD, RD, Division of Diabetes & Nutritional Sciences School of Medicine King's College, London

Heidi Chan BSc(Hons) RD, Senior Specialist Metabolic Dietitian National Hospital for Neurology and Neurosurgery, London

Keynes Chan BSc (Hons) RD, Macmillan Oncology Dietitian, South London Healthcare Trust, The Princess Royal University Hospital, Orpington, Kent

Wynnie Yuan Yee Chan BSc PhD RPH, Freelance Nutritionist and Health Writer, Hong Kong

Mary Foong Fong Chong BSc(Hons) PhD, Singapore Institute of Clinical Sciences, Brenner Centre for Molecular Medicine, Singapore

Thushara Dassanayake BSc PGDip RD, Specialist Renal Dietitian, Imperial College Healthcare NHS Trust, London

Zelalem Debebe BSc RD, Adult and Lead Paediatric Dietitian, Hounslow & Richmond Community Health Care, West Middlesex University Hospital, Isleworth, Middlesex

Maclinh Duong BSc(Hons) RD, Primary Care Nutrition Care Dietitian, Community Services Wandsworth, St John's Therapy Centre, London

Mandy Fraser BSc(Hons) RD, Public Health and Sports Nutrition Post Graduate Certificate Specialist, Paediatric HEF Dietitian, Central London, Community Healthcare NHS Trust Westminster, Woodfield Road Medical Centre, London

Fumi Fukuda BSC RD Community Dietitian, British Forces, Germany Medical Centre, Hammersmith Barracks, Herford

Eulalee Green BSc MSc RD Dietitian, Health Development Manager, Maternal & Child Nutrition, Ealing, London

Kalpana Hussain BSc RD, Paediatric Dietitian, Porters Avenue Health Centre, Romford, Essex

Rose Jackson BSc(Hons) RD MSc, Diabetes Specialist Dietitian, Queen Mary's Hospital, Roehampton

Bushra Jafri BSc RD, Renal Dietitian, Lister Hospital, Stevenage, Hertfordshire

Susanna Johnson BSc RD, Senior Dietitian, Hounslow & Richmond Community Health Care, West Middlesex University Hospital, Isleworth, Middx

Ruth Kander BSc(Hons) RD, Specialist Renal Dietitian, Imperial College Healthcare NHS Trust, Hammersmith Hospital, London

Maureen Lee, Health Visitor, Kensington and Chelsea Primary Care Trust, London

Renuka McArthur BSc MSc RD DDPHN DHA PGCE, Consultant Dietitian and Health Educator, Diabetes Specialist Centre, Gulf State, Dubai

Christina Merrifield BSc (Hons) RD, Lead Dietitian, Cromwell Hospital, London

Kashena Mohadawoo BSc (Hons) RD, Community Dietitian, Community Services Wandsworth, St John's Therapy Centre, London

Afsha Mugha BSc (Hons) RD, Paediatric Dietitian, The London NHS Trust, King George's Hospital, Goodmayes Redbridge, London

Rabia Nabi BSc RD Intermediate Care Dietitian, Hainault Health Centre, Hainault, Essex

Lindy Parfrey BSc RD, Dietitian, South Australia

Damyanti Patel SRN, National Diversity Coordinator, Macmillan Cancer Support, London

Ruple Patel BSc(Hons) RD, Specialist Renal Dietitian and Master NLP Practitioner, St Helier Hospital, Carshalton, Surrey

Shamaela Perwiz BSc (Hons) RD MSc, Community Dietitian, London

Stavroulla Petrides BSc(Hons) PGDip RD, Specialist Dietitian in Chronic Disease, Enfield Primary Care Trust, Enfield

Rupindar Sahota BSc RD, Diabetes Specialist Dietitian, Hounslow & Richmond Community Health Care, West Middlesex University Hospital, Isleworth, Middlesex

Tahira Sarwar, Specialist BSc(Hons) ADDP RD, Diabetes Dietitian, Community Nutrition and Dietetics Department, Nottingham

Vanitha Subbu BSc PgDip RD, Community Specialist Dietitian, Northwick Park Hospital, Harrow, Middlesex

Natalie Sutherland BSc RD, Dietitian for Stroke, South London Healthcare NHS Trust, London

Elzbieta Szymula MSc PGDip RD, Specialist Cardiovascular Disease Dietitian, Central London Community Healthcare, Lisson Grove Health Centre, London

Ravita Taheem BSc PGDip RD, Community Development Dietitian, Southampton University Hospitals Trust, Southampton, Hants

Angela Telle BSc RD, Nutrition Consultan, Illumina Lifestyle Consulting, Hornchurch, Essex

Aruna Thaker BSc PgDip RD, Retired Chief Dietitian, Wandsworth PCT, London

Deborah Thompson BSc RD, Dietitian, The Princess Royal University Hospital, Orpington, Kent

Sunita Wallia MSc RD PGDip ADP, Specialist Community Dietitian, NHS Greater Glasgow and Clyde, Glasgow

Ghazala Yousuf BSc MSc RD, Specialist Paediatric Dietitian The Portland Hospital, London

Rita Žemaitis BSc RD, Dietitian, Westminster Primary Care Trust, London

Acknowledgements

The editors are grateful to following people for their assistance with coordinating the contents of the multipart chapters.

Arit Ana MSc BSc PGDip RD, Freelance Consultant in Public Health Nutrition, Trainer and Writer, Luton, Beds

Auline Cudjoe BSc(Hons) RD Primary Care Prescribing Lead Dietitian, Community Services Wandsworth, St John's Therapy Centre, London

Shahzadi Uzma Devje BSc PGDip MSc RD, Mississauga Diabetes Centre, Mississauga, Ontario, Canada

Eulalee Green BSc RD MSc, Dietitian, Health Development Manager, Maternal & Child Nutrition, Ealing

Dr Yvonne Jeanes BSc PhD RD, Senior Lecturer,Clinical Nutrition Health Sciences Research Centre, Department of Life Sciences, Roehampton University, London

Sema Jethma BSc RD, Nutrition Consultant, Hainault, Essex

Deepa Kariyawasam BSc(Hons) RD, Senior Renal Dietitian, King's College Hospital, Denmark Hill, London

Thomina Mirza BSc RD, Children Centres Dietitian, St Bartholomew's Hospital and the London NHS Trust, London

Tahira Sarwar, Specialist BSc ADDP RD, Diabetes Dietitian, Community Nutrition and Dietetics Department, Nottingham

Jevanjot Kaur Sihra BSc RD, Food Development Dietitian, Sandwell Primary Care Trust, West Midlands

Sarah Toule BSc(Hons) MSc, Project Manager African Caribbean Communities, Prostate Cancer Organization, London

Emma Tsoi BSc MSc PGDip RD, Specialist Dietitian for Continuing Care, Central London Community Healthcare, Soho Centre for Health & Care, London

Tahira Sarwar, Specialist BSc(Hons) ADDP RD, Diabetes Dietitian, Community Nutrition and Dietetics Department, Nottingham

Eulalee Green BSc MSc RD Dietitian, Health Development Manager, Maternal & Child Nutrition, Ealing, London

The editors and contributors gratefully acknowledge the following for reading and usefully commenting on their sections in this volume:

Karishma Desai BSc, London

Rathika Howarth BSc MA DDPHN, Research and Community Development Consultant, London

Mrs Jagpoonia BA PGDip, Ethnic Dimension, London

Naomi Joseph BSc(Hons) RD, London

Nicholas S Kempton BA(Hons), Hartshill, Warwickshire

Sajeda Malek BSc(Hons), Surrey

Rabbi David Meyer MBA NPQH, London

Dr Gita Patel PhD, Senior Clinical Research Associate, London

Shehlata Patel BCom, Devon

Dr Pushpa Ranjan MD, Wijesinghe Ministry of Health Care and Nutrition, Colombo, Sri Lanka

Christopher Reynolds, Editor, London

Foreword

It is a pleasure to write the Foreword to this *Multicultural Handbook of Food, Nutrition and Dietetics*. As the editors say in their Introduction, they and their several contributors from many different backgrounds 'had a vision that culturally appropriate dietary information was needed..'. Some 30 years ago, there was virtually no systematic nor clear realisation in Britain or other European countries of what 'culturally appropriate' meant, and certainly little practical dietary information for specific peoples of any background. So this text brings together, probably for the first time, comprehensive portraits of regional and local ethnic and geographic food patterns and what is known of their relationship to the emergence of 'chronic disease' in respective populations. Having authors from many of those backgrounds write their relevant chapters adds key value, where outsiders would have been less able to grasp subtleties needed to understand food choice and dietary behaviour.

The editors should be congratulated on choosing appropriate authors, as should be the authors on delivering their effective texts. Each chapter begins with a brief historical outline, of how migration developed to Britain and more globally, who migrated, and where possible a sketch of how ties with original countries were maintained, helping reinforce trading to allow continued traditional diets to persist. Dietary variation *within* South Asian origin communities has been the most neglected aspect of the considerable work now available, summarised elegantly in Chapter 1. In some settings, notably for African-origin people across the western hemisphere, the mortality on transport ships and conditions under slavery meant little direct connection with original western African roots could persist. Traditional foods faded for African-Americans, lost historically via forced transit only through the Caribbean, and with different climates for growing such crops. However, yams, sweet potato, edoes, occasionally cassava, and then green bananas and especially for Jamaicans, breadfruit still form a main focus of many Caribbean-origin households at home and abroad. While household soups remain strong features, dietary patterns are generally quite distinct from most directly west African peoples' diets. Hence the term 'African-Caribbean' is confusing – and should not include people of direct West African, and of Caribbean origin of African, descent under one heading. Chapter 6 outlining data from Ghana and Nigeria redresses that balance.

Throughout, the text is 'flavoured' intriguingly with historical vignettes, as in Chapter 2 on the West Indies, that shows that the word 'barbeque' may have originated from the conquered Arawak or Taino Indians when the Caribbean islands were first colonised by Europeans. Chapter 3 on east Asia, and notably Chinese migration, both historically and now short-term, is of great relevance with so many current Chinese government-funded projects globally, not least as dietary patterns change rapidly and for concerns over the traditionally high salt intakes both from popular Chinese cooking, and also in Japan. In both these dynamic nations and their migrants, high stroke rates from elevated blood pressure may be related to excess salt intakes, and rising smoking habits, which change dietary preferences but have often been minimised by religious restrictions elsewhere. There are also major opportunities in China itself to test whether formal trials, and/or local and regional government and tax initiatives, can cut that high salt content, and the over-consumption of both food and drink that goes with it. The authors bring out important results from Hong Kong, showing that short sleeping hours in a large survey was associated with higher BMI and presumably over-eating. Then a particularly welcome Chapter 5 contains important data on people of Eastern Mediterranean mainly of Arab origin, including Yemenis and Somalis, long-neglected but growing groups often but not just originally refugees, following the ravages of war and civil disruption. The fascinating account in Chapter 7

from among large UK groups of people from Polish, Greek and Turkish backgrounds and these original countries, plugs an important gap, at least in my reading. The final chapters set all this work into their maternal and child health & more clinical context.

The scientific basis generally remains wanting to link reliably particular food patterns, respective nutrient intakes, and their biochemical translation with most chronic 'disease' outcomes. In part, this is because the phenotypes of, for example, (high) blood pressure, almost as variable as food patterns in its measurement, and type 2 diabetes lack precision, except as related to excess body fat and less muscle mass. While basic and clinical science grapple with those issues, this book offers both general and more specialist readers insights into improving the measurement and understanding of diet among many of the world's major populations who migrated to Europe and beyond. It will be a very useful reference for any modern, properly informed health practitioner.

Kennedy Cruickshank
King's College & King's Health Partners, London
December 2011

Introduction

The UK is now a multicultural society and so dietitians and other health and food providers need to be aware not only of the medical aspects of a patient's condition but also their cultural requirements in terms of religion and traditional food choices.

In the 20th century, young men from different ethnic groups arrived in the United Kingdom from the former British colonies. These men arrived for work and had varying skill levels from unskilled to professional workers. Many of these men subsequently settled permanently with their families in this country. Research has shown that the traditional diets of their country of birth can, in most cases, be relatively healthy. However, following migration, lifestyle changes occur which can bring detrimental effects to their health. The incidence of chronic illness has been shown to dramatically increase in these minority groups, especially among the first generation of migrant workers.

In the western world there are increasing levels of obesity, cardiovascular disease and diabetes affecting all ethnic groups. It is important when developing strategies to address these issues and also when seeing individual clients to ensure that the messages are culturally acceptable.

Many registered and student dietitians have admitted that they have limited knowledge of the cultural requirements of the ethnic minorities they do not come into contact with regularly. When a patient or client is referred to them there are few resources to consult to ensure that any dietetic treatment takes into account their religious or cultural needs and habitual food choices.

The editors and contributors had a vision that culturally appropriate dietary information was needed. And it was as a result of discussions with colleagues and students wishing to expand their knowledge that this vision was realized in this handbook.

The aim of this multi-contributor volume is to take this vision a step forward and provide in-depth dietary information on well-established as well as recently migrated ethnic groups.

The book is divided into nine main chapters:

1 South Asian Sub-continent
2 West Indies
3 East Asia
4 Israel
5 Eastern Mediterranean Region
6 West Africa
7 East and South East Europe
8 Maternal and Child Nutrition
9 Nutritional Management of Disease

In each of these chapters there are sections that relate to particular cultural groups from that region. It is envisaged that if you want information about a particular group you can go directly to the relevant section; however, you may find links to other chapters where more detail is available.

The authors of each section are experienced registered dietitians, mainly from the cultural group they are writing about. Each contributor not only has expert dietetic knowledge, but also long and varied experience of the traditional diets and diets on migration of the ethnic group. This makes the text highly practical. The editors have also contributed from their own experience and from the limited research data available for ethnic groups. The editors and contributors acknowledge that there are many lacunae in the literature as often different cultural groups are grouped together in research studies, which makes generalization difficult.

This book offers practical information about traditional diets, how they have changed on migration and the impact this will have on migrants' health. It gives much needed insight into the foods commonly eaten in traditional diets and suitable alternatives available in the UK. It also provides best practice information and, where possible, what support is available from well-established voluntary organizations.

It is hoped that this resource will be valuable not only to dietitians and students who are presently working with different black and minority ethnic groups but also to other professionals who want deeper understanding of the needs of different ethnic groups.

Many people have played a part in the creation of this handbook and the editors would like to thank them all for their very valuable contribution.

Aruna Thaker and Arlene Barton
October 2011

1

South Asian Sub-continent

Sema Jethma, Ruple Patel, Aruna Thaker (Gujarat), Renuka McArthur, Jevanjot Sihra, Rupinder Sahota, Ravita Taheem, Sunita Wallia (Punjab), Zenab Ahmad, Bushra Jafri, Afsha Mughal, Rabia Nabi, Shamaela Perwiz, Tahira Sarmar, Ghazala Yousuf (Pakistan), Kalpana Hussain, Thomina Mirza (Bangladesh), Thushara Dassanayake, Deepa Kariyawasam, Vanitha Subhu (Sri Lanka)

The cultural groups from Gujarat, Punjab, Pakistan, Bangladesh and Sri Lanka have migrated from the South Asian subcontinent to the United Kingdom from different regions over last 60 years, mostly due to economic and political upheavals, and made the UK their home. As a result of the vast distances between the countries there were many differences in their cultural, traditional beliefs and diets but also many similarities as well. The reasons for these changes are many, but lifestyle changes, especially dietary changes, have had the greatest impact on health. The traditional diets which they were following were much healthier, more in line with what is currently recommended, but inclusions of some of the host country's unhealthy foods are having detrimental effects. This is now highlighted in scientific research; however, much of this is generic to those of South Asian origin rather than related to specific cultural groups. In this book, for the first time, an attempt has been made to provide detailed information on each of group. There is information on migration, traditional diets and changes in migration, religious influences and on dietary considerations for specific diseases, such as obesity, diabetes and cardiovascular disease.

1.1 Gujarati Diet

Sema Jethma, Ruple Patel, Aruna Thaker

1.1.1 Introduction

The South Asian sub-continent comprises India, Pakistan, Bangladesh and Sri Lanka. Four per cent of the total UK population is classified as 'Asian' or 'Asian British' and this group makes up 50.2% of the UK minority ethnic population (UK Census, 2001).

'South Asian' defines many ethnic groups, with distinctive regions of origin, languages, religions and customs, and includes people born in India, Bangladesh, Pakistan or Sri Lanka (Fox, 2004).

Multicultural Handbook of Food, Nutrition and Dietetics, First Edition. Edited by Aruna Thaker, Arlene Barton.
© 2012 Blackwell Publishing Ltd. Published 2012 by Blackwell Publishing Ltd.

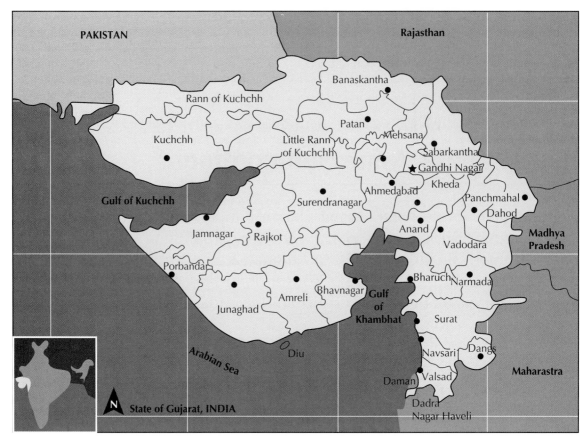

Figure 1.1.1 Map of Gujarat

Gujarat state is situated on the west coast of India and boasts a 1,600 km-long coastline. The Arabian Sea sweeps the western and south-western frontiers. The state extends from Kutch in the west to Daman in the south, with Pakistan to the north-west and the state of Rajasthan to the north and north-east. To the east is Madhya Pradesh and Maharashtra (Figure 1.1.1). This state celebrated the 50th anniversary of its formation on 1 May 2010.

Gujarat is one of the prime developing states of India and is known for its vibrancy and colourful profile. Traditionally, the population has engaged in agriculture as their principal occupation. It is the main producer of tobacco, cotton, peanuts (groundnuts) and other major food crops (rice, wheat, sorghum (*jowar*), millet (*bajra*), maize, red gram dal (*tuvar dal*) and whole pulses); crops account for more than half of the total land area. Animal husbandry and dairy farming also play a vital role in the rural economy. Dairy farming – primarily milk production – is run on a cooperative basis and has more than a million members; it is one of the best examples of cooperative enterprise in the developing economy so that Gujarat is now the largest producer of milk in India. 'Amul' (Anand Milk Union Limited), formed in 1946, is based in Anand and is Asia's biggest dairy. Its products are well known throughout India.

The state is currently experiencing rapid urbanization, with 37.67 per cent of the population living in 242 urban areas according to the 2001 census. Over the last four decades it has become an industrial powerhouse, thereby reducing its dependence on agriculture. Oil, fertilizers, chemicals and textiles production attract many outsiders from across India.

The population of Gujarat state was 50,671,017 according to the 2001 census. Some 89.1% of the population are Hindus, Muslims account for 9.1%, Jains 1.0% and Sikhs 0.1%. The density of population is 258 persons per km^2, which is less than that of other Indian states.

Gujarati is one of the 14 main languages of India and is spoken by an estimated 47 million people worldwide making it the 26th most commonly spoken language in the world. In Gujarat 71% speak Gujarati; the rest (29%) speak Hindi. Almost 88% of the Muslims speak Gujarati while the other 12% speak Urdu. In addition to Gujarati, Kutchi is widely spoken in Kutch District. Almost all Jains speak Gujarati and a few speak Marwardi as well. Gujaratis form the second largest of the British South Asian-speaking communities, with important communities in Leicester and Coventry, in the northern textile towns and in Greater London.

Migration to the United Kingdom

Britain has had commercial links with Gujarat since the early seventeenth century when the British East India Company first set up a trading post in Surat in 1612.

Migration was common from Gujarat during the 18th century. When the winds were favourable, people travelled in dhows (traditional Arab sailing vessels) to East Africa, especially Zanzibar, for cloves and other spices.

In 1896, when Kenya, Uganda and Tanzania were part of British East Africa, migration from Gujarat and Punjab started for the construction of the railway from the Kenyan port of Mombasa to Kampala in Uganda to provide a modern transportation link to carry raw materials out of Uganda and to import manufactured British goods to East Africa. After the construction was completed many of these workers remained in East Africa and established substantial Indian minority communities. Their numbers may have been as high as 500,000 in the 1960s. Apart from being employed to manage the railways, they ran businesses which were, and in some cases remain, the backbone of the economies of these countries. These ranged from small rural grocery stores to sugar mills. In addition, Indian professionals – doctors, teachers, engineers and civil servants – in privileged positions played an important role in the development of these countries. After independence from Britain in the 1960s, the majority of East African Asians migrated or were expelled from these countries (in the 1970s from Uganda). Most moved to Britain, India or other popular destinations like the United States (USA) and Canada as they had acquired British citizenship.

The first Gujaratis to come to UK were students in the late nineteenth century for further studies, especially in law. Notable among them was Mohandas Karamchand Gandhi, born in Porbandar on the western coast of Saurashtra. He was the pre-eminent political and spiritual leader of India during the independence movement, pioneering *satyagraha* (resistance to tyranny through mass civil disobedience), a philosophy firmly founded on *ahimsa* (non-violence), which inspired civil rights movements and demands for freedom across the world.

Prior to Indian independence in 1947 small numbers of students, sailors and emissaries migrated to the imperial capital by exercising the right of all colonial subjects to study, travel and settle in UK. This was followed by different types of migration during the postwar period of decolonization, as the British government began recruiting labour from its former colonies to fill vacancies in its industrial sectors.

Later the main growth of Gujarati communities in UK came when their experience in the textile and steel industries was welcomed at a time of labour shortages. These South Asian workers typically followed an arrangement known as 'chain migration', which involved men from villages and districts (generally in Gujarat, Bengal and the Punjab) migrating temporarily to industrialized inner cities and sharing dormitory-style accommodation while searching for employment as semi-skilled labourers. When the government began to restrict entry into Britain in the 1960s, many of these men decided to stay permanently, sponsoring their immediate families and establishing their lives in different parts of UK.

Current UK population

There are 300,000 Gujarati language speakers in the UK, including East African Gujaratis, many of them in Leicester, Coventry, Bradford and the London boroughs of Wembley, Harrow and Newham.

1.1.2   Religion

The majority of Gujaratis are Hindus. Hindu religion is believed to be the oldest religion in the world; it is nearly 5,000 years old. It can be seen as a 'way or interdependence of life' which gave rise to other religions – Jainism, Buddhism and Sikhism. Hindus avoid eating meat and eggs or food prepared from animal products (e.g., cheeses that contain rennet and gelatin). They believe that if they consume animal flesh, they will accumulate karma – the spiritual load we accumulate or relieve ourselves of during our lifetime – which will then need to be redressed through good actions in this life or the next. Approximately 80% of Gujaratis are lacto-vegetarians (i.e., dairy products, including milk, yoghurt, butter and ghee [clarified butter], are included in their diet).

- Hindus do not eat beef or beef products as cows are considered sacred (this is also the case with Zoroastrianism). The cow has been a symbol of wealth since Vedic times (1500–500 BC), possibly because the largely pastoral Vedic people and subsequent generations relied heavily on dairy products and bullocks for tilling the fields. The milk of a cow is believed to promote *sattvic* (purifying) qualities. The ghee from cow's milk is used in ceremonies and in preparing religious food. Hindus still use cow dung for various purposes; the burning of cow dung repels mosquitoes and the ash formed is used as a fertilizer.
- Although many Hindus are lacto-vegetarian, proscribed animal products tend to vary from one country or region to the next. For example, meat and poultry may be consumed in one geographical location, while fish may be a staple food for people living in the coastal areas.

Foods such as onions and garlic are avoided or restricted as they are thought to inhibit Hindus' spiritual quest.

Religious dietary restrictions

The *Bhagavad Gita* is the holy Hindu scripture and comprises of 18 chapters. In chapter 17, verses 2–22 healthy eating habits are recommended. Food is classified into three major categories:

- *Sattvik* (nutritious) food is the most desirable. Non-irritating to the stomach and purifying to the mind, it includes milk, fruit, vegetables, nuts and whole grains. These foods are believed to produce calmness and nobility, or what is known as an 'increase in one's magnetism'.
- *Rajasi* food is believed to produce strong emotional qualities, passions and restlessness of the mind. This category includes meat, eggs, fish, spices, onions, garlic, hot peppers, pickles and other pungent or spicy foods.
- *Tamasi* food is leftover, stale, overripe, spoiled or otherwise impure food, and is believed to produce negative emotions, such as anger, jealousy and greed.

Many Hindu families have a room set aside for a shrine where deities are worshipped; it is treated as a holy place. Some devotees will refuse to accept any food that is not offered first to the deities. They do this is by placing freshly cooked food garnished with few holy basil leaves (*tulsi*) before the deities and reciting *shlokas* (prayers). Once the food has been offered to God, it is eaten as *prasad* (blessed). Before starting any meal some devout Hindus will first sprinkle water around the plate as an act of purification. Five morsels of food are placed on the side to acknowledge the debt owed to the *devta runa* (divine forces) for their benign grace and protection. This is then given to birds and animals.

There are rituals entrenched in Hindu religion which are associated with food. Food is essential for survival so it is treated with respect from the time it is cultivated, how it is cooked and disposed of. Wasting food is discouraged so food is either served or placed on the table for family members to help themselves to whatever they want to eat. Women takes immense pride in preparing and serving food and hospitality is part of the culture and tradition norms. 'Atithi devo bhava' is a Sanskrit phrase which means 'a guest is divine'. This is very apparent and especially when guests are treated with the same devotion, love and respect accorded to God. Frequently, it happens that people drop in unexpectedly and stay for lunch or dinner. If there is not enough food to go round, then a meal will be prepared for them.

Fasting

Hindus practise fasting on special occasions, such as holy days, new moon days and festivals. A fast is different from a hunger strike: a fast is a personal act of devotion, while a hunger strike is a public act, most often used to highlight an injustice. A fast is also different from anorexia nervosa: it is a 'disciplined' diet, not total abstention from food. Hindus fast in various ways, depending on the individual: they may choose not to eat at all during the fasting period, or eat only once a day or eat only 'pure' foods, such as fruits, nuts and milk. Women and older members of the family fast more regularly then younger family members, but on certain religious days the whole family may fast.

Fasting is believed to help reinforce control over one's senses and is seen as a way of staying close to God and achieving close mental proximity to Him, suppressing earthly desires and guiding the mind to be poised and at peace. Hindus believe that when there is a spiritual goal behind fasting, it should not make the body weak, irritable or create an urge to indulge later. A change of diet during the fasting period is considered to be very good for the digestive system and the entire body.

The Jain community

Gujarat is a stronghold for the Jain community. Jainism was founded as an offshoot of Hinduism in the sixth century BC. Jains preach non-violence to all living creatures and practise a unique concept of restricted vegetarianism. The Jains have also heavily influenced the cuisine of Gujarat with the Gujarati *thali* containing different lacto-vegetarian dishes along with *rotli* (flatbread) and *chaas* (yoghurt drink). They do not consume root vegetables such as potatoes, garlic, onions, carrots, radishes, cassava or sweet potatoes. However, they do consume rhizomes such as dried turmeric and dried ginger. The reason behind this restricted diet is that vegetables grown underground *Kandmul* are believed to contain far more bacteria, and hence are alive than other vegetables. Most Jain recipes substitute potatoes with plantain. Some Jains also avoid *brinjal* (aubergine) owing to the large number of seeds they contain, as a seed or bean sprout is taken to be a form of life. Strict Jains do not consume food which has been left overnight, such as yoghurt, and have their meals before sunset because large amounts of bacteria grow overnight when there is no ultraviolet light from the sun to destroy them.

Religious festivals, celebration and public holidays

Gujarat is known as the land of festivals, making it popular throughout India as well as the rest of the world for its spirit of festivity associated with special dishes. Every festival brings with it the joy of the festival and also ceremonious food that is looked forward to all year long. These festivals have been celebrated in the region for millennia. People observe these festivals strictly as they choose to keep to their age-old customs and traditions. Dates of the festivals vary every year as Hindus follow the lunar calendar. Gujaratis are proud of their rich heritage and this can be seen in the way they celebrate.

Makar Sankranti and the kite-flying festival (January)

The kite-flying festival takes place in mid-January and marks the time when the sun's rays reach the Tropic of Capricorn after the winter solstice. It is celebrated with folk music and dance as well as kite flying. People gather on terraces to fly kites of various colours to celebrate Makar Sankranti or Uttrayana. The glass-reinforced threads of the Indian fighter kites are pitted against each other in the air, and the kite fighter who cuts the other's thread is the winner. At night, kites strung with Chinese lanterns are flown. Food such as *undhiyu* (a mixture of seasonal vegatables), sugar cane juice and sweets are prepared to celebrate the day.

Maha Shivratri (February/March)

Maha shivratri marks the birthday of Lord Shiva. Traditionally, a fast is observed from dawn to dusk, and only pure foods (e.g., milk, fruit, nuts, yoghurt, potatoes and sweet potatoes) are eaten. Some people abstain from all solid food and consume fluids only.

Holi (March)

Holi is a spring festival and is celebrated at the end of winter by people throwing coloured powder and coloured water at each other.

Ram navmi (March/April)

Ram navmi is the birthday of Lord Ram. A fast is observed or one meal a day can be taken.

Mahavir Jayanti (April)

This marks the birth of Lord Mahavir and is one of the biggest Jain festivals in India.

Shravan (July/August)

This is a holy month when devotees attend a temple on specific days or, if possible, for the whole month to worship Lord Shiva. Devotees fast for the whole month or on specific days, during which they consume just one meal a day.

Rakshabandhan (August)

This festival marks the special bond between brother and sister. On this day a sister ties a *rakhee* (wrist band) on her brother's wrist and in return he buys her a gift. A festive meal is prepared and includes snacks such as *bhajiya* and Indian sweets or puddings.

Janmashtmi (August/September)

Janmashtami is the birthday of Lord Krishna. A fast is observed on this day. He was born at midnight so the next day his birthday is celebrated and *mal puda* (pancakes made from whole wheat flour, sugar and ghee) and *rabadi* (sweet thickened milk) are served with other elaborate dishes.

Navratri (September/October)

Navratri is the principal festival of Gujarat. It is celebrated not only in Gujarat but in different parts of India and around the world where Gujaratis have migrated. These celebrations are a part of a nine-day festival before Dussehra, which celebrates the nine manifestations of the Mother Goddess. During these nine days, people observe fasts and visit temples to pray to the Goddess.

At night, the festive mood overtakes everybody. The young and old celebrate the festival alike. The main attraction is Dandia Ras (a dance with decorated sticks) and Garba (a regional dance wearing traditional dress) performed in groups by huge crowds in the open. People joyfully dance to drum beats and folk songs while carrying *diva* (tea candles). The festival is a true blend of devotion,

dance, drumming and colourful dress. The dance continues all through the night with great zeal. Today Gujaratis are proud to hear their drumbeats and see their attire on international catwalks.

Sharad Purnima

This is a harvest festival celebrated on the first full moon after Navratri by having dinner with milk (*doodh*) and pava (*rice flakes*) by moonlight.

Diwali (October/November)

Diwali (the festival of light) is celebrated over four days and on each day a religious ceremony is performed in every home. Specific dishes are prepared for each day. In the evening *diva* (oil-filled lamps to signify the triumph of good over evil) are lit and placed in front of the house.

New Year

The fourth day is celebrated as New Year. On this day devotees go to the temple to pray, meet and greet family and friends and to see the display of sacred *Annakut*, an array of hundreds of lacto-vegetarian dishes arranged in tiers before the deities. Business people also mark the end of the fiscal year when a sacred ceremony is performed on the new account books after which the fast is broken.

1.1.3 The traditional diet and eating pattern

Gujarati lacto-vegetarian cuisine has evolved over hundreds of years and contains dishes made from cereals, pulses, vegetables (*shaak*), and side-dishes such as pickles, chutney, papadoms (*papad*), *raita* (yoghurt mixed with shredded cucumber/vegetables) or salad (*kachumber*) and *chaas*.

Northern Gujarat, Kathiawad, Kutch and southern Gujarat are the four major regions of the state and each has its own cuisine. Many Gujarati dishes are distinctively sweet, salty, sour and spicy at the same time and can vary widely depending on the family or region. This harmony, derived from the mix of the sweet with the salt, sour and spices, is what makes the cooking of lacto-vegetarian dishes of this state different from the rest of the Indian subcontinent.

Meals are usually served in a *thali* and include flatbread *rotli*, rice, whole pulses or dal, or yoghurt soup (*kadhi*) and *shaak*, with *papad* or *raita*. Different accompaniments and sweet dishes are served depending on the menu and occasion. The cuisine changes with the seasonal availability of vegetables. Fresh fruits are normally eaten between meals or sometimes served with the meal. In summer, when mangoes are widely available, *keri no ras* (fresh mango pulp) is often an integral part of the meal.

There are also simple meals of rice and dal known as *khichadi*, served with *kadhi* or with lightly spiced *chaas* and *shaak*.

Cooking methods are handed down from one generation to the next and these cooking styles are followed even though sometimes the main ingredients differ according to the country in which they are prepared. First-generation South Asians are likely to follow traditional eating patterns and habits (Thomas & Bishop, 2007). People who migrated from East Africa were able to maintain their religious festivals and cultural and traditional diet, but they also included cassava (*mogo*) and green banana (*matoke*).

Atta (whole wheat/whole meal flour) is the main ingredient of most varieties of breads on the South Asian subcontinent. Traditionally, *chakki atta*, which is creamy-brown in colour, is made by stone-grinding wheat. This process imparts a characteristic aroma and flavour to the breads.

Atta is made from wheat which has a high gluten content so dough made from this flour is strong and can be rolled out very thin.

Since nothing is removed from *atta*, all of the wheat grain is preserved. *Atta* available in the UK varies in its fibre content from very low to around 12%. The high bran content of *atta* makes it rich in dietary fibre; it also contains significant quantities of starch, protein, vitamins and minerals.

When South Asian communities migrated to UK the *atta* they were used to was not available. In 1962 Elephant Atta 'medium flour' was launched and today it is widely used by this community. However, as the fibre content of this flour is 7.1% this has resulted in a reduction in the fibre content of their diet.

Now different brands of *chakki atta* are widely available in UK but people from the South Asian communities are reluctant to change, as over the years they have acquired a taste for medium *atta* and also because *chakki atta* is more expensive.

Indian breads

Different types of unleavened, round, soft breads are flattened by rolling and baked in a *tava* (frying pan). They vary in size and thickness in different regions and are called by different names.

Plain flatbread is traditionally referred to as *roti*, but also commonly known as *chapatti*. If possible it is served piping hot. A small piece of bread is torn off and used to scoop up a vegetable dish or folded into a loose cone to scoop liquid dishes like dal that form part of the meal.

Rotli or *phulka* is made from a firm but pliable dough. Some people add salt and/or oil. The dough is rolled out into circles 15–18 cm in diameter. The rolled rotli is then placed on a preheated *tava* and partly cooked on both sides, and then directly put on a medium flame, which makes it puff up like a balloon when hot air cooks the *rotli* rapidly from the inside. Finally, ghee is spread on it.

Double *pud* in *rotli* follows the same method as above, but two small balls are loosely joined with oil and flour, rolled together and then cooked. When it is slightly cold they are separated and ghee is spread on it. This type of *rotli* is served with freshly squeezed mango pulp.

Plain *paratha* is one of the most popular breads, made from firm dough shallow-fried in a *tava*.

Layered or puffed *paratha* are made by rolling out the dough in circles approximately 15 cm in diameter and then ghee or cooking oil and a sprinkling of flour is spread over it. It is then folded and rolled again and shallow-fried over a low heat. The *paratha* can be round, square or triangular.

Spicy *paratha* are made following the same method but salt, chilli powder, turmeric and cumin are added before rolling and cooking.

Sweet *paratha* are made following the same method but sugar or jaggery (unrefined cane sugar) is added.

Stuffed *paratha* are usually filled with vegetables such as boiled potatoes, radishes, cauliflower or *paneer*, seasoned with herbs, spices and other seasonings. The stuffing is made into a small ball and placed in the middle of the dough and sealed. This is then rolled quite thin and shallow-fried.

Bhakhari is a thicker, crisper flatbread cooked without oil over a very low heat.

Thepla is a shallow-fried, spiced flatbread made with wheat and chickpea flour dough. It usually contains shredded vegetables or leftover cooked rice to which salt, chilli powder, turmeric, cumin and sesame seeds are added.

Puran puri (vedmi) is made with a sweetened *tuvar dal* or *mung dal* filling following the same method as stuffed *paratha* but cooked at a low temperature and spread with ghee.

Puri: plain *puri* made with whole wheat flour or semolina and deep-fried. Spicy *puri (tikkhi)* is made with salt, chilli powder, turmeric and *ajmo* (carom seeds).

Bajri no rotlo is made from *bajri atta* and cooked without oil or ghee.

Jawar no rotlo is made from *jawar atta* and cooked without oil or ghee.

Makai no rotlo is made from *makai* (maize) *atta* which is cooked without oil or ghee.

Khakhra is a very thin flatbread made from moth bean flour, wheat flour and oil and cooked on a hot tava. There are several types such *methi, jeera* and different *masala* flavours. It is mostly eaten as a snack by the Jain community.

Khichadi is a mixture of rice and *tuvar dal* or *mung dal* with a little ghee. It is a very popular dish and regularly cooked in most homes, typically on a busy day due to its ease of cooking.

Kadhi is a mixture of yoghurt, chickpea flour, salt, turmeric, crushed ginger, chillies and garlic simmered over a slow heat and stirred continuously. *Vaghar* of ghee, mustard seeds, cumin, fenugreek seeds, curry leaves and asafoetida is added. It is garnished with chopped coriander leaves and served hot.

Rice: There are hundreds of varieties of rice but most prized is Basmati rice. It is a staple of the diet and plain boiled rice is eaten at least once a day. It also has a symbolic importance as it is needed for all the religious rites, including wedding ceremonies.

Vegetable rice (*pilau*) is made by adding a mixture of different vegetables (e.g., peas, spinach and onions).

Pulses and dals: There are many varieties of pulses and dals and most are available in the UK.

Apart from soya beans, pulses contain 20–25% protein by weight, twice the protein content of wheat and three times that of rice. For this reason, pulses are called 'vegetarian meat'. The digestibility of pulse protein is high but it is relatively poor in the essential amino acid methionine. However, as they are commonly consumed with grains (high in methionine, but deficient in lysine, which is found in pulses) the two foods complement each other, forming a complete protein. In Gujarati cuisine a combination of three parts rice to one part dals is used in the preparation of most dishes.

Pulses and dals have been part of the South Asian diet for generations and the skills of cooking delicious dishes has been passed on from one generation to another and make the lacto-vegetarian diet unique but also nutritious.

Whole pulses

All pulses grow in a pod. Green tender pods with seeds are used as vegetables and cooked with aubergine. Tender pods with seeds are sold fresh or frozen: e.g., french beans, pink beans (*valor*), haricot beans (*surti papdi*).

Seeds (*lilva*): They are sold fresh, frozen or tinned: e.g., peas, broad beans, black-eyed beans, soya beans, *chana* (chickpeas), red gram (*tuvar lilva*).

Dried whole pulses
When they are fully mature, the crop is harvested and the seeds are sun-dried. They are cleaned and sold as whole pulses which are soaked, boiled and cooked in different ways. They are also sold in tins, which reduces the cooking time.

- Plain boiled pulses are eaten as a snack or cooked as a dish.
- Whole pulses are deep-fried and consumed as a snack (e.g., Bombay mix).
- They are dry-roasted in cast-iron wok in hot sand. Roasted Bengal gram (Chana) are a most popular snack.
- They are boiled and mashed and used as snack (e.g., *Bengal gram chana chor garam*).

Most pulses can be sprouted (e.g., sprouted mung or moth). Sprouting has both nutritional and practical advantages:

- Germination increases the content of folic acid and other B vitamins.
- Tannins and phytates, which adversely affect bioavailability, are broken down by germination.
- The breakdown of phytic acids allows more absorption of calcium and iron and generation of vitamin C also helps in the absorption of iron.

- As they become soft, digestibility is increased and they can be eaten raw in salad.
- Cooking time is reduced as they are stir-fried.

Split whole pulses are called dals and are eaten with or without the skin.

Cooking methods
Depending on the menu, dal can be cooked into different textures: liquid, semi-liquid or dry.

Dals are deep-fried and used as a snack. Dals are also made into *vadi* like soya chunks and cooked with vegetables.

Dals without skin is ground into flour.

Chickpea flour
This is one of the most versatile of the pulse flours and is used in a variety of ways:

- as a thickening agent (e.g., added to yoghurt in preparation of *kadhi*);
- to prepare sweet or savoury dishes;
- added to wheat flour to make Indian bread;
- to make *puda* (pancakes).

Black gram flour or mung flour
Papadoms are mostly made from black gram flour or mung flour with the addition of different spices. They are rolled very thin and dried in the sun, then dry-roasted over low flame or deep-fried.

Moth dal flour
Mathiya are prepared in the same way as papadams but deep-fried and prepared on special occasions and especially for the festival of Diwali.

Dal and rice flour
These are used in fermented dishes, e.g., steamed – *dhokra/khaman/muthiya*; or baked – *ondhwa*.

Nuts and oilseeds
Nuts, such as almonds, cashews, pistachios and walnuts, are widely used in cooking.

Oilseeds are rich in fat. Groundnuts (peanuts) and sesame seeds are commonly used:

- Dry-roasted in a cast iron wok over a low flame (e.g., peanuts).
- Deep-fried as snacks.
- Sesame seeds used to garnish dishes.
- Crushed into powder and used in cooking, especially stuffed vegetables, and added to sweet dishes and puddings.

- Sweetmeats: e.g., sesame snaps (*chikki*). In Gujarat *chikki* is prepared with nuts or oilseeds and jaggery.

Vegetables
In the tropics, seasonal vegetables are very cheap and they are bought and cooked fresh for each meal. These include both green leafy vegetables and root vegetables. Potatoes are considered as vegetables rather then starchy food as in the UK.

Methods of cooking vegetables

- dry vegetables (*koroo shaak*);
- vegetable in sauce (*rasa varoo shaak*);
- deep-fried vegetables (*tareloo shaak*);
- stuffed vegetables (*bhareloo shaak*);
- stir-fried vegetables (e.g., cabbage, carrots and green chillies [*sambharo*]);
- vegetables cooked with dal;
- steamed dishes made with vegetables (e.g., *patra*, *muthiya*);

Tropical fruits are delicious and are seasonal.

Fresh fruits are included in the diet (e.g., fruit salad, fruit juices, milkshake). Fruits are also made into pickles.

Milk and dairy foods
Traditionally, throughout India (including in Gujarat) full-fat cow or buffalo milk is boiled before it is consumed. As the milk cools a layer of cream (*tor/malai*) forms and this is skimmed off and reserved. When enough cream is accumulated a small amount of yoghurt is added and left overnight. Next morning this mixture is churned with the addition of water and this process separates the fat from the cream. The fat is called 'white butter'. The liquid that remains is called *chaas* and is used in cooking. White butter is placed in a pan and brought to the boil at a low temperature. It is stirred until all the water has evaporated. When it is cool it is sieved through muslin to remove any remaining sediments. This pure fat is called ghee and is used in religious ceremonies and in cooking.

In the UK commercial butter is used to make ghee at home; alternatively, ready made ghee can be bought from groceries.

Milk is used in beverages, as a milky drink, in milkshakes, for making milky puddings, yoghurt and *paneer* (unsalted white cheese).

Yoghurt is mostly made at home, but in the UK commercially made yoghurt is widely available. It is used in cooking, for making sweet dishes, *kadhi* and *raita* (see Table 1.1.1).

Beverages

- Masala tea (*chai*) is made by brewing leaves, sugar and milk with a mixture of aromatic spices (e.g., dried ginger, black pepper, cloves, cardamom, cinnamon and nutmeg) and herbs (e.g., basil or mint).
- *Limbu pani* (sweetened and spiced lime juice).
- Fruit juice (sweetened and unsweetened).
- Carbonated drinks (e.g., cola or Lucozade).
- *Chaas* made with natural yoghurt and water.

Accompaniments

- *Raita*: Made with yoghurt, chopped fruit, aubergine or grated vegetables. Added to this mixture are fresh chopped green chillies, coriander leaves, salt, sugar and cumin powder or mustard powder.
- *Bharatu*: Made with yoghurt and roasted aubergine. Added to this mixture are fresh chopped green chillies, coriander, salt, sugar and cumin powder.

- *Papdi*: Like papadam but made from seasoned rice flour which is steamed then rolled quite thin and sun-dried. *Papdi* can be cooked over a low flame or deep-fried.
- *Rice sev*: Made from rice flour cooked in the same way as above but prepared by squeezing through a special press and sun-dried. Rice *sev* is deep-fried.
- *Vadi* (rice flour): Like soya chunks; it is deep-fried.

Pickles and chutney

- Mango pickles (sweet or spicy).
- Lemon pickles (sweet or spicy).
- Green chilli pickles.
- Mixed vegetables pickle made with mustard powder and lemon juice.
- Herbs preserved in brine or vinegar.
- Tamarind chutney (tamarind and dates).
- Green chutney (coriander and mint).
- Mango chutney.
- Red chutney (red pepper, red chillies and tomatoes).
- Coconut chutney.
- Mint and tomato chutney.

Table 1.1.1 Description of Gujarati foods

Food groups	Description of foods	Gujarati name
Bread, rice, potatoes, pasta and other starchy foods	Wheat atta (flour)	*Ghau no lot*
	Vermicelli	*Ghau ni sev*
	Semolina	*Soji*
	Plain flour	*Maido*
	Millet	*Bajri*
	Sorghum	*Jowar*
	Maize	*Makai*
	Rice	*Chokha*
	White rice boiled/steamed	*Bhaat*
	Pilau rice (cooked with vegetables)	*Pulav*
	Rice pudding	*Kheer*
	Rice flour	*Chokha no lot*
	Rice flakes (pounded rice)	*Pava*
	Puffed rice (made by heating rice in a sand-filled oven)	*Mumara*
	Potato	*Batata*
	Sweet potato	*Shakkaria*
	Sago	*Sabu dana*
	Yam	*Suran*
	A mixture of rice and dal flour is used to make different snacks	

Table 1.1.1 (*cont'd*)

Food groups	Description of foods	Gujarati name
Vegetables and fruits	Amaranth tender	*Tanjurdo*
	Aubergine	*Ringun*
	Bitter gourd	*Karela*
	Bottle gourd	*Dudhi*
	Black-eyed beans	*Chora*
	Broad beans	*Fafda papdi*
	Cluster beans	*Guvar*
	Cauliflower	*Ful kobi*
	Cabbage	*Kobi*
	Carrot	*Gaajar*
	Colocasia leaves	*Arvi/Salia na pan*
	Drumstick	*Saragavo*
	Green peas	*Vatana/Matar*
	Fenugreek leaves	*Methi ni bhaji*
	Fennel leaves	*Sava ni bhaji*
	French beans	*Funsi*
	Mint	*Fudino*
	Okra (ladies' fingers)	*Bhinda*
	Onion	*Doongari*
	Other gourds	*Parval,Gheloda, Kankoda*
	Pink beans	*Valor*
	Pumpkin	*Kollu*
	Radish	*Moora*
	Radish leaves	*Moora ni bhaji*
	Ridge gourd	*Turia*
	Snake gourd	*Gulka*
	Spinach	*Bhaji*
	Sweet corn	*Makai*
	Apple	*Sufferjan*
	Banana	*Kela*
	Custard apple	*Sitaful*
	Dates	*Khajoor*
	Figs	*Anjeer*
	Grapes	*Draksh*
	Guava	*Jamfal*
	Jackfruit	*Phanas*
	Lime	*Limbu*
	Mango	*Keri*
	Melon	*Tarbooch*
	Orange	*Mosumbi*
	Pears	*Nashpati*
	Pawpaw	*Papaya*
	Pomegranate	*Daddam*
	Pineapple	*Ananus*
	Tangerine	*Suntra*
	Sapodilla (Sapota)	*Chikku*

(*Continued*)

Table 1.1.1 (*cont'd*)

Food groups	Description of foods	Gujarati name
Meat, fish, eggs, beans and other non-dairy sources of protein (i.e., pulses/dals, nuts and seeds)	Meat	*Mass*
	Chicken	*Moorghi*
	Eggs	*Inda*
	Fish	*Maachli*
	Bengal gram/dal/flour	*Chana/Chana ni dal/lot*
	Black gram/dal/flour	*Urad/urad in dal/lot*
	Black-eyed peas/dal	*White chora/dal*
	Field beans/dal	*Val/val in dal*
	Green gram/dal	*Mung/Mung ni dal*
	Lentil/dal	*Masoor/Masoor ni dal*
	Turkish gram/dal	*Moth/Moth in dal*
	Red gram/dal	*Tuvar/Tuvar ni dal*
	Peas	*Vatana/Matar*
	Almonds	*Badam*
	Cashews	*Kaju*
	Dried coconut	*Copru*
	Fresh coconut	*Naliyer*
	Dates	*Khajur*
	Pistachios	*Pista*
	Peanuts (groundnuts)	*Sing danna*
	Walnuts	*Akhrot*
Milk and dairy foods	Milk	*Doodh*
	Milk powder	*Doodh no powder*
	Yoghurt	*Dahi*
	Buttermilk	*Chaas*
	(Reduction of milk in an open wok until it is thickened to fudge-like consistency but not caramelized)	*Maavo*
	Unsalted white cheese (can be made at home)	*Paneer*
Foods and drinks high in fat and/or sugar	Pre-packed tropical fruit juices	
	Indian sweets and puddings	*Ladwa, Burfi, Jallebi, gulab-jambu, kulfi, ice cream*
Sugar and sugary foods	Sugar	*Sakker*
	Jaggery	*Gor*
Fats and oils	Corn oil	*Makai nu tel*
	Sunflower oil	*Suryamukhi nu tel*
	Peanut oil	*Sing nu tel*
	Sesame seed oil	*Tul nu tel*
	Rapeseed oil	*Canola/rapeseed oil*
	Butter	*Maakhan*
	Clarified butter	*Ghee*

How herbs and spices are used in cooking

Herbs and spices are an integral part of South Asian cooking and apart from flavouring the food they also have medicinal properties. The making of masala is traditionally done on grinding stones. Nowadays, people use an electric blender or grinder and ready-made masala are widely available in the UK. Each person makes their masala to their own recipe, hence dishes taste different depending on the household. For example, people from northern Gujarat use dry red chilli powder, whereas people from southern Gujarat prefer green chillies, ginger, garlic and coriander. Gujarati Jains (and many Hindus) avoid garlic and onions.

Traditionally, dried (whole and ground) and fresh herbs and spices are used in the Gujarati diet. They are an excellent way to add flavour to foods when reducing the salt and/or sugar content of the diet (see Table 1.1.2).

Table 1.1.2 Use of herbs and spices in Gujarati diet

Ingredients	Gujarati name	Comments
Asafoetida	Hing	Used in vegetable/pulse cooking
Bay leaves	Tejpatta	In rice dishes
Coriander leaves	Lila dhana/Kothmeer	For garnish/in chutney
Curry leaves	Mitho-limbdo	In yoghurt dishes
Coriander seeds	Dhana	Used for making coriander powder
Cumin seeds	Jeeru	As seasoning
Cinnamon	Taj	Whole stick and powder used in cooking
Cardamom	Elchi	In tea, whole in cooking, crushed in pudding
Cloves	Laving	Used whole in cooking
Green chillies	Lila marcha	In cooking, pickles, chutney
Garlic	Lasan	In cooking, crushed
Ginger	Adhu	In tea. In cooking, crushed or grated
Dried ginger	Sunth	In tea
Fenugreek	Methi	In cooking, in pickles
Mint	Fudino	In tea, in chutney
Mustard seeds	Rai	In cooking, pickles
Nutmeg	Jaifal	In pudding
Poppy seeds	Khus khus	For garnish
Peppercorns	Kara mari	In tea, in cooking
Red chillies, whole	Lal mircha	In vaghar
Red chilli powder	Mirchu	In cooking, garnish
Sesame seeds	Tal	For garnish, crushed, used in cooking, sesame snaps
Saffron	Kasar	In pudding and sweets
Turmeric powder	Harder	In cooking
Tamarind	Amli	In chutney and in pulses
Sesame seeds	Tal	For garnish, crushed used in cooking, Sesame snaps
Fennel seeds	Variyali	In cooking
Carom seeds	ajmo	In vaghar for cooking vegetables and pulses
Cocum	Kokum na phool	In dal dishes

Cooking methods and food preservation

Cooking is mostly done over an open flame. A pressure cooker is used initially to cook pulses or dals. It is also used for cooking vegetables and rice dishes.

Steaming, shallow frying, baking and dry roasting are common cooking methods, but most of the dishes are deep-fried in oil.

Sun drying: This is a common way of preserving food.

Vaghar

Vaghar is essential when spices and herbs are added one at a time to hot oil or ghee and this tempering is either done as the first step in the cooking process, before adding the vegetables or as the last, pouring the tempered oil over dal. The oil extracts and retains all the sharp flavours of the mustard seeds (*rai*), *mitho-limbdo* (curry leaves), cumin seeds (*jeera*), asafoetida (*hing*), etc., and coats the entire dish.

Therapeutic use of foods

The use of ayurvedic (traditional) medicine has been shown to be more common among Indians than in any other ethnic groups (Sproston & Mindell, 2006).

- Hot and cold foods: 'Hot' foods, such as mangoes and ginger, are thought to promote an increase in body temperature; conversely, 'cold' foods, such as potatoes, are believed to reduce temperature (Thomas & Bishop, 2007). It is believed that hot foods should be avoided in hot conditions, such as pregnancy (Hawthorne *et al.*, 1993) and cold foods avoided in cold conditions, such as lactation. For health professionals it is important to be aware of such beliefs, especially if they have nutritional implications, for example, a pregnant women suffering from nausea and vomiting and not meeting her nutritional needs may be avoiding ginger, yet anecdotally ginger can be helpful in sickness and may help her to increase her oral intake and meet her requirements.
- Joint pain: Sour foods, such as lemon or tamarind, may be avoided by older people or those with joint problems as it is believed that these

foods may exacerbate joint pain and arthritis (Hamid & Sarwar, 2004).
- During pregnancy and postnatally: Women who have recently given birth may be given *katlu*, an Indian sweet made from nuts, herbs, spices and jaggery, as it is thought to aid convalescence, increase lactation and reduce back pain. The consumption of pulses and beans may be discouraged if a mother is breastfeeding as such foods are thought to induce colic in the baby (Hamid & Sarwar, 2004).

Paan and mukhvas

Mukhvas is mostly eaten after a meal. It is made with dry-roasted split coriander seeds, fennel seeds and sesame seeds.

Mukhvas is added to betel nut *paan*.

The use of chewing tobacco (*paan* or *gutka*) is common in the South Asian subcontinent. Research looking at *paan* and *gutka* use by Gujaratis living in the USA showed that the use of *paan* had fallen but the use of *gutka* had increased (Changrani *et al.*, 2006).

The use of chewing tobacco is a risk factor for oral cancer, however it is a strong cultural habit for many and the safe use of these products is being promoted (Carlisle, 2002). A patient quoted in an article by Sproston and Mindell (2006) highlights this: 'You can take tobacco out of the *pan* but not *paan* away from the community'.

Smoking

Research looking at cigarette smoking in ethnic minority groups versus the general population has shown that self-reported smoking levels for Indian men is less than the general population in UK (20% versus 24%) and also for women from ethnic minority groups versus women in the general population in UK (Sproston & Mindell, 2006).

Alcohol

Drinking alcohol is forbidden and the majority of first-generation migrants avoided it. However, with exposure to western culture, and as alcohol is widely available, alcohol consumption is quite common among the younger generation.

1.1.4   Traditional eating patterns and changes in migration to UK

Migration is likely to result in dietary changes. In the USA nearly 57.7% of Gujarati subjects surveyed reported dietary changes since immigration. Their total energy intake was as follows: carbohydrates – 57%; protein – 12%; total fat 33% (Jonnalagadda & Diwan, 2002). Problems with maintaining the traditional diet can include the increased cost and reduced availability of ingredients, leading to more use of host country vegetables such as potatoes (Thomas & Bishop, 2007). Also, women are more likely to be in paid work, leading to less time available to prepare traditional foods and more reliance on convenience foods (Thomas & Bishop, 2007). The drawback of increasing the intake of convenience foods may be an increased energy intake and consequent weight gain. A study of Gujaratis in the USA showed that 20% of individuals were overweight or obese (Jonnalagadda & Diwan, 2002). Comparison between Gujaratis in the UK and those in India shows that those in the UK have a higher BMI, energy and fat intake. Patel *et al.* (2006) also reported that Gujaratis in the UK had higher lipid and blood pressure levels.

Stone *et al.* (2005) found that extended family networks are common and are used for information on health and diet.

Traditional cooking is done from scratch and is time-consuming and labour-intensive. Although working women have the option of buying ready-made meals, these are high in fat and sugar (see Tables 1.1.3 and Table 1.1.4).

1.1.5   Healthy eating

Key points

- The traditional Gujarati lacto-vegetarian diet is high in fibre and low in fat and should be encouraged as part of a healthy eating diet.
- The Gujarati diet is influenced by religion and can range from being strictly lacto-vegetarian for orthodox Hindus, to including meat, fish and alcohol.
- After migration the first generation tries to maintain their traditional eating patterns but the children who are born or brought into the country of migration will adopt western-eating habits as they are more exposed to processed foods.
- Traditional cooking methods are time-consuming and women who go to work may rely instead on fried and convenience foods which are high in fat and sugar.
- Some traditional ingredients may not be readily available or are expensive.
- Health promotion education should be targeted in which traditional healthy eating habits are encouraged with the inclusion of healthy local foods.

Introduction

Traditional diets are passed from one generation to the next and, over the years, people have adapted to these foods. The traditional Gujarati lacto-vegetarian diet is very healthy because it contains plenty of cereals, varieties of fresh vegetables/fruits, whole pulses/dals, milk and dairy products, all of which provide the nutrients the body needs, but there are only small quantities of fat and sugar. Food is cooked with different condiments and spices, which not only give a delicate flavour, but also provide beneficial nutrients and have medicinal properties. In the right proportions, this diet is a very healthy option. The traditional diets are closer to dietary recommendations for dietary fat and fibre than those for the general UK population (Health Education Authority, 1991). However, with migration to the UK the balance has changed, resulting in an increase in sugar and fat consumption and a reduction in fibre intake (see Table 1.1.5 pages 19-20).

Recent evidence of good practice to promote healthy eating

A report by Fox (2004) highlights initiatives in the UK to promote healthy eating. These include a 'five-a-day' scheme in Coventry, involving providing weekly vouchers to residents to buy fruit and vegetables at reduced cost and links with a local delivery service, so fruits and vegetables can remain accessible for residents with mobility difficulties.

Table 1.1.3   Traditional eating pattern and changes in Gujarati diet on migration to UK

Meal	Traditional meal	Dietary changes on migration to UK	Healthier alternatives
Breakfast	Nasto, e.g., *Chevdo, ganthia, sev-mumara puri* or *paratha* with tea	Nasto, e.g., *Chevdo, ganthia, sev-mumara* *Puri* or *paratha* with Tea/coffee Cereal with full-fat milk Toast with butter	High-fibre breakfast cereal with semi-skimmed milk Whole meal toast with low-fat spread Tea/coffee
Lunch	(Main meal) *Rotli* with ghee Vegetables/dal Plain yoghurt Salad/pickles Papaddom (*papad*) *Chaas* made with semi-skimmed milk, salt	Leftovers from the night before, e.g., *rotli*/rice with vegetables/dal Sandwich Chips, pizza	*Rotli* made with whole wheat flour, no ghee Boiled rice Vegetables/dal cooked with measured amount of oil Salad *Chaas* made with low-fat yoghurt and small amount of salt Fruit Sandwich made with whole meal bread
Evening meal	As lunch *Puri/paratha/thepla* with vegetables Sweet pickles Dhokra, chutney	(Main meal) *Rotli* Chapatti/rice Vegetables/dal Plain yoghurt Salad/pickle Pizza/pasta	As lunch *Rotli*/boiled rice Vegetables/dal Low fat yoghurt Homemade pickles (made with less oil and sugar/or in vinegar)
Puddings/ Desserts	Indian sweets and puddings, e.g., *jallebi, shrikhand* Fruit	Indian sweets and puddings, e.g., *jallebi, shrikhand* Ice cream, fruit	Fruit Canned fruit in natural juice Fruit salad
Drinks	Water, *chaas* Tea with sugar Fruit juice (special occasions) Fizzy drinks	Water, *chaas* Tea/coffee with sugar Fruit juice, sweetened Fizzy drinks (e.g., cola) Soft drinks (e.g., orange squash, Ribena)	Water, *chaas* Tea/coffee with sweetener Unsweetened fruit juice Diet/low-sugar fizzy/soft drinks
Snacks	*Chevdo, ganthia, sev mumara* *Thepla/puri* (if leftover). *Kachori, dhokra, patra batatavada, samosas* Fruit	*Chevdo, ganthia, sev mumara, bhajiya, kachori, samosas* Cakes, biscuits. Chocolates, nuts, crisps, sweets	Dry-roasted nuts and chana Popcorn Dry-roasted *papad, papdi* Rice cakes, oat biscuits

Table 1.1.4 Glossary of Gujarati foods

Foods	Description
Farsaan	Cooked fresh and served with a meal or as a snack.
Nasto	Deep fried snacks mostly eaten at breakfast or teatime.
Mithai	Indian sweets and puddings.
Ladwa	Made from whole wheat flour, ghee and milk or water are added to make a firm dough. This is then rolled into small balls and deep-fried in oil or ghee until golden-brown. When they are cold they are ground, added to sugar or jaggery syrup, crushed cardamom mixed together and small balls of ladwa are made. They are garnished with poppy seeds.
Shiro	Made with whole wheat flour or semolina which is cooked in ghee over a low flame until golden-brown, then milk and sugar are added. It is cooked until all the milk is absorbed. Garnished with chopped almonds and crushed cardamom.
Lapsi	Made with cracked wheat and raisins which is cooked in ghee over a low flame until light brown. Water and sugar are added and cooking continues until the ghee starts oozing out. Garnished with blanched chopped almonds and pistachios.
Sukhadi	Cooked whole wheat flour in ghee and jaggery. This is leavened and left to set. Served cut into small squares.
Mal puda	Made from whole wheat flour which is fermented overnight by adding a little yoghurt and jaggery or sugar to make them sweet. Before frying, fennel seeds and a few crushed black peppers are added to the batter which is then prepared like crepes to golden brown. Garnished with poppy seeds.
Furshi puri	Made from plain flour and semolina dough and seasoned with salt, cumin and crushed black pepper. Small balls of the dough are rolled like puri, scored and then deep-fried until crisp. Eaten as snacks.
Dal dhokori	A complete dish made with tuvar dal. Spiced wheat flour is kneaded into dough and rolled into thin rotli which are cut into small pieces. These are dropped into boiling dal and cooked until soft. Garnished with coriander leaves and served warm. Frozen peas or tuvar lilva may also be added.
Dhebara	Shallow-fried spiced flatbread made with a mixture of flours, or millet flour. Mostly fresh finely chopped fenugreek leaves are added and cooked with oil.
Batata pava	Made with potatoes and rice flakes and lightly spiced.
Papdi no lot	Made with steamed spiced rice flour.
Khichi no lot	Same as above but made with mung dal flour.
Puda	Made from spiced chickpea flour batter, like pancake. It can be plain or with added chopped methi leaves, onions or shredded vegetables.
Batata-vada	Deep-fried spicy chickpea flour batter balls stuffed with mashed potato fresh herbs and spices.
Methi na gota	Made with chickpea flour and finely chopped fenugreek leaves, seasoned and deep-fried.
Bhel	Mixture of sev mumara, boiled/sprouted pulses, boiled chopped potatoes and onions. Served with chutneys.
Sev usad	Boiled dried peas or black-eyed peas seasoned and served with sev, chopped onions and chutney.
Chevdo	Known as Bombay mix in UK. It includes deep-fried, potato, chana dal and rice flakes (pava). This is then seasoned.
Bhajiya	They are made of different vegetables which are cut into thin slices and dipped into spiced chickpea flour batter and deep-fried.
Fuli ganthia	Deep-fried, spicy, star-shaped noodles made from seasoned chana dal flour which is pressed through a special press directly into hot oil.
Sev	Deep-fried noodles of different thickness made from seasoned chana dal flour. Same cooking method as above.
Sev mumara	A mixture of spicy dry ingredients such as puffed rice, sev and peanuts. It is a very light, healthy dish.

(continued)

Table 1.1.4 (*cont'd*)

Foods	Description
Magash	Cook coarse chickpea flour in ghee and caster sugar on a low flame. This is leavened, garnished with chopped almond and cardamom and left to set. Served cut in small squares.
Undhiyu	Made with layers of diced potatoes, yam, raw bananas, small *brinjals*, *papdi* seeds cooked with *muthiya* and seasoned with salt, turmeric and a paste of garlic, green chillies, ginger and finely chopped coriander. It is served hot decorated with grated coconut. (*Muthiya* is chickpea flour deep-fried dumplings with added fenugreek leaves (*methi*), crushed ginger, green chillies and salt to taste.)
Ondhwa	Baked dish made from rice and *tuvar dal* flour fermented with yogurt. Shredded vegetables are added and seasoned.
Muthiya	Steamed dish made from rice and *chana dal* flour to which shredded vegetables are added and seasoned.
Kachori	Deep-fried spicy balls of semolina pastry stuffed with crush green peas or soaked *mug dal*, grated coconut and spices.
Samosa	Triangle-shaped deep-fried spicy pastry of plain flour stuffed with green peas and potatoes and spices.
Dahi vada	Made from *urad dal* soaked overnight and ground into smooth batter. Crushed herbs and seasonings (salt, black pepper, green chillies and ginger) are added to taste. Small batter balls are deep-fried to golden brown then put in cold water for 2–3 minutes and the water squeezed out. They are served with spiced yoghurt and tamarind chutney garnished with chopped coriander.
Dhokra	Made from chickpea flour which is fermented with yoghurt for 4–5 hours. Herbs and spices (salt, crushed green chillies and ginger) and baking soda are added and then they are steamed for about 15 minutes in a flat dish and cut into pieces. A *vaghar* of oil mustard and sesame seeds is poured over it for extra spiciness. They are garnished with coriander and usually served with green chutney.
Khaman	Same as above but instead of chickpea flour *chana dal* is soaked for 4–5 hours and then liquidized and fermented with yoghurt, seasoned and steamed.
Vada	Made from different *dals* (mung, lentil or mixed) which are soaked and liquidized to a batter; seasonings are added and small batter balls are deep fried.
	In India 'Maavo' is used to make sweets described below but as it is not available in UK, full-fat milk powder is used instead.
Penda	Made from full-fat milk powder, which is cooked in ghee on a low flame until light brown. Sugar and cardamom is added. Small round palates are made.
Gulab Jambu	Made with full-fat milk powder dough. Small balls are then deep-fried in ghee or oil on medium flame until light brown. These are dipped into sugar syrup.
Burfi	Sweet made with full-fat milk powder and sugar. Many varieties, including coconut, pistachio and chocolate.
Shrikhand	A creamy dessert made from strained yoghurt. Sugar is added and then it is flavoured with saffron, cardamom and nuts. Chopped fresh fruit or candied fruit can be added for extra flavour.
Doodh pak	Made from milk and rice. Sugar and cardamom are added and garnished with chopped almonds.
Rice Kheer	Rice cooked in milk and sugar to which crushed cardamom is added. Garnished with chopped almonds.
Rabdi	Made from milk until condensed. Sugar and cardamom is added and garnished with chopped almonds.
Jallebi	Made from fermented plain flour batter which is made into cartwheels over hot fat and dipped into sugar syrup.

Table 1.1.5   Healthier alternatives for Gujarati diet

Food groups	Healthier alternatives
Bread, rice, potatoes, pasta and other starchy foods	Try using whole wheat flour to make Indian breads.
	Make *rotli* and *bhakhari* without adding oil to the dough and spread ghee or butter on them vary sparingly.
	Try to cook *paratha, thepla, dhebara* in non-stick frying pan, and use as little oil in cooking as possible.
	Have fried bread, such as *puri*, only as a treat.
	Try whole meal/granary rolls/brown instead of white varieties and low-fat spreads instead of butter.
	Choose high-fibre breakfast cereals rather than those coated with sugar or honey.
	Try brown rice and avoid adding extra ghee or butter to rice or *khichadi*.
	Try whole meal pasta.
	Use millet/maize/jowar flour more often.
	Potatoes, sweet potatoes, yams, cassava, green banana are all good sources of carbohydrates, but use them on their own rather than with Indian breads and rice.
	Leave the skin on potatoes when cooking.
Vegetables and fruits	Wash vegetables before chopping and avoid peeling.
	Do not cut into very small pieces where possible.
	Include traditional vegetables such as okra (*bhinda*), spinach (*palak*), peas (*matter*), cauliflower (*ful gobi*), but also try local vegetables and fruits as they are cheaper, fresher and can be just as nutritious.
	Frozen vegetables and tinned fruits in their own juices.
	Limit sweetened fruit products such as tinned mango pulp.
	Use only small amounts of oil in cooking.
	Make *raita* with low-fat yoghurt.
	Eat salad every day, using lemon juice instead of dressing.
	Eat 3–4 pieces of fruit daily, and eat them with the skin where possible.
	Avoid oily pickles.
	Try using more green chutney.
Meat, fish, eggs, beans pluses dals, nuts and seeds	Use more boiled pulses dishes rather than deep fried (e.g., *bhel/sev usad*).
	Try dals with skins on where possible.
	Use more shallow-fried dishes rather than deep-fried, e.g., *puda*.
	Try to cook more steamed and baked dishes, e.g., *dhokra, patra, muthiya, ondhwa*.
	Use sprouted pulses at least three or four times a week cooked or raw in salad.
	Cut down on deep-fried snacks, e.g., *chevdo, ganthia*.Try dry roasted chick peas.
	Restrict intake of nuts to occasional use. Try dry-roasted peanuts instead of deep-fried nuts.
	Make more use of sesame seeds as they contain calcium and iron.
	If non-vegetarian, trim fat off meat, take skin off chicken and include oily fish, such as salmon and sardines in the diet.
Milk and dairy foods	Make milky puddings such as *kheer* with semi-skimmed milk and less sugar.
	Instead of full-fat milk choose semi- or skimmed milk.
	Try making yoghurt/milkshakes with semi-skimmed milk.
	Try low-fat plain yoghurts for cooking and for making *raita/chaas*
	Try low-fat varieties of cheese such as Edam or cottage cheese.
	Try making *paneer* with semi-skimmed instead of whole milk.
	Try low-fat varieties of ice cream.
	Cut down on cream in cooking,
Foods and drinks high in fat and/ or sugar	Have Indian sweets as treats, e.g., *barfi* and *ladwa*.
	Cut down intake of pies, pastries, sausage rolls, cake, biscuits English sweets, chocolates and all convenience foods.

(Continued)

Table 1.1.5 (cont'd)

Food groups	Healthier alternatives
Sugar and sugary foods	Gradually cut down on sugar in tea and coffee. Use less sugar and jaggery when making Indian sweets and pickles. Try to restrict eating Indian sweets, biscuits, cakes, chocolates and ice cream to special occasions. Avoid fizzy drinks containing sugar. Try 'no added sugar' varieties of squash, and diet fizzy drinks. Buy tinned fruit in natural juice, not syrup. Buy unsweetened fruit juices. Reduce jaggery intake.
Fats and oil	Cut down on deep-fried foods such as *chevdo, sev, ghthiya*, chips, crisps, samosas. Shallow-fry rather than deep-fry. Spread butter/margarine sparingly on bread. Avoid adding oil when making Indian breads. Use low-fat spread instead of ghee. Steamed dishes are healthier options – *muthiya, patra, dhokra, khaman*. Make more use of microwave, oven, grill, pressure cooker and slow cooker. Invest in non-stick, thick-bottomed saucepans as they require less oil in cooking, and prevent food from sticking or burning.
Salt	Cut down on salt in cooking. Do not add salt at the table. Reduce intake of salty snacks such as crisps, tinned and convenience foods, nuts. Cut down on oily pickles. Use herbs and spices to flavour foods.

Another initiative is a community farm in London to encourage women to grow traditional and indigenous vegetables, and a cookery class, particularly useful for giving health information for chronic conditions such as diabetes.

Suggestions for the way forward

- Working more closely with religious and local voluntary organizations, which are now well established within the local community and are already providing religious and cultural needs.
- Introducing the 'Cook and Eat' model, which has been used successfully in many parts of the UK. The main aim is to discuss and demonstrate simple changes to the diet and different cooking methods.
- Further research looking at the health needs and dietary intake of the Gujarati population in the UK as this would aid health professionals in providing individualized, culturally appropriate information.

- Compiling nutritive values and suitable portion size of foods used by the South Asian communities in the UK.
- The development of appropriate resources.
- Cookery competitions which aim to demonstrate the use of traditional and seasonal indigenous ingredients which are high in fibre and cooked using less fat.

1.1.6   Nutritional deficiencies

Iron deficiency anaemia

Research suggests that anaemia is more prevalent among Indian women than the general population (Sproston & Mindell, 2006). Lacto-vegetarians should consume a variety of foods rich in iron and vitamin C at each meal (see Table 1.1.6).

Vitamin B$_{12}$ deficiency

A low intake of vitamin B$_{12}$ (folate), which has been shown to result in increased homocysteine levels

Table 1.1.6 Sources of iron in Gujarati lactovegetarian diet

Cereals	Vegetables	
Whole wheat flour	Amaranth	
Bajri (millet flour)	Colocasia leaves	
Whole meal bread	Mustard leaves	
Wholegrain breakfast cereal	Spinach	
Rice Flakes	Radish leaves	
Puffed Rice	Fenugreek leaves	
Sugary foods	Cluster beans	
Jaggery	Mint leaves	
	Fennel leaves	
	Bitter gourd	
	Leeks	
	Tomatoes	

Whole pulses and dals	Seeds and nuts	Fresh and dry fruits
Whole chana dal (chickpeas)	Sesame seeds	Citrus fruits and unsweetened fruit juices
Roasted chana	Peanuts	Dates
Black-eyed beans dal	Dried coconut	Blackcurrants
Whole urad dal (black gram)	Pistachios	Figs
Whole mung dal	Almond	Raisins
Sprouted pulses	Cashew nuts	Apricots
		Prunes/prune juice

and increased cardiovascular risk, and Vitamin B_6 has been reported among Asians (Jonnalagadda & Diwan, 2002).

According the American Dietetic Association (ADA) lacto-vegetarians should increase their consumption of dairy products, fortified breakfast cereals, soy milk and yeast extract to ensure a sufficient intake of vitamin B_{12}.

Strict vegetarians or vegans, however, may need to supplement their diet by taking a vitamin B_{12} (cobalamin) supplement of no more than 100% of the recommended daily value. Some Jains are vegans and will avoid dairy products, so they will need a B_{12} supplement.

Vitamin D deficiency

Low calcium has been shown among Asian women, a risk factor for osteoporosis (Jonnalagadda & Diwan, 2002). Insufficient vitamin D status and

corresponding low bone mineral density has also been identified in Gujaratis living in UK (Hamson et al., 2003). Research conducted in the USA looking at older Gujarati immigrants found that they were meeting government nutritional guidelines for carbohydrates and vegetables, but not for dairy foods, meat and fruits (Jonnalagadda et al., 2005).

Advantages of a vegetarian diet

The ADA is just one example of a major health organization that recognizes that a well-planned vegetarian/vegan diet can reduce the risk of many chronic conditions, such as heart disease, obesity, diabetes, asthma, high blood pressure and cancer. Because vegetarians are less susceptible to major diseases, they can live healthier, longer and more productive lives, with fewer visits to doctors, fewer dental problems and lower medical bills.

Here are some additional health benefits of the vegetarian diet:

- Food is easier to digest, provides a wider ranger of nutrients and requires less effort to purify the body from its wastes.
- Vegetarians' immune systems are stronger, their skin is less flawed and their bodies are more pure and refined.
- Meat is expensive compared to fruit and vegetables so a vegetarian diet can also have advantages for low-income populations. Unfortunately, lack of access to food stores that sell good quality fresh produce continues to be a serious problem among disadvantaged communities (www.betterhealth.vic.gov.au).

1.1.7 Diabetes

Introduction

When talking about Gujarati diets, it is important to make a distinction between the typical urban lacto-vegetarian diet and the non-vegetarian Gujarati diet which has become more westernized, both in large South Asian cities in India and abroad.

In India, the diet of the rural lacto-vegetarian farmer with diabetes appears to be very sound, judging by the current recommendations of Diabetic Associations. The diet is high in carbohydrate and fibre, with cereals and pulses forming the staple. In contrast, the Gujarati person with

---

Key points

- The traditional Gujarati diet is well balanced, high in fibre and low in fat.
- Following urbanization and migration, most Gujaratis adopt western eating patterns/ habits while maintaining some traditional eating habits.
- Adoption of unhealthy western eating patterns and changes in lifestyle have resulted in an increase in diabetes among Gujaratis.
- Cultural beliefs, dietary habits, religious and family influences play a key role in self-care management.
- Some Gujaratis rely on complementary medicine, and asking about the use of these remedies should be an important part of the history, assessment and management of these patients.
- Dietary guidance for people with type 1 and 2 diabetes should be based on a healthy eating framework and current evidence base for the nutritional management of diabetes.
- The principles of dietary management in respect of diabetes for the Gujarati community are no different from those for any other population, but they do have to be applied in a culturally appropriate way.
- Dietitians need to make a careful individual assessment of where a client is in the process of acculturation before tailoring dietary advice.
- For effective health promotion, it is essential to work closely with the local Gujarati community and religious and voluntary organizations.

---

diabetes living in a city or abroad is more likely to eat fat-rich snacks and fast foods. These Gujaratis also use more oil in food preparation and eat more fat than carbohydrate. This, combined with a sedentary lifestyle, results in an unusually high proportion of body fat, which makes them more insulin resistant.

Prevalence of diabetes

Diabetes is one of the most common chronic disorders and affects about 2 million people in the UK, equivalent to about 4% of the population. The incidence, particularly of type 2 diabetes, is rising rapidly and it was estimated there would be nearly 3 million people with diabetes living in the UK by 2010. Globally, the number of people with diabetes is projected to rise from 171 million in 2000 to 366 million in 2030 (Wild *et al.*, 2004).

The reasons for this increase are population growth, ageing, urbanization and the increasing prevalence of obesity and lack of physical exercise (Wild *et al.*, 2004). With regard to South Asian people, the World Health Organization (WHO) estimated that by 2030 around one third of all people with diabetes will reside in the Indian subcontinent.

The risk of South Asians developing type 2 diabetes is about 4–5 times that of Europeans and around 1 in 4 South Asian adults over the age of 50 have diabetes. Over the course of their lifetime, South Asians have about a 1 in 3 chance of developing diabetes. The condition also tends to develop earlier and complications of diabetes, such as kidney disease and heart disease, develop much more frequently compared to Europeans (Chowdhury, 2007).

A high prevalence of diabetes has been found in South Asians from the Indian subcontinent both in their country of origin and in the countries to which they have migrated when compared to the local resident population (McKeigue *et al.*, 1991; Ramachandran *et al.*, 1992). Diabetes is more prevalent among the less affluent and its incidence may be 1.5 times greater among the more deprived population. Currently, approximately 2–5% of people in India's urban areas are reported to have diabetes (Pawa, 2005).

South Asians, including Gujaratis, are more likely to develop diabetes at a younger age than people of European origin. Increased central obesity plays a role in its increased prevalence in this group in UK (Burden *et al.*, 1992). The Health Survey for England (Joint Health Surveys for England, 2001) indicated that the prevalence of diagnosed diabetes in Indians was 10% for men and 7% for women. According to The Health Survey for England (2004), after adjusting for age, diagnosed diabetes was almost 2.5–3 times more prevalent in Indians compared with the general population. The prevalence of undiagnosed diabetes did not differ between different minority groups in men.

The UK Prospective Diabetes Study (1994) showed that Asian people had a more sedentary lifestyle and a higher prevalence of family history of known diabetes than other groups. Both environmental and genetic factors could thus explain the high prevalence of diabetes among the Asian population. The trend for a higher prevalence across all age bands implies significant public health implications for resource planning and allocation. A concerted global initiative is required to address the diabetes epidemic.

Risk factors and treatment

At all ages, mortality rates are higher in people with diabetes than in their non-diabetic counterparts (Laing *et al.*, 1999). Diabetes has major implications in terms of morbidity and mortality, not only from the acute effects of the disease itself but also because it significantly increases the risk of cardiovascular disease and damage to the microcirculation of the kidneys, nerves, eyes and limbs. As a result, diabetes is a major contributor to heart disease, stroke, renal failure, blindness, gangrene and amputations. It also tends to exacerbate the effects of other risk factors for cardiovascular disease (CVD), such as dyslipidaemia, hypertension, smoking and obesity (Laing *et al.*, 1999).

To minimize the risk of complications, people with diabetes require diet and lifestyle measures which help achieve near-normal levels of glycaemia and reduce CVD risk factors. Type 1 diabetes requires treatment with insulin. Ensuring that carbohydrate intake balances insulin action is a major dietary objective in order to maintain tight glycaemic control without hypoglycaemia. Type 2 diabetes is commonly associated with obesity and features of metabolic syndrome. Weight management by means of diet and exercise is a priority for many patients. Prevention of overweight and obesity is the key to prevention of type 2 diabetes. Effective self-care is essential to good diabetes management. Structured education, follow-up and support are essential from diagnosis onwards (Thomas & Bishop, 2007).

Complications associated with diabetes

Although some deaths occur from the acute effects of diabetes (mainly ketoacidosis), most result from the chronic complications associated with the disease. These include diabetic retinopathy, neuropathy, nephropathy and CVD (Thomas & Bishop, 2007). The prevalence of CVD and renal disease is higher in people of South Asian origin than among the European population (Chowdhury *et al.*, 2003). The risks of developing diabetic complications are also much greater due to early presentation and the large number of undiagnosed cases.

In renal disease, the principal aim of dietary management is to provide optimal nutritional support. Fluid, salt, potassium and phosphate are restricted according to the cause and degree of renal impairment. Protein and energy requirements are increased among people on haemodialysis and peritoneal dialysis.

There is now indisputable evidence from long-term prospective trials that meticulous control of blood glucose can prevent or delay the onset of microvascular complications in people with type 2 diabetes (UKPDS, 1998).

Dietary modification

Unfortunately, the management of Asian people with diabetes is often both inadequate and ineffective (Cruickshank, 1989). Patients often lack knowledge about the disease, its complications and the importance of self-management, problems which stem from poor communication, provision of inadequate or culturally inappropriate information, and a lack of educational material in minority languages (Goodwin *et al.*, 1987; Hawthorne 1990; Close *et al.*, 1995). To some extent, the situation will have improved following the implementation of the National Service Framework for Diabetes and the development of translated literature by organizations such as Diabetes UK (2006). However, delivery of appropriate care to this patient group remains variable.

Carbohydrates

The rural Gujarati diet provides 60–70% of the total energy intake from carbohydrates (Raghuram *et al.*, 1993). Slow-absorbing carbohydrates are a standard part of the diet, and include cereals such as rice, whole wheat, sorghum, millet and maize. Consumption of cereals seems to decrease with increasing income of the household, while that of pulses, milk, meat/fish, vegetables, fats and oils increases (Food and Agriculture Organization,

2004). The more affluent also consume more refined white flour (*maida*) and carbohydrates in the form of sweetmeats, desserts, cakes, biscuits and preserves. The Indian Diabetes Association recommends a diet high in complex carbohydrates, providing up to 60–70% of energy (this is higher than the Diabetes UK of 45–60% guideline). The consumption of refined carbohydrates is discouraged. The distribution and type of carbohydrates in the diet should be tailored to individual habits.

In people with type 2 diabetes, choosing lower glycaemic index (GI) foods may help to reduce postprandial glycaemia and insulinaemia. Quantitative guidance on carbohydrate intake (e.g., the amount typically needed at a main meal, late night snack or to prevent/treat hypoglycaemia) may be helpful for some patients. It is therefore essential that dietitians should have a thorough knowledge of several models for carbohydrate management. For overweight patients, weight management is a priority, particularly with the increasing incidence of central obesity in those with type 2 diabetes. Newly diagnosed patients with type 2 diabetes should be encouraged to attend Diabetes Education and Self Management for Ongoing and Newly Diagnosed (DESMOND) which are offered by their local Primary Care Trust (PCT).

The introduction of short-acting analogues, the basal-bolus system and insulin pumps has allowed greater flexibility in the timings of meals for people with type 1 diabetes (Nutrition Subcommittee of Diabetes UK, 2003). This has enabled knowledgeable patients to vary their carbohydrate intake at any mealtime. The Dose Adjustment For Normal Eating (DAFNE) structured education programme teaches carbohydrate counting and flexible insulin adjustments to match carbohydrates on a meal-by-meal basis. Those on two fixed daily injections need to choose foods with a similar glycaemic effect in order to balance the prescribed insulin profile. They have better glycaemic control if they achieve day-to-day consistency in the amount and source of the carbohydrate content of their diets (Wolever *et al.*, 1991).

Dietary fibre

Diets high in carbohydrate and fibre improve glucose metabolism without increasing insulin

secretion. The benefits of a high-fibre diet are numerous. Soluble fibre which is present in fruit, vegetables and legumes is encouraged. An intake of 25 g of dietary fibre each day is considered to be optimal (Raghuram *et al.*, 1993) (see Table 1.1.7).

Glycaemic index

Different carbohydrates raise blood glucose levels to variable extents, so the glycaemic index (GI) has a value in planning diets for people with diabetes. Diets with a low GI are generally rich in fibre as in the typical lacto-vegetarian Gujarati diet. Another approach to increase the fibre content is by the addition of purified fibre supplements such as wheat bran, guar gum, tragacanth, oatmeal and ispaghula. It is not only the GI, but also the quantity of the glycaemic load (GL) of carbohydrate influences the metabolic response to the ingestion of carbohydrate.

There is insufficient evidence of the long-term benefit to recommend the use of low GI diets as a primary strategy in meal planning (Franz *et al.*, 2002). Although the value of GI in the management of diabetes remains controversial, it can be a useful pointer to carbohydrate food choice in order to minimize glycaemic peaks (see Table 1.1.8).

Protein

Protein is essential for growth and tissue repair. It is generally recommended that 15–20% of total energy is derived from protein. Cereals, pulses and dairy products provide most of the protein requirements of the lacto-vegetarian Gujarati diet. Non-vegetarians can also meet their protein requirements from meat or fish. Studies in India have shown that the protein and energy content of diets increase with increasing income (National Institute of Nutrition, 1992).

In India, it is generally believed that proteins from vegetable sources are better than those from animal sources as they do not contain saturated fat and also add fibre to the diet (Raghuram *et al.*, 1993). Diabetes UK recommends lean meats, the consumption of oily fish twice a week and the inclusion of more beans/lentils in the diet. People with diabetes should be discouraged from consuming high-protein, low-carbohydrate weight management diets.

Table 1.1.7 Dietary fibre of some common South Asian foods

Foods	Total dietary fibre (100g raw)	Foods	Total dietary fibre (100g raw)
Cereals and millet		**Roots and tubers**	
Bajri (millet)	11.3	Potato	1.7
Jowar (sorghum)	9.7	Sweet potato	3.9
Maize, dry	11.9	Yam	4.2
Rice	4.1		
Wheat	12.5	**Fruits**	
		Banana	1.8
Pulses and legumes		Guava (jamphal)	8.5
Bengal gram, whole (chana)	28.3	Mango	2.0
Bengal gram, dal (chana ni dal)	15.3	Sapodilla (Sapota) (chikku)	10.9
Black gram, whole (urad)	20.3		
Black gram, dal (urad ni dal)	11.7	**Vegetables**	
Green gram, whole (mung)	16.7	Amaranth (tanjurdo)	4.0
Green gram, dal (mung ni dal)	8.2	Aubergine (ringun)	6.3
Lentil, whole (masoor)	15.8	Bitter gourd	4.3
Lentil, dal (masoor ni dal)	10.3	Broad beans	8.9
Red gram, whole (tuvar)	22.6	Bottle gourd (dudhi)	2.0
Red gram, dal (tuvar ni dal)	9.1	Cluster beans	5.7
Soya bean	23.0	Colocasia green	6.6
		Fenugreek	4.7
Nuts and oilseeds		Spinach (palak)	2.5
Peanuts (groundnuts)	11.0	Ridge gourd (turia)	1.9
Sesame seeds	16.8	Snake gourd (gulka)	2.1

(Narasinga et al., 1991)

Fat

Fats are concentrated sources of energy and an excess intake increases body fat and leads to obesity. Obesity is increasing in India among western Gujarati diabetics and makes them more vulnerable to hypertension, cardiovascular disease and other related ailments. A recent study suggests that even Gujaratis who appear thin may face a similar risk, as they may have a lot of fat inside the body, in vessels, around organs and in the blood, despite the appearance of healthiness (Joshi et al., 2007). Exercise has to be encouraged as part of the lifestyle for a sedentary Gujarati, whereas for the average rural farmer it is their lifestyle.

It is recommended that 15–25% of the total energy should be derived from fat. Since serum lipids are generally raised in people with diabetes, they have to be careful about the amount and nature of the fats consumed. It is recommended that saturated fatty acid sources such as ghee, butter, *vanaspati* (hydrogenated vegetable fat) and coconut oil are taken in small quantities only. It is suggested that monounsaturated (MONO) and/or polyunsaturated (PUFA; e.g., sunflower, safflower, groundnut and olive oil) vegetable fats are used instead. Obese people with diabetes should restrict their total fat consumption.

1.1.8 Exchange system

It is rare that the rural farmer will ever see a dietitian for diabetes dietary advice. However, for the more affluent Gujarati, a diet is prescribed in terms of exchange lists. In India, it is the general belief that the quantity of food and the total calorie intake of a person with diabetes should not vary markedly from day to day. For this purpose, a food

Table 1.1.8 Glycaemic index of some common South
Asian foods

Foods	Glycaemic index	Foods	Glycaemic index
Cereal products		**Fruits**	
Bread	70	Apple	39
Millet	71	Banana	69
Rice (white)	72	Orange	40
Breakfast snacks		**Vegetables**	
Pongal	55	Brown beans	79
Pasarattu	60	Frozen beans	51
Upma	75	Potato	70
Idli	80	Yam	51
Chola	65	Beetroot	64
Sprouted green gram	60	**Dried legumes**	
Dairy products		Kidney beans	29
Milk	33	Bengal gram	47
Ice cream	36	Green gram	48
Curds	36	Black gram	48
Miscellaneous		**Sugars**	
Peanuts	13	Sucrose	59
Potato chips	51	Fructose	20
Tomato soup	38	Glucose	100
		Maltose	105
		Honey	87

(Raghuram et al., 1993)

exchange system is used in which foods providing almost the same amount of energy, carbohydrates, proteins and fats are grouped together.

The food exchange system helps the patient:

- To restrict their food intake according to the insulin prescription for better glycaemic control.
- To have variety in the diet while maintaining the desired daily energy intake.
- To learn the principles of the diet easily.

There are seven food groups used in the exchange system:

- Vegetable exchange.
- Fruit exchange.
- Cereal exchange.
- Legume and pulse exchange.
- Meat/fish exchange.
- Milk exchange.
- Fat exchange.

The foods have been carefully chosen and placed in each group because they contain approximately the same nutritive value when they are eaten in the amounts listed. Notice that it takes different amounts of food to contain the same amount of carbohydrate and energy. For instance, in a vegetable exchange, 90 g onion or 105 g carrot provide 10 g carbohydrate and 50 kcal.

Each exchange list provides a number of food items which can be interchanged within the group. All groups of food exchanges make a specific contribution to a good diet, and none of the exchange groups can itself supply all the nutrients needed for a well-balanced diet (Raghuram et al., 1993).

Particular emphasis may need to be placed on:

- The timing of meals, particularly for those on insulin or oral hypoglycaemic drugs. It is sometimes necessary to remind patients of the importance of taking medications at the specified times and in the prescribed doses.
- The need for starchy cereal foods throughout the day, which is appropriate for any hypoglycaemic therapy given.
- The need to avoid rich sources of sugars, particularly sweetmeats and sugar-containing carbonated drinks, which are often consumed in large quantities.
- The need to reduce fat consumption (principally by using less during cooking) and to reduce the intake of deep-fried snacks.
- The importance of weight loss for those who are overweight (via restriction of energy intake, primarily from fat, and by increased physical activity).
- Those choosing to fast for religious purposes being advised regarding their diet and any medication (especially insulin/oral hypoglycaemic drugs).

Herbal remedies

Many Asians with diabetes either bring traditional/ herbal preparations back with them after holidaying in their native country or use such remedies on the suggestion of family members. These preparations are commonly used either on their own or in conjunction with other therapeutic agents and have hypoglycaemic effects. They are available in South Asian shops and grocery stores in the UK and worldwide. Asking about these remedies should be an important part of the history, assessment and management of patients with diabetes (Pawa, 2005).

Fenugreek

The medicinal qualities of fenugreek seeds (*trigonella foenum graecum*) have been known since ancient times, and the seeds are commonly used as a condiment for seasoning in South Asian homes. The seeds are high in fibre (mucilaginous fibre and total fibre of 20% and 50% respectively). In addition, it contains trigonelline, an alkaloid known to reduce blood sugar levels.

There are several trials available for fenugreek in type 2 diabetes; however, most are non-controlled (Madar *et al.*, 1988). Of the available randomized controlled trials, they are generally poorer quality studies with small numbers and from a single investigator group. Nonetheless, these trials, including a single trial in type 2 diabetes, have reported improved glycaemic control using seed powder added to unleavened bread (Sharma & Raghuram, 1990). In another series of trials, whole raw seeds, extracted seed powder, gum isolate of seeds and cooked whole seeds seemed to decrease postprandial glucose levels, whereas degummed seeds and cooked leaves did not (Sharma *et al.*, 1986). No adverse effects were reported in any of these trials. There is some preliminary evidence for the efficacy of fenugreek, which suggests further studies may be warranted.

In Gujarati families, fenugreek preparations may be used as supportive therapy to anti-diabetic treatment. The use of fenugreek seeds in the management of diabetes is advocated by the National Institute of Nutrition in Hyderabad in India (1991). The quantity of fenugreek seeds to be taken daily depends on the severity of the diabetes. The doses vary from 25 g to 50 g. Initially, 25 g of fenugreek seeds is recommended in two equal parts (approximately two teaspoons each) with lunch and dinner.

The seeds can be taken whole after soaking in water overnight or in powder form in water or butter milk 15 minutes before a meal. Fenugreek seed powder can be incorporated in preparations such as chapatti, rice, dal and vegetables. The preparations can be made salty or sour according to individual taste (Raghuram *et al.*, 1993).

Karela (*momordica charantia; bitter melon gourd*)

Karela is indigenous to tropical areas and as the English name suggests, it tastes bitter. The glycaemic effect of karela is well known within the Gujarati community. Reported preparations of the herb range from injectable extracts to fruit juice. Processed bitter gourd in the form of capsules or tablets is commonly advertised and sold, or can be ordered online.

The active components of karela are thought to be charantin, vicine and polypeptide-p (an unidentified insulin-like protein similar to bovine insulin). Some, albeit limited, data suggest a potential effect of karela in diabetes, with no adverse side-effects reported. However, further information from RCTs is needed (Yeh *et al.*, 2003).

Many Gujaratis with diabetes will cook and eat karela as part of a meal or drink karela juice for its hypoglycaemic effect. For these to have a clinical effect karela need to be taken every day, but most people eat them on an ad hoc basis. This may have implications as it is often taken as well as oral hypoglycaemic drugs and therefore has a doubling effect on the dose. Medical staff may not be aware of this and as a result the severity of the diabetes may be misjudged. Some people with diabetes use this opportunity to indulge by consuming inappropriate foods, but still have control of their diabetes (Hamid & Sarwar, 2004).

Diabetes UK has issued a warning with regard to the use of karela, because it is not yet known what dose is safe when taken with other anti-diabetic agents, and there is a lack of information on other potential bioactive components of the capsule (Diabetes UK, 2006).

Yoga and spiritual healing

Yoga and spiritual healing play an important part of the Gujarati lifestyle. It has been observed that some Gujaratis have stopped using anti-diabetic drugs after adopting a yogic lifestyle and diet (Shankardevananda, 2002).

It is important to note that Gujarati fasts do not involve total abstinence from food. Pure foods can be taken regularly throughout the day. If the individual wishes to fast, they should do so as safely as possible and may need to modify their diabetes medication/insulin during this period. The dietitian should be able to advise on timely foods/ snacks in line with treatment. Patients are encouraged to monitor their diabetes more closely. If they are feeling unwell, they should be encouraged to break their fast.

Suggestions for the way forward in diabetes

Access to healthcare services by South Asians tends to be poor, particularly in older age groups or for whose command of the English language is limited. These issues are beginning to be addressed at both national and local levels by targeted programmes of outreach and health improvement.

Although the aims of dietary management are the same for South Asians as for anyone else, the nature of the advice given must be culturally appropriate and local resources should reflect this. A number of organizations such as Diabetes UK, the British Dietetic Association and British Nutrition Foundation have developed resource material for people from ethnic minorities with diabetes. Information in Gujarati may be helpful, although some of the older generation may be illiterate. Alternative resources such as audiotapes, CDs and DVDs should also be available in different languages (Thomas & Bishop, 2007).

In order to improve compliance, the health professional must first ascertain dietary food patterns and customs, the hierarchy within the family, social pressures within the house and other socioeconomic factors. A skilled interpreter/link worker/health advocate is an essential part of a healthcare team which has among its clients patients with little command of English. Guidance in pictorial form and cookery demonstrations can be an effective way of getting the message across.

The Diabetic Association of India also acts as an advisory body for people with diabetes and provides support for its members. Many Gujaratis living in the UK have their own social clubs (e.g.,

Asian Women UK), which provide support and good networking in the community.

1.2   Punjabi Diet

Renuka McArthur, Jevanjot Sihra, Rupinder Sahota, Ravita Taheem, Sunita Wallia

The South Asian subcontinent comprises India, Pakistan, Bangladesh and Sri Lanka. Four per cent of the total UK population are classified as 'Asian' or 'Asian British' and this group makes up 50.2% of the minority ethnic group population in the UK (UK Census, 2001).

'South Asians' is 'a term which defines many ethnic groups with distinctive regions of origin, languages, religions and customs and includes people born in India, Bangladesh, Pakistan or Sri Lanka' (Fox, 2004).

1.2.1   Introduction

Punjab is located in the north-west of India and occupies 1.54% of the area. The word Punjab is a hybrid of the Persian words *panj* (five) and *āb* (water), that is, it is the land of five rivers, and it is so fertile that it has come to be known as the food basket of India, providing at least 40% of the country's rice and 60% of the country's wheat requirement (see Figure 1.2.1).

Worldwide, there are 25.8 million Sikhs and approximately 75% of Sikhs live in Punjab, where they constitute about 61% of the population, 37% are Hindus and the rest a small Muslim population still living there after the partition of India in 1947 when the Punjab province of British India was divided between India and Pakistan.

Language

It was estimated from the 1991 census that the British population included 840,000 people from India, of whom 51% were Sikh, and 477,000 people from Pakistan, of whom 48,000 had Punjabi as their main language. In fact, Punjabi is the most common language among British Asians and has become the second language in Britain, used by an estimated 1.3 million people. Punjabi is spoken by Muslims who write it in the Arabic script, whereas

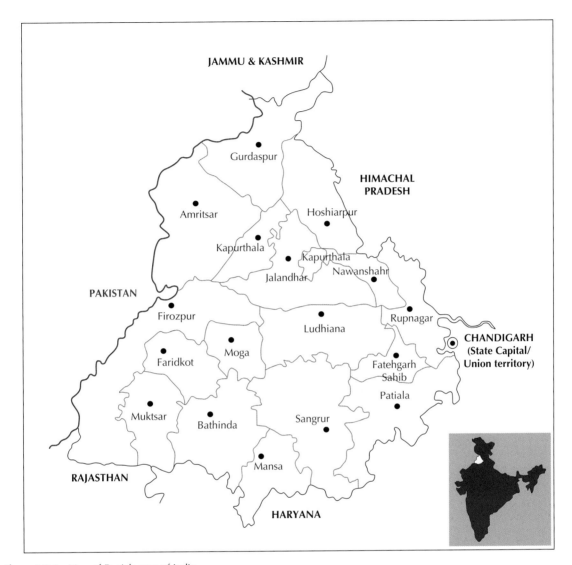

Figure 1.2.1   Map of Punjab area of India

the Sikhs and Hindus of Punjab write it in the Gurmukhi (language of the Gurus) script. It has very many letters in common with Hindi and shares similar vowel marks but the sound systems of Hindi and Punjabi are different. Older generations are concerned that English is becoming the first language for younger generations, who are thereby losing their linguistic heritage.

Migration to the United Kingdom

By the end of the nineteenth century Great Britain had colonized parts of East Africa – Tanzania,

Uganda, Kenya, Zambia and Malawi. Skilled workers from the Punjab and Gujarat were brought to the area to construct the railway line from Mombassa to Kampala and also work in government administration in these countries.

The main settlement of Indian families in these countries took place between 1890 and 1935 and again between 1945 and 1960. Because of their history as traders and junior administrators many established successful businesses or professional careers. However, when the East African countries became independent after 1960, they were given the option to become citizens of these countries or remain British. Most chose to exercise their rights to choose British citizenship. The largest exodus of South Asians to UK occurred in 1972, when Uganda expelled them in line with the government's policy of Africanization. All South Asians families with British passports were expelled to the UK.

People also migrated directly to UK from Punjab in the 1950s not only to work in industry to fill the labour shortages but also to escape the unrest that resulted from the partition of India.

Current UK population

The 2001 census recorded 366,000 Sikhs in the UK (this number excludes the Hindu Punjabi population). Slough has the highest percentage of Sikh residents in the country according to the 2001 census where they make up 9.1% of the population, more than in any other local authority. Many live in Southall, which is primarily a South Asian residential district, sometimes known as 'Little India'. In 1950, the first group of South Asians arrived in Southall, reputedly recruited to work in a local factory owned by a former British Indian Army officer. This population grew, due to the proximity to expanding employment opportunities such as Heathrow Airport. The most significant cultural group to settle in Southall are Asians. According to the Commission for Racial Equality, over 55% of Southall's population of 70,000 are Indian/Pakistani, with less than 10% White British. There are 10 Sikh Gurdwaras in Southall and one of them won the Ealing Civic Society Architectural Award in 2003. The Gurdwara Sri Guru Singh Sabha, which opened in 2003, is one of the largest Sikh Gurdwara outside India.

1.2.2   Religion

Most people from Punjab follow the Sikh religion and the most notable sign of a Sikh man is the wearing of a turban. There are also many Punjabis in the UK who follow the Hindu religion and they call themselves Hindu Punjabi.

The Sikh religion is based on the teachings of 10 Gurus. The Sikh holy scriptures, *Guru Granth Sahib Ji*, were first compiled by the fifth Guru, Guru Arjan Dev Ji, and contained teachings from the first five gurus and other holy saints of that time. These teachings were then complemented by scriptures from the last five gurus.

Religious beliefs

Naam Japna
A Sikh is to engage in the daily practice of meditation and prayers (*nitnem*) by reciting and chanting God's name.

Kirat Karni
To live honestly and earn by one's physical and mental effort while accepting God's gifts and blessings. A Sikh has to live as a householder carrying out his or her duties and responsibilities to the full.

Vand Chakna
Sikhs are asked to share their wealth within the community and outside by giving (*dasvand*) and practising charity (*daan*), 'sharing and consuming together'.

Kill the Five Thieves
The Sikh Gurus tell us that our mind and spirit are constantly being attacked by the Five Evils – *kam* (lust), *krodh* (rage), *lobh* (greed), *moh* (attachment) and *ahankar* (ego). A Sikh needs constantly to combat and overcome these five vices.

Positive human qualities
The Gurus taught the Sikhs to develop and harness positive human qualities which lead the soul closer to God and away from evil. These are *sat* (truth), *daya* (compassion), *santokh* (contentment), *nimrata* (humility) and *pyare* (love).

Sikhs undergo the initiation ceremony (*amrit shakh*) at any point during their lifetime. After this ceremony they strictly follow the Sikh philosophy and beliefs, and wear the five K's:

Kesh: uncut hair, symbolizing a movement away from physical appearance and towards spirituality.
Kara: a steel bracelet symbolizing the infinite God.
Kanga: a comb representing the importance of cleanliness and neatness.
Kacha: cotton underwear, symbolizing modesty and chastity.
Kirpan: a dagger or sword, symbolizing the defence of truth and against injustice.

Gurdwara

The gurdwara (temple) is a holy place for the Sikh community where the scriptures are kept and also where all religious, social and cultural activities take place.

One of the holiest of Sikh shrines, the Sri Harmandir Sahib Ji or Golden Temple, is in the city of Amritsar. The Golden Temple culturally is the most significant shrine and one of the oldest Sikh gurdwara in the world.

Within the gurdwara, the *Guru ka langar* (Guru's community kitchen) serves free meals for all. The institution of the *langar* was started by the first Sikh Guru, Guru Nanak. It was designed to uphold the principle of equality among all people regardless of religion, caste, colour, creed, age, gender or social status, a revolutionary concept in the caste-ordered society of 16th-century India where Sikhism was founded. In addition to the ideals of equality, the tradition of the *langar* expresses the ethics of sharing, community, inclusiveness and the oneness of all humankind.

People from all classes are welcome at the *langar*. Only lacto-vegetarian food is served to ensure that all people, regardless of their dietary restrictions, can eat as equals. The *langar* is open to Sikhs and non-Sikhs alike. Food is normally served twice a day, on every day of the year. Each week one or more families volunteer to provide and prepare the *langar*. This is very generous, as there may be several hundred people to feed, and caterers are not used as it is considered a form of *sewa* (voluntary community service). All the preparation, cooking and washing-up are also done by volunteers, who are known as *sewadars*. In the UK most *langar* food is cooked and served at least twice a week and on religious days.

Religious dietary restrictions

Sikhs who have been initiated and have undergone the religious Amrit ceremony become lacto-vegetarian and so avoid meat, fish and eggs, and products containing these, and do not drink alcohol. Non-practising Sikhs are not usually vegetarian but do avoid beef and beef products and *halal* meat, preferring animals to be slaughtered with one stroke (the *jatka* method). Some Sikhs also avoid pork and pork products.

Religious festivals

Vaisakhi (also known as *Baisakhi*) is celebrated in the second week of April. It is an ancient harvest festival in the Punjab region, which also marks beginning of the new solar year and the foundation of the Khalsa.

Diwali (festival of light)

This is celebrated during October/November.

Sahib (birthday of Guru Nanak, founder of Sikhism)

One of the most important festivals, Sahib is celebrated on 15 November.

1.2.3 Traditional diet and eating pattern

Traditional Punjabi food is rich in texture and flavour and is characterized by a profusion of dairy products in the form of *malai* (cream), *paneer* (white cheese), butter, ghee and curds (yoghurt) as these food products are readily available. The cuisine is so versatile that sometimes Indian food is associated with Punjabi cuisine.

- *Makke di roti*: maize/cornflour *roti*.
- *Sarson ka saag*: spinach curry is something of a delicacy simply because of the time it takes to prepare as the dish is cooked on a slow fire for hours with a minimum of spices so that the fresh taste can be retained. In fact, the longer it takes to cook, the better it tastes. It is traditionally served with small pieces of white butter which is made at home using cream.
- Whole pulses and dal: black gram, green gram and bengal gram are simmered on a slow fire, often for hours, until they turn creamy and then are flavoured with herbs and spices. *Malai* (cream) is added at the end of cooking process for a rich finish before serving.
- *Chola bhatura*: chickpea curry served with small fried *puri* made from plain flour.
- *Mah ke dal*: Dal made from yellow split peas.
- Stuffed *parathas*: One of the most popular unleavened flatbreads made by pan-frying whole wheat flour in a *tava* (frying pan). The *paratha* dough usually contains ghee or cooking oil. *Parathas* are usually stuffed with spiced vegetables (e.g., potatoes, cabbages, radishes, cauliflowers) or *paneer*. They can be eaten on their own, with pickles or with *raita*.

Traditional meal pattern

The traditional Punjabi diet is a healthy one based on starchy foods, lentils and vegetables. The daily diet consists of roti or rice dal (lentil curry) *sabji* (mixed curry) with some *achar* (pickle) or natural (homemade) yoghurt. *Lassi* (a sweet or savoury yoghurt-based drink) is mainly consumed during the summer season. It can be sweetened and flavoured with rose water or mango, or served plain. Food is usually served in a regular plate with little helpings of the pre-

pared dishes. Fresh fruit or a sweet dessert may follow. Most Indian meals include different types of flatbread, which is traditionally used to scoop up or roll vegetables. Dals can be eaten with a spoon or scooped with flatbread. Traditionally, Indians in Punjab eat their main meal at midday, preferring a light evening meal. People either bring their midday meal to work or use a lunch packing service (tiffin) which delivers traditional hot meals to the workplace. If possible, many Indians like to come home for the midday meal (see Table 1.2.1).

Table 1.2.1 Traditional eating pattern and dietary changes in Punjabi diet on migration

	Traditional meal	Dietary changes on migration to UK	Healthier alternatives
Breakfast	Plain or stuffed *paratha* (potatoes/radish/cauliflower) made with ghee or butter, pickle, yoghurt, milky tea	Cereal or porridge with milk Toast with omelette Biscuits English tea or coffee	Whole meal cereal with semi-skimmed milk and fruit Whole meal toast with low-fat spread Tea with sweetener
Lunch	Chapatti (rotli) with ghee or butter/rice Vegetable/meat/fish/scrambled egg curry/whole pulses/dal Salad, pickle *Boondi*, cucumber yoghurt Plain yoghurt or *lassi* made with yoghurt	Leftover *sabji* with *roti*, e.g., chapatti with ghee or butter, rice Vegetable/meat/fish/scrambled egg *sabji*/whole pulses/dal Sandwiches, pizza chips, pasta, jacket potato	Chapatti, whole meal flour no butter or ghee; use low-fat spread Boiled rice Vegetable/meat/fish/scrambled egg curry/dal (measure amount of oil in cooking) Salad, pickle *Boondi*, cucumber yoghurt Poppadum – grilled or dry-roasted Sandwich of whole meal bread and low-fat filling Fruit
Snacks	Samosa, *pokora*, spring rolls Indian snacks and sweet meats with tea	Biscuits and cakes Indian snacks and sweet meats with tea	Biscuits and cakes with tea Unsalted, dry-roasted *chana* or nuts
Evening	Same as lunch May have pudding *Halwa/kheer*/semolina pudding/*sevia*/sweet rice	Chapatti with ghee or butter/rice Vegetable/meat/fish/scrambled egg/*kadhi* (yoghurt curry)/dal/kidney beans Salad, pickle *Boondi*/cucumber yoghurt Papadom Fruit juice/fizzy drinks Pizza/fish and chips/pasta/ready-meals/noodles	Chapatti, wholemeal flour no butter or ghee or use of low-fat spread/boiled rice Vegetable/meat/fish/scrambled egg curry/*kadhi* (yoghurt curry) dal/kidney beans (measure amount of oil in cooking) Salad, pickle *Boondi*, cucumber yoghurt papadom

Cooking methods

The custom of cooking in community ovens or tandoors prevails in rural areas and tandoori dishes are popular all over the country. There is a variety of both non-vegetarian and vegetarian dishes and one of the main features of Punjabi cuisine is its diversity. Almost all dishes are cooked on a slow fire to achieve a robust taste. The basic sauce used for vegetables and meat dishes is a combination of onion, tomato, garlic and ginger.

Herbs and spices

Herbs and spices (masala) are an integral part of Punjabi cooking. Freshly ground garlic, ginger and green chillies are commonly used. Spices are used individually (e.g. *haldi* (turmeric), chilli powder, cumin, cinnamon or peppercorns) or in specific combinations (e.g. garam masala). 'Curry powder' as used in Britain is not comparable. Different combinations of spices are used and often only with certain foods. Many spices are thought to have special digestive and medicinal qualities. Salt (*nimak*) is also used. Black salt is good for the digestion and used on fruit or in drinks. Less spicy foods may be given to children and invalids.

Hot and cold foods

This bears no relationship to the spiciness of a food or the temperature at which it is served but is regarded as an inherent property of the food itself and one which affects the body's balance and state of health. It is believed that foods can affect the individual physically, emotionally and spiritually.

'Hot' foods are thought to increase the body temperature, stimulate the emotions and increase activity. 'Cold' foods are considered to reduce the body temperature and impart strength and cheerfulness. Normally, a diet containing a mixture of hot and cold foods is consumed. However, hot foods may be restricted during 'hot' conditions (e.g., mangoes/papaya are restricted during pregnancy). The intake of cold foods is controlled during 'cold' conditions (e.g., potatoes are con-

sumed only in small amounts during lactation). It is mainly the older generation from the South Asian community that follow this advice during illness and during hot and cold weather. This belief can have nutritional implications if important sources of nutrients are restricted in vulnerable people. For example, dairy product consumption may be reduced in people who have arthritis and the consequent lower calcium intake may be significant for the elderly.

There is also anecdotal evidence that many people attribute asthma and coughs to the use of oils and margarines instead of ghee. Ghee is considered a pure food and has religious significance (Dhina, 1991).

Dietary manipulations based on 'hotness' and 'coldness' tend to have less influence on the diets of people originating from the Indian subcontinent than on those from Far East Asian countries such as China. There is also much more variation among different South Asian groups as to which foods are considered 'hot' and 'cold', and the younger generation may not follow these practices at all (see Table 1.2.2).

Alcohol

A community survey of Sikh, Hindu, Muslim and White men in the West Midlands showed men living in Britain born of Indian origin have higher than expected rates of alcohol-related disorders. According to the study, older Sikh men consumed more alcohol than younger men (Cochrane & Bal, 1990). Sikhs were more likely to be regular drinkers, followed by Whites, then Hindus; very few Muslims drank. Greater levels of alcohol consumption were reported by Sikhs and Hindus born in India than Sikhs and Hindus in Britain (Cochrane & Bal, 1990).

Smoking

According to Johnson *et al.* (2000), South Asians had very little knowledge on health-related issues and the impact of smoking on heart disease. In the South Asian community smoking habits vary

Table 1.2.2   Classification of South Asian hot and cold foods

Food group	Hot	Cold
Cereals		Wheat, rice
Green leafy vegetables	Fenugreek	All others
Root vegetables	Carrots and onions	Potatoes
Other vegetables	Capsicum peppers, aubergine or brinjal	Most other vegetables, including cucumbers, beans, cauliflower, marrow, okra, gourds
Fruit	Dates, mango, papaya	
Animal products	Meat, including chicken, mutton, fish	
Dairy products	Eggs	
Milk products		Milk and cream, curd or yoghurt, buttermilk
Pulses	Lentils	Bengal gram or chickpeas, green gram, peas, red gram
Nuts		All types, including groundnuts (peanuts), cashew nuts
Spices and condiments	Chilli, cinnamon, cloves, garlic, ginger, hing (asafoetida), mustard, nutmeg, pepper	Coriander, cumin, cardamom, fennel, tamarind
Oils	Mustard	Butter, ghee, coconut oil, ground oil
Miscellaneous	Tea, coffee, honey, *gurr* (jaggery), brown sugar	White sugar

British Diabetic Association, Asian diet information pack

significantly. Women rarely report smoking, however this is changing among the younger generation. Higher rates of smoking in certain groups can be attributed to social acceptance (Bush, 2003). It has been suggested that the heterogeneity of South Asians is an important consideration in the development of any health programme (Bhopal, 1999). Many health professionals regard South Asians as a homogeneous community; however, there are many sub-groups in terms of religion, traditions, education, language, beliefs and attitudes. Therefore, it is important to take account of heterogeneity when designing health promotion programmes (Bhopal, 1999).

Physical activity

On the Indian subcontinent physical activity is part of daily life, however, this is declining with modernization and affluence. In the UK South Asian men and women from all ethnic groups are less likely to take part in physical activity than the general population (Fischbacher *et al.*, 2004). Younger generations of South Asians in the UK may access gym facilities, but this is uncommon among older generations.

1.2.4   Eating patterns in the United Kingdom

Findings from a qualitative study, using focus group discussions and individual interviews, about diet and cuisine among family members from a range of South Asian origins in Scotland found that South Asians are more likely to eat South Asian meals in the evening; other meals tend to be based on British cuisine (Wyke & Landman, 1997). This implies that a change of eating habits may be taking place. The widest ranges of cereal, pulse and vegetable foodstuffs were associated with South Asian-style cuisine; British cuisine was more likely to be associated with convenience foods (see Table 1.2.3). Older and younger generations were very strongly committed to South Asian eating habits (Wyke & Landman, 1997). The National Food Survey (2003), which records food purchases, suggests a lower total fat intake, higher total polyunsaturated fatty acid and a higher polyunsaturated saturated fatty acid intake ratio in South Asians than in British Whites. However, the survey fails to take into account the diversity of South Asian diets.

1.2.5   Healthy eating

Key points

- After migration, most people adopt western eating habits while maintaining their traditional eating habits.
- Liberal use of oil/butter/ghee in cooking may result in a high intake of saturated fat and calories.
- Traditional vegetables and pulses are easily obtained in major cities but can be expensive.
- Potato may be a major component of a vegetable curry and accompanied by a large serving of rice or chapatti. The carbohydrate content of a main meal can therefore be very high.
- Poor cooking facilities and skills may make traditional cooking methods of difficult, resulting in a greater reliance on fried and convenience foods.
- Women are more likely to work and have less time for traditional, time-consuming methods of food preparation.

The traditional Punjabi diet is rich in starchy cereal foods, pulses and vegetables, and in principle could be made a very healthy one, resulting in a diet high in complex carbohydrate and fibre and low in fat (see Table 1.2.4).

Due to the heterogeneity of diets consumed by Punjabis it is impossible to generalize about the nutritional implications as these will vary from person to person depending on the nature of the diet and the extent to which it meets individual nutritional needs and provides an overall dietary

balance. The younger generation is increasingly moving away from traditional dietary practices in favour of western eating habits (Thomas & Bishop, 2007).

The government's consumer insight summary (2008) reports that mothers in younger families from a Punjabi and Gujarati background are confident in preparing both western and traditional cuisines and generally do so for their families.

There may be a number of nutritional problems with the diets of Punjabi population in the UK. For those on low incomes an inadequate intake of energy and micronutrients may be due to ignorance. For others, often younger people, it is becoming increasingly common to consume high-fat, convenience and snack foods in preference to fruit, vegetables and starchy cereal foods, a diet that is energy-dense and nutritionally unbalanced. The range of nutritionally related health problems within the Punjabi community is similarly wide, extending from malnutrition, anaemia and rickets to obesity, diabetes and heart disease.

Specific guidance on modification of traditional recipes (e.g., in terms of the quantity and type of oil and fat used), cooking methods and meal patterns may also be advisable. Portion sizes may need to be reviewed as they tend to be large.

1.2.6   Coronary heart disease and stroke

Key points

- Coronary heart disease (CHD) has a high mortality rate, incidence and prevalence among Indian, Pakistani and Bangladeshi communities in the UK, indicating the need for effective prevention initiatives for these communities.
- There is a need to develop effective, culturally focused CHD prevention interventions for these groups by addressing identified barriers, including deeply held cultural beliefs.

Introduction

The South Asian community is approximately 50% more likely to die prematurely from CHD than the

Table 1.2.3   Glossary of Punjabi foods

Punjabi name	English name	Punjabi name	English name
Commonly used pulses		Palak	Spinach
		Payaz	Onions
Chola	White chickpea	Phalli	Green leaves
Lobia	Black-eyed beans /cow peas	Phul gobi	Cauliflower
Masur dal	Red lentils	Saag	Mustard leaves
Matar	Peas	Salad	Lettuce
Mung	Green gram	Sarson-ka saag	Mustard leaves
Rajma	Kidney beans	Shakarkund	Sweet potato
Toor	Red gram (pigeon peas)	Tamater	Tomato
Urad	Black gram		
		Commonly eaten fruits	
Most commonly used vegetables		Aam	Mango
Aloo	Potato	Amrud	Guava
Aloo saag	Potato and spinach	Ananas	Pineapple
Baingan	Aubergine (brinjal)	Angoor	Grapes
Band gobi	Cabbage	Karbooja	Sweet melon
Bindi	Ladies' fingers (okra)	Karbooja	Water melon
Gajar	Carrots	Kela	Banana
Hara dhania	Coriander leaves	Narial	Coconut
Kadoo	Pumpkin	Nashpati	Pear
Karela	Bitter gourd	Nimbu	Lemon
Khira	Cucumber	Papita	Papaya
Matar	Peas	Saib	Apple
Methi saag	Fenugreek leaves	Santra	Orange
Mooli	Large white radish		

general population. The death rate is 51% higher for women and 46% higher for men. Currently, the death rates compared to the rest of the population is increasing (DH, 2004). The reasons for the risk of CHD are not understood. It may be due to the South Asian community being genetically predisposed to CHD or factors associated with its development, such as insulin resistance or central obesity.

Prevalence

The high prevalence of type 2 diabetes is known to be a major contributory factor to CHD mortality; other risk factors are low levels of physical activity and a diet high in fat and low in fruit and vegetables (DH, 2004). The relatively disadvantaged socioeconomic status of the South Asian population has also been suggested as an explanatory factor (DH, 2004).

Other key risk factors requiring control are diabetes, which is up to six times more common in South Asians than in the general population, high cholesterol levels and hypertension (DH, 2004). There is evidence to suggest that Asian communities tend to be diagnosed at a more advanced stage of disease and have poorer survival rates (DH, 2004). For example, Punjabis living in Southall had mean serum cholesterol of 6.5 mmol/l compared with 4.9 mmol/l for their siblings in Punjab, India (Bhopal et al., 1999), i.e., their cholesterol concentration showed a marked rise (about 1.6 mmol/l) after migration. Rapid risk factors of this magnitude may be very important (Bhopal et al., 1999). Although we cannot fully explain why there is increased incidence of CHD in South Asian communities, it is important to address the inequalities. According to Bhopal and colleagues (1999), among the South Asian communities there are important differences between them for many

Table 1.2.4   Healthier alternatives for Punjabi diet

Foods	Healthier alternatives
Indian flatbreads *Roti* or chapatti	Encourage use of whole meal flour *Roti* is also be made from millet flour (*bhajra*), maize/cornmeal (*makke*) or gram flour (*basan*).
Fat added to dough (oil/butter), i.e., *roti*	Try not to add any to the dough. Keep *rotis* soft by covering with a tea cloth.
Butter/margarine/ghee spread on chapatti	Have dry *roti* or try low-fat spreads or reduce the amount of spreads used.
Plain *paratha* made with wheat flour with butter spread inside, folded and shallow-fried on a hot griddle Can also be made sweet or stuffed (with meat or vegetables)	Reduce amount of fat in preparation, and try not to add any after cooking. Try to use whole meal flour instead of plain flour. Use small amount of oil while shallow-frying, cook on dry hot griddle – it's the stuffing that provides most of the flavour.
Puris are deep-fried can be spicy or sweet	Very high in fat so only on special occasions.
Bhatura, deep-fried in oil/ghee (made for special occasions)	Try not to have often (e.g., only on special occasions or weekends).
Bread and breakfast cereals	
Bread	Try to have whole meal or granary bread.
Breakfast cereals	Try wholegrain cereals or low-sugar variety.
Rice	
White rice is mainly consumed	Best type for diabetes control is white basmati as it has a low glycaemic index. Brown basmati is also available. Try to boil, steam or microwave.
Pilau rice (fried rice with cumin and onions)	High in fat. Cut down on the oil used.
Biriyani, meat or vegetable	High in fat. Try to use low-fat cooking methods.
Potatoes	Cook with skins on when added to curry. Avoid deep-frying (e.g., chips).
Meat, fish and alternatives	
Meat/chicken curried, kebab or tandoori	Try to remove all visible fat. Use low-fat cooking methods. Skim fat from surface when dish is made. If eaten daily, try to encourage reducing frequency and portion sizes and substitute some days with dal/vegetable curry.
Fish (white or oily) may be deep- fried (masala fish), curried or steamed	Try not to fry; instead bake in foil. Use yoghurt and tandoori paste as a marinade. Try to include oily fish 1–2 times a week.
Eggs	Boiled, poached, scrambled. Cut down on oil when cooking omelettes or fried eggs.
Pulses and dals (60 different varieties, whole or split, e.g., *chola* (white chickpeas), kidney beans). Dals can be boiled, mashed, dry- roasted or fried. Dals can be ground into flour and used as a thickening agent and to make pancakes.	When cooking dal cut down on oil used (1–2 tablespoons of oil). Try low-fat cooking methods. Avoid adding any butter at the table before eating. If vegetarian, try to have dal every day for protein and iron. To help absorption of vitamin C have pure fruit juice or fruit after meal.
Milk and dairy products	Encourage 2–3 servings per day.
Milk used in sweet dishes, tea or *khoya* (or *maavo*), a solidified full-fat milk.	Do not use gold top, evaporated or condensed milk. Try semi-skimmed or skimmed milk. Mention that semi- or skimmed milk tastes thinner but is still full of goodness.

(Continued)

Table 1.2.4 (cont'd)

Foods	Healthier alternatives
Yoghurt	Try low-fat or use semi-skimmed milk to make yoghurt at home. *Raita* – try using cucumber, carrots and tomato instead, or *boondi* (small deep-fried gram flour balls).
Paneer (white cheese)	Add to curries shredded or cut into cubes without frying. Make *paneer* with semi-skimmed milk. Try low-fat varieties (e.g., cottage cheese).
Vegetables and fruit	
Vegetables (aubergine, spinach, tomato, okra, peas and cauliflower). Can be made with a sauce, deep-fried, stuffed or steamed.	Encourage low-fat vegetable curry (*sabji*); try not to overcook or reheat vegetables as this reduces vitamin content, especially spinach (*saag*). Encourage salad with meals. Store vegetables in a cool, dark place and use while fresh.
Fruit	Encourage all fruit but for diabetes be cautious of very sweet fruits (e.g., mangoes, grapes). Small portions only. Generally recommend three a day and spread these out. Where possible, eat with the skins. Try to have dried fruit as a snack or add to breakfast cereals. Try to have tinned fruit in natural juice rather than syrup. Avoid *chaat* (fresh fruit with added salt or salty spice mixes).
Fruit juice	Try not have sweetened juice drinks. Only small glass of pure juice if taken, as still high in natural sugars. Best to take with food to slow down absorption.
Snack foods	
Biscuits, cakes, pastry	Avoid sweet rusks. Try to reduce the frequency of biscuits and cakes.
Bhajis, pakoras, samosas, poppadum (*papad*) (fried or roasted)	Cut down, as these are very high in fat and salt. Best to have fresh fruit. Limit fried foods. If frying, shallow-fry instead of deep-fat frying and remove excess fat, or bake samosas in the oven. Try tea cakes, toast and crumpets, or oven-baked *aloo tikki* (spicy potato cake) and *chola* (chickpea curry) and salad or small portion of oven-baked chilli *paneer* served with salad.
Chevra (Bombay mix), nuts (dry-roasted or deep-fried)	Try to have dry-roasted nuts (chickpeas, peanuts or popcorn) instead of high-fat snacks (*chevra, gathiya, sevia* or crisps).
Sugary foods	
Indian sweetmeats (*barfi, jallebi* and *ladoo*)	High in fat and sugar. Try to avoid Asian sweets – save these for special occasions. Try to have fruit instead.
Puddings: *Sevia* (made with milk, fine noodles and sugar), *kheer* (rice pudding), *halva* (semolina pudding), *phirni* (made with milk, rice flour and sugar) *gajar halwa* (carrot pudding), sweet rice	*Kheer* – use semi-skimmed milk. Use sweetener for taste or dried fruit, sultanas and raisins. In puddings, try margarine instead of ghee and reduce the quantity. Save for special occasions. If not overweight, can have puddings made with low-fat milk and artificial sweetener.
Squash/soft drinks/cordial	Diet or low-calorie, even if only having occasionally; try sugar-free drinks.
Sweet *paan/paan* masala	Avoid. Have savoury version instead.

Table 1.2.4 (*cont'd*)

Foods	Healthier alternatives
Sugar, honey, *gurr*, in sweet or savoury foods. Glucose drinks	Try to cut down on these, or use artificial sweetener.
Tea. *Chai* (Indian tea) usually prepared with milk, sugar and a blend of ginger, nutmeg, cinnamon, cloves, fennel seeds and cardamom). Coffee.	Check the amount and type of milk used. Advise low-fat milk. Check if sugar, *gurr* or honey is added. If necessary, use artificial sweetener.
Fats	
Butter, margarine, ghee	Use mono- or polyunsaturated, rapeseed or olive oil, sunflower or corn oil instead of ghee or butter. Measure the amount of oil used and try to reduce the quantity. Aim for one teaspoon per person in curries. Avoid frying; try to grill, bake, steam or microwave.
Takeaways, weddings, parties, weekend, temple/ place of worship	Check type of food eaten and how often. Advise to be sensible and only eat small quantities of high-fat and sugar foods.
Pickle	High in fat and salt, drain oil before eating. Or try to make pickle with lemon juice or vinegar or have chutneys (tomato, mango or mint).

CHD risk factors. The belief that South Asians have lower risk factors for CHD is incorrect and may be the result of combining ethnic sub-groups and a narrow range of factors (e.g., insulin resistance; Bhopal *et al.*, 1999).

Risk factors

- Age.
- Male gender.
- A family history of heart disease.
- Obesity.
- Diabetes and insulin resistance.
- Hypertension.
- Stress.
- A high saturated fat diet.
- High LDL and low HDL cholesterol.
- Socioeconomic factors.
- Smoking.
- Lack of physical activity.

Physical activity

People who engage in little physical activity have almost double the risk of dying from coronary heart disease than active people. Thirty minutes or more of at least moderate-intensity physical activity a day on at least five days a week significantly reduces the risk of cardiovascular disease and has general health benefits (DH, 2000). The recommended levels of activity can be achieved either by doing all the daily activity in one session, or in several shorter bouts (e.g., 10 minutes) of activity. The activity can be lifestyle activity or structured exercise or sport, or a combination of these (DH, 2000). It is known that South Asian men and women from all ethnic groups are less likely to take part in physical activity than the general population (Fischbacher *et al.*, 2004).

Treatment

The National Service Framework for Coronary Heart Disease set national standards of treatment and care for preventing and treating CHD, with the aim of improving the standard of care and reducing inequalities (DH, 2000). Standards were set for better, faster treatment of patients who have had or are suspected to have had a heart attack, faster diagnosis of heart disease and shorter waiting times for heart surgery (DH, 2004).

1.2.7 Diet modification

Fruit and vegetables

Eating at least five portions of a variety of fruit and vegetables a day could lead to an estimated reduction of up to 20% in overall deaths from chronic diseases, such as heart disease, stroke and cancer (DH, 2004). It is found that each increase of one portion of fruit and vegetables a day lowered the risk of CHD by 4% and the risk of stroke by 6% (DH, 2004).

Fat

Other dietary changes that would help to reduce rates of CHD include a reduction in consumption of fat, particularly saturated fat. A survey that focused on the health of minority ethnic groups asked about the frequency of consumption of a range of foods, including fruit and vegetables and a number of high-fat and high-sugar foodstuffs. The results show considerable variation in eating habits by ethnic group (Health Survey for England, 1999). As there is limited nutritional intake data for the South Asian population these findings should be interpreted with caution. It does appear that second-generation South Asians have adopted British dietary patterns, increasing fat and reducing fruit and vegetable consumption (Landman & Cruickshank, 2001).

Fish and omega 3 fatty acids

Research by the UK Food Standards Agency (2003) suggests that the Sikh population, and other Asian groups, could significantly reduce their risk of heart disease by increasing the amount of oily fish they eat. The study found that Sikh men and women consumed less fish oil and more vegetable oils than White men and women in the UK. After a moderate intake of fish oil (4 g a day for 12 weeks), the levels of beneficial fatty acids in the body increased in the Sikh group to levels similar to those of the White men and women studied. Results also showed that taking fish oil supplements reduced the risk of heart disease by changing levels of fats in the blood. Eating at least two portions of fish a week, one of which should be oily fish such as salmon or mackerel, could significantly help reduce the risk of heart disease in Asian communities.

This recommendation applies to pregnant and breastfeeding women, but they should limit oily fish consumption to no more than two servings a week and avoid marlin, swordfish and shark because of potential exposure to methyl mercury which accumulates in these fish. The FSA also advises pregnant women that the amount of tuna eaten should be limited to no more than two tuna steaks a week or four medium-sized cans a week, again because tuna may contain mercury, which at high levels can harm the foetus's developing nervous system.

In line with guidelines from the Food Standards Agency a diet high in fruit and vegetables, including two portions of oily fish and low in saturated fat, reduces the risk of CHD (Bhopal *et al.*, 1999).

Plant-based source of omega 3 fatty acids

For patients who are following a lacto-vegetarian diet, omega 3 fatty acids can be derived from:

- Rapeseed or canola oil (most blended vegetable oils contain rapeseed oil).
- Walnut oil.
- Olive oil-based margarine.
- Soya beans, soya chunks/mince, soya milk/ yoghurt, soya flour, soya oil and tofu.
- Nuts (walnuts, pecan, almonds).
- Peanuts.
- Ground flax (linseed) seeds and flax (linseed) oil.

The International College of Nutrition India recommendations for the prevention of CHD are that, in this population, a BMI > 23 kg/m^2 should be considered overweight and that an intake of 440 g/ day fruit and vegetables and 25 g/day mustard oil or soybean oil instead of hydrogenated fat, coconut oil or butter is advised (Singh *et al.*, 1996). Moderate physical activity, smoking cessation and moderate alcohol intake are also recommended (Singh *et al.*, 1996).

1.2.8 Suggestions for way forward

A study of South Asians in Tyneside found that 35% did not understand the term heart disease,

19% were unable to provide any description of it, 14% could not give a single cause and 16% could not suggest a preventative measure (Rankin & Bhopal., 2001). This highlights that education and intervention for the South Asian community are needed.

1.3 Pakistani Diet

Zenab Ahmad, Bushra Jafri, Afsha Mughal, Rabia Nabi, Shamaela Perwiz, Tahira Sarmar, Ghazala Yousuf

1.3.1 Introduction

The South Asian subcontinent comprises India, Pakistan, Bangladesh and Sri Lanka. Four per cent of the total UK population is classified as 'Asian' or 'Asian British' and this group makes up 50.2% of the minority ethnic group population in the UK (UK Census, 2001).

'South Asians' is 'a term which defines many ethnic groups, with distinctive regions of origin, languages, religions and customs and include people born in India, Bangladesh, Pakistan or Sri Lanka' (Fox, 2004).

Pakistan is situated in the west of the Indian subcontinent, with Afghanistan and Iran to the west, India to the east and the Arabian Sea to the south. The name Pakistan is derived from the Urdu words *pak* meaning pure and *stan* meaning country (see Figure 1.3.1).

The British ruled the Indian subcontinent for nearly 200 years – from 1756 to 1947. After a revolt in 1857, the British initiated political reforms, allowing the formation of political parties. The Indian National Congress, representing the overwhelming majority of Hindus, was created in 1885. The Muslim League was formed in 1906 to represent the Muslim minority. When the British introduced constitutional reforms in 1909, the Muslims demanded and acquired separate electoral rolls.

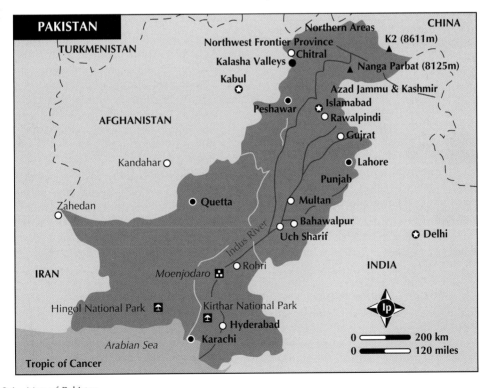

Figure 1.3.1 Map of Pakistan

This guaranteed them representation in the provincial as well as national legislatures until independence in 1947 (Hamid & Sarwar, 2004). The British decided on partition and on 15 August 1947 power was transferred to Pakistan and India. For almost 25 years following independence Pakistan consisted of two separate regions, East (now known as Bangladesh) and West Pakistan, but now it is made up only of the western sector. Both India and Pakistan have laid claim to the Kashmir region; this territorial dispute has led to four wars and remains unresolved (www.infoplease.com/ipa/A0107861.html).

Migration has been a constant in the history of Pakistan. From its inception, its people have been moving in migratory waves. This migration of people started with the movement of millions of people from India into Pakistan when the two nations gained independence in 1947. Muslims moved to Pakistan in the hope of a better life, not just economically but also socially and for religious freedom (www.yespakistan.com).

- Languages: Urdu 8%, English (both official); Punjabi 48%, Sindhi 12%, Siraiki (a Punjabi variant) 10%, Pashtu 8%, Balochi 3%, Hindko 2%, Brahui 1%, Burushaski, others 8%.
- Religions: Islam 97% (Sunni 77%, Shiite 20%); Christian, Hindu and other 3% (http://www.infoplease.com/ipa/A0107861.html).

Migration to the United Kingdom

Large-scale immigration to the UK began in the 1950s, when Britain encouraged migration from its former colonies to fill its labour shortages following the Second World War. Many Pakistanis were economic migrants from rural areas of the country and most intended to return to Pakistan once they had earned enough money in Britain. Throughout the 1960s and 1970s their numbers increased. Men came first, followed by their wives, children and other dependants. By the 1960s and 1970s many Pakistanis believed it would be difficult to return home due to the higher living standards in the UK, the need to maintain new businesses, their children's education and political instability in Pakistan. Therefore the community settled and expanded.

Current UK population

The total minority ethnic population was 4.6 million in 2001 or 7.9% of the total population. Pakistanis were the second largest ethnic minority group with a population of 747,285, or 1.3% of the UK population, making up 16.1% of the minority ethnic group (www.statistics.gov.uk).

1.3.2   Religion

The main religion of Pakistan is Islam, which comes from the Arabic word meaning submission. Sunni Muslims comprise the largest denomination of Islam. Approximately 77% of Pakistanis are Sunni and 20% are Shia Muslim. The word Sunni comes from *sunnah* which means the words and actions or example of the Prophet Muhammad (peace be upon him). Shia is a shortened version and means the followers of Ali. Sunni Muslims and Shia Muslims differ regarding various beliefs in Islam.

All Muslims acknowledge the obligation to express their submission in terms of the 'five pillars of Islam'.

- Belief: Allah (the Arabic word for God) is the only God and Mohammed is his true messenger.
- Prayer: Muslims should pray five times a day at set times throughout the day.
- *Zakat*: Muslims should give 2.5% of their wealth (*zakat*) to the poor and needy. This is not a tax but a purification of their wealth through sharing. *Zakat* is normally paid during Ramadan.
- Fasting: In Islam, fasting means complete abstention from eating and drinking from dawn to sunset during Ramadan. Muslims rise before sunrise (*sehri*) to have a meal similar to breakfast and break their fast at sunset (*iftari*). Ramadan occurs in the ninth month of the Islamic year. It is considered one of the highest forms of worship as it enables people to practise self-discipline and helps them to appreciate and share the experiences of the poor and hungry. Fasting is also a way of purifying oneself spiritually and physically, a process of detoxifying to allow rest and recuperation for the body, mind and spirit (see Table 1.3.1).

Table 1.3.1 Exemptions from fasting

Persons exempt from fasting	Others exempt for certain periods but are supposed to make up for the missed fasts later
Young children (below the age of puberty)	The sick
	The frail and elderly
Those with a life-threatening or chronic disease	Women during menstruation
	Pregnant and lactating women
	People travelling on a long journey

Other than eating and drinking the fast can be broken by:

- engaging in any sexual pleasure or indulging in unclean thoughts;
- smoking;
- taking any kind of medicine;
- displaying anger or using foul language.

For those unable to fast they should feed a needy person, preferably a fasting person, with the same quality and quantity of food they would eat, for every day they do not fast.

- Pilgrimage (*hajj*): Once in a lifetime, a Muslim should make a pilgrimage to Mecca, if they can afford it. The *hajj* formally begins on the eighth day of Dhul-Hijjah, the 12th month of the Muslim lunar calendar. The *hajj* consists of several ceremonies, meant to symbolize the essential concepts of the Islamic faith and to commemorate the trials of Prophet Abraham and his family. It is a magnificent form of worship, combining prayers (*salat*), physical effort, long hours of meditation, supplication and glorification of Allah. *Hajj* results in the largest gathering of Muslims in any one place (Hamid & Sarwar, 2004).

Religious festivals and celebrations

The two main festivals of Islam mark the ending of Ramadan (*Eid-al-Fitr*) and the climax of *hajj* (*Eid-al-Adha*).

Eid-al-Fitr

The holiday follows the month of Ramadan falls on the first day of Shawwal, the 10th month of the Islamic calendar. Fasting is forbidden on this day. Muslims must pay *zakat-ul-fitr* (a charitable donation) for the month of Ramadan.

Eid-al-Adha

This feast of sacrifice is observed at the end of *hajj* and is celebrated over a number of days. The celebration is in commemoration of the command given by Allah to Prophet Abraham to sacrifice his son. Abraham's willingness to obey this noble command signified his faith in Allah. Today Muslims offer animals such as goats, sheep, lambs and cows as a symbol of sacrifice. Some of this meat is given to the poor and the rest is shared among family and friends. The Islamic New Year starts three weeks after *hajj*.

Religious dietary restrictions

In Islam, all wholesome things may be used for food and the general rule is that every food is lawful (*halal*) unless it is declared unlawful (*haram*).

Unlawful foods are:

- Foods and food products from pig meat.
- All other meat which has not been ritually slaughtered by reciting the name of Allah as the animal is slaughtered, the blood being allowed to drain. Kosher meat may be acceptable.
- Foods containing ingredients or additives derived from the pig, or from any animal which has not been ritually slaughtered or from any *haram* source. In practice, this means that a wide range of manufactured foods containing gelatine, animal fats or emulsifiers derived from animal sources will be avoided.
- Shellfish or fish without fins and scales.
- Alcohol, including that used in cooking or for medicinal purposes (Thomas & Bishop, 2007).

1.3.3   Traditional diet and eating patterns

The cuisine of Pakistan can be described as a fusion of cuisine from two Asian regions: Central Asia and the Middle East. Pakistani cuisine is known for its use of a variety spices and richness.

Breads

- *Roti* or chapattis are the most common bread made at home. The flat round bread (*roti*) is a staple part of the daily diet. They are thin, unleavened and made from whole wheat flour.
- *Tandoor* bread made with white flour: Different varieties of breads are prepared in a clay oven (tandoor). They are extremely popular in Pakistan and are consumed with just about anything, most commonly with shish kebabs. Restaurants usually cook these or if people have a clay oven, they might make these themselves.
- *Naan*: Naans are slightly thicker than chapattis, typically leavened with yeast and mainly made with white flour. They may be sprinkled with sesame seeds (*kulcha*). They are often served with *sri paya* and *nihari* for breakfast.
- *Roghni naan*, made from white flour: This is a naan sprinkled with sesame seeds and covered with a minute amount of oil. It is usually round and thicker than the standard *roti*.
- *Sheermal naan*, made from white flour and prepared with milk and butter: It is often sweetened and is particularly enjoyed by children.
- *Taftan* made from white flour: It is leavened and flavoured with saffron and cardamom powder and baked in a clay oven.
- *Puri*: It is deep-fried and is typically eaten with *halwa* or *bhujia* (made from chickpeas and potatoes). *Halwa purian* or *bhujia* with *puri* (now commonly known as *poorian*) has become a typical breakfast in Pakistan. They are also sold from makeshift carts or otherwise in breakfast stores.
- *Paratha*, a flat, multi-layered chapatti separated by ghee (similar to pastry dough). It is commonly eaten for breakfast and may be served with a variety of stuffings. It can be made from white or whole meal flour.

Rice

Basmati is the most popular variety rice consumed in Pakistan. Dishes made with rice include many varieties of pilau. *Biryani*, a very popular dish made with red meat or chicken, is always served at weddings and most parties. *Yakhni pilau* is made from meat stock, meat and rice. *Tahiri* is a vegetarian biryani and is made with rice and potatoes. *Matar pilau* is made with the additions of pea and, occasionally, corn and carrots.

Meat

An average Pakistani consumes three times more meat than an average Indian (Speedy, 2003). Of all the meats, the most popular are beef, goat, lamb and chicken.

Fish

Fish (e.g., sardines, prawns, tuna and cod) is generally not consumed in large quantities, though it is popular in the coastal areas.

Pulses and dals

Various kinds of pulses also make up an important part of the Pakistani dishes.

Lentils (dal) are considered an inexpensive food source and hotel/restaurants may only offer a limited variety of these dishes. Lentil dishes are also typically not served to guests or on special occasions. The main exception is *haleem*, which contains a variety of lentils, rice, wheat and barley. Vegetables may be added.

Beverages

Tea or coffee.

Accompaniments

Chutneys
Coconut chutney
Onion chutney
Tomato chutney
Coriander leaves chutney
Mint chutney
Tamarind chutney (Imli chutney)
Mango chutney (made from unripe, green mangos)
Garlic chutney made from fresh garlic, coconut and groundnut

Achars (pickle)
Mango achar
Lemon achar
Carrot achar
Green chilli achar
Pickle achar
Green chilli yoghurt is made with plain yoghurt, grounded garlic, green chilli and ground chilli powder
Raita (yoghurt) can also be made with cucumber, cumin seeds and oil
Aubergine *raita*

Although, traditionally, home-cooked meals are preferred, those who live in cities are becoming more inclined to eat fast foods. Furthermore, as a result of lifestyle changes, ready-made masalas are becoming increasingly popular (see Tables 1.3.2 and 1.3.3).

Typical meal pattern

Traditional food is cooked fresh from scratch and Pakistanis living in the UK will cook at least two or three main dishes, excluding accompaniments. Food for Pakistanis is a means by which the whole family gets together in preparation as well eating together.

The main course usually consists of meat curry (with or without vegetables) or vegetable curry (*sabzi*) and/or bean/whole pulses/lentils or dal curry, which is served with *roti* or boiled rice (basmati rice is mainly used). An example of dal is red lentils and *roti* is made from wheat flour, usually whole meal.

Meat plays a dominant role in Pakistani diet compared to other South Asian cuisines. Vegetables are added to meat curry (e.g., potatoes, spinach, courgettes, tomatoes, peas, aubergine, cauliflower and cabbage).

Salad is generally served with the main course.

Assorted fresh fruit or desserts are consumed and sweet dishes are cooked and served on special occasions (see Table 1.3.4 and Table 1.3.5).

Cooking methods

- Barbecue dishes are extremely popular and are a specialty of various cities. All barbecue dishes

are marinated with variety of herbs and spices and are therefore very flavourful rather than being just dominated by chilli. Among the well-known dishes are chicken tikka, mutton tikka, shish kebab and bihari kebab. These specialties are usually cooked on special occasions or for dinner parties.

- One-pot (*handi*) cooking means that all the ingredients are cooked together on top of the cooker.
- Ovens are mainly used in this country to cook stuffed pastries but not meals.
- Tandoori meat dishes are a healthy way of cooking as fat drips into the fire.
- Grills are used for grilled chicken and kebabs.
- Pressure cookers are widely used as less oil is needed and the meat cooks more quickly.
- Rice cookers are also used occasionally.

Paan

Paan is a South Asian tradition which consists of chewing betel leaf combined with the areca nut. *Paan* is chewed as a palate cleanser and a breath freshener. It is also commonly offered to guests and visitors as a sign of hospitality and as an ice-breaker to start conversation. It also has a symbolic value at ceremonies and cultural events. *Paan* makers may use tobacco as an ingredient in their *paan* fillings. Although most types of *paan* contain areca nuts, some do not. Other types include sweet *paan*, where sugar, candied fruit and fennel seeds are used. Although the term *paan* is generally used to refer to the leaves of the betel vine, the common use of the word refers mostly to the chewing mixture wrapped in the leaves. Pakistanis who have migrated to the West generally do not chew *paan* as often as they would have in Pakistan (Panesar *et al.*, 2008).

Alcohol

Alcohol is forbidden for Muslims so the majority of Pakistanis do not drink it, however some do and others may do but not admit it. Therefore it is best always to ask patients and not to make assumptions.

Table 1.3.2   Description of Pakistani foods

Food group	Description of foods	Urdu name
Bread, cereal, rice, potatoes and other starchy food	Wheat,	*Gehon*
	Wheat flour	*Gehon ka atta*
	Rice	*Chawal*
	Semolina	*Suji*
	Potatoes/chips/crisps	*Alu*
	Sweet potatoes	*Shakarkandi*
	Turnips	*Shalgam*
Meat, fish, egg, beans, nuts, seeds	Mutton/lamb	*Bakeka ka gosh*
	Minced meat	*Keema*
	Beef	*Gai ka gosh*
	Chicken	*Murga*
	Fish	*Machli*
	Chickpeas, white	*Chola*
	Kidney beans	*Rajma,*
	Lentil	*Masoor,*
	Black-eyed peas	*Lobia*
	Split pulses	*dal*
	Almonds	*Baadam*
Vegetables	Vegetables	*Sabzis*
	Green beans	*Faliya*
	Aubergine, cabbage,	*Bagan, kobi,*
	spinach, okra	*Palak, bhindi,*
	Karela, cauliflower	*Bitter gourd, Ful gobi*
Fruit, fresh or dried	Mangoes, oranges, lychees, pomegranates, bananas, papaya, apples, pears, dried apricots, dates	
Milk and dairy foods	Milk	*Doodh*
	Plain yoghurt	*Dahi*
	Paneer	*paneer*
	Milk-based drink made with yoghurt, milk, sugar or salt and ice cubes. There are three types of *lassi*: salted, sweetened or mango-based	*lassi*
Foods and drinks high in fat and sugar	Butter	*Maakhan*
	Ghee	*Ghee*
	Sugar	*Shaker*
	Sunflower oil/olive oil	*Sunflower oil/olive oil*
	Jaggery (unrefined sugar)	*Ghur*
	Regular fizzy drinks, concentrated tropical/fruit juices e.g. mango	
	Asian sweets and savoury dishes	*Ladoo, gulab jamun, rasmalai, garjur carrot) halwa*
		pakora, samosa, chevra, Cakes, biscuits and ice cream
	Cakes, biscuits and ice cream	

Table 1.3.3   Herbs and spices used in Pakistani cooking

English name	Urdu name
Asafoetida	Hing
Black cardamom	Bari elaichi
Black peppercorn	Kali mirch
Black salt	Kala namak or Sanchal
Carom seed	Ajwain
Chutney	Chutney
Cinnamon	Darchini
Cloves	Loonng
Coriander powder	Pissa dhania
Coriander seed	Sabut dhania
Cumin seed	Zeera
Dried fenugreek leaves	Kasoori methi
Emblica gooseberry	Aamla
Garam masala	Garam masala
Garlic	Lahsun
Ginger	Adrak
Green cardamom	Choti elaichi
Green chilli	Hari mirch
Green coriander	Hara Dhania
Mango powder	Amchoor
Mint	Pudina
Nigella seed	Kalonji
Nutmeg	Jaifal
Onion	Pyaz
Parsley	Jafari
Pickle	Achar
Pomegranate seed	Anaar dana
Rosewater	Gulab rus
Saffron	Kesar
Salt	Namak
Sesame seed	Til
Tamarind	Imli
Turmeric	Haldi

Smoking

Smoking prevalence is increasing, especially in the developing countries. In Pakistan, the sixth most populous country, there is a high prevalence of smoking. A study conducted in Karachi in 1983 reported a prevalence of 21% among male medical students with average age of commencement 17 years (Ali *et al.*, 2008). Another study conducted in 1995 reported a smoking prevalence of nearly 17% among male medical students as compared to 4% among female medical students in Karachi. It can be suggested that smoking among British

Pakistanis will be more prevalent in men than that in women (Rozi *et al.*, 2005). Similar to the general UK population 26% of Pakistani men smoke and 6% of Pakistani men and women reported tobacco chewing in *paan* (Rozi *et al.*, 2005).

1.3.4   Healthy eating

The traditional Pakistani diet can be very healthy because it often includes plenty of vegetables, starchy foods (e.g., rice and bread) and good sources of protein (e.g., meat, fish, beans and pulses). However, as large quantities of oil/fat are added it can have a high fat content.

Simple changes to the diet and cooking methods should be discussed (see Table 1.3.6 and Figure 1.3.2).

Evidence to promote healthy eating

There is evidence that the UK health services are not reaching South Asian communities effectively. Attendance rates at outpatient clinics are notoriously low and compliance with treatment and advice can be similarly poor. Some may be reluctant to approach health professionals because they feel their ignorance will be exposed, their lifestyle scrutinized and possibly ridiculed, and their culture neither understood nor respected.

In order to overcome these barriers it is necessary for health professionals to develop local initiatives where links are built with respected community leaders and health promotion work is conducted within the community itself. It is often more productive and hence time- and cost-effective to run specific healthy eating sessions, cookery classes and group sessions in a local centre or even someone's home. It is also important that health education is focused on specific ethnic groups rather than being targeted at 'South Asians' (Thomas & Bishop, 2007).

Interpreters may also be invaluable for group teaching sessions, for example when introducing a video presentation, especially if the group has a common language. If the group is mixed, Hindi is usually the most appropriate language to use since Indian films are produced in Hindi and these are

Table 1.3.4 Traditional eating pattern and dietary changes in the Pakistani diet on migration to the UK

Meal	Traditional meal	Dietary changes on migration to UK	Healthier alternatives
Breakfast	*Paratha* with curry (eggs and potato) or yoghurt Fried eggs/omelette *Halwa* (made with semolina) with *puris* Water or tea Leftovers from the night before	Cereals Toast (usually white bread) Fried eggs/omelette Fruit cake Tea or coffee	Whole meal bread or wholegrain cereal (with semi-skimmed or skimmed milk). Unsweetened fruit juice Tea or coffee
Lunch (Main meal)	Chapattis (rotis) Meat or vegetable curry Salad	Leftovers from the night before Chapattis (rotis) with curry (vegetable/meat) Chips, pizza, fish fingers	Chapattis (rotis) with meat or vegetable curry or boiled rice with curry or sandwich with low-fat filling (chicken, salad, egg) or baked potato with leftover curry or baked beans
Evening meal	Rice with curry (meat/vegetable) or chapattis with curry, chutney, salad, yoghurt, pickles (in oil)	Rice or chapatti (roti) with meat/vegetable curry, salad, yoghurt, chutney (green)	Chapatti (roti) with vegetable or meat curry or rice with dal curry, fish curry or grilled fish (oily fish – mackerel, salmon, pilchard), salad
Puddings/ Desserts	Rice pudding (*kheer*) *Sevian* (vermicelli) *Zarda* (sweet rice) *Halwa* made with semolina or carrots	Rice pudding Vermicelli Sweet rice Cakes Ice cream Tinned fruit in syrup	Fresh/tinned fruit in natural juice. Rice pudding or vermicelli (made with sweetener and semi-skimmed milk). Fruit salad. Fruit yoghurt (low-fat/low-sugar)
Drinks	Water. Tea (made with milk and usually sugar or salt). Coke. *Lassi* (sweet or salty). Home-made lemon cordial with sugar	Fizzy drinks (e.g., cola). Sweetened soft drinks (Ribena, orange squash, etc.). Fruit juices. Sweetened fruit juices	Water. Unsweetened fruit juices. Diet or sugar-free soft drinks. *Lassi* made with low-fat yoghurt, milk and sweetener. Tea made with less semi-skimmed milk and sweetener
Snacks	Fried samosas, *pakoras*, kebabs, Bombay mix, Asian sweets (*burfi, jalebi, sweet sev, halwa*)	Bombay mix, peanuts, crisps, chocolates, Asian sweets, biscuits, fruit cakes Fried snacks such as samosas, *pakoras*, kebabs	Oven-baked samosas, *chana* (chickpeas) and/or potato *chaat*, fruit *chaat*, pitta bread filled with salad or vegetable curry. Grilled kebab with pitta/naan bread, more fruit and vegetables

(Hamid & Sarwar, 2004)

generally widely understood (Thomas & Bishop, 2007).

In health promotion work, education sessions that use a respected and well-known community elder as an interpreter are likely to be particularly well received. However, it must not be forgotten that some people may not be prepared to reveal personal information in a public setting (Thomas & Bishop, 2007).

Suggestions for the way forward

The development of effective nutritional intervention strategies to meet the needs of any population group should take account of modifiable risk factors that can form the basis of intervention and understand relevant health behaviours or beliefs so that appropriate strategies can be designed (Thomas, 2002).

Table 1.3.5 Glossary of Pakistani foods

Name of food	Description
Aachar	Pickle mainly made from vegetable and fruit (e.g., mango, lime, green chillies).
Burfi	Dessert made from milk that has been reduced to fudge-like consistency. Flavoured with saffron, vanilla essence, cocoa, rosewater, etc. Sometimes coconut and nuts are added. Eaten and served in bite-sized pieces.
Chaat	Sweet and spicy spices mixed in fruit or chickpeas.
Chapatti/Roti	Unleavened flatbread made with wheat and water. Usually cooked on a *tava* (griddle).
Halwa	Sweet made from semolina and finely grated vegetables (e.g., carrots), with milk, sugar and flavoured with cardamom. Consistency of thick pudding.
Jallebi	Crisp round whirls, made from plain flour and water, deep-fried and then dipped in an orange-flavoured syrup.
Kheer	Rice pudding made with rice, milk, sugar, flavoured with cardamom. Sometimes nuts are added. Served hot or cold.
Kulfi	Sweet, aromatic ice cream made from cream, milk and sugar, flavoured with mango, pistachio, saffron, etc.
Lassi	Drink made from yoghurt, milk and water. Either salty or sweet.
Mathai	Asian sweetmeats (e g., *burfi, Jallebi*).
Pakora	Crispy and spicy snack served straight from the frying pan with coriander chutney. Slices of different vegetables are dipped in batter made from gram or chickpea flour and a few dry spices, then deep-fried.
Paneer	Home-made white cheese from full-fat milk.
Paratha	Whole wheat unleavened flatbread. Sometimes filled with ground meat or a vegetable mixture. Shallow-fried.
Puri	Deep-fried whole wheat flatbread. Usually 10 cm in diameter. They puff up when fried.
Samosa	Deep-fried pastry appetizers filled with vegetable or meat mixtures.
Sev	Thin, string-like fried snack made out of gram flour.
Zarda	Sweet rice.

(Hamid & Sarwar, 2004)

Table 1.3.6 Dietary modification of Pakistani diet to meet healthy eating guidelines

Foods	Discourage	Encourage
Staple foods: breads	*Paratha* *Sheermal* *Puri*	Chapatti (roti) made with whole meal flour Whole meal pitta bread
Vegetables	Frying or adding oil	Boiling and continue adding to curries
Fruit	Adding cream or sugar	Prepare fresh fruit salad
Meat	Fatty meats Excessive salt	Use lean meat. Incorporate more fish in the diet Use less salt
Lentils and pulses	Large amount of oil for *bargar* (added to dal)	No more than 1 teaspoon of oil in *bargar*
Fats and oils	Ghee, butter Limit fried snacks, e.g., *chevra*, samosa	Olive oil, sunflower oil, rapeseed oil Snack of fruit/dried fruit
Dairy	Making *keer* and other desserts with full-fat milk/condensed milk. Evaporated milk	Use semi-skimmed milk and sweetened using less sugar

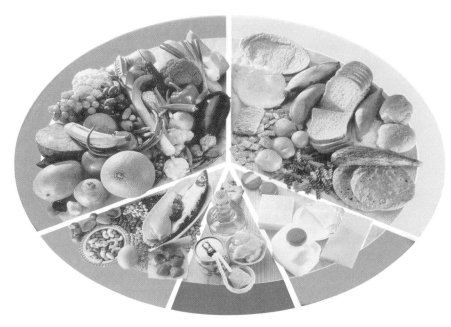

Figure 1.3.2   South Asian eat well plate model
© Aruna Thaker

Guidance in pictorial form (e.g., photographs or drawings of the foods that should be eaten more frequently or avoided) is particularly valuable because even if the client is fluent in English, other members of the family (who may be the ones who do the shopping or cooking) may not be. Other innovative methods such as cookery demonstrations can also be effective.

Written information in Punjabi Gurmukhi (a Punjabi dialect) can be useful, although it should be borne in mind that some people, especially older women, may be illiterate in their own language. In contrast, younger people often prefer to be given written information in English. Rather than make assumptions, it is usually better to ask the client (if necessary via an interpreter) which written language would be most helpful. Dietitians will also need an English translation to refer to. Alternative resources (e.g., audiotapes, CDs and DVDs) should be considered and made available in different languages.

For strategies focusing on risk factors to be effective, two key elements are required: first,

information needs to reach the right people; and second, the people need to commit to behavioural change.

Strategies need to take account of language, communication and cultural barriers and be targeted appropriately, and communities must be involved in their development.

People also need to have the opportunity to make healthier choices. Some communities do not have ready access to affordable healthy foods, safe, pleasant open spaces or affordable facilities for physical activity.

Information and knowledge need to be targeted to this community and services need to be made accessible.

Nutritional health groups should be established aimed at Pakistanis to educate them on healthy eating and the relationship between diet and disease.

More literature should be available in Urdu, including a website approved by British Dietetic Association (BDA) about nutrition and fact sheets in Urdu made available online.

1.3.5   Obesity

Key points

- The incidence and prevalence of obesity have continued to rise in the UK, which is a precursor for major diseases such as diabetes, coronary heart disease and certain types of cancer.
- Pakistani women living in the UK have been identified as having one of the highest rates of obesity.
- Being overweight or obese not only shortens life, it also reduces the years of life spent free of major illness and disability.
- As well as the emotional and psychological struggles, there is an immense toll on the NHS in treating as well as preventing obesity.

Introduction

Obesity is a major risk factor for cardiovascular disease, diabetes, hypertension and premature death. Body mass index (BMI) is a widely accepted measure of weight-for-height. Generalized obesity is defined as a $BMI > 30 \, kg/m^2$. However, BMI does not take account of the distribution of fat around the abdomen, which has been recognized as a risk factor in relation to chronic diseases. For this, the waist/hip ratio (WHR) is used, a measure of central obesity. Central obesity is defined as a WHR of 0.95 or greater in men, and of 0.85 or greater in women (www.statistics.gov uk).

Prevalence

According to the World Health Organization (1998), the global prevalence of obesity is in excess of 250 million people, and has been described as the single biggest public health issue in the western world. One in five adults in the UK are obese, an incidence which has nearly trebled over the past 20 years – the fastest rise in Europe, (National Audit Office, 2001). It is having a vast effect on health services, mainly due to related complications such as coronary heart disease (CHD), diabetes, hypertension and certain cancers (Andersen, 2003). Obesity is also increasingly affecting the emotional

and psychological health of those who are obese (DH, 2004a).

Aspects such as greater food production, cheaper high energy-dense foods, more disposable income, lack of positive exercise/activity messages from young age, lack of sports opportunities, advances in technology, and so on have all contributed to this situation (Laing, 2002).

In the UK, children, people of low socioeconomic status and South Asians (in particular women with a Pakistani origin) have all been shown to have high rates of obesity (NAO, 2001). The National Audit Office reported that women of Pakistani origin are suffering not only high rates of obesity compared to the rest of the population (NAO, 2001), but also CHD and diabetes (Vyas et al., 2003; DH, 2004b).

However, compared with the general population, levels of obesity are three times lower in Pakistani men compared to their White counterparts (London Health Observatory, 2003). British Pakistani girls have an increased risk of becoming obese and Pakistani boys an increased risk of becoming overweight than the general population (DH, 2001). Obesity is therefore increasing in this community. The UK is unique in that it has the largest population of Pakistanis outside of Pakistan. It has therefore been the first to encounter the health issues within this community outside of Pakistan, and perhaps it has taken many generations to settle in the UK in order for the health issues to present themselves. Public health now has the advantage of having this long-established community with whom it can work to tackle health issues such as obesity (Shaw, 2000).

Results from the National Health Survey in Pakistan found overweight/obesity to be generally higher in women compared to men in Pakistan, and higher in urban than rural areas; women aged 45–64 years had the highest prevalence (40% overweight/obese) (Nanan & White, 1999). In comparison, Shah et al. (2004) profiled a mountain population in Pakistan whose prevalence of overweight and obesity was 1.8% among men and 2.5% among women, dramatically lower than elsewhere in the country.

Although many lifestyle factors determine whether someone becomes obese, the government has recognized in the White Paper 'Saving Lives

– Our Healthier Nation' (DH, 1999) that certain vulnerable groups are more at risk of suffering from poorer health due to inbuilt inequalities. High obesity levels among low socioeconomic status and ethnic minority groups suggest that these groups are experiencing health inequalities (Phillips, 2005).

There is a vast array of information on obesity from dedicated books and journals to websites (Garrow, 2000; Bessen & Kushner, 2001; National Obesity Forum, 2003). However, there is very little research, in particular qualitative research, specifically related to obesity and South Asians, or Pakistanis. There is therefore a huge gap, which is of particular concern as obesity is an emergent issue among those of Pakistani origin.

BMI and waist circumference

'Obesity is a condition, in which body fat stores are enlarged to an extent which impairs health' (Garrow, 2000). WHO recommends a BMI classification in order to diagnose overweight and obesity, where obesity is determined by a BMI > 30 kg/m². This is the most targeted or at-risk group, as they are likely to have the most serious medical and psychological problems (WHO, 1998). Although it has limitations, the BMI is useful for diagnosing and indicating the degree of severity of the obesity (Thomas, 2001).

The increase in the average BMI in the UK is graphically illustrated by the fact that aeroplane designers have had to increase the assumed weight of each passenger by over 9 kg, designers of clothes, beds, chairs and cars are all acknowledging that this increase in girth is not a temporary deviation in the statistics (Prentice, 1997).

Dietary modification

The National Institutes of Health review of 48 randomized controlled trials found strong and consistent evidence that weight loss can be achieved by reducing fat as part of a low-energy diet. However, both diet and physical activity are essential components of any weight loss programme (Mulvihill & Quigley, 2003).

Surgery for obesity is now used more frequently in the NHS, although it should be considered a last resort for severe and intractable obesity (Kopelman, 2001).

Physical activity

Physical activity is one of the key determinants of good health. A physically active lifestyle delivers significant physical and mental health benefits, notably helping to reduce cardiovascular disease and osteoporosis. Current guidance recommends that adults should take part in 30 minutes or more of moderate physical activity at least five times a week. Twenty-nine per cent of Pakistani men met the guideline whereas only 16% of women did. Traditionally, Pakistanis are accustomed to walking to markets or to visit relatives. However, in the West these things are harder to do and the weather conditions can act as a deterrent, therefore decreasing levels of activity and increasing health risks.

Physical activity is an important component of long-term weight control (Jakicic & Otto, 2005). As well as benefiting the internal functions of the body, it has been shown that it can also vastly improve mental health (Brownell & Kramer, 1994). There are clear differences in exercise behaviour and the effects of exercise across different cultural groups. Among African-Caribbeans aged 16–74 years, 62% of men and 75% of women do not participate in enough physical activity to benefit their health. Similar statistics are true of South Asians in the same age group. Activity levels in women vary: 83% of Indians, 86% of Pakistanis and 82% of Bangladeshis do not take enough exercise to benefit their health, while the figures for men are 67%, 72% and 75% respectively. About half of all South Asian women are sedentary compared to about 45% of South Asian men (DH, 2001). The exercise rate among South Asians is low (Fischbacher et al., 2004) and factors such as lack of encouragement for sports (especially with females) and older women preferring not to leave the house alone, may partly explain this. Many said that they are lazy, especially due to habits adopted from Pakistan (too much rest/not enough exercise). This can only be related to the higher social classes, as much of the population in Pakistan lives in poverty (Nanan & White, 1999). A comparison was made with Indians, who are more active, with traditional dancing. Culturally, Pakistanis take pleasure in eating and entertaining (Shaw, 2000). Sports and exercise have not been dominant aspects of the culture, perhaps partly due to the lack of women-only facilities in Britain and Pakistan and free mixing of males and females is not encouraged (Shaw, 2000). The sports culture in Pakistan is very much based around the male-dominated sport of cricket, with other world championship status in hockey and squash. However, this does not mean that women cannot have their own teams. Pakistani women have represented Pakistan in the world athletic games, marathon (*Jang*, 2005) and, more recently, in tennis.

Behavioural changes

Over the last decade the importance of behaviour modification as part of any weight loss programme has increased (Bagozzi & Edwards, 2000). Cognitive behavioural therapy has been shown to increase motivation and positive thinking and help people to change difficult aspects of their lives, whether this is smoking, drugs, alcohol or eating behaviour (Armitage & Conner, 2002). Behavioural treatment is an approach used to help individuals develop a set of skills to achieve a healthier weight and identify how to change (Garaulet *et al.*, 1999). Foster *et al.* (2005) evaluated the weight loss of a dietary/behavioural weight reduction programme in 90 overweight patients. Treatment included behavioural therapy, nutritional education and physical activity. Forty-three per cent of patients completed the treatment, with a mean weight loss of 9 kg. It is known that many aspects can affect the behaviour of an individual, especially with regard to health. It is believed that behaviours are the result of complex psychological factors, including habits, emotions, attitudes and beliefs, and that any attempt to change behaviour must therefore be targeted at these factors (Marks *et al.*, 2004).

The reasons why an individual or group follow a particular diet or exercise pattern include upbringing, family habits, culture, religion, education, knowledge and location (Brown, 1991). There is little research on health behaviour, obesity and ethnicity, although these have been highlighted in recent years (Alexander, 1999; London Health Observatory, 2003).

In Pakistan, social and environmental changes are occurring rapidly, with increasing urbanization, changing lifestyles, energy-dense diets and less physical activity. There has been a vast expansion of the food industry, with many new restaurants and fast-food outlets as eating out has become very popular (Nanan, 2002). However, awareness of obesity is increasing, especially among the younger generation who are taking their body image more seriously (Anwar, 1998). The leisure industry in Pakistan is developing rapidly, with more gyms, parks and other leisure activities (Nanan, 2002). However, this tends to be targeted at the wealthy who can afford to use these services, thus highlighting inequalities within Pakistan itself.

Many of the most significant, social and pleasurable activities in human experience are centred on eating and drinking, and thus are common to all people, (Beardsworth & Keil, 1997). However, eating and drinking are also social activities that are rich in symbolic, moral and cultural meaning (Marks *et al.*, 2004) which shapes the individual's experiences with food (Mela & Rogers, 1998).

Eating patterns may be influenced by religious beliefs, cultural background, availability of traditional foods and adaptation to a western lifestyle. Culture is the major determinant of what and when we eat and, to a lesser degree, how much we eat, and is embraced with pride and not readily altered. Thus, food habits and preferences are among the last characteristics of a culture to be lost following migration to a new culture (Marks *et al.*, 2004).

In some cultures, including the South Asians', obesity has been admired as a symbol of wealth and success, and fatness regarded as physically attractive. For example, in Africa and the Pacific Basin, in the past, obesity was perceived as attractive or a symbol of power and status (Brown, 1991; Marks *et al.*, 2004). Brown (1991) found that 81% of the societies for which there were sufficient data rated 'plumpness' or being 'filled out' as an attribute of beauty in females. Ethnicity is an important variable for understanding the distribution of obesity, but it brings with it the danger of stereotyping – the mistaken notion that all members of a group are alike.

Studies show that migrant groups who move to the UK become more overweight than the general UK population due to a combination of poor social conditions, little physical activity and a sharp increase in the amount of fat in the diet, linked to western influences on the traditional South Asian diet (Chowdhury *et al.*, 2003).

Prescott-Clarke and Primatests (1998) reviewed the influence of socioeconomic status on obesity around the world. They concluded that in industrialized countries, obesity tends to be more prevalent among the lower socioeconomic groups, whereas in poorer countries it is more common in the upper social groups, because only the relatively affluent have the opportunity to get fat. Poverty, inner-city living, poor housing and unemployment remain harsh realities for Pakistanis, Bangladeshis and African-Caribbeans (National Audit Office, 2001).

Recent evidence of good practice

There is a dearth of research and data to suggest the best evidence-based solutions in addressing obesity within this community, as well as others (Maryon-Davis Giles & Rona, 2000).

Perwiz (2005) explored the key issues and concerns of a sample of obese Pakistani women in London to identify the barriers that prevented this group from generating any sustained weight loss. Twenty-six participants were recruited from two local community groups. Overall, the subjects felt that aspects surrounding their own behavior, such as lack of motivation and time, rather than specific inequalities acted as the barriers. However, recurrent issues expressed by the subjects included a lack of appropriate weight management services, resources, support and awareness. Over half of the respondents said that they would go to a commercial slimming group, but only if there were other Asian women there and if it was not expensive. Groups such as Weight Watchers and Slimming World are successful because there is a need for such a service for the obese population (Thomas, 2001). However, such groups have not made concerted efforts to target ethnic minority groups. The fact that it is not a free service may prove to be an issue for those who are affected by wider inequalities. These results indicate that the main reasons for the increase in obesity in this community are diet and exercise. This and other factors, such laziness, are not exclusive to this community but affect the wider obese population too (Garrow, 2000).

Suggestions for the way forward

The lack of positive psychosocial support for the obese population and public health services/ initiatives sensitive to the needs of this community must be addressed in order to tackle this epidemic, as well as the absence of extensive qualitative research, especially within the more deprived areas.

The Faculty of Public Health Medicine states that improving access to effective weight management programmes and health and leisure services by such groups needs to be addressed (Maryon-Davis et al., 2000). The current situation of 'too little and (often) too late' cannot be allowed to continue. Only in this way will the obesity epidemic witnessed in South Asians be arrested and reversed (Chowdhury et al., 2003).

It appears that local councils, Primary Care Trusts and government have to make full use of the opportunities available to increase the commitment to raising awareness. At the same time, the community needs to increase their awareness and support within the community.

Rankin and Bhopal (2001) state that there is an urgent need for health education within South Asian communities, as they found that for both heart disease and diabetes two-thirds of respondents in their study understood too little about the conditions and how to prevent them.

1.3.6   Diabetes

Prevalence

In 2009 the prevalence of diabetes in the adult population across UK was 5.1% in England, 4.5% Northern Ireland, 4.6% in Wales and 3.9% in Scotland. The average prevalence of diabetes in UK was estimated to be 4% (Diabetes UK, 2010).

Not all diabetes is diagnosed. The Health Survey for England (DH, 2004c) suggests that 3.1% of men and 1.5% of women aged 35 and over have undiagnosed diabetes. For both men and women, the proportion of people with diabetes increases with age. The Health Survey for England (DH, 2006) suggests that around 1% of men aged 16–34 years have diagnosed diabetes compared with 13.5% of those aged 75 and over. The pattern is similar in women, although rates are slightly lower at most ages than for men. Prevalence rates of diabetes in the UK are average for developed countries. In general, developed countries have higher rates than developing countries. The prevalence of diabetes in 2004 was much higher among some ethnic minority communities than in the general population. The prevalence for Pakistani women was 2.5 times that of the general population (www. heartstats.org).

Almost 10% of the adult population of Pakistan suffer from diabetes (Staines *et al.*, 1997; Shah, 2004). The very low incidence of children aged up to 16 years with type 1 diabetes in Karachi contrasted with the substantially higher incidence among migrants, which supports the view that environmental factors are the major determinants of variations in the incidence of this condition between populations.

In the UK, people of South Asian origin are four times more likely to develop type 2 diabetes than Europeans (Mather & Keen, 1985). A more recent survey in inner city Manchester, where around 30% of the population is South Asian, showed that among individuals aged 35–79 years, 30% of Pakistani men and 36% of Pakistani women had previously known or newly diagnosed diabetes (Riste *et al.*, 2001).

The Health of Minority Groups Report 1999 (DH, 2001) stated that South Asian men and women had the highest rates of diabetes. Pakistanis of both sexes were more than five times as likely as the general population to have diabetes (www. statistics.gov.uk).

Diabetes substantially increases the risk of coronary heart disease (CHD). Men with type 2 diabetes have a 2–4-fold greater annual risk of CHD, with an even higher, 3–5-fold risk in women. Diabetes not only increases the risk of CHD but also amplifies the effect of other risk factors for CHD, such as raised cholesterol levels, raised blood pressure, smoking and obesity.

Diabetes causes severe morbidity (www. heartstats.org, 2009).

Complications of diabetes can be divided into three categories:

- Metabolic complications: low blood glucose levels (hypoglycaemia) and high blood glucose levels (hyperglycaemia). Diabetic coma is one such metabolic complication and is particularly severe.
- Microvascular complications: damage to small blood vessels leading to damage to the retina (retinopathy), kidneys (nephropathy) and nerves (neuropathy).

- Macrovascular complications: damage to the arteries leading to the brain (resulting in stroke) or to the heart (resulting in coronary heart disease) or to the legs and feet (causing peripheral vascular disease).

Data from South Asia and from areas with high concentrations of South Asian immigrants (Indians, Sri Lankans, Pakistanis and Bangladeshis) suggest that the diagnosis of type 2 diabetes among this ethnic group is increasing rapidly. Type 2 diabetes presents around a decade earlier in South Asians than indigenous Chinese, Japanese and UK populations. Cardiovascular complications of diabetes are more common among South Asians, with a 50% higher mortality compared to Caucasians. Similarly, renal disease is three times more common among South Asian diabetics than Europeans (Chowdhury & Hitman, 2007).

Type 1 diabetes requires treatment with insulin to achieve a balance between carbohydrate intake and insulin action. The overall aim is to establish good glycaemic control and prevent hypoglycaemic episodes. Although it is not yet possible to prevent type 1 diabetes, much can be done to prevent or delay the onset of type 2 diabetes. The development of type 2 diabetes is closely associated with obesity. Diabetes UK (2005) discusses how diabetes is approximately three times more common in people who have gained around 10 kg in weight during adulthood than in those who remain the same weight. There is increasing evidence that effective weight management and an active lifestyle can delay its onset.

Diet and lifestyle measures, including physical activity and ceasing smoking, are necessary if people with diabetes are to achieve near-normal blood glucose control and reduce cardiovascular risk factors.

Dietary modification

The South Asian eatwell plate (Figure 1.3.2) should be followed for healthy eating principles for diabetes management (see Table 1.3.7).

Those choosing to fast for religious purposes need to be advised on how to manage their diet and drug treatment, especially those taking insulin or oral hypoglycaemic drugs (Thomas & Bishop, 2007).

Table 1.3.7   Dietary modification for diabetes

- The timing of meals, particularly for those on insulin or oral hypoglycemic drugs. It is sometimes necessary to remind patients of the importance of these medications being taken at the specified times (and in the specific amounts).
- The need for an even and relatively constant distribution of starchy cereal foods throughout the day, and which is appropriate for any hypoglycemic therapy given.
- The need to avoid rich sources of sugars, particularly sweetmeats and sugar-containing fizzy drinks, which are often consumed in large quantities.
- The need to reduce fat consumption (principally by using less in cooking) and to reduce the intake of deep-fried snacks.
- The importance of weight loss for those who are overweight (via restriction of energy intake, primarily from fat and from increased physical activity).

Table 1.3.8   Glycaemic index of South Asian foods

Foods	Glycaemic index
Cereal products	
Chapatti	59–67
Basmati rice	58
Potato	70
Vegetables	
Karela	65
Saag (spinach)	0
Pulses and lentils	
Chickpeas	28
Mung beans	31
Red lentils	21
Chana dal	12
Fruit	
Banana	51
Mango	56
Water melon	72
Dates (dried)	45

Several prospective observational studies have shown that the long-term consumption of a diet with a high glycaemic load (GL; GI × dietary carbohydrate content) is a significant independent predictor of the risk of developing type 2 diabetes and cardiovascular disease. More recently, evidence has been accumulating that a low-GI diet may also protect against obesity (Foster-Powell et al., 2002) (see Table 1.3.8).

Herbal remedies

Karela (bitter gourd)

Karela is commonly consumed by the Pakistani population as it is believed to have a positive impact in reducing blood glucose levels. Pawa (2005) discusses how Indo-Asian people with type 2 diabetes may use traditional/herbal remedies for their perceived hypoglycaemic effects In the UK, karela capsules and juice are consumed, or added to curry. However, some people believe these can be taken as a substitute for oral medication so it is important that this is discussed by health professionals. Pawa (2005) recommends that asking about the use of these remedies should be an important part of the history, assessment and management of patients with diabetes.

Fenugreek

Fenugreek (trigonella foenum graecum) has been used for a variety of medicinal and other purposes, and may be used in the treatment of diabetes. Fenugreek is a member of the Leguminosae, or Fabaceae, family and grows well in India, Egypt and elsewhere in the Middle East. The part used medicinally is the seeds.

Fenugreek seeds contain alkaloids, including trigonelline, gentianine and carpaine compounds. The seeds also contain fibre, 4-hydroxyisoleucine and fenugreekine, a component that may have hypoglycaemic activity. The mechanism is thought to delay gastric emptying, slow carbohydrate absorption and inhibit glucose transport. Fenugreek may also increase the number of insulin receptors in red blood cells and improve glucose utilization in peripheral tissues, thus demonstrating potential anti-diabetes effects in the pancreas and other sites. The amino acid 4-hydroxyisoleucine in the seeds may also directly stimulate insulin secretion (Sharma et al., 1996).

The lipid-lowering effect of fenugreek seeds was studied in 60 non-insulin-dependent diabetic subjects. Isocaloric diets without and with fenugreek were given for 7 days and 24 weeks respectively.

Ingestion of an experimental diet containing 25 g fenugreek seed powder resulted in a significant reduction of total cholesterol, low density-lipoprotein (LDL) and very low-density lipoprotein (VLDL) cholesterol and triglyceride levels. These results indicate the beneficial effect of fenugreek seeds in diabetic subjects (Sharma *et al.*, 1996).

Cinnamon

Cinnamon is the inner bark of an evergreen tree native to India and Sri Lanka. It has insulin-like properties, which decrease blood glucose levels as well as triglycerides and cholesterol, all of which are important, especially for type 2 diabetes patients. Just half a teaspoon of cinnamon powder in the daily diet of a person with diabetes can significantly reduce blood glucose levels. The results of a study by Khan *et al.* (2003) demonstrated that intake of 1 g, 3 g or 6 g of cinnamon per day reduces serum glucose, triglyceride, LDL cholesterol and total cholesterol in people with type 2 diabetes and suggest that the addition of cinnamon to the diet of people with type 2 diabetes reduces risk factors associated with diabetes and cardiovascular disease.

By taking cinnamon, reduction in fasting blood levels was 18–29%, triglycerides was 23–30%, LDL cholesterol was 7–27% and total cholesterol was 12–26%.

Fasting

The Pakistani population mostly follows Islam. Fasting during the month of Ramadan is one of the five pillars of Islam (see introduction). Patients with a chronic condition are exempt from fasting on medical grounds, however many people with diabetes may choose to fast. With appropriate guidance and counselling some patients with diabetes may be able to fast quite safely.

Shaikh *et al.* (2001) discussed those who should not fast. They include:

- Type 1 or type 2 diabetics with poor glycaemic control.
- Individuals known to be non-compliant with diet or medication.
- Those with serious concurrent disease, including unstable angina or uncontrolled hypertension.
- Patients with a recurrent diabetic ketoacidosis.

- Pregnant women.
- Patients with intercurrent infections.
- Patients with renal impairment of any severity because of the risk of dehydration and uraemia.
- Elderly patients with reduced alertness.
- Those that have previously experienced severe deterioration in glycaemic control during Ramadan.

Suggestions for the way forward

- Unfortunately, the management of Asian people with diabetes is often inadequate and ineffective (Cruickshank, 1989).
- Patients often lack knowledge about the disease, its complications and the importance of self-management, problems which stem from poor communication, inadequate or culturally inappropriate information and the lack of availability of educational material in minority languages (Goodwin *et al.*, 1987; Hawthorne, 1990; Close *et al.*, 1995).
- To some extent, the situation will have improved following the implementation of the National Service Framework for Diabetes and the development of translated literature by organizations such as Diabetes UK. However, delivery of appropriate care to this patient group remains patchy.

1.3.7   Coronary heart disease/stroke

Key points

- The incidence of CHD is higher among South Asians than the general population.
- The main risk factors are poor diet, physical inactivity, smoking, high blood pressure, obesity, type 2 diabetes, age and socioeconomic deprivation.
- Many support groups are working to ensure equal access to treatment and services.

Prevalence

The British Heart Foundation shows that CHD is the UK's single biggest killer. One in four men and one in five women die from the disease.

South Asians living in the UK are 50% more likely to die prematurely from coronary heart disease than the general population. The death rate is 46% higher for men and 51% higher for women. The difference between South Asians and the rest of the population is increasing because the death rate from CHD is not falling as fast in South Asians as it is in the general population. 'From 1971 to 1991 the mortality rate for 20–69 year olds for the whole population fell by 29% for men and 17% for women, whereas in people born in South Asia it fell by 20% for men and 7% for women' (Coronary Heart Disease Statistics, 2008). By reducing the incidence of CHD, other arterial diseases, especially stroke, will also fall.

Cardiovascular disease (CVD) can affect anyone, but it is more prevalent in certain ethnic minorities. Pakistani men had rates of CVD about 60–70% higher than men in the general population. The picture was similar for women (British Cardiac Society, 2008).

Risk factors and treatments

It is not understood why South Asians suffer more from heart disease than other groups. Several explanations have been suggested (WHO, 2002). When several risk factors coexist, the risk of CHD is greatly increased.

Risk factors

- Age.
- A family history of heart disease.
- Economic deprivation.
- Diet and low fruit and vegetable intake.
- Low HDL cholesterol and elevated triglycerides.
- Diabetes.
- Smoking.
- Hypertension.
- Inadequate exercise.

Certain risk factors are more common among South Asians, but vary between communities.

Diabetes

Diabetes is a chronic condition that occurs when the pancreas does not produce enough insulin or when the body cannot effectively use the insulin it

does produce. There are two forms of diabetes: type 1 – people with this type of diabetes produce very little or no insulin; and type 2 – people cannot use insulin effectively. Most people with diabetes have type 2 (WHO, 2002).

People with diabetes are at increased risk of developing CHD than the general population. Men with type 2 diabetes have a 2–4-fold greater annual risk of CHD. However, women face a greater risk, with a 3–5-fold risk of type 2 diabetes (Garcia et al., 1974). Similar results were seen in The Interheart study (2004), which estimated that 15% of heart attacks in Western Europe are due to diagnosed diabetes; therefore, those who suffer from diabetes were at three times the risk of heart attack.

The Health Survey for England (1999) found South Asian men and women had the highest rates of diabetes. Pakistanis and Bangladeshis of both sexes were more than five times as likely as the general population to have diabetes, and Indian men and women were almost three times as likely.

Hypertension

The 2004 British Hypertension Society guidelines are that optimal blood pressure treatment targets are a systolic blood pressure of less than 140 mmHg and a diastolic blood pressure of less than 85 mmHg (and lower still, at 130/85 mmHg, for people with diabetes). People with high normal blood pressures (130–139/85–89 mmHg should be assessed annually). Data from the Health Survey for England show that in 2004 the proportion of Pakistani men with high blood pressure was two-thirds that of the general population. Pakistani women had half the levels of high blood pressure than women in the general population. In addition, the prevalence of untreated hypertension was lower among Pakistani men and women than in the general population.

Diet modification

To reduce the risk of CHD the British Nutrition Foundation recommend the following: maintain a healthy body weight; eat five or more portions of fruit and vegetables a day; reduce intake of fat, particularly saturated fat; reduce salt intake; eat at least two portions of fish, of which one should be

Table 1.3.9   Dietary modification of Pakistani diet for treatment for coronary heart disease

Food group	Encourage	Discourage
Carbohydrates	Whole meal bread or wholegrain cereal, chapatti (roti) made with whole meal flour, boiled rice	*Parathas, puri,* fried toast
Protein	Meat or chicken curry, dal (using small amounts of oil and choosing lean meats). Fish curry using oily fish (mackerel, trout, kippers, pilchards, salmon, sardines, herring, sprats) Boiled eggs Boil/steam/grill-meat/fish	Fried egg/omelette. Fatty meats and fried meat/fish
Dairy	Semi-skimmed or skimmed milk	Full-fat milk, cream, evaporated milk
Desserts	Fresh or tinned fruit in natural juice Rice pudding or vermicelli (made with semi-skimmed milk). Fruit salad Fruit yoghurt	*Halwa* (made with carrots or semolina), *zarda* (sweet rice)
Snacks	Oven-baked samosas. *Chana* (chickpeas) and/or potato *chaat,* fruit *chaat.* Grilled kebab with pitta/naan bread with salad. More fruit and vegetables	Fried samosas, pokoras, chips. Bombay mix, crisps. Asian sweets (*jalebi, halwa, burfi*)
Drinks	Water, unsweetened fruit juices. Diet or sugar-free soft drinks. *Lassi*	Fizzy drinks. Sweetened soft drinks. Sweetened fruit juices
Fats and oils	Reduce fats and oils	Ghee, butter

oily fish, a week. This is consistent with general healthy eating guidelines (see Table 1.3.9).

Increased consumption of fruit and vegetables has been shown to be associated with a reduced risk of CHD. The general population consumption of fruit and vegetables is less than three portions a day, however by increasing just one portion of fruit and vegetables the risk of CHD is lowered by 4% and the risk of stroke by 6% (Heart Disease and South Asians). The Health Survey of England (1999) found considerable variation in eating habits among ethnic groups. The Pakistani community had the lowest levels of vegetable consumption, with just 7% of men and 11% of women eating vegetables on six or more days a week. The survey also showed that about half of South Asians (Pakistanis 53%) perceived their traditional diets to be healthier than western diets. In addition, 79% of Pakistani people reported that traditional foods constituted a major component of the diets eaten at home.

Dietary restrictions for cultural or religious reasons were widespread among Indian (80%), Pakistani (97%) and Bangladeshi (97%) people (Health Education Authority, 1999). The survey also reported less understanding of key terms used in healthy eating messages, such as 'starchy foods', 'dietary fibre' and 'saturated fat', though this varied widely among South Asians. Among those who said they understood dietary terms, knowledge of foods high in starch, dietary fibre, fat and saturated fat was patchy and often poor across all ethnic groups.

Smoking

It is estimated that the average male smoker loses about 13 years of life and the average female smoker about 14 years of life. Stopping smoking is the single most important thing an individual can do to avoid a heart attack. Some studies have shown that 5–15 years after quitting smoking the risk of stroke is reduced to the level of a non-smoker, and 15 years after quitting the risk of coronary heart disease is the same as a non-smoker's. South Asian men and women on average smoked fewer cigarettes than men and women in the wider population. The reported rate of current cigarette smoking was very low in women (1%) but higher among men (Health Education Authority, 1999). However, knowledge about the main diseases linked to smoking was low among men and women in all groups. The serious illness most likely to be linked to cigarette smoking was lung cancer, but knowledge about the links between smoking and other respiratory diseases, heart disease and throat and mouth cancers was very low.

Physical activity

The government confirms that at least 30 minutes of at least moderate physical activity a day on five or more days a week (45–60 minutes a day for children and 60 minutes for young people) significantly reduces the risk of premature death from cardiovascular disease (DH, 2004c).

There is evidence to show that an inactive lifestyle has a sustainable negative effect on health (DH, 2004d). Estimates have shown that 37% of CHD deaths can be attributed to physical inactivity. This compares to 13% attributable to high blood pressure (Britton & McPherson, 2002).

South Asian men and women from all ethnic groups are less likely to take part in physical activity than the general population (British Heart Foundation, 2001). Compared with the general population, Indian, Pakistani, Bangladeshi and Chinese men and women were less likely to meet physical activity recommendations.

The second health and lifestyle survey found several barriers for individuals not participating in exercise. Religion played an important role, though the desire to maintain modesty or avoid mixed-sex activity and fear of going out alone were not confined to Muslims. It was also found that Pakistani men were more likely to identify taking regular exercise as health-enhancing than Pakistani women. Other barriers may be due to lack of knowledge about recommended levels of physical activity. Fear of racism may affect people's willingness to exercise in public places, and socioeconomic disadvantage or lack of money or transport to attend facilities is commonly cited as a barrier to participation in sport and leisure activities.

Recent evidence of good practice

Evidence of good practice can be difficult to find as some support groups have only recently been set up or there is insufficient evidence for the Pakistani population.

The Khush Dil is a primary care-led, NHS Lothian-funded, community health project that offers a culturally sensitive framework for the identification and management of CHD risk factors. Staff include a health visitor, dietitian, two South Asian community health workers and an administrator. The nurse/health visitor provides a one-to-one cardiac health assessment designed for Asian patients. This helps build a picture of their individual heart health profile and identify any risk factors. In addition, the dietetic clinic provides one-to-one support to promote healthy eating using a South Asian diet. Community programme activities are also available for South Asians and include aerobic exercise for women, circuit training for men, walking and jogging groups. The Khush Dil project has found it difficult to formally evaluate the effectiveness of these changes in the group session. However, they did find it reassuring that healthy changes can be made without changing the taste of food. 'The local Asian community is enthusiastic about the project and anecdotal evidence suggests health and social outcomes have been improved for many Khush Dil attendees.'

In Birmingham Heartlands and Solihull NHS Trust interpreters play a vital role in ensuring that patients understand their condition. If needed the interpreters have the support of an Equal Access Facilitator. In addition, software packages in Urdu and Bengali are available. The resources available for Asians include a video, *Help Yourself to a Healthy Heart*, which is available in several Asian languages. The video covers what happens when you have a heart attack, medication and advice on exercise and diet. Later the Trust employed a CHD Asian Link Nurse who speaks Punjabi, Hindi and Urdu and as a result is able to check patients' understanding of their condition and what they need to follow. All patients attend the same rehabilitation programme; however, classes are given in different languages to different groups. Useful resources in different languages, as well as employing a suitable candidate for the role, have led to increased take-up of cardiac rehabilitation and compliance with the programmme.

Similar to the above Trust, the New Cross in Wolverhampton has a dedicated heart disease nurse who speaks Punjabi and Hindi. A common problem highlighted was patients failing to take medication or follow treatment and rehabilitation programmes. Since the nurse was recruited she has been able to work with patients to provide a better understanding of their medical condition and ways to improve their quality of life. As a result attendance at rehabilitation and heart failure clinics by Asian patients has greatly increased, compliance with medication is up and patients appear more satisfied with the information provided.

Support groups

Many initiatives are working specifically to break down barriers to health inequalities and some particularly focus on minority ethnic groups and people living in areas of high deprivation. Below are some examples of organizations working to improve heart disease services for South Asians.

Improving access

- The South Asian Living with Heart Disease project was set up to examine and improve equal access to primary care services between South Asian and non-South Asian with CVD.
- Using ethnic profiling to improve services for BME (black and minority ethnic) communities with CHD. The aim was to improve the percentage of DNAs (did not attends) for patients with CHD attending the GP practice. Following ethnic profiling the practice provided appropriate bilingual services which resulted in fewer DNAs.

General prevention

- QUIT: The British Heart Foundation (BHF) and Diabetes UK have teamed up to promote healthy lifestyle messages to a large number of Asian families at venues such as summer *melas* (community fairs), as well as providing imams and other religious leaders with training in basic prevention of heart disease.
- Project Dil: a Leicester-wide primary care and health promotion programme, which aims to increase understanding of CHD and improve primary and secondary prevention of CHD in the South Asian community.
- Rochdale Healthy Living Centre is running initiatives to break down barriers to health infor-

mation and services, with their main focus on general healthy eating advice as well as CHD and diabetes.
- Khush Dil Happy Heart Project is a primary care-led, NHS Lothian-funded, community health project which aims to prevent CHD in South Asian communities. Core project staff include a health visitor, dietitian, two South Asian community health workers and an administration worker based in Leicester.

Rehabilitation

- Fair and equal access to cardiac rehabilitation in Leicester was the aim of the project, in addition to helping patients understand their illness, its treatment and promoting their return to a full and normal life.
- Planning and delivering an equitable cardiac rehabilitation service in Newham – a two-year project delivering cardiac rehabilitation services to minority ethnic groups.
- Action CHD (Dil Ke Baat): the aim of the two-year project was to reduce deaths from CHD in South Asians by developing an education programme covering secondary prevention and cardiac rehabilitation.
- The CADISAP (Coronary Artery Disease in South Asian Prevention) study: the aim was to improve the uptake of and adherence to cardiac rehabilitation among South Asians through culturally specific interventions.
- Bengali Bridge Project: addresses chronic health conditions in the Bengali population in Euston.

Treatment

- The 3 Cities Project: covers Sheffield, Leicester and Nottingham, where multi-language health information can be accessed using touch-screen computers.
- The Ealing Coronary Risk Prevention Programme is nurse-led programme focusing on men and women aged 35–75 years and assessing risk of CHD from the participating practices.
- Birmingham Heartlands and Solihull NHS Trust: the Trust has employed interpreters which staff in any department can book at short notice; they also carry out ward rounds. In

addition, the trust has a CHD Asian Link Nurse. This has resulted in an increased take-up of cardiac rehabilitation and compliance with the programme.

- The New Cross Heart Disease Asian Link Nurse increases take-up of services.
- The Manchester Heart Centre Cardiac Liaison Team provides advice at every stage of the patient journey from point of listing through to follow-up support after discharge. In addition, booklets for patient in Urdu, Hindi and Punjabi are available, and 50 audio tapes are available in each language.
- Improving care for South Asian cardiac patients in Bradford to improve the care of heart failure patients. This was achieved by employing a bilingual community cardiac worker as part of the CHD team.

Diet and nutrition

- The Coventry 5-a-Day Scheme provides people with £2 vouchers to spend on fruit and vegetables.
- The Coriander Club, Spitalfields City Farm is a group of Bangladeshi women who get together to grow vegetables. The group has two weekly gardening days and a weekly healthy cookery class.
- The Birmingham Food Net began in August 2000 to promote a cardio-protective diet in a specified area of Birmingham, including some areas with a high South Asian polulation.
- The Bradford Trident Healthy Living Project weight management programme is a 12-week programme and groups meets on a weekly basis as it has been identified that health ine-qualities are significantly higher in this area, as are rates of CHD and type 2 diabetes.
- Dietary intervention in high-risk families with CHD in Ealing – a family-based programme, where a cardio-protective diet is emphasized.

Physical activity

There are now over 700 GP exercise referral schemes prescribing physical activity to improve health and well-being. Pilot projects, such as LEAP and the Walking the Way to Health initiative, are trialling different approaches for increasing access to and levels of physical activity.

- Walking for Health in Wolverhampton is a local scheme that provides regular, free, led walks, map-packs of short local walk routes and general health information on walking.
- SITARA is a women-only projct, staffed by women for women, in Batley, West Yorkshire.
- Hamara Healthy Living Centre in Leeds pro-motes physical activity as a preventative measure for CHD.
- Al-Badr Health & Fitness is a fitness centre in East London, serving the entire Muslim community.

Suggestions for the way forward

The National Service Framework on coronary heart disease suggests: 'Adopt[ing] broadly-based strategies that focus on established risk factors, taking account of language and cultural needs.'

- Smoking cessation, which has been relatively neglected, needs to be targeted at Bangladeshi and Pakistani men and all South Asian teenagers.
- Other key risk factors requiring vigorous control include diabetes, hypertension, obesity, raised cholesterol and triglycerides values and lack of physical exercise.
- Disease registers and practice lists may need an ethnic code so services can be appropriately targeted.

Other suggestions

- Identify barriers experienced by the ethnic community in accessing the service, by patient involvement.
- Create a local network of organizations working as partners in health care to increase awareness of CHD and its prevention.
- Integrated work between primary and second-ary care.
- Improve awareness among patients of CHD risk factors and their prevention. Care profes-sionals created a local network of organizations working as partners in health care to increase awareness of CHD and its prevention.
- Recruit and train community health educators from minority ethnic men and women who live in their respective communities to carry out particular health education sessions with members of their communities.

- Community educators must be bilingual, have some cultural understanding of their own communities and be able to deliver quite complex information in an accessible manner.
- Community involvement to devise effective implementation of policies and ensure that South Asians are well informed about their risk of CHD (BHF fact file, 2000).

1.3.8 Cancer

Key points

- Cancer is a consequence of complex and multiple factors, involving the environment and genetics.
- Tobacco use is the principal causative factor for cancer.
- Dietary modification and regular physical activity are significant elements in cancer prevention and control.
- Diets high in fruit, vegetables and fibre may reduce the risk for various types of cancer, whereas high intake of preserved and/or red meat, salt, alcohol and fat are associated with increased cancer risk.
- Overweight and obesity are both serious risk factors for cancer in both the general population and the Pakistani community in the UK.

Introduction

Cancer is the second leading cause of death in developed countries and becoming a significant cause of death in developing countries. Evidence suggests that cancer rates change as populations move between countries and adopt different lifestyles. Currently, little information is available about cancer in the Pakistani population due to lack of data from cancer registries in the UK.

Prevalence

There is little information on ethnic differences in the incidence of cancer and cancer mortality among adults in the UK, especially the Pakistani population, mainly due to the lack of reliable ethnicity data in cancer registries (Lees & Papadopoulos, 2000; Moles *et al.*, 2008) and lack of published data

on the Pakistani population both in Pakistan and the UK (Winter *et al.*, 1999). Due to a recent trend in collecting data about ethnic minorities by health care services only some data are available, which show that cancer incidence rates and mortality are lower in minority groups compared to the general population (Winter *et al.*, 1999; Lane *et al.*, 2007).

This might underestimate the true extent of the prevalence of cancer in the Pakistani population as the main reason accountable for this difference is a the younger age structure of the ethnic minority groups compared to the White population and cancer incidence increases with age. It is estimated that more than half the ethnic minority population are under 16 years of age (National Statistics, 2002). This could partly be explained by the fact that some members of the ethnic minority return to their country of origin after retirement (Lodge, 2001). Another important reason to explain the underestimation of the cancer burden is lack of reporting by some members of this population as they rely on alternative therapies or traditional interventions for their disease.

However, when compared to cancer incidence rates in the Indian subcontinent, the migrant Asian populations have higher cancer rates. This suggests that changes in lifestyle or greater exposure to a carcinogenic environment have occurred within this population group which has changed the incidence rates from the country of origin to that of the country of residence (Winter, 1999).

Breast and lung cancers are the most common cancers among ethnic minority groups in the UK (Lodge, 2001). However, although they are at a lower risk of most cancers, the South Asian population, including Pakistani people, have increased risks of oral and pharyngeal cancers relative to the general British population. This mirrors similar trends in the Indian subcontinent (Winter, 1999; Merseyside Regional Head and Neck Cancer Centre, 2007).

Among the other main cancers, Hodgkin's lymphoma in males and cancer of the tongue, mouth, oesophagus and thyroid and myeloid leukaemia in females are significant. Cancer of the hypopharynx, liver and gall bladder are prevalent in both sexes (Winter, 1999).

Another study suggested that on the basis of the number of cases, breast, lung and neoplasm of the lymphatic system were the three main cancers for adults in the ethnic minority in the UK, whereas cancers of the gall bladder, liver and oral cavity were considered to be the three predominant cancers, based on the standardized mortality ratio (Bhopal & Rankin, 1996).

Risk factors and treatments

It is yet to be established what the exact mechanism is that leads to the development of cancer. It appears to be a series of complex factors. Some of these, such as environmental influences, which are thought to be accountable for 95% of cancers, can be modified, whereas a genetic predisposition cannot, but the aetiology of such cancers remains complex and with genetic influence the development of the disease is not definitive.

Due to the scope of this chapter only environmental factors are discussed in the following sections.

Tobacco and smoking

Tobacco use is one of the most recognized risk factors in the development of cancer. Not only smoking but chewing tobacco is associated with this disease (Critchley & Unal, 2003). As in other South East Asian populations, both smoking and chewing tobacco are common in the Pakistani population, with an estimated 29% of Pakistani men compared to 24% of men in the general population smoking (DH, 2004d). The prevalence of tobacco chewing increases with age, especially among women. Betel quid mixed with tobacco is the most commonly used tobacco product (DH, 1999).

Mouth, throat, oesophagus, lung, stomach, kidney and bladder cancers are all related to tobacco exposure. Passive smoking is also a risk and studies show that there is a 25–50% increase in the risk of developing lung cancer in people exposed to secondhand smoke (Boffetta, 2002; Jamrozik, 2005; Vineis et al., 2005). This could be of particular importance among the Pakistani population, as they have large families and live in an extended family environment (National Statistics, 2002), thus exposing more people to passive smoking.

Environmental pollution and fuel smoke are other possible factors in the development of predominantly lung cancer (Fullerton et al., 2008). The International Agency for Research on Cancer iden-

tified biomass smoke as a probable carcinogen and coal as carcinogenic to humans (Straif, 2006). This could be a particularly important risk factor for the first-generation Pakistani population who were frequently exposed to smoke from household use of solid fuels. Data from India, Mexico and China have recognized domestic coal smoke and biomass fuel smoke as significant risk factors for the development of lung cancer (Du et al., 1996; Hernandez-Garduno et al., 2004; Behera & Balamugesh, 2005; Zhao, 2006).

Betel quid (paan) and areca nut (chalia)

Betel quid or *paan* consists of areca nut, lime and catechu wrapped in a betel leaf to which tobacco is often added (Centres for Disease Control and Prevention, 2007). The habit of chewing betel quid is widespread in South-East Asia, especially in the Indian subcontinent. This habit is also common in migrants from these countries (Gupta & Warnakulasuriya, 2002; Cancer Research UK, 2009).

There is evidence to show that chewing betel quid containing tobacco is carcinogenic (Gupta et al., 1992; Gupta & Ray 2003, 2004; IARC, 2004; Nair et al., 2004; Centres for Disease Control and Prevention, 2007). In 2004, the International Agency for Research on Cancer (IARC) declared betel quid and areca nut to be group 1 carcinogens.

Oral cancers, predominantly cancers of the lip, mouth, tongue, and pharynx and oesophageal cancer, are associated with betel quid use (Gupta & Ray, 2003, 2004; IARC, 2004; Nair et al., 2004; Centres for Disease Control and Prevention, 2007). Much of the evidence for such an association comes from Indian studies, however this research can also be implied for the Pakistani population due to similar cultural and geographical characteristics.

Diet

After smoking and tobacco use, diet is considered to be the most attributable cause of cancer (Cancer Research UK). Dietary factors are thought to cause about 30% of all cancers in western countries and up to 20% in developing countries (WHO, 2004). Alcohol, salt, meat and fat are some of the dietary factors which have well-established links to cancer risk.

The traditional Pakistani diet tends to be high in carbohydrates, fibre, fruit and vegetables, legumes, lentils and dairy products and low in meat, poultry and fish. The Pakistani diet is also high in fat, in particular saturated fat (mainly from full-fat dairy products, ghee and butter), as well as high in salt and sugar (Pakistan manual). However, due to adopting of western eating pattern and habits, and an increase in socioeconomic status, the Pakistani diet is depicting trends of more modern but unhealthy choices. This is especially true of the migrant Pakistani population in western countries (Winter *et al.*, 1999). The Health Survey for England (2004) shows poor health and lifestyle choices among the Asian community in general and Muslim community in particular. Women tend to make better lifestyle choices than men, but report more illness or poor health when compared with Pakistani men.

Fat

High fat intake, especially saturated fat, has been linked predominantly with breast cancer by various studies; however, there is no conclusive evidence for this. It is not clear whether it is saturated fat, dairy products in general or the resultant obesity which is increasing the risk of cancer (Thomas, 2001). There is clear evidence of high fat intake among the Pakistani population, which was also observed in the Health Survey for England in 2004. It was found that women of all other ethnic minorities apart from Pakistani women had lower mean consumption of fat. However, female fat consumption is considered to be lower than their male counterparts: 84% of women had a low fat intake as compared to 72% of men in the general population. Health promotion messages aimed at the Pakistani population should focus on decreasing fat consumption for its associated links with heart disease and diabetes, which are also prevalent in this ethnic minority group.

Salt

High salt intake has been linked with stomach cancer, however most of the evidence comes from countries with high salt intake which makes it unclear to what extent salt can cause stomach cancer in other populations (Cancer Research UK). Salt may either increase the sensitivity of the lining of the stomach to carcinogens or directly cause damage to mucosa and inflammation. It was found that the pattern of salt intake in the Pakistani popu-

lation was similar in both genders, however in comparison with the general population the amount of salt used in cooking was higher in ethnic minorities (DH, 2004a). This finding was comparable with the traditional Pakistani diet, which consists of significant salt intake in both cooking and at the table. Accompaniments like pickles and chutneys which are used on daily basis also contribute large quantities. However it was found that both Pakistani men and women were using less salt in cooking as well as on the table in the 2004 Health Survey compared with 1999. This could be attributable to health messages especially aimed at ethnic minorities regarding excessive salt intake and related health risks such as high blood pressure, stroke, heart disease and some cancers.

Fruit and vegetables

A combination of fibre, antioxidants, folate and a range of phytochemicals make this food group protective against the development of cancers. Hence the government's current advice is in line with the World Health Organization's (2004) – five portions of fruit and vegetables a day. High intakes are linked with a reduced risk of oral, oesophageal, larynx, stomach, lung and bladder cancers. Some 33% of Pakistani men and women eat the recommended five or more portions of fruit and vegetables a day as compared with 14% of the adult general population (DH, 2004a). The ratio of women eating recommended fruits and vegetable was higher than men. This is also true for the general population. These findings are based on self-reports of the consumption of fruit and vegetables. That does not necessarily take into account the cooking or preparation methods which can result in substantial losses of nutrients and hence reduce the protective effects of fruit and vegetables.

Fibre

Some evidence suggests that a high fibre intake is protective against some forms of cancer (e.g., bowel and pancreas). Studies show that it is particularly protective in people with high consumption of red and processed meat. However, it is important not to link only one aspect of food with the development of cancers as other factors (e.g., physical activity, drinking alcohol, smoking, high consumption of red and processed meat and salt) are also strongly linked with the development of bowel and pancreatic cancers. Therefore, the focus should be on promoting general healthy eating guidelines (Thomas *et al.*, 2005).

Two mechanisms are linked with the protective effects of fibre: first, fermentation of fibre in the bowel produces short-chain fatty acids, which may have anti-proliferative properties; second, fibre contributes to maintaining gut health by increasing the transit time of stool, thereby decreasing the exposure of the intestine to possible harmful substances. There were no data available on the fibre intake of the Pakistani population from the Health Survey of Minority Ethnic Groups in 2004. The Department of Health recommended an average intake of 18 g a day for the general population; however, the average individual daily intake of fibre in the UK is 14 g (DH, 1991).

Red and processed meat

Some evidence suggests that people with a high intake of red and processed meat have a high risk of bowel cancer (Larsson & Wolk, 2006). Two possible mechanisms relating high intake of meat to cancer include an exposure to carcinogens like heterocyclic amines produced during cooking or increased production of nitrosamines in the gut. There are no data on the meat intake in the Pakistani population, but it is generalized that red meat intake is rising in this group, whereas processed meat intake remains low (Pakistani Manual).

Alcohol

Alcohol is well established as a cause of cancer and its risk is greatly increased in combination with smoking. Cancers of the upper respiratory-digestive tract, bowel and liver are especially linked with alcohol consumption (Cancer Research UK, 2009). Alcohol is prohibited for Muslims, so there is less consumption among the Pakistani population when compared with other minority groups and the general population, but it is not totally uncommon. An estimated 89% of Pakistani men and 95% women are non-drinkers as compared to 8% of men and 14% of women in the general population (DH, 2004a).

Body weight and physical activity

Obesity and lack of physical activity are both linked with the development of a number of diseases including cancer (WHO, 2002). The main cancers associated with excess body weight are cancers of the colon, breast, endometrium, kidney, oesophagus, gastric cardia, gall bladder and pancreas (Cancer Research UK, 2009).

The prevalence of obesity is increasing in the South Asian ethnic group. Although mean body mass index (BMI) for men was lower when compared with the general population, Pakistani women were most obese after Black Caribbean and Black Africans women and were also more obese than women in general population. Similar trends were observed in Pakistani children, with Pakistani girls at a high risk of being obese and boys of being overweight (DH, 2004c).

Central obesity is considered to be more accurate in determining the risk of obesity-related diseases as compared to the BMI. The Health Survey of England (2004) showed an increase in central obesity in the Pakistani population (37% men and 39% in women as compared to 33% and 30% respectively in the general population).

Research also suggests that overall participation in sport and activity is clearly lower in the Pakistani population as compared to other ethnic minority populations. Figures on sports show that participation of Pakistani population is lower (31%) as compared to the national average of 46% (Rowe & Champion, 2000).

The thresholds for BMI, waist circumference and WHR used in the Health Survey of England (2004) are intended for White European populations and growing evidence suggests that they might not apply to those of non-European descent (Deurenberg *et al.*, 2000; Dudeja *et al.*, 2001). This could lead to an underestimation of the actual prevalence of obesity in the South Asian, in particular the Pakistani, population (Lovegrove, 2007). The World Health Organization Expert Consultation in 2004 highlighted that the health risks can considerably increase, particularly in South Asian populations, below the cut-off point of $25 \, \text{kg/m}^2$ for there is significant evidence to suggest that associations between BMI, percentage of body fat and body fat distribution differ across populations (Seidell *et al.*, 2001; Misra *et al.*, 2005, 2006).

(For further reading on obesity and ethnic-specific cut-offs for BMI and waist circumference see the section on Obesity.)

Table 1.3.10 Dietary guidelines for cancer prevention

- Maintain weight within healthy BMI range.
- Eat at least five portions of fruit and vegetables of a wide variety each day.
- Eat more starchy foods and mainly high-fibre varieties.
- Eat red or processed meat only within the UK's average intake (90 g/day).
- Drink alcohol in moderation.
- Do not take high-dose supplements of beta-carotene or other micronutrients.
- Avoid excess salt.

Dietary modification

Although there is a strong association between dietary influences and the prevention or development of cancer, focusing on one aspect of diet and its relationship with a particular cancer is not advisable. Therefore the COMA working party (DH, 1998) recommended dietary guidelines for the prevention of cancer, which are summarized in (Table 1.3.10) and are in accordance with WHO (2002) and the Food Standard Agency's recommendations. However, these guidelines should be used in conjunction with the healthy eating principle.

Dietary management of cancer is not a straightforward process due to the involvement of a number of interlinked, and to some extent complex, factors. These can range from health promotion for cancer prevention to specific aspects of dietary management before, during and after cancer treatment. It can also extend to addressing psychological and emotional issues associated with diagnosis, treatment and prognosis. In addition, due to the extended family structure, dietetic intervention will be further complicated with meeting expectations of the family members as well as the patient.

In the Pakistani population group, the language barrier also plays an important role, especially as risk of cancer increases with age and therefore the group at a higher risk of cancer development are the first-generation migrants who encounter language and cultural barriers the most.

Dietetic modification involves nutritional assessment with particular importance to the following aspects:

- Weight changes and present nutritional intake.
- Changes in appetite or taste.
- Difficulty in eating and/or swallowing.

Table 1.3.11 Main cancer treatments and their nutritional implications

Surgery	Increased nutritional requirements
	Delay in nutritional intake
	Surgery induced side-effects, e.g., ineffective digestion and absorption
Radiotherapy	Anorexia, nausea, sickness
	Increased risk of infections of mouth and throat
	Mucositis, painful and sore mouth and throat
	Abdominal cramps and diarrhoea
	Loss or change in taste
	Xerostoma
	Dysphagia
	Difficulty in speech
	Tiredness
Chemotherapy	Nausea, vomiting
	Taste changes
	Stomatitis
	Mucositis
	Oesophagitis
	Diarrhoea
	Constipation
	Poor appetite

- Nutritional implications of specific types of cancers.
- Nutritional implications of treatment related side-effects.
- Requirement of oral or enteral nutrition support.

However, it is important to note that spirituality and religion also play a vital role in the lives of people from this cultural group as well as use of herbal and alternative therapies. Reliance on tales, myths and personal beliefs about specific foods or treatments can pose a real challenge for dietary management. Therefore, it is essential that all members of the healthcare team are aware of the need to look for specific cultural issues when treating this group (see Table 1.3.11).

Recent evidence of good practice

There is little information on the evidence of good practice on cancer in the ethnic minority population. The main focus of cancer care is on increasing awareness and improving the take-up of screening services. Another important area of work is targeting health messages at this population group. That is being done in conjunction with other diseases related to lifestyle factors, such as heart disease and diabetes.

Suggestions for the way forward

There is increasing evidence suggesting that healthcare provision for ethnic minority groups is poorer than for the majority population and same trend is found in cancer care (Lodge, 2001; Elkan *et al.*, 2007). The main issues highlighted in the literature are communication barriers, lack of awareness and failure of providers to accommodate religious and cultural diversity. Dietary management should take into account the cultural and religious needs of the Pakistani population.

Evidence highlights health inequalities among ethnic minority groups in the UK. Lack of knowledge about cancer and cancer services leads to a low uptake of screening and preventative services.

Language and communication barriers are significant causes of the low uptake of health service in the Pakistani population.

Improvement in socioeconomic factors, the importance of cancer awareness and screening with targeted health promotion and regular monitoring are ways forward in cancer care in this population group.

Traditional intervention strategies are mostly designed for the majority White population and do not necessarily accommodate the needs of the ethnic communities. Therefore, intervention strategies should be devised, such as stopping smoking and chewing tobacco services, improving the use of screening services, education on cancer, targeted health promotion messages especially translated in Urdu with the use of audiovisual aids when necessary.

Further research about cancer in this group with systematic collecting and recording of data in cancer registries will help to develop good practice in the UK (Lodge, 2001; Thomas, 2001).

Resources in different languages and how to obtain them

Cancer Equality is a registered charity, which with the funding from the Department of Health estab-

lished the National Black and Minority Ethnic Cancer Resource Centre in 2003. This is the first resource of its kind and has produced a directory of various cancer-related information resources in different languages for both health professionals and people affected by cancer. The directory is available at ethnicminoritycancerdirectory.pdf 590.64 Kb.

1.3.9 Maternal and child nutrition

Introduction

Many of the Pakistani immigrants and nationals living in the UK have largely retained their cultural and religious practices, some of which are reflected in their diet. This is particularly true of maternal and infant nutritional practices. Despite some dietary acculturation, dietary transition appears to be minimal between the first- and second-generation Pakistani communities, which may be attributed to the cohesive nature of the community (Parsons *et al.*, 1999).

It is important to note that family, cultural traditions and religious beliefs have a powerful influence on maternal nutrition and weaning practices within the Pakistani community (James & Underwood, 1997).

Pre-conception and pregnancy beliefs

Many myths and traditions regarding nutrition and pregnancy/post-pregnancy are practised and widely advocated in many parts of Pakistan, some of which may be followed by the UK Pakistani population as well. Many women rely on the experience, knowledge, support of their friends and family to guide them through their pregnancy as well as rearing their children. However, often the advice given is not supported by any scientific evidence and may often contradict the advice and recommendations specified by local and international health professionals or governing bodies such as the Department of Health or WHO.

The following gives a brief insight into the typical traditions and practices within some of the Pakistani communities, however it is important to note that this is largely based on reported observations and variances may occur within the community.

During the first trimester of pregnancy, due to the increased risk of miscarriage, certain dietary recommendations are advocated to ensure the latter is avoided. Women during this period are recommended to abstain from the consumption of 'hot' foods and the intake of 'cold' foods is recommended. The latter does not refer to the temperature of the foods, but to its energy properties (Homans, 1983). There are many intricacies attached to the two categories, some of which neatly map onto western medicine and some of which do not. One of the basic distinctions is between cold and heat, the logic behind it being that you consume cold and cooling foods when you are hot and consume hot and warming foods when you are cold. Pregnancy is thought of as a 'hot' condition therefore 'hot' food such as meat, fish, nuts, seafood and eggs are not recommended initially whereas 'cold' foods such as yoghurt, milk and some fruits and vegetables are encouraged (Caplan, 1997).

There are certain beliefs surrounding the association between nutrition and its contribution to the appearance and physical features or attributes of the child. Having a child who is fair-skinned is a generally desired attribute within some communities across the South Asian populations. It is perceived that if you drink light-coloured drinks – milk, water, fruit juice, etc. – this will result in a fairer baby, whereas the consumption of darker drinks – tea, coffee, cola, etc. – will result in a darker complexion. The latter are thus avoided. In addition, some women may choose not to take iron supplements as it is believed that iron can result in dark stools, and may have a similar effect on the skin tone of the child. However, there is no documented evidence to support these theories.

Iron deficiency anaemia

Iron deficiency anaemia is highly among pregnant women in Pakistan (Hassan et al., 1992; Hayat, 1997). This may be explained by the fact that iron-rich foods such as meat, fish and eggs are excluded from the diet in the initial stages of pregnancy. This may further be compounded by the fact that many women requiring iron supplementation as we have seen fail to take it. In addition, lengthy Asian cooking processes can result in loss of vitamins and minerals, particularly vitamin C, which can inhibit iron absorption (Alvi et al., 2003).

After giving birth, women are often recommended by family members to have a diet high in

calories, protein and calcium in order to maintain energy levels throughout breastfeeding as well as to aid with recovery following labour (Ingram et al., 2003).

Panjiri, a Punjabi dish made from whole wheat flour fried in sugar and ghee, heavily laced with dried fruits and herbal gums, is often offered to nursing mothers as it is categorized as a hot food and is thought to promote the production of breast milk and restore the energy that the mother loses during labour (Laroia & Sharma, 2006). The seeds contained in this dish are a good source of protein and minerals, and so have many health benefits for the mother (Firdous & Bhopal, 1989; Laroia & Sharma, 2006). However, as the diet following a pregnancy can be high in sugar and fat, it is possible that many mothers will find returning to a healthy weight challenging.

It is also believed that the nature of cravings experienced during pregnancy can be an indication of the sex of the child: cravings for sweet foods indicate that the baby is female, whereas cravings for savoury foods indicate a male. However there is no scientific evidence to support this.

There is a lack of peer-reviewed evidence exploring many of the practices within the Pakistani community, many of which have evolved and have been unquestioningly practised over the centuries. However, it is clear that the appropriateness as well as the impact of food exclusions and dietary manipulations dictated by these practices may need to be further explored.

Vitamin D deficiency

It is thought that a significant number of the UK population have a low vitamin D status. This is particularly prevalent in the South Asian and East African Asian communities (Brooke et al., 2005). Although vitamin D deficiency in Asians originating from India, Pakistan and Bangladesh living in the UK was reported 30 years ago (Ford et al., 1972) and despite many successful campaigns to tackle this problem, there appears to be resurgence in vitamin D deficiency in this group over the last few years. Vitamin D deficiency has been implicated as a risk factor for diabetes, ischaemic heart disease and tuberculosis (Awumey et al., 1998; Shaw & Pal, 2002).

Most vitamin D comes from exposure to sunlight. Ethnic Pakistani women as well as those from other South Asian groups are at greater risk of vitamin D deficiency because many cover themselves for cultural and religious reasons (Alfaham *et al.*, 1995). They may also lack an adequate intake of dietary vitamin D and supplements are indicated (Shaw & Pal, 2002).

Newborn infants depend on foetal stores of vitamin D obtained from their mother (Clements & Fraser, 1988). Following delivery their vitamin D status is 60–70% of measured maternal vitamin D concentrations. Low maternal vitamin D may adversely affect the foetal brain. In addition to the known paediatric problems of infantile rickets, dental enamel hypoplasia, hypocalcaemic fits and congenital cataracts in early life, vitamin D deficiency has also been shown to affect postnatal head and linear growth (Brunvand *et al.*, 1996).

Reliance on vitamin D supplements for infants or the amounts in infant formula is inadequate to overcome the impact of maternal vitamin D deficiency (Shaw & Pal, 2002). Supplementing all Asian women at risk of vitamin D deficiency may be a simpler way to improve maternal vitamin D status. However, there may be issues with compliance, particularly if supplements are recommended to be taken daily. The latter was demonstrated by a health programme in Norway, where women of Pakistani origin failed to achieve reduced vitamin D deficiency despite provisions of free supplements and advice (Brunvand *et al.*, 1996). It is evident that there is a need for a renewed public health campaign to tackle this problem.

Low birth weight and childhood obesity

In the UK, low birth weight babies are particularly common in the South Asian populations, in particular in the Pakistani, Bangladeshi and Indian populations. Although generally babies born in the UK to mothers from South Asia have a birth weight greater than that of babies born in the South Asian subcontinent, it is still lower than that for the general UK population by about 300 g (Chetcuti *et al.*, 1985; Margetts *et al.*, 2002).

Low birth weight babies have an increased risk of developing type 2 diabetes, cardiovascular disease and obesity (Gillman *et al.*, 2003). The latter has been illustrated by the rise in overweight/obesity in children of Pakistani origin in the UK (Ridler *et al.*, 2009). It is thought that a small size

at birth can result in an acceleration of linear and adipose growth, a process described as catch-up growth (Tanner & Whitehouse, 1975). Studies also demonstrate that foetuses that experience intrauterine growth retardation tend to show higher levels of adiposity than their peers during mid-childhood (Rogers *et al.*, 2006).

Breastfeeding

Contrary to the custom of their native country, many mothers of Pakistani origin living in the UK adopt the habit of formula feeding instead of breastfeeding. Sarwar (2002) found that 73% of mothers in Pakistan breastfed their infants, whereas only 23% of mothers of Pakistani origin in the UK breastfed theirs. A study carried out in Cardiff observed that many women of Pakistani origin initiated and favoured breastfeeding, however more than half discontinued before the infant was three months old (Burton-Jeangros, 1995). This could be attributed to the fact that infant formula is readily available and accessible and support is available to individuals of even a low socioeconomic status in the UK.

Ingram *et al.* (2003) highlighted importantly that many South Asian women are very private and Muslim mothers in particular are required to be appropriately covered. Ingram *et al.* (2003) observed that while many South Asian women were exclusively breastfeeding at home, the majority use a dummy or bottles of water when outside. This may also be one of the reasons why many of the women in Hartley's audit (2003) discontinued breastfeeding while still in hospital, as even being behind a curtain may not provide the amount of privacy they require.

Mitra *et al.* (2004) illustrated that many Pakistani women are not fully aware of the benefits of breastfeeding.

There may be many plausible explanations for why women of Pakistani origin fail to initiate and continue with breastfeeding. Many live within a joint/extended family system, therefore pressures of housework and caring for other members of the family mean that breastfeeding may often be seen as a time-consuming chore. A survey by the Department of Health (1997) found that while 76% of Pakistani mothers in the UK initiated breastfeeding, only 36% continued and the most frequent reasons given for discontinuing were due to perceptions that the milk was insufficient or difficulties in latching on.

A recent study looking at the relationship between breastfeeding and maternal mental well-being in the Pakistani and Bangladeshi populations found that mothers that breastfed exclusively were able to enjoy everyday activities and had better sleep and mood patterns in comparison to mothers that were formula feeding (Sayeda & Rousham, 2008). However, it indicated that there is a lack of support for breastfeeding mothers from a Pakistani origin living in the UK (Sayeda & Rousham, 2008).

Many mothers may experience problems in obtaining advice from health professionals, due to inaccessibility of appropriate primary health care services, language or cultural difficulties (Scheppers et al., 2006). Often the dietary knowledge of health professionals is inadequate and conflicting and many may lack the knowledge of cultural practices within certain communities. If the mothers are not approached in a sensitive manner, many may feel patronized or inadequate; as a result they perceive health professionals as inapproachable (Garret et al., 1998).

Although there appears to be an increased awareness of the benefits of breastfeeding as well as support networks (i.e., breastfeeding counsellors within the community), it is clear that advice needs to be tailored to meet the needs of Pakistani mothers, thus encouraging and providing them with confidence and conveying the benefits of breastfeeding (Dyson et al., 2006; Meddings & Porter, 2007).

Weaning practices

Weaning practices depend principally on the knowledge, beliefs, attitudes and resources of the infant's parents. Although common to all groups, ethnic minority groups are likely to experience particular challenges (Williams et al., 1989).

The recommendations for weaning in Pakistan are the same as those advocated by the WHO and the UK Department of Health, namely exclusive breastfeeding or formula feeding until six months, with the introduction of solids not recommended before four months (Shamim, 2005). However, generally food is introduced by the age of four months, commencing usually with semi-solids and gradually progressing to solids at or after six months. Sarwar (2002) found that women living in Pakistan and mothers living in the UK of a Pakistani origin commenced weaning between three and four months. However some infants within these populations were not weaned until seven months or later as mothers perceive breast milk to be an adequate source of nutrition. Delayed weaning can lead to many feeding difficulties caused by the lack of opportunity to develop chewing skills, becoming accustomed to different tastes and textures and overall poor feeding skills (Northstone et al., 2001). In addition, delayed weaning may result in a delay in speech and language development (Hutchinson, 2001). Research by Shamim (2005) demonstrated that poor weaning practices are a public health issue in many parts of the country.

Common first weaning foods are baby rice, cereal, boiled mashed eggs, banana, rice and yoghurt as well as expensive cereals given in diluted form (e.g., Cerelac). Cerelac is commonly used as a weaning food in the UK South Asian population and is particularly favoured within the Pakistani community. Following on, infants living in Pakistan are likely to progress to fruits and vegetables and eventually family foods. In contrast, in the UK, in addition to fruit and vegetables infants are likely to progress to meat and convenience foods, particularly the sweeter varieties (Sarwar, 2002). Many have observed that it is difficult to progress to family foods as a result of late introduction, a pattern observed with older children as well. In the latter case where family foods are refused or where infants are more difficult to feed, parents may offer sweet foods, which infants usually have a natural preference for (Godson & Williams, 1996).

Although many mothers commence weaning between the ages of three and four months, milk often remains the principal source of nutrition in the infant's diet and can be so until the age of two years. As a result many children are at risk of iron deficiency anaemia (Harbottle & Duggan, 1992). In addition, many mothers may give their children traditional tea made with water and milk, where tannins contained in the tea can inhibit iron absorption (Lilly, 1995).

Many infants of Pakistani origin in the UK and particularly in the Muslim community (Bedi, 1989) are offered and weaned on a diet of convenience foods and drinks high in sugar. This has been shown to have potential adverse effects on dental health (Shahid *et al.*, 2009). Sarwar (2002) found that some mothers in Pakistan gave their children chapatti and rusks in a bottle as many found that offering solids in this manner was easily accepted by the child. However, the latter is discouraged and it is recommended that non-milk drinks should be given from a cup or a feeder to avoid the risk of dental decay (Watt, 2000).

Suggestions for the way forward

Following appropriate weaning guidelines and practices is imperative. There is a clear need to provide better and more accessible information for mothers which is sensitive to their culture, beliefs, attitudes, knowledge and expectations as well as their economic status. Many mothers newly arrived in the UK may find it difficult to obtain foods they are familiar with and be influenced by mass advertising for baby foods and infant formulas. In addition, they may experience difficulty in learning new ways of preparing the foods they are encountering for the first time. Language can also be a barrier in effectively conveying appropriate advice (Horsfall *et al.*, 2003).

Hence it is important to ensure health professionals are aware of family dynamics and have detailed knowledge of the background and culture of ethnic minority groups. It is also essential that all health professionals involved in providing advice on nutrition are consistent and in line with national/international recommendations. Health professionals that do not have a nutrition background (community nursery nurses, health visitors, etc.) involved in providing dietary advice need to ensure adequate training is accessed and received from appropriate professionals (i.e., registered dietitians).

Vitamin D deficiency in the Pakistani population was highlighted earlier and it is clear that measures need to be taken to increase awareness of this within this population. This can be achieved by ensuring women at risk are identified and supplemented appropriately. Local policies may need to be implemented on maternity units to ensure women at risk of vitamin D deficiency are receiving and taking supplements (Sharma *et al.*, 2009).

There are many opportunities for women to access support groups and receive advice in the community. Many of these are channelled through the National Children Centre programme, which is in place as part of the Every Child Matters Initiative (Department for Education and Skills, 2002). However, specific to the Pakistani community, efforts need to be made to identify issues within this population and strong links need to be built with the community to ensure better health outcomes.

More research needs to be conducted into the feeding practices, attitudes, family dynamics and beliefs within this community to enable health professionals to understand better what motivates many of their practices. It is also important to note that there are few studies looking at the differences in attitudes, beliefs and practices with regard to maternal and infant nutrition between the first- and second-generation Pakistanis. Many studies conducted on the latter where undertaken in the 1990s. Research on present trends would give us a better insight into the current degree of acculturation and dietary transition.

1.4 Bangladeshi Diet

Kalpana Hussain, Thomina Mirza

1.4.1 Introduction

The South Asian subcontinent comprises India, Pakistan, Bangladesh and Sri Lanka. Four per cent of the total UK population are classified as 'Asian' or 'Asian British' and this group makes up 50.2% of the minority ethnic group population in the UK (UK Census, 2001).

'South Asians' is 'a term which defines many ethnic groups with distinctive regions of origin, languages, religions and customs, and include people born in India, Bangladesh, Pakistan or Sri Lanka' (Fox, 2004).

Bangladesh is located on the northern coast of the Bay of Bengal, bordering India. It also shares a border with Myanmar in the south-east. The country is low-lying riverine land criss-crossed by the many branches and tributaries of the Ganges and Brahmaputra rivers. Tropical monsoons and frequent floods and cyclones inflict heavy damage in the delta region (see Figure 1.4.1).

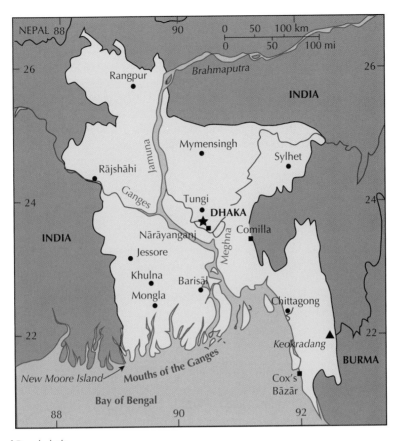

Figure 1.4.1   Map of Bangladesh

What is now called Bangladesh is part of the historic region of Bengal, the north-east area of the Indian subcontinent. Bangladesh consists primarily of East Bengal (West Bengal is part of India and its people are primarily Hindu) plus the Sylhet district of the Indian state of Assam.

The Bengali people are the ethnic community of Bengal (now divided between Bangladesh and India) in South Asia with a history dating back four millennia. They are an eastern Indo-Aryan people, who are also descended from Austro-Asiatic and Dravidian peoples, and closely related to the Oriya, Assamese, Biharis and other East Indians, as well as to Munda and Tibeto-Burman peoples. As such, Bengalis are a homogeneous but considerably diverse ethnic group with heterogeneous origins.

Bangladesh has a population of about 127 million; 124 million of these are Bengalis and almost 1 million are tribal or indigenous people. Of the Bengalis, 88.3% are Muslim, 10.5% Hindus and 1.2% Buddhist, Christian or animist (www.idex.org, 2002).

History

Bangladesh came into existence in 1971 after the Indo-Pakistan war and is now one of the poorest nations in the world. Before its existence, Bangladesh used to be part of India which was a colony of the British Empire. Present-day Bangladesh had a turbulent colonial history, which affected many features of the country, among them the culture, economy and a large population. There is little modernization of towns and villages and as a result it has a predominantly rural environment (Hillier & Rahman, 1996). The delta consists of many small rivers, creeks and streams, thus making fishing a popular livelihood and fish an important part of the diet. Agriculture is another principal means of living and hence many Bangladeshi migrants have an agricultural background.

Language

The official language is Bengali, however many dialects are spoken. These vary from region to region and depend on geographical location. The three most commonly spoken languages are Bengali, Sylheti and English. Some people speak Urdu. Sylheti is a dialect of Bengali and is not written. Those who have access to education in Bangladesh can read and write standard Bengali (Hamid & Sarwar, 2004).

Migration to the United Kingdom

Adams (1994) notes that many Bangladeshis opted to migrate to the UK in search of work because Bangladesh used to be a part of the British Empire. Initial migration was during between the 1940s and 1960s, when mostly single men from small landowning families sought employment in the UK as workers in factories or the clothing trade. Almost 95% of the Bangladeshi migrants in the UK came from the Sylhet region and so speak the Sylheti dialect. During these years they maintained close ties with their country of origin by making frequent trips to Bangladesh throughout the year. The introduction of strict immigration legislation in the 1970s meant that the men had to choose to bring their wives and children into the UK or risk permanent separation; therefore during the 1970s–1980s immigration peaked as wives joined their husbands in the UK with their children. During this period, migrants from other countries also entered the UK. As a consequence 5.5% of the UK population are now composed of ethnic minority groups. The population of South Asian ethnic minorities in the UK tends to be younger than the general population, with the number of 65 year olds among migrants being the lowest for those of Pakistani and Bangladeshi origin (Landman & Cruickshank, 2001).

The UK has a particularly strong tradition of what the general population call Indian cuisine which is in fact a misnomer as the restaurants in question are mainly run by people of Bangladeshi origin. In the second half of the 20th century there

was a burgeoning in the development of so-called Anglo-Indian cuisine, as families from countries such as Bangladesh (particularly from the Sylhet region) migrated to London to look for work. Some of the earliest restaurants were opened in Brick Lane in the East End of London, a place still famous for this type of cuisine and is now popularly known as 'Bangla Town', with even the street signs bilingual (wikipedia.org/wiki/East_End_of_London).

In the 1960s, a number of inauthentic 'Indian' foods were developed by British Bangladeshi chefs, including the widely popular chicken tikka masala. This tendency has now been reversed, with subcontinental restaurants being more willing to serve authentic Indian, Bangladeshi and Pakistani food, and to offer their regional variations.

Bangladeshi food has become a staple of the British national cuisine. Until the early 1970s more than three-quarters of Indian restaurants in Britain were identified as being owned and run by people of Bengali origin. Most were run by migrants from East Pakistan, which became Bangladesh in 1971. Bangladeshi restaurateurs overwhelmingly come from the northern district of Sylhet. Until 1998, as many as 85% of Tandoori restaurants in the UK were Bangladeshi but by 2003 this figure declined to just over 65%. Currently the dominance of Bangladeshi restaurants is generally declining in some parts of London and the further north one travels. (en.wikipedia.org/wiki/Sylhet).

The cuisine of Bangladesh is popular, as Bangladeshi restaurateurs have established themselves by creating new businesses throughout Britain. The number of Bangladeshi-owned restaurants has increased rapidly over the years. In 1946 there were 20 restaurants, today there are 7,200 owned by Bangladeshis out of a total of 8,500 Indian restaurants in the UK. Surveys show that Bangladeshi curries are among the most popular of dishes.

Current UK population

A high proportion of Bangladeshi migrants settled in Tower Hamlets, an inner city borough of London, one of the most deprived areas in the UK. Here the largest Bangladeshi community lives, with 33% of the population being of Bangladeshi origin and 42% White British (UK Census, 2001). Deprivation adversely affects standards of living – a significant proportion of council housing in Tower Hamlets does not meet government standards. Poor housing, which is also usually associated with overcrowding, can lead to poor health (The Tower Hamlets Partnership, 2006). The rest of the UK Bangladeshi community is largely settled in the London borough of Camden, and in the North.

1.4.2   Religion

The majority of Bangladeshis are Sunni Muslims and follow the dietary laws stipulated in the Qu'ran (the holy book of Islam) and the Hadith, a collection of the sayings and actions of the prophet Muhammad (Kassam-Khamis *et al.*, 1999).

Islam

Religious dietary restrictions
Muslims are required to eat only permitted (*halal*) food that has been earned lawfully and are expected to avoid eating any prohibited (*haram*) foods and drinks. In order for any meat to be *halal*, it must be prepared according to the Islamic laws of slaughter (Khan, 1982). Lawful foods include the flesh of any animals that are cloven hoofed and those that chew the cud. Fruits, vegetables, rice, wheat, cereals, pulses, milk, milk products and eggs are also permitted and do not require any special preparation other than ensuring that they are clean and safe to consume. All fish with fins and scales are also lawful. The flesh of pigs, blood, carrion and foods offered to idols or deities except God (Allah) are forbidden. All carnivorous animals and birds of prey are prohibited, as well as land animals without ears such as frogs (Fieldhouse, 1995).

Consumption of alcohol is prohibited. In a survey looking at the health of South Asians, Nazroo (1997) found low consumption of alcohol among Bangladeshi men – only 3% drank alcohol – and virtually no consumption of alcohol among Bangladeshi women – less than 1% – compared to 56% of White men drinking alcohol once a week or more in the UK. As alcohol consumption is related to cultural and religious practice, Aspinall and Jacobson (2004) point out that Muslims who do drink alcohol are unlikely to admit it, thus highlighting that a level of under-reporting may exist.

Fasting
All Muslims are expected to fast during Ramadan, the ninth month of the Islamic calendar. Ramadan usually lasts for 29 or 30 days and the fast involves abstinence from food and water between sunrise and sunset. Eating and drinking are permitted during the night and a pre-dawn meal is eaten before the daytime fast begins. The fast is broken at sunset with a meal called *iftar*.

Although one of the aspects of Ramadan is moderation of food and drink, due to the number of social engagements with family and friends during this month, there is usually an abundance of foods prepared, especially fried snacks such as samosa and *pakora* and Indian sweets. Indian sweets are prepared using a combination of sugar, ghee, fullcream milk powder, nuts, chickpea flour and sweetened condensed milk, and thus are very energy dense and high in fat and sugar. These foods are also eaten on other special occasions and festivities such as weddings and *Eid* (Kassam-Khamis *et al.*, 1999).

Religious festivals and holidays

Eid ul Fitr: The end of Ramadan is signalled by the sighting of the new moon and is celebrated with a festival called *Eid ul Fitr*, which is associated with the serving of sweet foods and engaging in many social events with family and friends (Fieldhouse, 1995).

Eid-ul-Adha: A celebration marking the pilgrimage (*hajj*) to Mecca. Sheep or goats are sacrificed in remembrance of Prophet Abraham's willingness to sacrifice his son to Allah.

Hinduism

Hinduism is the second largest religion in Bangladesh, and is followed by a little over 9% of the population. Hindus believe in the principle of *ahimsa* (avoidance of violence) and this is universally observed. Therefore some Bangladeshi Hindus are vegetarians, but abstinence from all kinds of meat is regarded as a higher virtue so high-caste Bangladeshi Hindus, unlike their counterparts elsewhere in South Asia, ordinarily eat fish and chicken. The same is found in the Indian state of West Bengal, which being climatologically similar to Bangladesh, has led Hindus (regardless of caste) to consume fish as it is the only major source of protein.

Durga Puja

A giant named Durg had acquired such terrifying psychic powers that he threatened to turn the whole of creation upside down. The Gods then appealed to the Goddess Parvati, and each of them donated a special divine power to her. Armed with these powers, depicted as a number of hands, the Great Mother mounted her 'vehicle', the lion, and attacked the monster. As the demon's name was Durg, the triumphant Mother Goddess took the feminine form of the name, Durga. Nine of her ten arms hold various weapons. Images of her four children – the warrior-God, Kartik, the benign, elephant-headed Ganesh. the Goddess of wealth, Lakshmi, and the Goddess Saraswati – are also featured. The biggest festival of the Hindu community continues for nine days, the last three days being the culmination with the idol of the Goddess Durga immersed in rivers. The festival occurs in September/October (www.indiantravelportal.com).

National holidays

Pahela Baishakh: The advent of the Bengali New Year is joyously observed throughout the country. The day (in mid-April) is a public holiday.

Bhasha Andolon Dibosh: Language Movement Day or Language Revolution Day is a national day to commemorate protests and sacrifices to protect Bengali as a national language during the Pakistani regime in 1952.

Independence Day: Independence is celebrated on 26 March.

1.4.3 Traditional diet and eating pattern

The traditional Bengali cuisine consists of vast range of rice dishes with various preparations of freshwater fish and or vegetables cooked in a spicy sauce. Green leafy vegetables are seasonal and locally grown and they form part of the daily diet. Fruit is only eaten when it is in season (and never in large quantities). Imported fruits such as apples and grapes are expensive. Fruits such as strawberries are now grown in Bangladesh, though peaches, plums, kiwis and cherries are not usually found. Pulses such as split yellow lentils dal and plain rice (*bhat*) are popular Kwan, 2005. Meat, eggs and milk are expensive and their consumption depends on their affordability. Unlike some Asian cultures, milk and dairy products are not part of the traditional diet. Milk is expensive in Bangladesh and it is mainly only affluent farming households that have access to it. Fresh cow's milk is always boiled before consumption. Due to the limited supply of milk most families use imported powdered milk. Adults tend to have milk in tea (*chai*) only (Kwan, 2005); otherwise it tends to be seen as suitable for babies or very young children. Milk is also viewed as a high-energy food leading to weight gain. Yoghurt is not regularly eaten, although it is occasionally used in cooking dishes such as korma on special occasions (Zannath & Edholm, 2004). Oil is used very sparingly and processed foods such as cakes, biscuits, crisps and chocolates are not part of the traditional diet.

Bangladeshi puddings and desserts are creamy, sweetened with sugar and flavoured with nuts, saffron or cinnamon. One of the most popular is a sweet rice pudding called *kheer* (Kwan, 2005). As alcohol is prohibited, cold drinks include fresh lime sodas and tender coconut water *dub*; (Kwan, 2005). Almost all food is prepared and cooked at home and is often eaten with the fingers. Village people tend to eat that way. Middle-class urban people may or may not use cutlery. It is considered polite and a mark of respect to use the right hand when giving or receiving anything, particularly food. You might hold a glass of water with your left hand, or use both hands to break bread, but food goes into your mouth from your right hand only (Kwan, 2005) (see Tables 1.4.1 and 1.4.2).

Herbs and spices

A wide variety of herbs and spices are now available in the UK and there has been an increase in the use of ginger, garlic and chillies. These fresh herbs are ground together into green masala and added to dishes in addition to ground coriander, ground cumin and turmeric power. Other spices used are cardamom, cinnamon, bay leaves, fenugreek seeds, black onion seeds, cloves and fennel seeds. Ready-made pastes are also used to marinade meat and fish at home, but different colourings are mainly used in the restaurants.

Paan

Chewing *paan* is a very common habit in Bengali society, practised by both men and women, and is easily available in Britain. The heart-shaped betel leaf, or piper betel, is preferably picked when it is still young and tender and its taste is at its best. Betel is slightly sour but is a popular mouth freshener. It is often used as an aromatic stimulant and anti-flatulent. One of the most important ingredients of a betel preparation is the areca nut (a seed),

Table 1.4.1 Traditional meal pattern and dietary changes in Bangladeshi diet on migration to the UK

Meal	Traditional meal	Dietary changes on migration to the UK	Healthier alternatives
Breakfast	Tea with sweet biscuits and/or sweet bread Sometime rusks are eaten or leftover curry or with rice. On special occasions *shemai, shuji* with *paratha* or *muri* with tea	Cereal with milk (e.g., Rice Krispies or a sugar-coated variety). Chocolate-coated breakfast cereals are popular with children. Fried bread or crumpets with fried eggs Tea with rusks or *muri*	High-fibre cereal with low-fat milk Whole meal bread/toast with poached/boiled egg. Tea
Lunch	Boiled rice (no ghee) with dal, fish/meat/chicken curry (seasonal)	As traditional meal Fish and chips, potato fritters Kebabs in naan bread Burgers, sandwiches, pizzas	Boiled rice with curry (made with minimal oil) Curries to include vegetables. One curry per meal. Salad to accompany the meal Grilled kebab with naan bread and salad Baked potato and salad
Evening meal	Rice (boiled, biryani, kedgeree), dal, vegetables, fish and meat/chicken curry, pickle, salad, naan bread	As traditional meal, Fish and chips Potato fritters Kebabs in naan bread Burgers, sandwiches, pizzas	Boiled rice with curry (made with minimal oil) Curries to include vegetables. One curry per meal. Salad to accompany the meals Grilled kebab with Naan bread and salad Baked potato and salad
Puddings/Desserts	Asian sweets (*burfi, gulab jaman shandesh, ras malai,ras gulla, cham cham, raskadam, sevian* (milk pudding) orange-flavoured sweet rice (*zarda*), fruit	Traditional sweets Ice cream Cakes	Fresh fruit/fruit salad
Snacks	*Nimki, shingara* (samosas)	As traditional snacks Chocolates biscuits, cakes	Oven-baked samosas, nuts, fruit Asian sweets eaten only on special occasions
Drinks	Water, tea, *lassi*, soft drinks, milk	Water, tea, soft drinks, fruit drinks, fruit juice, squash	Water, tea Unsweetened fruit juice, diet soft drinks, *lassi* made with low-fat milk and yoghurt and sweetener

the fruit of the areca palm, areca catechu (*katha*). The orange-coloured conical fruit is enjoyed both as a raw and a soft fruit. Seed (locally known as *supari*) is the most popular ingredient in a *paan*. Its narcotic value is appreciated by all who chew *paan* and is produced when lime is added. Its stimulating effect increases the more it is chewed (www.indiaprofile.com). The ingredients of *paan* vary according to individual preference and may contain other seeds, nuts and herbs. The leaves can be plain or sugar-coated. It is usually eaten after meals. Adults often add tobacco to the mixture. The ingredients are often grown at home, so *paan* is easily available and cheap. When chewed, the mixture turns a brilliant red colour, staining the teeth. The colour is considered attractive on the lips of young women. Betel nut is addictive and can cause dizziness and perspiration; it may also be linked to diabetes. Chewing tobacco has the added risk of causing cancer of the mouth, throat and stomach.

Smoking

Cigarette smoking is common among men, both older and younger generations. The Bangladeshi ethnic group has the second highest rate of smoking, with over 50% of Bangladeshi men reporting to smoke. Smoking among Bangladeshi women, however, is low, with fewer than 1% reporting it (Nazroo, 1997). The Health Survey for England (1999) reported similar findings, with 44% of Bangladeshi men smoking compared to 27% of men in the general population (Erens *et al.*, 2001). In a survey researching health in ethnic minorities in Britain, 17% of Bangladeshis described their health as poor – the highest figure to be reported in comparison to other ethnic groups (Nazroo, 1997). Smoking through water pipes (*shisha*) has become popular among the Bengali community, especially since the increase in the number of *shisha* cafés and bars.

Table 1.4.2   Glossary of Bangladeshis foods

Bengali name	English name	Bengali name	English name
Aam	Mango	Chuun	Lime added to the *paan* leaf
Adda	Ginger	dal	Red spilt peas
Amloki	Indian gooseberry	dal Chana	Pulses
Amra	Hog plum	Dhalim	Pomegranate
Anaras	Pineapple	Derish/Bindi	Okra (ladies' fingers)
Ata Fol	Custard apple	Doi	Sweetened homemade creamy yoghurt, mainly shop-bought in the UK
Bandhakopi/ Kopi	Cabbage		
Bangon	Aubergine		
Bel	Indian apple	Doniya	Coriander
Bhaat	Plain white/brown boiled rice	Dood	Milk
		Gajor	Carrots
Borfi	Indian dry sweets	Guyr Mangsho	Beef
Boroi	Indian jujube	Hilsa	Herring
Cha	Tea	Jambura	Grapefruit
Chalta	Elephant apple	Jamrul	Star apple
Chana	Chickpeas	Jorda	Sweetener used in *paan* making
Cheeni	Sugar		
Chitol	A large fish with a very soft oily stomach or frontal portion	Kalajam	Blackberry
		Kamla	Orange
		Kamranga	Carambola

Table 1.4.2 (cont'd)

Bengali name	English name	Bengali name	English name
Kathal	Jackfruit	Paani/ Jol	Water
Kathbel	Wood apple	Papaya	Papaya
Kechuri	Soft, watery rice pudding, cooked with fried onions, ghee or butter. Given to help with ill health. Also eaten during iftaar	Paratha	Sweet or savoury chapatti cooked in oil
		Payara/Shofri	Guava
		Peetha	Steamed rice cakes, often deep-fried with onions or wheat flour
Kerela	Kerala		
Kheer/Finni	Sweet rice pudding	Peyaz	Onions
Kodu	Marrow	Phol Peyaz	Spring onions
Kola	Banana	Phulkopi	Cauliflower
Lebu	Lemon	Roshun	Garlic
Lichu	Lychee	Shada	Tobacco used in paan making
Maas	Fish		
Mamlet	Omelette	Shak Shobzi	Vegetables
Mangsho	Lamb	Shalgom	Turnip
Masala	The mixture in curry made with oil, onions, salt and spices	Shemai	Sweet vermicelli milky pudding. Ghee and milk can be added
Meeta Kudo	Sweet potatoes	Shingara	Samosas. .
Mola	Mooli	Shuji	Semolina pudding made with ghee and sugar. Sometimes with milk. Can be eaten with parathas
Morich	Chillies		
Motorshuti	Peas		
Muki	Eddos	Shupari	Betel nut
Murgi/Moorug	Chicken	Sofeda	Sapodilla
Muri	Puffed rice	Tarcarry	Curry
Naga	Chilli peppers	Tarmuj	Watermelon
Narikel	Coconut	Tomato	Tomatoes
Nimki	Flour crackers	Urie	Snow beans

1.4.4 Healthy eating

Key points
- Migration to the UK has resulted in an increase in oil and meat consumption, and a reduction in fruit and vegetable intake.
- Fruit in season is often eaten fresh and as a snack.
- Fruits are also preserved using spices and molasses, but not consumed commonly in this form.
- Processed foods are very popular among the young population.
- Salt is added to all foods.

Introduction

The traditional in Bangladesh is generally quite healthy as it is rich in complex carbohydrate (brown rice), fish, pulses and vegetables (added to curries)(see Table 1.4.3).

Table 1.4.3   Traditional Bangladeshi diet and healthier alternatives

	Traditional diet	Diet in the UK	Healthier alternatives
Bread, rice, potatoes and other starchy foods	Boiled brown and/or white rice, with no fat Chapattis *roti* on occasions	Boiled white rice, with no fat Basmati rice on special occasions (often in the form of *akhne* or *pulau*, oil or ghee is added)	Basmati rice is a healthier alternative and is low GI. However basmati rice is expensive even when bought in bulk. Also there is a difference in taste. Some people associate basmati rice with meat rather than fish
	Potatoes – added to curries as a vegetable, eaten as chips Sweet bread and sweet rusk, often taken with tea as breakfast Puffed rice (*muri*) – dried grains of uncooked rice, which is deep fried, the rice puffs into a white fluffy shape. Salt is added for flavour. Often eaten with tea at breakfast or as a snack with tea and biscuits. *Muri* can also be eaten on its own as a snack	Potatoes – added to curries as a vegetable, eaten as chips, Potatoes are also bought in bulk therefore they are often the King Edward type. Potatoes are not baked or boiled before adding to the curries. Chips are often either bought ready cooked from a take–away, or bought frozen and fried at home Potatoes are very rarely baked Bread – white is preferred toasted with butter or jam *Roti* – fried with butter served with fried egg Crumpets – fried with butter and served with fried egg Croissants – toasted, served with butter. Some add processed cheese Sugar-coated breakfast cereals or refined rice-based cereals are preferred. The older generation do not like breakfast cereals, especially the wholegrain varieties. Those who have been raised in the UK are accustomed to cereals. Rusk and sweet bread are imported and sold in Bangladeshi grocery shops. *Muri* is imported or prepared at home. Some people have *muri* for breakfast while others have it as a snack.	If potatoes are added to curries, then there needs to be a reduction in the amount of rice eaten. Chips to be kept to a minimum. Try thicker cuts of chips or potato wedges Baking the chips and potato products should be encouraged rather than frying Toast – whole meal bread. Avoid frying bread and egg Scrambled/poached egg Avoid using processed cheese Encourage breakfast cereals with a reduced amount of added sugar. Children should be encouraged to try healthier alternatives rather than sugar-coated cereals. Avoid rusk and sweet breads as they are high in saturated fats (made with ghee) and contain a lot of sugar. Alternatives include rich tea, digestives, low-fat /low-sugar crackers. Try wholegrain cereals as an alternative
Meat, fish and beans	Fish – mainly freshwater. Fish is never frozen, but bought fresh and cooked and eaten on the same day. Oily fish – *koi, chitol, ayre, rohi, pangash, elisha, mirka.* Non-oily fish – *katla, bual.*	The fish in the UK is imported and therefore not fresh. Fish is expensive. Fish is fried and added to curries. Traditional Bengali vegetables are commonly cooked with fish curries. Fish is also soaked in brine to increase its freshness.	Avoid soaking fish in brine Avoid frying the fish before adding the fish to curries and also use less oil in the curries Try to include oily fish in the diet as a good source of calcium and omega 3 Reduce the amount of spices and chilli especially if suffering from peptic ulcers

Table 1.4.3 (*cont'd*)

Traditional diet	Diet in the UK	Healthier alternatives
Can be fried before adding to a curry masala. Frying is not essential. After the fish is prepared, it may be left in brine for a few minutes. Small fish, e.g., *rani, keski*, similar to sardines in size. Cooked whole, with minimal oil and vegetables. Cheaper than bigger fish Dried fish (*shutki*) are sun-dried or oven-dried. The dried fish is boiled and the broth is added to boiling vegetables. No oil is added to this curry. Dried fish is very popular among the rural populations and especially women. It is customary to have the curry very hot and spicy	Small fish are also imported from Bangladesh and bought frozen. The method of cooking is no different Dried fish is also imported from Bangladesh and the cooking method is the same. Children born in the UK often do not like this curry European fish (tuna, mackerel, salmon, sardines, cod) are not found in Bangladesh. They can be cooked in curry or as dry curry. Fish are often fried first Fish fingers are very common among the younger population and are often fried	The quality and source of the dried fish is questionable, therefore there has been a reduction in supply from Bangladesh. Due to the fall in supply the price has increased. Try to avoid frying the fish, if frying to prepare the dry curry then shallow fry with minimal oil. Grill or bake fish fingers
Prawns are a delicacy and are popular. Prawns can be fried or added to other fish curries	There is a higher consumption of prawns in the UK especially due to its popularity in restaurants. The cooking method is the same.	Avoid frying the prawns and use less oil in the curries
Lamb/goat/beef are eaten, mainly on special occasions	Lamb is more commonly eaten and often bought in bulk. Lamb is mainly cooked in a curry. Grilled lamb chops and kebabs are often shop-bought. Lamb mince (*keema*) is used for samosas and meat balls. Beef and goat are eaten less. Beef burgers are available frozen and at fast food out lets. Beef/lamb burgers are often fried at home.	Reduce consumption of red meat. Trim off all fat and reduce oil when cooking curries. Try to use other vegetables as an alternative to potatoes. Grill meats and kebabs. Use chicken mince instead of lamb mince. Grill burgers rather than frying.
Chicken is more commonly consumed	Chicken is commonly eaten. Chicken in curries and fried chicken with chips from fast food retailers. Chicken nuggets, and other products are very popular snacks. Chicken frankfurters are also popular with young children.	Try to limit fried chicken snacks. Try grilling meat. Use less oil in curries. Avoid fried chicken products.
Eggs are often fried or boiled and then added to curry. Eggs are cheap but are ranked with meat. Hen's eggs and fish (seafood) never eaten together. Roe is expensive and a delicacy. Often eaten in a curry	Eggs are commonly eaten more frequently for breakfast and used in curries. The attitude towards roe is the same.	Limit consumption of fried eggs.

(Continued)

Table 1.4.3 (cont'd)

	Traditional diet	Diet in the UK	Healthier alternatives
	Yellow split peas (*dal*), *mossor dal, chana dal* and *chana* (chickpeas) are common pulses. Cooked as curries, eaten with rice as part of the main meal or as a snack	The same pulses are cooked in the UK, but the frequency has reduced. Chickpeas are now mainly eaten during Ramadan as part of the fast-breaking meal (*iftaar*) Baked beans are also popular, can be fried but often reheated in the microwave	Increase intake of pulses, but reduce oil when cooking.
Fats and oils	Vegetable oil and ghee	Vegetable, corn and sunflower oil are sold in barrels and cheaply available in the UK Butter and margarines are popular to cook with, especially with bread and used as spreads Ghee is used to cook *pilau* or *akhne*. Not used in everyday cooking	Olive oil is not commonly used in large quantities and is not very palatable in curries due to its after-taste when heated. Using less oil is the main message Use low-fat spreads and avoid ghee. Margarines can be used as an alternative
Fruits	Mango, papaya, guava, pineapple, jackfruit, banana, pomegranate, lychee, grapefruit, melon, hog plum, coconut, star fruit, Indian apple, custard apple, wood apple, sapodilla, elephant apple, carambola, Indian gooseberry, tangerines, oranges, grapes. Fruits are eaten after meals	Almost all of the fruits from Bangladesh and other Asian countries can be found in the UK. Due to their seasonal element, European fruits such as apple, pears strawberries and different varieties of banana; grapes are also eaten, along with exotic fruits like kiwi. Fruit is often sliced and one fruit is shared rather than eaten whole. Fruits are sprinkled with salt. The consumptionof fruit is reduced in the UK	Try to increase the intake of fruit
	Chutneys are made with sour fruit (unripe mango, grapefruit, oranges). They are mixed with garlic, fresh coriander and salt and eaten as a snack	Making chutneys is still common among some families	Reduce salt (and chilli if suffering from peptic ulcers)
Vegetables	Kerela, okra, onions, tomatoes, carrots, cabbage, spring onions, mooli, eddos, peas, snow beans, marrow, sweet potatoes, garlic, ginger, coriander, chillies, peppers, aubergine, cucumber and cauliflower	Most of the vegetables are available fresh in the UK and are relatively cheap. European vegetables such as sweet corn, lettuce, cress, squash, capsicum, broccoli are also used in cooking or in salads. Most people prefer to cook the Bengali vegetables with fish and use the European vegetables with meat dishes. Potatoes are thought to be a vegetable and therefore is the most common vegetable eaten	Try to avoid frying vegetables. Include a variety of vegetables in all curries Try to experiment with vegetables
	Chutneys are made with raw vegetables like tomatoes. Salt and coriander is added to sautéed onions. This chutney would be eaten with rice	Chutneys are not commonly made in the UK	
	Vegetable curry (*bhaji*) often eaten	Vegetable curries are often an accompaniment with other dishes	Try to steam vegetables and not overcook them, before adding them to the masala Use less oil in the curries

Table 1.4.3 (cont'd)

	Traditional diet	Diet in the UK	Healthier alternatives
Milk and dairy foods	Dried whole milk powder Sweet yoghurt – often shop bought Fresh milk	Fresh whole cow's milk is cheap and readily available Cow's milk is boiled and the skin removed before adding to tea Whole cow's milk is also given to children to drink and taken with breakfast cereals Adults do not commonly drink milk Children are often partial to the portion-sized yoghurts. The elder generation prefer natural yoghurt. Yoghurts are eaten on special occasions (weddings and parties) Cream, yoghurt and fresh whole milk are popular with a fruit and sweet rice dish, especially during Ramadan and during the summer months. Some people like to use whole milk powder in tea and desserts	Try semi-skimmed milk. Avoid boiling, there is no need to reheat pasteurized milk. Children to try low-sugar/ low-fat yoghurts
Alcohol	Muslims in Bangladesh do not drink, some Hindu and other faiths may do. Alcohol is not widely available in Muslim areas	Those who have migrated or were raised in the UK may drink alcohol but will not always admit to it. Alcohol tends to be beer rather than wine, as it is more common for boys to drink than girls. Some girls also drink alcohol	Drink within the legal limits

1.4.5   Obesity

The mean body mass index of Bangladeshi men ($24.7\,\text{kg}/\text{m}^2$) is lower than that in the general population ($27.1\,\text{kg}/\text{m}^2$). Bangladeshi men are almost five times less likely to be obese than men in the general population. However, Bangladeshi men and women are more likely to have bigger waist circumference than the general population (Health Survey for England, 2004).

Bangladeshi men and women are less likely to participate in sports and exercise and less likely to meet the physical activity recommendations of at least 30 minutes of moderate or vigorous exercise on at least five days a week than the general population (37% of men, 25% of women). Bangladeshi men were, on average, shorter than men in the general population. Women in minority ethnic groups were on average shorter than women in the general population.

Other indicators of poor health include obesity and low physical activity levels. Studies examining the body composition in South Asian ethnic groups have found that South Asians have a tendency for central fat deposition. Research has identified that central fat deposition is associated with insulin resistance and a greater risk of developing coronary heart disease (Knight et al., 1992; Bush et al., 1995). Other studies have found that South Asian women tend to have a higher BMI than their European counterparts and a high waist circumference and a high waist/hip ratio (WHR), with higher measures among the longer resident South Asians (McKeigue et al., 1991; Bose, 1995). According to Bose (1992), a high WHR is correlated with impaired glucose tolerance, raised insulin levels, hypertension and high triglyceride levels and is associated with central obesity.

Exercise and physical activity levels appear to be very low in the Bangladeshi ethnic group, which is a cause for concern as it is another predisposing factor to poor health. The Health Survey for England (1999) found that both Bangladeshi men and women did not meet the recommended guidelines for participation in physical activity and that the Bangladeshi ethnic group had the lowest figures for physical activity levels and exercise patterns of all ethnic groups (Erens *et al.*, 2001). Rudat (1994) reported similar findings in the Health and Lifestyle survey, which found that only 45% of Bangladeshi men and 29% of Bangladeshi women participated in health-promoting activities. Studies have reported that the low levels of physical activity and regular exercise may pose a greater risk of developing obesity, cardiovascular diseases and other circulatory diseases (Rudat, 1994; Acheson, 1998).

1.4.6 Diabetes

Diabetes mellitus is a cause of both morbidity and mortality and a risk factor for a number of other diseases such as cardiovascular disease, renal failure, neuropathy and retinopathy. Numerous studies have ascertained that the prevalence of diagnosed type 2 diabetes among South Asians is reported to be over four times greater than among the White population (McKeigue *et al.*, 1989). Mather *et al.* (1995) found that South Asians with diabetes attending the same clinic as Europeans had poorer glycaemic control, increased retinopathy and a higher prevalence of microalbuminuria. According to Raleigh (1997), mortality directly associated with diabetes among South Asian migrants is 3.5 times greater than that in the general population. Among the South Asian ethnic groups, Bangladeshis are reported to have the highest rates of diabetes and poor prognoses (Cappuccio *et al.*, 1997; Nazroo, 1997). Aspinall and Jacobson (2004) showed that the age at presentation of type 2 diabetes is much earlier in South Asians than the general population, thus placing them at greater risk of developing complications.

Bangladeshi migrants also have a much higher premature mortality due to diabetes than those originating from India and Pakistan (Balarajan & Raleigh, 1995). Within a generation of migration to Britain, research has shown that diabetes had become widespread among Bangladeshis living in East London. The Health Survey for England (2004) reported diabetes among Bangladeshi men was almost four times as prevalent as men in the general population. Among women, diabetes was at least three times as likely in Bangladeshis com-

pared with women in the general population. The ratio of type 2 diabetes among Bangladeshi men and women was higher than the general population. High levels of impaired glucose tolerance and high levels of insulin resistance were reported in this ethnic minority group (Kassam-Khamis *et al.*, 1999). Studies suggest that insulin resistance may be a contributory factor responsible for the higher rates of coronary heart disease seen among South Asians (McKeigue *et al.*, 1989). Hypertension is another common health problem among all ethnic minorities, and is more common in South Asians with diabetes (Mather *et al.*, 1995).

1.4.7 Coronary heart disease and stroke

> **Key points**
>
> - There is a higher risk and incidence of stroke among the Bengali community mainly due to a higher rate of hypertension and diabetes.
> - The traditional diet of Bangladesh is high in fruit and vegetables, complex carbohydrates, fish and pulses, and low in fat and processed foods.
> - Diet should be promoted as a natural way of preventing and treating hypertension in combination with medication and physical activity.
> - Health promotion strategies need to be specific to the Bengali community as their cardiovascular risk factors differ from the general population.

Studies have established that high rates of increased incidence of coronary heart disease, angina, stroke, hypertension, arrhythmia and diabetes are prevalent in all South Asians, but the rates are particularly high for Bangladeshis (Rudat, 1994; Karmi, 1996; Primatesta & Brooks, 2001). This may be related to the fact that Bangladeshi men and women are more likely to consume both red meat and fried foods frequently than adults from other ethnic groups. Bangladeshi adults were also found to have the lowest levels of fruit consumption, with only 15% men and 16% women consuming fruit six or more times a week (Health Survey for England, 1999; www.dphpc.ox.ac.uk). This is a particular concern as the causes of this are not clearly understood. Stress has been identified as another contributory factor, as psychosocial stress associated with migration and racial tensions are realities that have to be faced by most South Asians. Other contributory stress factors include unemployment, long working hours from shift work, lack of social support and the widening generation gap between migrant parents and British-born children (Kassam-Khamis *et al.*, 1999). Further research into the health of Bangladeshi migrants in the UK established high mortality rates from coronary heart diseases, a high proportional mortality ratio from ischaemic heart disease and that cardiovascular disease was more prevalent in the Bangladeshi community than any other South Asian ethnic group (Balarajan *et al.*, 1984; Wild & McKeigue, 1997). Data from The Tower Hamlets Partnership (2006) also illustrate that high mortality rates from circulatory diseases and cancer were observed in Tower Hamlets in both men and women. HSE (2004) reports that mean systolic blood pressure (SBP) was lower in South Asian men, particularly Bangladeshi men, compared with men in the general population. Bangladeshi men were significantly less likely to have high blood pressure (hypertension) than men in the general population. However, Bangladeshi women were significantly more likely to have high blood pressure than women in the general population.

1.5 Sri Lankan Diet

Thushara Dassanayakem, Deepa Kariyawasam, Vanitha Subhu

1.5.1 Introduction

The South Asian subcontinent comprises India, Pakistan, Bangladesh and Sri Lanka. Four per cent of the total UK population are classified as 'Asian' or 'Asian British' and this group makes up 50.2% of the minority ethnic group population in the UK (UK Census, 2001).

'South Asians' is 'a term which defines many ethnic groups, with distinctive regions of origin, languages, religions and customs and include people born in India, Bangladesh, Pakistan or Sri Lanka' (Fox, 2004).

Sri Lanka is an island located about 31 km off the southern coast of India. It is approximately the size of Ireland, has a population of 20 million and a growth rate of 0.79% p.a. The majority of the population are Sinhalese (80%) with Tamils (10%),

Moors (8%), Burghers and Malay forming the remaining 2% (see Figure 1.5.1).

Sri Lanka's ethnic diversity, proximity to India and agriculture-based economy combined with the influences of colonization successively by Portugal, Netherlands and Britain all contribute towards its language, customs, culture and dietary variation.

Language

The official languages are Sinhalese and Tamil, although English is the preferred language for commerce and medicine. Adult literacy rates are 90%, with no gender variation.

Migration to the United Kingdom

Annual settlement figures for Sri Lankans in the UK have decreased in recent years, possibly due to political changes in Sri Lanka. Between 1996 and 2006 immigration rates decreased from 7,600 to 1,600 people a year, with the purpose of migration falling predominantly into the categories of labour migration and political migration. In general, Sinhalese people migrated for labour/economic reasons whereas Tamil people were more likely to have migrated for political reasons (Sriskandarajah, 2002). For this reason the proportion of English speakers may vary between the groups, with unplanned migrants being less likely to speak English than planned migrants.

Current UK population

It can be approximated that Sri Lankans comprise the majority of the 0.4% (248,000 people) of the UK population classified as 'Other Asian' in the national census data (UK Census, 2001). Of these, approximately 96% are known to be of Tamil origin (Sri Lankan Embassy in the UK).

1.5.2 Religion

The four main religions in Sri Lanka are Buddhism (followed by 69.1% of the population), Islam (7.6%), Hinduism (7.1%) and Christianity (6.2%) (2001 census provisional data, Sri Lanka). The majority of Sinhalese people are Buddhists, the Tamils tend to follow either Hinduism or Christianity, and the Moors follow Islam (see Table 1.5.1).

Table 1.5.1 Religion and dietary influences

Religious groups	Dietary influences
Buddhists	Some are vegetarians but most eat meat. The Buddhist ethos of no harm is reflected in generally lower than average meat consumption. Some Buddhists may fast (*sil*) for one day a month to coincide with the full moon (*poya*). Those fasting will not eat beyond noon on that day.
Muslims	Forbidden: pork, fish without fins or scales and alcohol. Muslims fast during Ramadan.
Hindus	Can be vegan, lacto-vegetarian, lacto-ovo-vegetarian or meat-eating. Forbidden: Beef. Hindus may fast at various times.
Christians	No dietary restrictions. Lent: Christians may abstain from certain foods during Lent.

Religious celebrations and holidays

The Sinhalese and Tamil New Year is usually celebrated by two national holidays in April. Additionally, each major religion is granted at least one officially recognized national holiday. Political holidays include National Day (4 February), May Day (1 May) and National Heroes Day (22 May). Because the Buddhist calendar is based on the moon's phases, every full moon day (*poya*) in Sri Lanka is also a public holiday. Tamil festivals include Deepawali (Diwali), Pongal (mid-January) and Thai Poosam (full moon, January/February).

Customs and culture

A close family unit is an integral aspect of Sri Lankan culture, in terms of the nuclear unit and also in maintaining close ties with the extended family. Parents expect to provide their children with all their basic needs until they are self-sufficient. Family elders are treated with deep respect. Younger family members often seek the advice and approval of their elders and children are obliged to care for their elderly parents, when necessary.

Women have increasingly more economic opportunities outside the home, while retaining most household responsibilities. Freshly cooked food remains the cultural norm and value is placed on fresh ingredients and culinary skill. These values are likely to be retained on migration, with families eating fresh meals cooked daily.

Greetings

The greeting in Sinhalese is 'Ayubowan' or 'Vannakkam' if they speak Tamil, which means 'May you be blessed with the gift of a long life' in both languages. 'Hello' is universally understood.

Titles are important to Sri Lankans, and it is proper to address clients or acquaintances formally by their titles. Among close friends and relatives, familial titles of brother, sister, auntie or uncle replace formal ones. Due to its colonial past some Sri Lankans have names that originate from the Netherlands or Portugal (e.g., Vandenberg or Fernando) and therefore consideration should be taken when booking translators without first meeting the patient. Tamil names can usually be distinguished from Sinhalese ones by their endings. Tamil surnames usually end in a consonant (e.g., Karunanathan) whereas Sinhalese names usually end in a vowel (e.g., Karnadhara).

Generosity and hospitality are valued in Sri Lankan custom, particularly in terms of treating guests. For example, a simple Sinhalese greeting translates as 'Have you eaten rice?' Visitors are customarily offered food, drinks or even meals by their hosts to show that they are welcome and taken care of. It is considered impolite to refuse such an offer, although one can ask for a substitute, such as water. It is traditional to bring small gifts

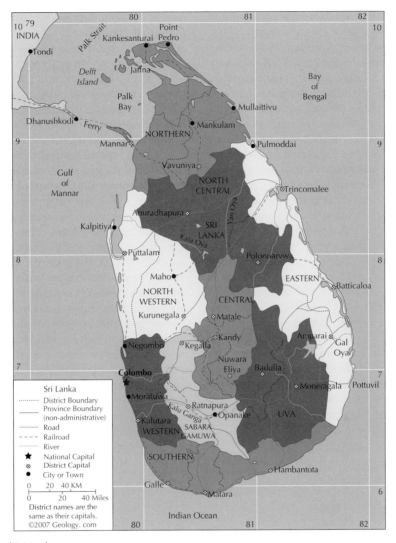

Figure 1.5.1   Map of Sri Lanka

(often food) when visiting. In some homes, people remove their shoes before entering.

1.5.3   Traditional diet and eating patterns

Sri Lankan cuisine has been influenced by most nationalities that have visited and traded over the years (e.g., Dutch, Portuguese, English, Arabs, Malays, Moors and Indians). Due to its tropical climate, fresh fruit, vegetables, coconut and spices are readily available and commonly used. Freshness

and home cooking are key aspects of the diet, with households regularly preparing 3–6 fresh dishes each day. After migration this is likely to reduce to 2–4 dishes.

Typical meal pattern

A typical Sri Lankan meal will include boiled rice and 2–4 of the following:

- *Kirata*: a mild yellow vegetable or fish curry cooked with milk.

- *Mirisata*: a hot and spicy meat, fish or vegetable curry, often orange or brown in colour.
- *Parrippu*: a pulse curry or dish.
- *Malloun*: shredded, half-wilted, *al-dente* greens or green vegetables or *sambol* (raw shredded greens/vegetables/onions/coconut dressed with lime juice), or salad.
- *Thel dhaala*: meat, seafood or vegetables pan-fried with onions and chilli.
- Pickles, chutneys, papadums, salty preserved dried chillies or lemons.

It is customary to eat only one meat or fish dish per meal.

Certain Sri Lankan dishes are intricate, labour-intensive and time-consuming. Hoppers (bowl-shaped fermented, rice flour pancakes) and string hoppers (rice flour dough piped into thin strings onto palm-sized circular mats and steamed), *pittu* (steamed wheat and coconut crumble), *dosai* and *idli* (steamed rice cake) are examples of foods that are served as staples instead of rice. On migration, due to their time-consuming preparation, consumption of these foods is likely to decrease.

Although it is a staple, rice also features in auspicious dishes such as milk rice (*kiributh*). This is a fatty, sticky, coconut-flavoured rice dish tradition-ally served to mark new beginnings – it is thus the first solid food given to a baby and a significant feature at weddings and New Year's Day.

Coconut plays an important role in traditional cooking. It is grated or reconstituted every day and used in *sambols* and vegetable dishes such as *malloun* (shredded wilted greens), and desserts. Sometimes coconut is dry toasted and added towards the end of cooking a curry to thicken it and add a toasted flavour. It is also squeezed to obtain a white cream which is added to curries. In the UK, powdered coconut, creamed coconut or fresh cow's milk may be used as a substitute.

As in many tropical countries, the salt content of the Sri Lankan diet tends to be high. Salt is added during cooking, used to preserve some fish and vegetables and even added to certain chopped fruit to temper acidity. Although a tropical climate may favour the metabolism of excess salt, a reduction of salt in the UK's temperate climate is advisable.

Sri Lanka grows a wide range of tropical fruit, which is commonly eaten as, or in place of, dessert and as snacks throughout the day. Traditional desserts are often fatty and sweet and tend to be reserved for celebrations and special occasions (see Tables 1.5.2 and 1.5.3).

Table 1.5.2 Description of Sri Lankan foods

Food group	Pronunciation/description and language	Pronunciation/description and language
	Sinhalese	Tamil
Bread rice potatoes pasta and other starchy foods		
Hoppers	*Appa* (made from white rice flour)	*Appam*
String hoppers	*Indi appa* (made from red rice or white rice flour)	*Idiyappam*
Pittu	Steamed rice flour and coconut mix	
Roti	Lightly griddled wheat flour (with or without coconut)-based flatbread	
Idli (Tamil dish)	Steamed *urid dal* and rice cakes	
Upma (Tamil dish)	Semolina flour with spices	
Dosai (Tamil dish)	Pancake with *urid dal* and rice flour	
Kottu roti	Chopped *roti* mixed with meat or vegetables	
Vegetables		
Spinach	*Nivithi*	*Pasalai kurai*

Table 1.5.2 (*cont'd*)

Food group	Pronunciation/description and language — Sinhalese	Pronunciation/description and language — Tamil
Potato	Ala	Orulai kizhangu
Cabbage	Go	Gosu
Aubergine	Vambotu	Kathirikai
Long beans	Maykarel	Payathang kai
Ladies' fingers (okra)	Bandaka	Vendakai
Ash plantain	Alu kehel	Valakai
Carrot	Carrot	
Green beans	Bornchi	
Bitter gourd (karela)	Karavilla	Pavakai
Capsicum (peppers)	Miris	Kodai milakai
Courgettes		
Drumsticks	Murunga	Murungai kai
Pumpkin	Vatakka	Posani, parangi
Sothi		Vegetable curry made with coconut milk and served with string hoppers
Sambar/sambol (Tamil dish)		Made from dal, coconut, okra, carrot, radish, pumpkin, potatoes, tomatoes, aubergine
Cassava/yam	Manioc	Maravelli kizhangu
Breadfruit	Del	Eera pilakai
Jackfruit	Kos	Pala pazham
Gotu kola		Valarai
Other English vegetables also eaten		
Fruit		
Mango	Amba	Mambazham
Papaya	Gasslabu	Papali pazham
Wood apple	Diwul	Vilam pazham
Avocado	Alligata pera	
Custard apple		Seetha Pazham
Other English fruits also eaten		
Meat, fish, egg, beans and other non-dairy sources of protein		
Lentils/dal	Parripu	Paruppu
Chickpeas	Kadhala	Konadai kadhalai
Maldive chips (dried fish flakes)	Umbalakada	
Salt fish	Karavula	Karuvadu
Coconut, onion and chilli sambol	Pol sambol	Thenga chutney
Spicy watery soup	Rasam	
Crème caramel-style pudding	Wattalapam (Sinhalese dish)	
Rice pudding made with coconut milk		Payasam

Table 1.5.3   Traditional eating pattern and healthier alternatives for Sri Lankan diet

Meal	Tamil	Sinhalese	Healthier alternatives
Breakfast	String hoppers or *Idli* or *dhosa* with *sambar* or *sambol*	Hoppers (rice flour pancakes, sometimes served with coconut milk) or milk rice (very thick rice pudding, cut into slices)	Traditional without coconut milk or cereal with semi-skimmed milk or bread, spread and jam Fruit
Lunch	Rice Vegetable curry Fish, meat or lentil curry Yoghurt	Rice Vegetable curry Fish or meat curry (beef often used as it is cheaper)	Traditional but without coconut milk and less oil Sandwiches, rolls with cheese or ham and salad Fruit
Evening meal	String hoppers or *pittu* *Sambar* or *sothi*	Rice (mainly) or string hoppers Vegetable or meat curry *Sambol*	Traditional without coconut milk If using oil, use 1 tablespoon monounsaturated oil
Puddings/ Desserts	Payasam fruit, especially mango, papaya, pomegranate	Rice pudding *Wattalappa* (caramel pudding with milk, egg, jaggery, sugar), jelly, trifle, cake	Fruit Milk pudding made with sweetener and semi-skimmed milk
Drinks	Tea/coffee (with milk) Water Fruit juice Yoghurt drinks Fizzy drinks	Tea/coffee (with milk) Water Fruit juice Yoghurt drinks Fizzy drinks	Tea/coffee (with semi-skimmed milk) Unsweetened fruit juice Low-fat yoghurt drink Water
Snacks	*Vadai* *murrukku* (*urad* and gram, shaped and deep-fried) *Bonda* (split chickpeas, boiled with sugar, coconut, in pastry and deep-fried)	Oil cakes (jaggery and rice flour, very difficult to make) Biscuits, cakes in general Crisps	Fruit Bread Plain biscuits

(Hamid & Sarwar, 2004)

Hot and cold foods

Some Sri Lankans observe the ayurvedic classification of foods into hot and cold categories. The classification of these foods has nothing to do with the temperature of the food or to any other observable or taste-related factor, but rather specifies the innate qualities of a food and its effect on the body.

The Sri Lankan rural study by Wandel *et al.* (1984) found that nearly everyone interviewed had some knowledge of the hot/cold system but did not always follow its guidelines. Hot foods are discouraged in conditions that are associated with too much heat in the body (e.g., skin allergies and inflammation). Alternatively, when the body is suffering from a 'cold' condition (e.g., phlegm or wheezing), cooling foods are avoided. Thus, it is during illness that particular emphasis is placed on the preventative and curative properties of this food classification system, and hence it may be prudent to ensure that, if appropriate, dietary advice is compatible with this categorization (see Table 1.5.4).

Table 1.5.4 Classification of hot and cold foods in South Asia

Hot	Cold
Chicken	Ghee
Tomatoes, mangoes and mushrooms	Cow's milk
	Bland vegetables
Powdered milk	Green, leafy vegetables
Some tuna, squid and shellfish	Some shark and most freshwater fish
Pork, beef and duck	Chicken and mutton
	Bananas and citrus fruits

Betel (paan) chewing

Betel (*paan*) is a leaf that is wrapped round an areca nut from the areca palm tree and chewed like gum. The lime reacts with compounds in the nut to produce alkaloids for a mild narcotic effect. Large amounts of red saliva are also produced, which chewers spit out. Betel nuts have been associated with oral malignancy (Trivedy *et al.*, 2002) and should therefore be discouraged. Betel took on symbolic meaning and was a central element of traditional marriage ceremonies. Among Malays, betel would be sent to the parents of a prospective bride and, if they accepted it, it meant they consented to the marriage.

Alcohol

A survey carried out in Sri Lanka in 2002–3 showed that 63% of people had never consumed alcohol, 20% consumed alcohol more than twice a week with 8% consuming alcohol daily. These levels may change on migration with ease of availability and relatively low cost. A popular spirit in Sri Lanka is Arrack made from fermented coconut sap. Arrack may be drunk neat or mixed like other spirits. On migration to the UK, local beers, lagers and other alcoholic beverages are likely to be taken instead of Arrack.

Smoking

A questionnaire was administered to 1,565 Sri Lankan adults living in Sri Lanka to identify the prevalence of smoking and to assess respondents'

attitudes to it. Of men, 41% were yearly smokers, 27.8% were monthly smokers and 21% were daily smokers. The corresponding figures for women were 3.4%, 2% and 0.6% respectively. Higher prevalence rates were observed among less educated, middle-aged men from underprivileged families (Perera *et al.*, 2005). The levels of smoking by Sri Lankans living in the UK may be different but there are no available data.

1.5.4 Healthy eating

Key points

- Traditional Sri Lankan diets are low in fat and should be encouraged as part of a healthy eating diet.
- The main staple food is rice.
- Sri Lankans may have a higher fat mass for any given BMI and therefore a lower BMI cut-off is advisable (Wickramasinghe et al., 2005).

The energy breakdown in a typical Sri Lanka diet is 72.4% energy from carbohydrate, 8.8% from protein and 18.8% from fat (FAO, 2004). This is in contrast to the 48% from carbohydrate, 16% from protein and 36% from fat in UK populations. Animal proteins play a small role in Sri Lanka due to cost, and most protein comes from vegetable sources. The consumption of fish is greater than meat primarily due to agricultural, cultural and religious reasons. The main staple consumed is rice which is predominantly grown in Sri Lanka and the second most commonly consumed staple is wheat, which is entirely imported. As meat is relatively cheap in the UK, the intake of meat on arrival to the UK may increase. The intake of fats also seems to increase with higher household income and therefore may increase on migration. Although there are no data showing the intakes of Sri Lankans in the UK, it is thought that with more household income and easy access to food, Sri Lankans living in the UK are likely to obtain energy in a similar way to those in the UK. From a nutritional point of view, the lower fat intake of the traditional diet should be encouraged. Carbohydrate intake can be high as the proportion of staple eaten differs greatly from the amounts in a typical balance of good health model (See Figure 1.3.2 page 50).

Traditionally, a rice or starch portion will constitute approximately two-thirds of a meal. Of the remaining third, vegetables, pulses or salad constitute approximately two-thirds of a meal (i.e., 2/9th of the whole plate) and meat or fish provide the rest (1/9th of the total plate). Healthy eating can be encouraged by advising a decrease in starchy foods and substitution with vegetable-based dishes (see Table 1.5.5).

Although there are not many studies looking at Sri Lankans food intake on migration, studies on Asian groups show that many Asians will eat a combination of native foods and Western foods (Smith *et al.*, 1993). Time and food availability are factors that are likely to have an impact on food choices made by Sri Lankans living in the West. Households in Sri Lanka tend to have home helps to help with food preparation and thus working families in Sri Lanka can still enjoy fresh foods cooked daily. Sri Lankan households in the UK tend to rely on the female member of the family to prepare meals and both sexes are equally likely to work. The person who cooks may thus need to fit this in with her work schedule and therefore may cook in bulk and reheat dishes. Sri Lankans should be encouraged to reheat quantities as required rather than reheating the same dish several times in order to maximize the nutritional content with respect to heat-labile vitamins.

A typical Sri Lankan diet can be high in salt. Most Sri Lankan households prepare food freshly, using herbs and spices in preference to ready-made pastes or sauces. Most dietary salt is therefore likely to be added during cooking and also added to salads and acidic fruit. Additionally, some Sri Lankans in the UK consume Indian pickles that contain fairly high amounts of salt. Traditional Sri Lankan pickles and chutneys can be made with less salt and therefore these should be encouraged as a substitute to ready-made Indian pickles. Other excessively salty foods used in Sri Lankan cooking is *karavela* (saltfish) or Maldive fish (dry salted fish flakes added to curries) .

Evolving and emerging nutritional health problems

Increasing urbanization, commercialization, higher exposure to western food and lifestyle and an

Table 1.5.5 Dietary modifications of Sri Lankan diet

	Limit	Try
Vegetable curries	Potato curries as an accompaniment to rice or other starchy food	Vegetable curry or dal (*parripu*) instead of high carbohydrate curries
Meat and fish curries	Fatty meats	Choose oily fish (mackerel, salmon sardines, fresh tuna) twice a week Choose lean meats
Cooking methods	Reheating whole dish	Reheating required amount only

increasingly sedentary lifestyle, together with the breakdown of traditional social frameworks, are starting to be reflected in a shift in Sri Lanka's nutrition-related health problems. There is a marked difference in major health problems between urban and rural areas, with the 'diseases of affluence' more prevalent in urban populations, while malnutrition and communicable diseases associated with rural areas. The Sri Lankan Ministry of Healthcare and Nutrition has identified the leading cause of death as ischaemic heart disease and that mortality due to non-communicable diseases is increasing. There are few migration studies relating specifically to the Sri Lankan population, however parallels can be drawn with the South Asian population in Britain, leading to the reasonable assumption that Sri Lankans are likely to be at higher risk of heart disease, diabetes and hypertension than the general population.

Obesity

Levels of obesity and overweight are similar to the UK and 24% of those living in Sri Lanka had a BMI > 25 and 5% had a BMI > 30. Those who were educated to O and A level and living in urban areas were more likely to be of a higher weight. Those from plantation estates were likely to be underweight and this may be due in part to the difficulties in obtaining adequate food on a limited income; also energy expenditure within the workers on plantation estates are greater.

Abdominal obesity levels are high in Sri Lanka (Arambepola & Fernando, 2005). An urban lifestyle and greater consumption of deep-fried foods and a lower consumption of wholegrain products were associated with higher levels of abdominal obesity.

The highest proportions of central obesity (waist/hip ratio [WHR] > 0.85) were observed among women from Sri Lanka (54.3%) and Pakistan (52.4%) as opposed to Turkey and Vietnam. For any given value of BMI, Sri Lankans and Pakistanis had higher WHR compared to those from Turkey, Iran and Vietnam (Kumar et al., 2006). They also had the lowest high-density lipoprotein (HDL) and the highest low-density lipoprotein of the groups (Glenday et al., 2006).

A similar study looking at Sri Lankan children born in Australia found that they have a higher fat mass in relation to their BMI. As central obesity leads to more health risks, it is important that weight gain is avoided. One study has also shown that Asians have cardiovascular risks at normal levels of BMI and waist circumference (Vikram et al., 2003) and Asians have also been found to have health risks at lower waist circumference cut-offs when compared to Caucasians. Misra et al. (2005) and Wickramasinghe et al. (2005) therefore suggest that different BMI cut-offs are produced for Asians. Migration may also affect the likelihood of developing obesity. Asian Indians in the UK and USA were also found to have a higher BMI, WHR and skinfold thickness compared to urban Indians living in India (Misra & Vikram, 2002). It is likely that Sri Lankans living in the UK will similarly have higher levels of obesity than their counterparts living in Sri Lanka.

Diabetes UK suggests that to avoid health risks, waist circumference should be less than 89 cm inches for South Asian men and 80 cm for South Asian women.

Dietary modification
A traditional low-fat diet should be encouraged but the traditional diet also consists of fairly high carbohydrate and therefore carbohydrate intake should be decreased and pulses increased.

The intake of fat can be quite high for those living in the UK as they may get fat from meats as well as from oil used for cooking and coconut added to dishes.

Coconut may be added to dishes in the form of coconut milk or fresh/dessicated coconut may be used to make sambols and mallung. The consumption of coconut should be limited due to its high saturated fat and energy content. Many Sri Lankans believe that coconut oil is beneficial but there is very little evidence for this (see Table 1.5.6).

Physical activity
Physical activity levels are lower in South Asians compared to Europeans. Some possible reasons for this are feeling uncomfortable about exercising in public and limited language skills. Older women also felt that spending time exercising was perceived as self-indulgent. South Asians with a family history of chronic diseases understood the benefits of exercise on health and also were aware of the benefits to body image (Sriskantharajah &

Table 1.5.6 Dietary modifications for weight reduction diet

	Limit	Try
Meat curries	Fatty meats Fried meat/fish	Lean meats Boil/steam/grill meat/fish
Coconut milk-based dishes	Coconut milk-based dishes	Semi-skimmed milk as an alternative to coconut milk
Accompaniments	Coconut-based sambols/chutney	Mallung or onion-based sambols, e.g., onion sambol, katta sambol
Snacks	Fried foods: vadai, cutlet, samosa, muruku, pakoda	Fruits, plain biscuits, unsalted roasted chickpeas
Food preparation	Reduce fats and oil	Cooking in non-stick pan

Kai, 2007) and therefore this awareness should be used to encourage physical activity. Another study found that the level of physical activity outside of work was lowest in South Asians and therefore this is a possible area to target for change (Pomerleau et al., 1999). Barriers to physical activity must be considered when encouraging physical activity. Single-sex exercise classes or activity that can be incorporated into daily life may be of benefit.

Diabetes

The prevalence of type 2 diabetes in Sri Lanka is approximately 5%, with a similar proportion having impaired glucose tolerance. Of those diagnosed as part of research, 21% were not aware they had diabetes (Wijesuriya, 1997).

In Sri Lanka a study has shown that smoking, low family income, BMI > 25, older age, duration of diabetes and diastolic blood pressure > 90 mmHg were significantly associated with the development of long-term complications. Peripheral diabetic neuropathy (25.2%) was the commonest complication among the study population with complications, followed by diabetic retinopathy and diabetic nephropathy (Amarasinghe et al., 2004).

Dietary modification

The dietary management of diabetes should consist of regular meals with complex carbohydrates and low simple sugars. Low glycaemic index foods such as basmati rice and pulses should also be encouraged. GIs of other rice has also been measured but the colour of the rice does not necessarily indicate a low GI (Hettiarachchi et al., 2001). The lowest GI Sri Lankan rice was parboiled red rice.

Some popular Sri Lankan drinks such as Necto (a squash-based drink) and Milo (a malted chocolate drink drunk hot or cold) are not always available in sugar-free versions, so patients should be advised to switch to an alternative. Soft drinks popular in the UK (e.g., cola, lemonade and orangeade) are also taken by Sri Lankans in the UK and while abroad. Diet versions should be encouraged and are available in Sri Lanka.

Herbs and ayurvedic treatments

Herbal and ayurvedic (traditional healthcare native to India and other parts of south Asia) treatment to help with diabetes control may be used by some Sri Lankans. Sri Lankans may take karivilla (bitter gourd) to help control blood glucose, as Indian communities do. Salacia oblonga has also been found to reduce postprandial glycaemia. S. oblonga seems to work by inhibiting alpha-glucosidase (Hertzler et al., 2007).

Renal failure

Those approaching or at end-stage renal failure may need to limit potassium- and phosphate-rich foods. Phosphate-rich foods in the Sri Lankan diet are similar to the phosphate-rich foods in the western diet (i.e., dairy foods, offal and seafood). Potassium-rich foods vary due to the different fruits and vegetables people eat and other foods that need to be restricted are those with significant amounts of coconut (e.g., pol sambol). Clients who eat meat/fish and have lentils at the same meal may need to decrease the amount of lentils or meat/fish as both are high in potassium. Vegetarians can have a generous serving of lentils as they are not having the potassium contributed by meat/fish. Other potassium-rich foods that need to be considered are nuts and chickpea snacks (kadala).

Cardiovascular disease and stroke

The energy breakdown in a typical Sri Lankan diet is carbohydrate 72.4%, protein 8.8% and fat 18.8%. Despite these figures the recent estimates for mortality from cardio- and cerebrovascular diseases (CVD) for Sri Lanka – 524 deaths per 100,000 – is higher than that observed in many western economies. With regard to the type of fat consumed, the ratio of saturated to polyunsaturated fat is 9:1 compared to the current recommendations of 1:1. This low PUFA intake combined with a high carbohydrate intake may contribute to high triglyceride levels and low LDL cholesterol levels (Abeywardena, 2003).

South Asians tend to have acute myocardial infarctions (MI) eight years earlier than ethnic groups that develop MI the latest, but when compared to the average person, Sri Lankans have MI only one year earlier. The main risk factors were current and former smoking status, a high $ApoB_{100}$/Apo-I ratio, a history of hypertension and a history of diabetes (Joshi et al., 2007). Low daily consumption of fruits and vegetables, lack of regular exercise and high WHRs observed among native South Asians compared with individuals from other countries may also contribute to the higher rates of coronary heart disease observed in South Asians. South Asians tend to have low folate intake possibly due to prolonged cooking of vegetables and therefore Sri Lankans should be advised to include lightly cooked vegetables.

Dietary modification

As with regular dietary advice for the management of coronary heart disease, individuals should be guided towards achieving a normal BMI through energy restriction and increased energy expenditure. Energy restriction can be achieved by portion size reduction, particularly of starchy staples such as rice, which is usually eaten in larger than recommended amounts.

Sri Lankans should be advised to include lightly cooked vegetables and increase the amount of salads, *sambols* and fresh fruit that they consume. Coconut oil should be replaced with a polyunsaturated oil and fried food should be discouraged. Coconut products should also be limited.

Sri Lankans often cook large quantities of vegetables which are then reheated before eating and this may be done more than once. This practice should be discouraged and the advice given that only the desired amount of food for those eating should be reheated.

Exercise is also beneficial with respect to CVD and a study in India showed that daily moderate intensity exercise for 35–40 minutes was associated with a 50% risk of CHD (Rastogi *et al.*, 2004).

Oily fish is a common feature of a traditional Sri Lankan diet. The beneficial aspects of oily fish should be discussed and these should be encouraged with regard to cardiovascular health. *Balaya* (tuna), *thora* (Spanish mackerel), *thalapath* (swordfish) and *mora* (shark) are common types of oily fish in Sri Lanka of which the latter two should be avoided during pregnancy due to high levels of mercury.

Cancer

A study in Australia (Grulich *et al.*, 1995) showed that some rates of cancer on migration change to the levels found in Australia. Overall cancer incidence was lower in Sri Lankans living in Australia than in native Australians, and this difference reached significance in migrants born in China/Taiwan, the Philippines, Vietnam and India/Sri Lanka, and in male migrants born in Indonesia. For the majority of cancers, rates were more in line with those born in the Australia than to those in the countries of birth. For cancers of the breast, colorectum and prostate, rates were relatively low in the countries of birth, but migrants generally exhibited rates nearer those of the Australia-born. For cancers of the liver, cervix and oral cavity, in India- and Sri Lanka-born migrants the incidence was relatively high in the countries of birth but tended to be lower, nearer native Australian rates, in the migrants. For these cancers, environmental factors related to the migrant's adopted country, and migrant selection, appeared to have a major effect on the risk of cancer. For certain other cancers, the incidence was similar to that in the countries of birth. Melanoma had low rates in both the migrants and in those that were born and lived in Sri Lanka. For melanoma, it was probable that genetic or environmental factors acting prior to migration were important in causation (see Table 1.5.7).

Table 1.5.7   Cancer incidence and which types of cancer occur in levels similar to the country of residence

	Native levels	Migrant levels
Breast		√
Colorectum		√
Prostate		√
Cervix		√
Liver		√
Oral		√
Skin	√	

1.5.5   Nutrition support

Nutrition support may be necessary during periods of ill health when appetite and food intake may decrease. Food fortification can be considered as a first-line measure and foods such as coconut milk and other coconut products may be added to help increase calorie (energy) intake. Typical food fortification, such as adding milk, cream and butter to dishes, can also be encouraged.

In Sri Lanka 9% of the female population are severely underweight with a BMI value < 16 kg/ m², while 25% of the women have a BMI between 16 and 18.5 kg/m² and are therefore mildly–moderately underweight (Ramanujan & Nestel, 2005). Although the prevalence of severe under-nutrition is slightly lower in men (5%), overall 37% of men suffer from under-nutrition (BMI < 18.5 kg/m²). This low weight may resolve on migration, but some Sri Lankans may have a natural slim build despite eating well and do not need the same attention as those that are truly malnourished. Most of the underweight people in Sri Lanka are found within the plantation worker group. They are unlikely to be found in the UK and therefore the levels of malnutrition in Sri Lankans in the UK do not reflect the levels of malnutrition in Sri Lanka (see Table 1.5.8).

Points to consider when choosing nutritional supplements

Sri Lankans of Buddhist, Hindu and Christian Sri Lankans will take standard oral nutritional supplements but Muslims may request *halal*-approved oral nutritional supplements. It is advisable to contact individual manufacturers to find out which supplements are *halal*-approved. If a patient is a strict vegan, then many supplements with added vitamin D may not be suitable as it is derived from

sheep wool. Most Sri Lankans are not vegans and therefore many supplements on the market will be suitable. The same applies for enteral feeds.

1.5.6   Maternal and child nutrition

Exclusive breastfeeding is not carried out for long in Sri Lanka; a survey found that 96% of babies in Sri Lanka were being breastfed at three months but 32% of these had already started formula milk. This demonstrates that efforts should be made to allow mothers to breastfeed exclusively until at least the fourth month. Many in Sri Lanka start early supplementation as full-pay maternity leave ceases at three months. Take-up rates of breastfeeding are high as hospitals encourage it and while in hospital mothers are not allowed to feed from the bottle without doctor approval. Exclusive breastfeeding for the first four months is carried out only by about 24% of mothers, whereas in India approximately 51% exclusively breastfeed for the first four months. Rates of breastfeeding among Sri Lankans in the UK are not available but may be different due to differences in lifestyle and maternity leave.

Weaning foods

In Sri Lanka about 25% of mothers in urban areas commence semi-solid feeding after the fourth month. Faltering growth (in comparison with NCHS standards) is commonly observed around the fourth month, mostly relating to late complementary feeding. Reasons for mothers being reluctant to feed earlier are because of a traditional rice-eating ceremony around the end of the year or until teeth have erupted (Soysa, 1988). Care should be taken to educate Sri Lankan mothers regarding the importance of timely weaning.

Common first weaning foods are soft-boiled mashed rice, potatoes, carrots and lentils. As weaning progresses, a greater variety of vegetables, greens, fish, meat and spices is added and food is often fortified with butter or margarine. It is traditional to encourage a variety of fresh food, textures and seemingly strong flavours, as and when it is judged the child can tolerate them. Initially, weaning foods are prepared separately; however, by one year children are fed from the

Table 1.5.8   Dietary modifications for nutritional support

Energy-dense foods	Energy- and protein-dense foods
Pol sambol (shredded coconut with chilli) Thengai chutney as an accompaniment to a meal	Cashew curry (cadju curry/*munthiri*) as an accompaniment to a meal
Pol mallung as an accompaniment to a meal	Yoghurt and treacle (*Kiri pani*) as a pudding/dessert
Mallung/ Keerai Kuttu – fried greens with coconut	*Wattalapam* – pudding/dessert
Sweetmeats, e.g., *kaung, kokis, thala guli*	*Payasam* – pudding/dessert
	Kadhala – chickpea snack
	Bombay mix/nuts

milder dishes prepared for family consumption, and sometimes graduate to eating highly spiced foods at a relatively young age. As with the adult population, dairy foods (cheese and yoghurt) feature minimally in the traditional weaning diet, however this is likely to change on migration.

Increasing commercialization and media advertising have begun to influence Sri Lanka's weaning patterns, with more affluent families choosing to wean using commercially prepared baby cereals and weaning foods. On migration to the UK, Sri Lankans are likely to be influenced by the same health messages and lifestyle factors relating to weaning as the general population.

1.5.7 Nutritional deficiencies

Due to a difference in intake on migration, it is likely that most of these deficiencies are rarely found in Sri Lankans living in the UK but may need to be considered in recent migrants.

Vitamin D deficiency

A study investigating Sri Lankans who have emigrated found that vitamin D levels of Sri Lankans appear to be low. About 32% of men and women (in almost equal proportions) were vitamin D-deficient. The risk of vitamin D deficiency increases with age. Those who were taking cod liver oil supplements were less likely to be deficient and 23% of the Sri Lankans in this study were taking cod liver oil. Those having an increased intake of fatty fish also had higher levels of vitamin D and hence oily fish should be encouraged for this as well as for cardiovascular reasons.

Iron deficiency anaemia

About 45% of pre-school children, 58% of 5–11-year-old children, 36% of adolescents and 45% of non-pregnant women suffer from anaemia. Women aged 18–45 years seem to be the most affected. Iron deficiency anaemia may still occur if certain food groups (e.g., meat) are omitted from the diet (FAO Nutrition Country Profiles).

Iodine deficiency

Nearly 19% of the population in Sri Lanka were diagnosed as iodine-deficient in the past but this is improving as most Sri Lankans (approximately 90%) have access to iodized salt (FAO Nutrition Country Profiles).

Vitamin A deficiency

More than 30% of pre-school children have marginal serum values of vitamin A (FAO Nutrition Country Profiles).

Suggestions for the way forward

Research looking at Sri Lankan migrants is limited as they are a small group in the UK. With regards to food composition, it would be valuable if data were available for the traditional foods, especially where micronutrients are concerned (e.g., potassium content of fruits and vegetables commonly consumed by the Sri Lankan population). Although traditional fruits and vegetables are similar to those eaten by all South Asian communities, other food groups, such as starchy foods and sweets, have very different names and if a diet sheet aimed at the Asian community is given to Sri Lankans, it is worth checking to see if it includes the types of food the patient may consume.

Websites

Gujarati Diet

www.virtualcurriculum.com/N3225/spring2006/inderjit/template2.html
For barriers Diabetes South Asians

Punjabi Diet

en.wikipedia.org/wiki/Sikh_beliefs#cite_note-0
www.bbc.co.uk/religion/religions/sikhism/ataglance/glance.shtml
punjabgovt.nic.in/WELCOME.html
www.publications.parliament.uk/pa/cm199900/cmhansrd/vo000307/halltext/00307h0
en.wikipedia.org/wiki/Southall
en.wikipedia.org/wiki/Sewadar
www.bhf.org.uk
The British Heart Foundation website has a useful Health Professionals section, including a number of fact files giving clear, concise and up-to-date information on heart health issues.
www.heartstats.org

A comprehensive and up-to-date data source on the incidence, prevention, treatment and causes of heart disease in the UK, including information on minority ethnic groups.

Pakistani Diet

Association for the Study of Obesity: www.aso.org.uk
British Heart Foundation: www.bhf.org.uk
Cancer Research UK: www.cancerresearchuk.org
en.wikipedia.org/wiki/Shiite
en.wikipedia.org/wiki/SunniIslam
International Association for the Study of Obesity: www.iaso.org
International Obesity Taskforce: www.iotf.org
Minority Ethnic Communities and Health: www.minority health.gov.uk/index.htm
Muslim Health Network: www.muslimhealthnetwork. org
National Obesity Forum: www.nof.org
QUIT: www.quit.org.uk
The Ismaili Nutrition Centre: www.theismaili.org/ nutrition
www.Diabeteshealth.com
www.carbs-information.com
www.heartstats.org
www.infoplease.com/ipa/A0107861.html
www.statistics.gov.uk
www.virtualcurriculum.com/N3225/spring2006/ inderjit/template2.html
www.yespakistan.com

Bangladeshi Diet

www.virtualcurriculum.com/N3225/spring2006/ inderjit/template2.html.
www.theismaili.org/nutrition.

Resources

Pakistani Diet

Al-Badr Health & Fitness
2nd Floor, 453 Leabridge Road
London E10 7EA
Tel: 020 8558 8819 or 020 8556 3889
Bengali Bridge Project
Suhas Khanderia, Pharmaceutical Adviser Islington Primary Care Trust
Tel: 0207 853 5558
Email: suhas.khanderia@nhs.net

Birmingham Food Net
Eleanor McGee, Projects Lead, Birmingham Community Dietitians
Tel: 0121 446 1021
Email: eleanor.mcgee@easternbirminghampct.nhs.uk

Bradford Trident Healthy Living Project weight management programme
Rukhsana Khan, Project Coordinator, Bradford Trident Healthy Living Project
Tel: 01274 436186/7
Email: rukhsanak@bilk.ac.uk

Cancer Equality
18 Boardman House
64 Broadway
London E15 1NT
Email:info@cancerequality.or.uk

The Coriander Club
Lutfun Hussain
Coriander Club
Spitalfields City Farm
London
Tel: 0207 247 8762

Coventry 5-a-Day Scheme
Helene Heath, 5-a-Day Coordinator, Coventry Health Promotion Service
Tel: 024 7624 6095
Email: Helene.Heath@coventrypct.nhs.uk

Dietary Intervention in High-Risk Families with CHD In Ealing
Professor J.S. Kooner, Head of Department of Cardiology, Ealing Hospital
Email: j.kooner@imperial.ac.uk

Hamara Healthy Living Centre
Khurshid Butt
Hamara Healthy Living Centre
Tel: 0113 277 3330
Email: Khurshid@hamara.co.uk

Khush Dil Project
Gill Mathews, Project Coordinator, Khush Dil
Tel: 0131 537 4585/7

Natalie Field, Assistant Director of Public Health
Avon HImP Performance Scheme
Tel: 0117 9002445
Email: natalie.field@bristolswpct.nhs.uk

Project DIL
Mina Bhavsar, CHD/Diabetes and Renal Services Lead
Tel: 0116 2954120
Email: Mina.Bhavsar@elpct.nhs.uk

QUIT
Kawaldip Sehmi, Director of Health Inequalities, QUIT
Tel: 0207 251 1551
Email: k.sehmi@quit.org.uk

Rochdale Healthy Living Centre
Geraldine Meagher, Health Connections Team Manager
01706 745125
Email: gergeraldine.meagher@rochdhale.gov.uk

SITARA
Alison Morby, Head of Physical Activity Development
   Team
Cultural and Leisure Services, Kirklees Metropolitan
   Council
Tel: 01484 234088
Email: alison.morby@kirklees.gov.uk

South Asian Living with Heart Disease Project
Habib Naqvi, Research Associate
Avon HImP Performance Scheme
Tel: 0117 9002653
Email: Habib.Naqvi@bristolswpct.nhs.uk

Using Ethnic Profiling to Improve Services for Black and
   Minority Ethnic Communities
Sarah Pollard, CHD Prevention Specialist Nurse
Tel: 0114 2264752
Email: Sarah.Pollard@sheffieldn-pct.nhs.uk

Walking for Health in Wolverhampton
Hayley Scott, Health Promotion Officer
Walking For Health in Wolverhampton, HAZ
Email: Hayley.scott@wolvespct.nhs.uk

Caroline Fernandez, Local Food Project Coordinator
Tel: 0207 481 9004
Email: food@wen.org.uk

Support groups/organizations

Punjabi Diet

British Heart Foundation
14 Fitzharding Street
London W1H 6DH

South Asian Health Foundation
info@sahf.org.uk
Telephone: 020 8846 7284; Fax: 020 8846 7284

Further reading

Gujarati Diet

Akhtar, M.S., Ahar, M.A. & Yaqub, M. (1981) Effect of momordica charantia on blood glucose levels of normal and alloxan-diabetic rabbits. *Planta Medica*, 42, 205–21.

Baldwa, V.S., Bhandari, C.M., Pangaria, A. & Goyal, R.K. (1977) Clinical trial in patients with diabetes mellitus of an insulin-like compound obtained from plant sources. *Upsala J Med Sci*, 82, 29–41.

Basch E., Gabardi, S. & Ulbricht, C. (2003) Bitter melon (*Momordica charantia*): a review of efficacy and safety. *American Journal Health – Syst Pharm*, 60, 356–9.

Chandhalia, H.B. (1988) *Diabetes and You*. Cadilla Chemicals Pvt Ltd, Ahmedabad.

Dans, A.M.L. *et al.* (2007) The effect of *Momordica charantia* capsule preparation on glycaemic control in type 2 diabetes mellitus needs further studies. *Journal of Clinical Epidemiology*, 60, 554–9.

Day, C. (2005) Are herbal remedies of use in diabetes? *Diabetic Medicine*, 22, 1–21.

Dietary Guidelines for Americans (2005) US Department of Health and Human Services, US Department of Agriculture. www.healthierus.gov/dietaryguidelines.

Govindji, A. (1991) Dietary advice for the Asian diabetic. *Practical Diabetes*, 8 202–3.

Henry, C.J. (1999) Glycaemic index of common foods tested in the UK and India. *Br J Nutr*, 4, 840–5.

Joshi, S. (2002) *Nutrition and Dietetics*. 2nd edition, Tata McGraw-Hill, Delhi.

Judd, P.A., Kassam-Khamis, T. & Thomas, J.E. (2000) *The Composition and Nutrient Content of Foods Commonly Consumed by South Asians in the UK*. The Aga Khan Health Board for the United Kingdom, London.

Khajuria, S. & Thomas, J. (1992) Traditional health beliefs about the dietary management of diabetes– an exploratory study of the implications for the management of Gujarati diabetics in Britain. *Journal of Human Nutrition and Dietetics*, 5, 311–21.

Kochhar, A. & Nagi, M. (2005) Effect of supplementation of traditional medicinal plants on non-insulin-dependent diabetics: a pilot study. *Journal of Medicinal Food*, 8(4), 545–9.

Krawinkel, M.B. & Keding, G.B. (2006) Bitter gourd (*Momordica charantia*): a dietary approach to hyperglycaemia. *Nutrition Reviews*, 64(7), 331–7.

Kuppu Rajan, K., Srivatsa, A. *et al.* (1998) Hypolglycemic and hypotriglyceridemic effects of Methika churna (fenugreek). *Antiseptic*, 95, 78–9.

Leatherdhale, V.A., Panesar, R.K. *et al.* (1981) Improvement in glucose tolerance due to Momordica charantia (karela). *British Medical Journal*, 282, 1823–4.

Modak, M., Dixit, P. *et al.* (2007) Indian herbs and herbal drugs used for the treatment of diabetes. *Journal of Clinical Biochemistry Nutr*, 40, 163–73.

Mukherjee, P.K., Maiti, K., Mukherjee, K. & Houghton, P.J. (2006) Leads from Indian medicinal plants with hypoglycaemic potentials. *Journal of Ethnopharmacology*, 106, 1–28.

Pilkington, K., Stenhouse, E., Kirkwood, G. & Richardson, J. (2007) Diabetes and complementary therapies: mapping the evidence. *Practical Diabetes International*, 24(7), 371–6.

Simmons, D., William, D.R. & Powell, M.J. (1992) Prevalence of diabetes in different regional and religious South Asian communities in Coventry. *Diabetic Medicine*, 9(5), 428–31.

Srilakshmi, B. (2007) *Dietetics*. 5th edition. New Age International Ltd, Delhi. www.newagepublishers.com.

Srivastava, Y., Venkatakrishna-Bhatt, H., Verma, Y. & Venkaiah, K. (1993) Antidiabetic and adaptogenic properties of omordica charantia extract. *Phytother Res*, 7, 285–9.

www.vegetarian-diet.info/vegetarian-dietary-guide-lines.htm.

Tongia, A., Tongia, S.K. & Dave, M. (2004) Phytochemical determination and extraction of Momordica charantia fruit and its hypoglycaemic potentiation of oral hypoglycaemic drugs in diabetes mellitus (NIDDM). *Indian J Physiol Pharmacol*, 48(2), 241–4.

Punjabi Diet

Examples of good practice can be found on heart disease and South Asians delivering NHF for coronary heart disease (DH, 2004) available at www.dh.gov.uk.

Balarajan, R. (1995) Ethnicity and variations in the nation's health. *Health Trends*, 27, 114–19.

Chambers, J.C., Obeid, O.A. *et al.* (2000) Serum homocysteine and risk of coronary heart disease in UK Indian Asians. *Lancet*. 12 February, 355(9203), 512–13.

Executive Summary 3rd Report (2001) The National Cholesterol Education Programme (NCEP) expert panel on detection evaluation and treatment of high blood cholesterol in adults (Adult treatment panel III). *JAMA*, 285, 2486–7.

Farooqi, A., Nagra, D., Edgar, T. & Khunti, K. (2000) Attitudes to lifestyle risk factors for coronary heart disease amongst South Asians in Leicester: a focus group study. *Family Practice*, 17, 293–7.

Patel, K.C.R. & Bhopal, R. (2003) *The Epidemic of Coronary Heart Disease in South Asian Populations: Causes and Consequences*. South Asian Health Foundation, London.

Sandhu, D. & Heinrich, M. (2008) The use of health foods, spices and other botanicals in the Sikh community in London. *Phototherapy Research*, 19(7), 633–42.

Pakistani Diet

Balaram, P., Sridhar, H., *et al.* (2002) Oral cancer in southern India: the influence of smoking, drinking, paan-chewing and oral hygiene. *Int J Cancer*, 98(3), 440–5.

BBC News (2002) Asian Health 'Worsens in the West'.

Berkshire Primary Care Trust (2000) *Weight Management – A Strategy for Berkshire Focusing on Coronary Heart Disease and Cancer Prevention*. Berkshire Primary Care Trust, Reading.

Chapple, A. (1998) Iron deficiency anaemia in women of South Asian descent: a qualitative study, *Ethnic Health*, 3, 199–212.

Coveney, J. (2003) Why food policy is critical to public health – editorial. *Critical Public Health*, 13(2), 99–105.

Cruickshank, J.K. (1989) Diabetes: contrasts between peoples of black (West African), Indian and white European origin. In J.K. Cruickshank & D.G. Beavers (eds.), *Ethnic Factors in Health and Disease* (pp. 289–304). Wright, London.

De Stefani, E., Oreggia, F., Rivero, S. & Fierro, L. (1992) Hand-rolled cigarette smoking and risk of cancer of the mouth, pharynx, and larynx. *Cancer*, 70(3), 679–82.

Department of Health (2002) *Tackling Health Inequalities – Cross-cutting Review*. DH, London.

Department of Health (2003) *Chief Medical Officer Annual Report – Obesity: Defusing the Health Time Bomb. Health Check*. DH, London.

Helman, C.G. (2001) *Culture, Health and Illness*. 4th edition. Arnold, London.

Judd, P.A. Kassam-Khamis, T. & Thomas, J.E. (n.d.) *The Composition and Nutrient Content of Foods Commonly Eaten by South Asians in the UK*. Department of Nutrition and Dietetics, Kings College, London.

Kaplan, M.S. *et al.* (2002) Acculturation status and hypertension among Asian immigrants in Canada. *Journal of Epidemiology and Community Health*, 56, 455–6.

Karseras, P. & Hopkins, E. (1987) *British Asians Health in the Community*. John Wiley & Sons. Chichester.

Lee, C.H., Ko, Y.C. *et al.* (2003) The precancer risk of betel quid chewing, tobacco use and alcohol consumption in oral leukoplakia and oral submucous fibrosis in southern Taiwan. *Br J Cancer*, 88(3), 366–72.

Petersen, S., Peto, V. & Rayner, M. (2004) *Coronary Heart Disease Statistics*. British Heart Foundation, London. www.heartstats.org/publications.

Review of Dietary Intervention Black and Minority Ethnic Groups (March 2009) *Part 1: An Analysis of the BME Situation in Wales Part 2: A Review of Evaluated Dietary Interventions from the UK Targeting BME Groups*. Prepared for The Food Standards Agency Wales by Lynn Stockley & Associates Food and Nutrition Consultancy.

Thorogood, M., Hillsdon, M. & Summerbell, C. (2003) *Lifestyle Interventions for Sustained Weight Loss*. www.clinicalevidence.com/ceweb/conditions/cvd/0203/0203_I14.jsp#REF63.

Townsend, P. & Davidson, W. (eds.) (1992) The Black Report. In *Inequalities in Health*. Penguin, London.

Werbner, P. (1990) *The Migration Process: Capital, Gifts and Offerings among British Pakistanis*. Berg, New York.

Whitehead, M. (1992) The health divide. In *Inequalities in Health*. Penguin, London.

Yusuf, S., Hawken, S. *et al.* (2004) Effect of potentially modifiable risk factors associated with myocardial infarction in 52 countries (the INTERHEART study): case-control study. *Lancet*, 364, 937–52.

Bangladeshi Diet

Abraham, R., Campbell-Brown, M. *et al.* (1985) Diet during pregnancy in an Asian community in Britain – energy, protein, zinc, copper, fibre and calcium. *Human Nutrition: Applied Nutrition*, 39A, 2–35.

Acheson, E.D. & Doll, R. (1964) Dietary factors in carcinoma of the stomach: a study of 100 cases and 200 controls. *Gut*, 5, 126–31.

Anderson, A. & Lean, M.E.J. (1995) Healthy changes? Observations on a decade of dietary change in a sample of Glaswegian South Asian migrant women. *Journal of Human Nutrition and Dietetics*, 8, 129–37.

Anderson, S.A. (1986) Guidelines for Use of Dietary Intake Data. Life Sciences Research Office, Federation of American Societies for Experimental Biology, Bethesda, MD.

Beaton, G.H., Milner, J. *et al.* (1979) Sources of variance in 24 hour dietary recall data: implications for nutrition study design and interpretation. *American Journal of Clinical Nutrition*, 32, 2546–59.

Black, A.E., Bingham, S.A., Johansson, G. & Coward, W.A. (1997) Validation of dietary intakes of protein and energy against 24 hour urinary and DLW energy expenditure in middle-aged women, retired men and post-obese subjects: comparisons with validation against presumed energy requirements. *European Journal of Clinical Nutrition* 51(6), 405–13.

Bull, N.L. & Wheeler, E.F. (1986) A study of different dietary survey methods among 30 civil servants. *Human Nutrition: Applied Nutrition*, 40A, 60–6.

Bush, H.M., Williams, R. *et al.* (1998) Family hospitality and ethnic traditions among South Asian, Italian and general population women in the west of Scotland. *Sociology of Health and Illness*, 20(3), 351–80.

Bush, H., Williams, R., Sharma, S. & Cruickshank, K. (1997) *Opportunities for and Barriers to Good Nutritional Health in Minority Ethnic Groups*. Health Education Authority, London.

COMA (2001) *Dietary Reference Values for Food Energy and Nutrients for the United Kingdom*. Report of the Panel on Dietary Reference Values, Committee on Medical Aspects of Food and Nutrition Policy. HMSO, London.

Garrow, J.S., James, W.P.T. & Ralph, A. (2000) *Human Nutrition & Dietetics*, 10th edition. Churchill Livingstone, Edinburgh.

Gibson, R (1990) *Principles of Nutritional Assessment*. Oxford University Press, Oxford.

Hill, R.J. & Davies, P.S. (2001) The validity of self reported energy intake as determined using the doubly labelled water technique. *British Journal of Nutrition*, 85, 415–30.

Hill, S.E. (1990) *More than Rice and Peas. Guidelines to Improve Food Provision for Black and Ethnic Minorities in Britain*. The Food Commission, London.

Hoidrup, S., Andreason, A.H. *et al.* (2002) Assessment of habitual energy and macronutrient intake in adults: comparison of a seven day food record with a dietary history interview. *European Journal of Clinical Nutrition*, 56(2), 105–13.

Judd, P.A., Kassam-Khamis, T. & Thomas, J.E. (2000) *The Composition and Nutrient Content of Foods Commonly Eaten by South Asians in the UK*. Department of Nutrition and Dietetics, Kings College London.

Lip, G.Y., Malik, I. *et al.* (1995) Dietary fat purchasing habits in Whites, Blacks and Asian peoples in England – implications for heart disease prevention. *International Journal of Cardiology*, 48, 287–93.

MacCauley, D. & Mares, P. (1987) *Nutrition Education in a Multiracial Society*. Hugh Hillword Parker NEC.

McKeigue, P. & Marmot, M. (1988) Mortality from CHD in Asian communities in London. *British Medical Journal*, 297, 903.

Rasanen, L (1979) Nutrition survey of Finnish rural children VI. Methodology study comparing the 24 hour recall and the dietary history interview. *American Journal of Clinical Nutrition*, 32, 2560–7.

Review of Dietary Intervention in Black and Minority Ethnic Groups (March 2009). *Part 1: An Analysis of the BME Situation in Wales. Part 2: A Review of Evaluated Dietary Interventions from the UK Targeting BME Groups*. Prepared for the Food Standards Agency Wales by Lynn Stockley. Lynn Stockley & Associates Food and Nutrition Consultancy.

Satia-Abouta, J., Patterson, R.E., Neuhouser, M.L. & Elder, J. (2002) Dietary acculturation: applications to nutrition research and dietetics. *Journal of American Dietetic Association*, 102, 1105–18.

Sawaya, A.L., Tucker, K. *et al.* (1996) Evaluation of four methods for determining energy intake in young and older women: comparison with doubly labelled water measurements of total energy expenditure. *American Journal of Clinical Nutrition*, 63, 491–9.

Sevak, L., Mangtani, P. *et al.* (2004) Validation of a food frequency questionnaire to assess macro- and micronutrient intake among South Asians in the United Kingdom. *European Journal of Nutrition*, 43(3), 160–8.

Swan, G. (2004) Findings from the latest National Diet and Nutrition Survey. *Proceedings of the Nutrition Society*, 63, 505–12.

Todd, K.S., Hudes, M. & Calloway, D.H. (1983) Food intake measurement: problems and approaches. *American Journal of Clinical Nutrition*, 37, 139–46.

Warwick, P.M. & Reid, J. (2004) Trends in energy and macronutrient intake, body weight and physical activity in female university students (1988 to 2003), and effects of excluding under-reporters. *British Journal of Nutrition*, 92, 679–88.

Willet, W.C., Sampson, L. *et al.* (1985) Reproducibility and validity of a semi-quantitative food frequency questionnaire. *American Journal of Epidemiology*, 122, 51–65.

Sri Lankan Diet

Agampodi, S.B., Agampodi, T.C., Kankanamge, U. & Piyaseeli, D. (2007) Breastfeeding practices in a public health field practice area in Sri Lanka: a survival analysis. *Int Breastfeed J*, 2, 13.

Church, S., Gilbert, P. & Khokar, S. (2005) Synthesis Report No 3: Ethnic Groups and Foods in Europe, 1–68.

Global Nutrition: A Multicultural Pack (2004) Brent NHS Teaching Primary Care Trust and Westminster Primary Care Trust.

Henderson, L., Gregory, J., Irving, K. & Swan, G. (2009) *National Diet and Nutrition Survey: Adults 19–64 Years.* Food Standards Agency, London.

Kumarapelli, V. & Athauda, T.A. (2004) Comparison of the dietary pattern of adolescent schoolgirls in two defined urban and rural settings. *Journal of the College of Community Physicians of Sri Lanka*, 9, 13–15.

Mendis, S., Athauda, S.B., Naser, M. & Takahashi K. (1999) Association between hyperhomocysteinaemia and hypertension in Sri Lankans. *J Int Med Res*, 27(1), January–February, 38–44.

NICE Guidance CG43. *Obesity: Full Guideline, Section 2 – Identification and Classification: Evidence Statements and Reviews.* NICE, London.

References

Gujarati Diet

Burden, A.C., McNally, P.G., Feehally, J. & Walls, J. (1992) Increased incidence of end-stage renal failure secondary to diabetes mellitus in Asian ethnic groups in the UK. *Diabetic Medicine*, 9, 641–5.

Cappuccio, F.P., Cook, D.G., Atkinson, R.W. & Strazzullo, P. (1997) Prevalence, detection and management of cardiovascular risk factors in different ethnic groups in South London. *Heart*, 78, 555–63.

Carlisle, D. (2002) Tobacco: the Asian angle. *Health Development Today*, August/September, 19–22.

Census (2001) Office for National Statistics, London. www.ons.gov.uk/census/index.html.

Changrani, J., Gany, F.M. *et al.* (2006) Paan and gutka use in the United States: a pilot study in Bangladeshi and Indian-Gujarati immigrants in New York City. *Journal of Immigration and Refugee Studies*, 4(1), 275–91.

Chowdhury, T.A., Grace, C. & Kopelman, P.G. (2003) Preventing diabetes in south Asians. *British Medical Journal*, 327, 1059–60.

Chowdhury, T. & King, L. (2007) *Diabetes in South Asian People Explained: A Guide for Patients and Carers.* Altman Publishing, Herts.

Close, C.F., Lewis, P.G., Holder, R. & Wright, A.D. (1995) Diabetes care in South Asian and white European patients with type 2 diabetes. *Diabetic Medicine*, 12 619–21.

Cruickshank, J.K. (1989) Diabetes: contrasts between peoples of black (West African), Indian and white European origin. In J.K. Cruickshank & D.G. Beavers (eds.), *Ethnic Factors in Health and Disease* (pp. 289–304). Wright, London.

Diabetes UK (2006) *Healthy Eating for the South Asian Community.* London.

Food and Agricultural Organization (1994) *Indian Experience on Household Food and Nutjhrition Security.* Regional Expert Consultation, Thailand.

Fox, C. (2004) Heart Disease and South Asians: Delivering the National Service Framework for Coronary Heart Disease. Department of Health and British Heart Foundation, London. www.dh.gov.uk/en/Healthcare/NationalServiceFrameworks/Coronaryheartdisease/DH_4098644.

Franz, M.J. *et al.* (2002) Evidence-based nutrition principles and recommendations for the treatment and prevention of diabetes and related complications. *Diabetes Care*, 25, 148–98.

Goodwin, A.M., Keen, H. & Mather, H.M. (1987) Ethnic minorities in British diabetic clinics: a questionnaire survey. *Diabetic Medicine*, 4, 266–9.

Gopalan, C., Rama Sastri, B.V. & Balasubramanian, S.C., revised and updated by B.S. Narasinga Rao, Y.G.

Deosthale & K.C. Pant (1991), *Nutritive Value of Indian Foods*. National Institute of Nutrition, Indian Council of Medical Research, Hyderabad.

Hamid, F. & Sarwar, T. (2004) *Global Nutrition A Multicultural Pack A Resource Pack for Developing Multicultural Dietary Competencies*. Brent NHS Teaching Primary Care Trust and Westminster Primary Care Trust, London.

Hamson, C., Goh, L., Sheldon, P. & Samanta, A. (2003) Comparative study of bone mineral density, calcium and vitamin D status in the Gujarati and white populations of Leicester. *Postgraduate Medical Journal*, 79(931), 279–83.

Hawthorne, K. (1990) Asian diabetics attending a British hospital clinic: a pilot study to evaluate their care. *British Journal of General Practice*, 40, 243–7.

Hawthorne, K., Mello, M. & Tomlinson, S. (1993) Cultural and religious influences in diabetes care in Great Britain. *Diabetic Medicine*, 10, 8–12.

Health Education Authority (1991) *Nutrition in Minority Ethnic Groups: Asians and African Caribbeans in the United Kingdom*. HEA, London.

Joint Health Surveys (2001) *Health Survey for England. The Health of Minority Groups 1999*. The Stationery Office, London.

Jonnalagadda, S.S. & Diwan, S. (2002) Nutrient intake of first generation Gujarati Asian Indian immigrants in the US. *Journal of the American College of Nutrition*, 21(5), 372–80.

Jonnalagadda, S.S., Diwan, S. & Cohen, D.L. (2005) US guided pyramid food group intake by Asian Indian immigrants in the US. *Journal of Nutrition, Health, Aging*, 9(4), 226–31.

Laing, S.P. *et al.* (1999) The British Diabetic Association Cohort Study, II: cause-specific mortality in patients with insulin-treated diabetes mellitus. *Diabetic Medicine*, 16, 466–71.

Madar, Z., Abel, R., Samish, S. & Arad, J. (1988) Glucose-lowering effect of fenugreek in non-insulin dependent diabetics. *European Journal of Clinical Nutrition*, 42, 51–4.

Mather, H.M. & Keen, H. (1985) The Southall Diabetes Survey: prevalence of known diabetes in Asians and Europeans. *British Medical Journal*, 291, 1081–4.

McKeigue, P.M., Shah, B. & Marmot, M.G. (1991) Relation of central obesity and insulin resistance with diabetes prevalence and cardiovascular risk. *Lancet*, 337, 382–6.

National Institute of Nutrition (1991) *Nutrition in India*. UN ACC/SCN Country case study supported by UNICEF. National Institute of Nutrition Hyderabad, India.

National Institute of Nutrition (1992) *Nutrition Trends in India*. Indian Council of Medical Research, Hyderabad, India.

Nutrition Subcommitee of the Diabetes Care Advisory Committee of Diabetes UK (2003) The implantation of nutritional advice for people with diabetes. *Diabetic Medicine*, 20, 786–807.

Patel, J., Karadia, V. *et al.* (2006) CHD risk factors in UK Gujarati immigrants compared with their contemporaries in Gujarat, India. *British Journal of Cardiac Nursing*, 1(9), 431–6.

Pawa, M. (2005) Use of traditional/ herbal remedies by Indo-Asian people with type 2 diabetes. *Practical Diabetes International*, 22(8), 292–4.

Raghuram, T.C., Pasricha, S. & Sharma, R.D. (1993) *Diet and Diabetes*. 2nd edition. National Institute of Nutrition, Hyderabad.

Ramachandran, A., Snehalatha, C., Dharmaraj, D. & Viswanathan, M. (1992) Prevalence of glucose intolerance in Asian Indians. *Diabetes Care*, 15, 1348–55.

Shankardevananda, S. (2002) *Yogic Management of Asthma and Diabetes*. 3rd edition. Yoga Publications Trust, Bihar.

Sharma, R.D. & Raghuram, T.C. (1990) Hypoglycemic effect of fenugreek seeds in non-insulin dependent diabetic subjects. *Nutr Res*, 10, 731–9.

Sharma, R.D., Raghuram, T.C. & Rao, N.S. (1990) Effect of fenugreek seeds on blood glucose and serum lipids in type 1 diabetes. *J Clinical Nutrition*, 44, 301–6.

Sharma, R.D., Sarka, A. *et al.* (1986) Use of fenugreek seed powder in the management of non-insulin dependent diabetes mellitus. *Nutr Res*, 16, 1331–9.

Sharma, R.D., Sarkar, A. *et al.* (1996) Hypolipidemic effect of fenugreek seeds: a chronic study in non-insulin dependent diabetic patients. *Phytother Res*, 10, 332–4.

Sharma, R.D., Sarkar, A. *et al.* (1996) Toxicological evaluation of fenugreek seeds: a long term feeding experiment in diabetic patients. *Phytother Res*, 10, 519–20.

Sproston, K. & Mindell, J. (eds.) (2006) *Health Survey for England 2004: The Health of Minority Ethnic Groups – Summary of Key Findings*. The Information Centre. www.ic.nhs.uk/webfiles/publications/healthsurvey2004ethnicfull/HealthSurveyforEngland210406_PDF.pdf

Stone, M., Pound, E. *et al.* (2005) Empowering patients with diabetes: a qualitative primary care study focussing on South Asians in Leicester, UK. *Family Practice*, 22(6), 647–52.

Thomas, B. & Bishop, J. (2007) *Manual of Dietetic Practice*. 4th edition. Blackwell, Oxford.

UK Prospective Diabetes Study Group (1994) UK Prospective Diabetes Study XII: differences between Asian, Afro-Caribbean and White Caucasian type 2 diabetic patients at diagnosis of diabetes. *Diabetic Medicine*, 11, 670–7.

UK Prospective Diabetes Study Group (1998) UK Prospective Diabetes Study 33: Intensive blood glucose control with sulphonylureas or insulin compared with conventional treatment and risk of complications in patients with type 2 diabetes. *Lancet*, 351, 837–53.

Wild, S., Roglic, G. *et al.* (2004) Global prevalence of diabetes. *Diabetes Care*, 27(5), 1047–53.

Wolever, T.M. *et al.* (1999) Day-to-day consistency in amount and source of carbohydrate associated with improved blood glucose control in type 1 diabetes. *J Am Coll Nutr*, 18, 242–7.

Yeh, G., Eisenberg, D., Kaptchuk, T. & Phillips, R. (2003) Systematic review of herbs and dietary supplements for glycemic control in diabetes. *Diabetes Care*, 26(4), 1277–94.

Punjabi Diet

Bhopal, R., Unwin, N. *et al.* (1999) Heterogeneity of coronary heart disease risk factors in Indian, Pakistani, Bangladeshi and European origin populations: cross-sectional study. *British Medical Journal*, 319, 215–20.

British Diabetic Association (n.d.). *Asian Information pack. Available from Diet Information Service*. British Diabetic Association, London.

Bush, J., White, M. *et al.* (2003) Smoking in Bangladeshi and Pakistani adults: a community-based, qualitative study. *British Medical Journal*, 326, 962.

Census (2001) Office for National Statistics, London. www.ons.gov.uk/census/index.html.

Cochrane, R. & Bal, S. (1990) The drinking habits of Sikhs, Hindu, Muslims and white men in the West Midlands: a community survey. *British Journal of Addiction*, 85(6), 759–69.

Department of Health (2000) *National Service Framework for Coronary Heart Disease*. The Stationery Office, London.

Department of Health (2004) *Heart Disease and South Asians: Delivering the National Service Framework for Coronary Heart Disease*. DH, London. www.dh.gov.uk.

Dhina, P. (September 1991) Diet and Culture Bridging the Gap, A conference for primary care in multicultural communities. AGUDA conference report, Leicester (unpublished).

Fischbacher, C.M., Hunt, S. & Alexander, L. (September 2004) How physically active are South Asians in the United Kingdom? A literature review. *Journal of Public Health*, 26(3), 250.

Food Standards Agency (2003) www.food.gov.uk/news/pressreleases/2003/apr/asiansoilyfishpress.

Fox, C. (2004) Heart Disease and South Asians: Delivering the National Service Framework for Coronary Heart Disease. Department of Health and British Heart Foundation, London. www.dh.gov.uk/en/Healthcare/NationalServiceFrameworks/Coronaryheartdisease/DH_4098644.

Health Education Authority (1999) *Black and Minority Ethnic Group in England: The Second Health and Lifestyles Survey*. HEA, London. www.hda-onlineorg.uk/pdfs/healifesblacks.pdf.

Health Survey for England (1999) *The Health of Ethnic Minority Groups Joint Health Service Units 2001*. The Stationery Office, London. www.archive.officialdocuments.co.uk/documents/do/survey99/hse99/htm.

Health Survey for England (2004) The Stationery Office, London.

Johnson, M.R., Owen, D. & Blackburn, C. (2000) *Black and Ethnic Minority Groups in England: The Second Health and Lifestyle Survey*. HEA, London.

Landman, J. & Cruickshank, J.K. (2001) A review of ethnicity, health and nutritional-related diseases in relation to migration in the UK. *Public Health Nutrition*, 4, 647–57.

National Food Survey (2003). statistics.defra.gov.uk/esg/publications/nfs/default.asp.

Rankin, J. & Bhopal, R. (2001) Understanding heart disease and diabetes in the South Asian community: cross-sectional study testing the 'snowball' sampling method. *Public Health*, 115, 253–60.

Singh, R.B., Mori, H. *et al.* (1996) Recommendations for the prevention of CHD in Asians: a scientific statement of the international college of nutrition. *J Cardiovascular Risk*, 3, 489–94.

Thomas, B. & Bishop, J. (2007) *Manual of Dietetic Practice* (ed. Briony Thomas). Blackwell Science, Oxford.

Thomas, J. (2002) Nutrition intervention in ethnic minority groups. *Proc Nutr Soc*, 61, 559–67.

Wyke, S. & Landman, J. (1997) Healthy eating? Diet and cuisine amongst Scottish South Asian people. *British Food Journal*, 99(1), 27–34.

Pakistani Diet

Alexander, Z. (1999) *Study of Black, Asian and Ethnic Minority Issues*. Department of Health, London.

Alfaham, M., Woodhead, S., Pask, G. & Davies, D. (1995) Vitamin D deficiency: a concern in pregnant Asian women. *British Journal of Nutrition*, 73, 881–7.

Ali, S., Ara, N. *et al.* (2008) Knowledge and practices regarding cigarette smoking among adult women in a rural district of Sindh, Pakistan, *Journal of the Pakistan Medical Association*, 58(12), 664–7.

Alvi, S., Khan, K.M. *et al.* (2003) Effect of peeling and cooking on nutrients in vegetables. *Pakistani Journal Nutrition*, 2(3), 189–91.

Andersen, R.E. (2003) *Obesity, Aetiology, Assessment, Treatment and Prevention*. Human Kinetics Europe Ltd, Leeds.

Anwar, M. (1998) *Between Cultures – Continuity and Change in the Lives of Young Asians*. Routledge, London.

Armitage, C.J. & Conner, M. (2002) Reducing fat intake: interventions based on the theory of planned behaviour. In D. Rutter & L. Quine (eds.) *Changing Health Behaviour*. Open University Press, Buckingham.

Awumey, E.M., Mitra, D.A. & Hollis, B.W. (1998) Vitamin D metabolism is altered in Asian Indians in the Southern United States: A clinical research study. *Journal of Clinical Endocrinology Metabolism*, 23, 173–7.

Bagozzi, R.P. & Edwards, E.A. (2000) Goal setting and goal pursuit in the regulation of body weight. In P. Norman, C. Abraham & M. Conner (eds.) *Understanding and Changing Health Behaviour – From Health Beliefs to Self-Regulation*. Harwood Academic, Amsterdam.

Beardsworth, A. & Keil, T. (1997) *Food, Family and Community. Sociology on the Menu – An Invitation to the Study of Food and Society*. Routledge, London.

Bedi, R (1989) Ethnic indicators of dental health for young Asian school children resident in areas of multiple deprivation. *British Journal of Dentistry*, 166, 331–4.

Behera, D. & Balamugesh, T. (2005) Indoor air pollution as a risk factor for lung cancer in women. *J. Assoc. Physicians India*, 53, 190–2.

Bessen, D.H. & Kushner, R. (2001) *Evaluation and Management of Obesity*. Hanley & Belfus Inc, USA.

Bhopal, R.S. & Rankin, J. (1996) Cancer in minority ethnic populations: priorities from epidemiological data. *Br J Cancer* (Suppl.), September, 29, S22–32.

Black and Minority Ethnic Groups in England (1999) *The Second Health and Lifestyles Survey*. Health Education Authority, London.

Boffetta, P (2002) Involuntary smoking and lung cancer. *Scand J Work Environ Health*, 28 (Suppl. 2), 30–40.

British Cardiac Society (2008) *Trends for Coronary Heart Disease and Stroke Mortality Among Migrants in England and Wales, 1979–2003: Slow Declines Notable For Some Groups*, 94(4), 463–70.

British Heart Foundation Factfile (04/2000) *South Asians and Heart Disease*. www.bhf.org.uk/professionals/uploaded/apr00.pdf.

British Heart Foundation (2001) Statistics website.

Britton, A. & McPherson, K. (2002) *Monitoring the Progress of the 2010 Target for CHD Mortality: Estimated Consequences on CHD Incidence and Mortality from Changing Prevalence of Risk Factors*. National Heart Forum, London.

Brooke, O.G., Brown, R.F., Cleeve, H.J.W. & Sood, A. (2005) Observations on the vitamin D state of pregnant women Asian women in London. *BOGJ: An International Journal of Obstetrics and Gynaecology*, 88(1), 18–26.

Brown, P.J. (1991) Culture and the evolution of obesity. *Human Nature*, 2, 31–57. Cited in Brown, P.J. and Bentley-Condit, V.K. (1998) Culture, evolution and obesity. In G.A. Bray, C. Bouchard & W.P.T. James (eds.) *Handbook of Obesity*. Marcel Dekker, New York.

Brownell, K.D. & Kramer, F.M. (1994) *Behavioral Management of Obesity*. Chapman and Hall, New York.

Brunvand, L., Henriken, C. & Haug, E. (1996). Vitamin D deficiency among pregnant women from Pakistan. How best to prevent it? *Tidsskr Nor Laegeforen*, 116, 1585–7.

Brunvand, L, Quigstad E., Urdhal, P. & Haug, E. (1996). Vitamin D deficiency and fetal growth. *Early Human Development*, 45, 27–33.

Burton-Jeangros, C (1995) Breastfeeding among mothers of Pakistani origin living in the UK. *Health Visitor*, 68(2), 66–8.

Cancer Research UK (2009) info.cancerresearchuk.org/cancerstats/causes/lifestyle/tobacco.

Caplan, P. (1997) *Food, Health and Identity: Glaswegian Punjabi Women's Thinking About Food*. Taylor and Francis, Routledge, London.

Census (2001) Office for National Statistics, London. www.ons.gov.uk/census/index.html.

Centres for Disease Control and Prevention (2007) Fact Sheet: Betel Quid with Tobacco.

Chetcuti, P., Sinha, S.H. & Levene, M.I. (1985) Birth size in Indian ethnic groups born in Britain. *Arch Dis Child*, 60, 868–70.

Chowdhury, T.A. & Hitman, G.A. (2007) Type 2 diabetes in people of South Asian origin: potential strategies for prevention. *Br J Diabetes Vasc Dis*, 7(6), 279–82.

Chowdhury, T.A., Grace, C. & Kopelman, P.G. (2003) Preventing diabetes in south Asians – Too little action and too late. *British Medical Journal*. 327, 1059–60.

Clements, M.R. & Fraser, R.D. (1988) Vitamin D supply to the rat fetus and neonate. *Journal of Clinical Investigation*, 81, 1768–73.

Coronary Heart Disease Statistics (2008) *Ethnic Differences in Mortality*. www.heartstats.org/publications.

Critchley J.A. & Unal, B. (2003). Health effects associated with smokeless tobacco: a systematic review. *Thorax*, 58(5), 435–43.

Department for Education and Skills (2002) *About Sure Start Children Centres*. www.surestart.gov.uk/about surestart.

Department of Health (1991) *Dietary Reference Values for Food Energy and Nutrients for the United Kingdom. Report of the Panel on Dietary Reference Values of the Committee on Medical Aspects of Food Policy*. Report on Health and Social Subjects 41. HMSO, London.

Department of Health (1997) *Infant Feeding in Asian Families: Early Practices and Growth*. HMSO, London.

Department of Health (1998) *Report of the Working Group on Diet and Cancer of the Committee on Medical Aspects of Food and Nutrition Policy. Nutritional Aspects of the Development of Cancer.* Report on Health and Social Subjects 48. The Stationery Office, London.

Department of Health (1999) *The Health Survey for England – The Health of Ethnic Minority Groups.* The Stationery Office, London.

Department of Health (1999) *Saving Lives: Our Healthier Nation.* The Stationery Office, London.

Department of Health (2001) *Health Survey for England: The Health of Minority Ethnic Groups '99.* The Stationery Office, London.

Department of Health (2004a) *At Least Five a Week: Evidence on the Impact of Physical Activity and its Relationship to Health. A Report from the Chief Medical Officer.* Department of Health Publications, London.

Department of Health (2004b) *Heart Disease and South Asians: Delivering the National Service Framework for Coronary Heart Disease.* Department of Health, London.

Department of Health (2004c) *The Health Survey for England – Health of Ethnic Minority.* Department of Health, London.

Department of Health (2004d) *Choosing Health: Making Healthier Choices Easier.* Department of Health, London.

Deurenberg-Yap, M., Schmid, T.G., Van Staveren, W.A. & Deurenberg, P. (2000) The paradox of low body mass index and high body fat percentage among Chinese, Malays and Indians in Singapore. *International Journal of Obesity and Related Metabolic Disorders,* 24, 1011–17.

Diabetes UK (2005) *Recommendations for the Provision of Services in Primary Care for People with Diabetes.* Diabetes UK, London.

Diabetes UK (2010) *Diabetes in the UK 2010: Key Statistics on Diabetes.* Diabetes UK, London.

Du, Y.X., Cha, Q. *et al.* (1996) An epidemiological study of risk factors for lung cancer in Guangzhou, China. *Lung Cancer,* 14(Suppl. 1), S9–S37.

Dudeja V., Misra A. *et al.* (2001) BMI does not accurately predict overweight in Asian Indians in northern India. *British Journal of Nutrition,* 86, 105–12.

Dyson, L., McFadden, A. *et al.* (2006) *Promotion of Breastfeeding Initiation and Duration: Evidence into Practice Briefing.* NICE Guidelines, 28–34.

Elkan, R., Avis, M. & Cox, K. (2007) The reported views and experiences of cancer service users from minority ethnic groups: a critical review of the literature. *Eur J Cancer Care,* 16(2), 109–21.

Firdous, R. & Bhopal, R.S. (1989) Reproductive health of Asian women: a comparative study with hospital and community perspectives. *Public Health,* 103, 307–15.

Fischbacher, C.M., Hunt, S. & Alexander, L. (2004) How physically active are South Asians in the United Kingdom? A literature review. *Journal of Public Health,* 26(3), 250–8.

Ford, J.A., Colhoun, E.M. *et al.* (1972) Rickets and osteomalacia in the Glasgow Pakistani community. *Archives of Disease in Childhood,* 51, 939–43.

Foster, G.D., Makris, A.P. & Bailer, B.A. (2005) Behavioural treatment of obesity. *American Journal of Clinical Nutrition,* 82(1 Suppl), 230S–235S.

Foster-Powell, K., Holt, S.H.A. & Brand-Miller, J.C. (2002) International table of glycemic index and glycemic load values. *American Journal of Clinical Nutrition,* 76(1), 5–56.

Fox, C. (2004) Heart Disease and South Asians: Delivering the National Service Framework for Coronary Heart Disease. Department of Health and British Heart Foundation, London. www.dh.gov.uk/en/Healthcare/NationalServiceFrameworks/Coronaryheartdisease/DH_4098644.

Fullerton, D.G., Bruce, N. & Stephen, B. (2008) Indoor air pollution from biomass fuel smoke is a major health concern in the developing world. *Trans R Soc Trop Med Hyg,* 102(9), 843–51.

Garaulet, M., Perez-Llamas, F., Zamora, S. & Tebar, F. (1999) Weight loss and possible reasons for dropping out of a dietary/behavioural programme in the treatment of overweight patients. *Journal of Human Nutrition and Dietetics.* 12(3), 219–27.

Garcia, M.J., McNamara, P.M. *et al.* (1974) Morbidity and mortality in diabetics in the Framingham population. Sixteen year follow up. *Diabetes,* 23, 105–11.

Garret, C.R., Treichel, C.J. & Ohmans, P. (1998) Barriers to health care for immigrants and non-immigrants: a comparative study. *Minn Medicine,* 81, 52–5.

Garrow, J.S. (2000) Obesity. In J.S. Garrow, W.P.T. James & A. Ralph, (eds.) *Human Nutrition and Dietetics.* 10th edition. Harcourt Medical, Chicago.

Gillman, M.W., Rifas-Shiman, S. *et al.* (2003). Maternal gestational diabetes, birth weight and adolescent obesity. *Paediatrics,* 111(3), 221–6.

Godson, J.H. & Williams, S.A. (1996) Oral health and health-related behaviours among three year old children born to first and second generation Pakistani mothers in Bradford, UK. *Community Dental Health,* 13(1), 27–33.

Gupta, P.C. & Ray, C.S. (2004) Epidemiology of betel quid usage. *Annals of the Academy of Medicine Singapore,* 33(Suppl), 31S–36S.

Gupta, P.C. & Ray, C.S. (2003) Smokeless tobacco and health in India and South Asia. *Respirology,* 8(4), 419–31.

Gupta, P.C., Hamner, J.E., III & Murti, P.R. (1992) *Control of Tobacco-Related Cancers and Other Diseases.* Proceedings of an international symposium, Bombay,

India: Tata Institute of Fundamental Research, Oxford University Press.

Gupta, P.C. & Warnakulasuriya, K.A. (2002) Global epidemiology of areca nut use. *Addict Biol*, 7, 77–83.

Hamid, F. & Sarwar, T. (2004) *Global Nutrition: A Multicultural Pack*. DH, London.

Harbottle, L. & Duggan, M.B. (1992) Comparative study of the dietary characteristics of Asian toddlers with iron deficiency in Sheffield. *Journal of Human Nutrition and Dietetics* 5, 351–61.

Hartley, D. (2003) *Breastfeeding Audit April 2002 to March 2003*. Sure Star Area (unpublished).

Hassan, K., Inam-ul-Haq, M. *et al.* (1992) Repeated pregnancies and early marriage are responsible for iron deficiency anaemia in the rural areas. *Journal of the Pakistan Institute of Medical Sciences*, 3, 140–4.

Hayat, T.K. (1997) Iron deficiency anaemia during pregnancy. *Journal of the College of Physicians and Surgeons Pakistan*, 17, 11–13.

Health Survey for England (1999) *The Health of Minority Ethnic Groups*. The Stationery Office, London.

Health Survey for England (2004) *The Health of Minority Ethnic Groups*. The Stationery Office, London.

Hernandez-Garduno, E., Brauer, M. & Perez-Neria, J.S. (2004) Wood smoke exposure and lung adenocarcinoma in non-smoking Mexican women. *Int. J. Tuberc. Lung Dis*, 8, 377–83.

Homans, H. (1983) A question of balance: Asian and British women's perception of food during pregnancy. In A. Murcott (ed.) *The Sociology of Food and Eating: Essays on the Sociological Significance of Food*, Gower, Aldershot.

Horsfall, A., Brook, G. *et al.* (2003) *Through Whose Eyes?* Bradford Teaching NHS Hospitals Trust, Bradford.

Hutchinson, H. (2001) Feeding problems in young children: report of three cases and review of the literature. *Journal of Human Nutrition and Dietetics*, 12(4), 337–43.

Ingram, J., Johnson, D. & Hamid, N. (2003). South Asian grandmothers' influence on breastfeeding in Bristol. *Midwifery*, 19, 318–27.

International Agency for Research on Cancer (2004) *Betel-Quid and Areca-Nut Chewing and Some Areca-Nut-Derived Nitrosamines*. Vol. 85. monographs.iarc.fr/ENG/Monographs/vol85/volume85.pdf.

Jakicic, J.M. & Otto, A.D. (2005) Physical activity considerations for the treatment and prevention of obesity. *American Journal of Clinical Nutrition*, 82(Suppl 1), 226S–229S.

James, J. & Underwood, A. (1997) Ethnic influences on the weaning diet in the UK. *Proceedings of the Nutrition Society*, 56, 121–30.

Jamrozik, K. (2005) Estimate of deaths attributable to passive smoking among UK adults: database analysis. *British Medical Journal*, 330(7495), 812.

Jang newspaper (February 2005) www.jang.com.pk.

Khan, A., Safdar, M. *et al.* (2003) Cinnamon improves glucose and lipids of people with type 2 diabetes. *Diabetes Care*, 26, 3215–18.

Kopelman, P.G. (ed.) (2001) Defining overweight and obesity. In *Management of Obesity and Related Disorders*. Martin Dunitz, London.

Kopelman, P.G. (ed.) (2001) An integrated approach to the management of overweight and obesity. In *Management of Obesity and Related Disorders*. Martin Dunitz, London.

Laing, P. (2002) Childhood obesity: a public health threat. *Paediatric Nursing*, 14(10), 14–16.

Lane, D.A., Lip, G.Y. & Beevers, D.G. (2007) Ethnic differences in cancer incidence and mortality: the Birmingham Factory Screening Project. *QJM*, 100(7), 423–31.

Laroia, N. & Sharma, D. (2006) The religious and cultural bases for breastfeeding practices among the Hindus. *Breastfeeding Medicine*, 1(2), 94–8.

Larsson, S.C. & Wolk, A. (2006) Meat consumption and risk of colorectal cancer: a meta-analysis of prospective Studies. *Int J Cancer*, 119(11), 2657–64.

Lees, S. & Papadopoulos, I. (2000) Cancer and men from minority ethnic groups: an exploration of the literature. *Eur J Cancer Care (Engl)*, 9(4), 221–9.

Lilly, R. (1995) The 1994 COMA report on 'weaning and the weaning diet': putting the theory into practice. *Professional Care Mother and Child*, 5, 41–5.

Lodge, N. (2001) The identified needs of ethnic minority groups with cancer within the community: a review of the literature. *Eur J Cancer Care (Engl)*, 10(4), 234–44.

London Health Observatory (2003) *Diversity Counts: Ethnic Health Intelligence in London: The Story So Far.* www.lho.org.uk/HIL/Ethnic_Health_Intelligence/Attachments/PDF_Files/Ethnic_Health_Intelligence_Report.pdf.

Lovegrove, J.A. (2007) CVD risk in South Asians: the importance of defining adiposity and influence of dietary polyunsaturated fat. Symposium: Nutrition Interventions in High-risk Groups. *Proceedings of the Nutrition Society*, 66, 286–98.

Margetts, B.M., Yusuf, M.S. *et al.* (2002) Persistence of lower birth weight in second generation South Asian babies born in the United Kingdom. *Journal of Epidemiology and Community Health*, 56, 684–7.

Marks, D.F, Murray, M., Evans, B. & Willig, C. (2004) Food and eating. In *Health Psychology; Theory, Research and Practice*. Sage, London.

Maryon-Davis, A., Giles, A. & Rona, R. (2000) *Tackling Obesity: A Toolbox for Local Partnership Action*. Faculty of Public Health Medicine of the Royal Colleges of Physicians of the United Kingdom, London.

Mather, H.M. & Keen, H. (1985) Southall Diabetes Survey: prevalence of known diabetes. *British Medical Journal*, 291, 1081–4.

Meddings, F. & Porter, J. (2007) Pakistani women: Feeding decisions: lecturers Fiona Meddings and Jan Poter of the division of midwifery and women's health at the School of Health Studies at the University of Bradford detail the difficulties faced by UK Pakistani women making informed choices in breastfeeding. *Royal College of Midwives Journal*, July–August.

Mela, D.J. & Rogers, P.J. (1998) *Food, Eating and Obesity – The Psychobiological Basis of Appetite and Weight Control.* Chapman and Hall, London.

Merseyside Regional Head and Neck Cancer Centre (2007) www.headandneckcancer.co.uk/showpage.asp?id=incidence&menu=2.

Misra, A., Vikram, N.K. *et al.* (2006) Waist circumference cutoff points and action levels for Asian Indians for identification of abdominal obesity. *International Journal of Obesity*, 30, 106–11.

Misra, A., Wasir, J.S. & Vikram, N.K. (2005) Waist circumference criteria for the diagnosis of abdominal obesity are not applicable uniformly to all populations and ethnic groups. *Nutrition*, 21, 969–76.

Mitra, A., Khoury, A. *et al.* (2004) Predictors of breastfeeding intention among low-income women. *Maternal and Child Health Journal*, 8(2), 65–70.

Moles, D.R., Fedele, S. *et al.* (2008) Oral and pharyngeal cancer in South Asians and non-South Asians in relation to socioeconomic deprivation in South East England. *British Journal of Cancer*, 98, 633–5.

.Mulvihill, C. & Quigley, R. (2003) *The Management of Obesity and Overweight – An Analysis of Reviews of Diet, Physical Activity and Behavioural Approaches.* Health Development Agency, www.hda.nhs.uk/evidence.

Nair, U., Bartsch, H. & Nair, J. (2004) Alert for an epidemic of oral cancer due to use of the betel quid substitutes gutkha and pan masala: a review of agents and causative mechanisms. *Mutagenesi*, 19(9), 251–62.

Nanan, D. & White, F. (1999) The National Health Survey of Pakistan. Review and discussion of report findings pertinent to selected risk factors for cardiovascular disease. *PCOR Digest*, 99, 6–11.

Nanan, D.J. (2002) The obesity pandemic – implications for Pakistan. *Journal of the Pakistan Medical Association*, 52(8), 342–6.

National Audit Office (2001) *Tackling Obesity in England.* The Stationery Office, London.

National Obesity Forum (2003) *Guidelines on the Management of Adult Obesity and Overweight in Primary Care.* www.nationalobesityforum.org.uk/NOF%20AdultGuidelines.pdf.

National Statistics (2002) *Minority Ethnic Groups in the UK.* London.

Northstone, K., Emmet, P., Nethersole, F. & ALSPAC Study Team, Avon Longitudinal Study of Pregnancy and Children (2001) The effect of age of introduction to lumpy solids on food eaten and reported feeding difficulties at 6 and 15 months. *Journal of Human Nutrition and Dietetics*, 14, 43–54.

Panesar, S.S., Gatrad, R. & Sheikh, A. (2008) Smokeless tobacco use by south Asian youth in the UK. *The Lancet*, 372(9633), 97–8.

Parsons, S., Godson, J.H.T., Williams, S.A. & Cade, J.E. (1999) Are there intergenerational differences in the diets of young children born to first and second generation Pakistani Muslims in Bradford, West Yorkshire, UK? *Journal of Human Nutrition and Dietetics*, 12(2), 113–22.

Pawa, M. (2005) Use of traditional/herbal remedies by Indo-Asian people with type 2 diabetes. *Practical Diabetes International*, 22(8), 292–4.

Perwiz, S. (2005) *An Exploration of the Barriers to Making Lifestyle Change Amongst Obese Pakistani Women Living in Redbridge.* MSc, Public Health with Health Promotion. School of Health Sciences, University of East London.

Phillips, C. (2005) Ethnic inequalities under new labour: progress or entrenchment? In J. Hills & K. Stewart (eds.) *A More Equal Society? New Labour, Poverty, Inequality and Exclusion.* Policy Press, Bristol.

Prentice, A.M. (1997) Obesity – the inevitable penalty of civilisation? 229–237 (In Finer, N. (ed.) *Obesity – A Series of Expert Reviews*). *British Medical Journal*, 53(2).

Prescott-Clarke, P. & Primatests, P. (1998) *Health Survey for England 1996.* The Stationery Office, London.

Rankin, J. & Bhopal, R. (2001) Understanding of heart disease and diabetes in a South Asian community: cross-sectional study testing the 'snowball' sample method. *Public Health*, 115, 253–60.

Ridler, C., Townsend, N. *et al.* (2009) *National Child Measurement Programme: Detailed Analysis of the 2007/08 National Dataset.* HM Government, London.

Riste, L., Khan, F. & Cruickshank, K. (2001) High prevalence of type 2 diabetes in all ethnic groups, including Europeans in a British inner city. Relative poverty, history, inactivity or 21st century Europe? *Diabetes Care*, 24, 1377–83.

Rogers, I.S., Ness, A.R. *et al.* (2006) Associations of size at birth and dual-energy X-ray absoptiometry measures of lean and fat mass at 9–10 years of age. *American Journal of Clinical Nutrition*, 84, 739–47.

Rowe, N. & Champion, R. (2000) *Sports Partnership and Ethnicity in England, National Survey 1999/2000 Headline Findings.* www.sportingequals.org.uk/Dynamic Content/Documents/BriefingPapers/Ethnic_minorities_physical_activity_and_health_bri(1).pdf.

Rozi, S., Akhtar, S. *et al.* (2005) Prevalence and factors associated with smoking among high school adolescent in Karachi, Pakistan, *Southeast Asian J Trop Med Public Health*, 36, 498–504.

Sarwar, T. (2002) Infant feeding practices of Pakistani mothers in England and Pakistan. *Journal of Human Nutrition and Dietetics*, 15(6), 419–28.

Sayeda, Z.N. & Rousham, E.K. (2008) Breast feeding and maternal mental well-being among Bangladeshi and Pakistani women in North-East England. *Public Health Nutrition*, 11, 486–92.

Scheppers, E., Dongen, E.V. *et al.* (2006) Potential barriers to the use of health services among ethnic minorities: a review. *Family Practice*, 23(3), 325–48.

Seidell, J.C., Kahn, H.S. *et al.* (2001) Report from Centers for Disease Control and Prevention. Workshop on use of adult anthropometry for public health and primary health care. *American Journal of Clinical Nutrition*, 73, 123–6.

Shah, M.A. (2004) Diabetes mellitus increasing at alarming rate. *The News*. 16 July.

Shah, S.M. Nanan, D. *et al.* (2004) Assessing obesity and overweight in a high mountain Pakistani population. *Tropical Medicine and International Health*, 9(4), 526–32.

Shahid, S.K., Williams, S.A., Malik, A. & Csikar, J.I. (2009) Parental control in caries prevention of young children of Pakistani and White origin: implications for oral health promotion – a pilot study. *International Journal of Health Promotion*, 43(1), 4–10.

Shaikh, S., James, D., Morrissey, J. & Patel, V. (2001) Diabetes care and Ramadan: to fast or not to fast? *The British Journal of Diabetes and Vascular Disease*, 1(1), 65–7.

Shamim, S. (2005) Weaning practices in peri-urban low socioeconomic groups. *Journal of the College of Physicians and Surgeons Pakistan*, 129–32.

Sharma, R.D., Sarkar, A. *et al.* (1996) Hypolipidaemic effect of fenugreek seeds: a chronic study in non-insulin dependent diabetic patients. *Phytotherapy Research*, 10(4), 332–4.

Sharma, S., Khan, N. *et al.* (2009) Vitamin D in pregnancy – time for action: a paediatric audit. *International Journal of Obstetrics and Gynaecology*, 116(12), 1678–82.

Shaw, A. (2000) *Kinship and Continuity. Pakistani Families in Britain*. Harwood Academic, Amsterdam.

Shaw, N.J. & Pal, B.R. (2002) Vitamin D deficiency in UK Asian families: activating a new concern, *Archives of Disease in Childhood*, 86, 147–9.

Speedy, A.W. (2003) Global production and consumption of animal source foods, *American Society for Nutritional Sciences*, 133, 4048S–4053S.

Staines, A., Hanif, S. *et al.* (1997) Incidence of insulin dependent diabetes mellitus in Karachi, Pakistan. *Archives of Disease in Childhood*, 76, 121–3.

Tanner, J.M. & Whitehouse, R.H. (1975) Revised standards for triceps and subscapular skinfolds in British children. *Archives of Disease in Childhood*, 50, 142–5.

Thomas, B. (2001) *Manual of Dietetic Practice*. 3rd edition. Blackwell Scientific, London.

Thomas, B. (2002) *Manual of Dietetic Practice*, eds. B. Thomas & J. Bishop. 4th edition. Blackwell Scientific, London.

Thomas, B. & Bishop, J. (2007) *Manual of Dietetic Practice*. 4th edition. Blackwell, Oxford.

Thomas, V.N., Saleem, T. & Abraham, R. (2005) Barriers to effective uptake of cancer screening among Black and minority ethnic groups. *Int J Palliat Nurs*, 11(11), 562, 564–71.

Vineis, P., Airoldi, L. *et al.* (2005) Environmental tobacco smoke and risk of respiratory cancer and chronic obstructive pulmonary disease in former smokers and never smokers in the EPIC prospective study. *British Medical Journal*, 330(7486), 277.

Vyas, A., Greenhalgh, A. *et al.* (2003) Nutrient intakes of an adult Pakistani, European and African-Caribbean community in inner city Britain. *Journal of Human Nutrition and Dietetics*, 16(5), 327–37.

Watt, R.G. (2000) A national survey of infant feeding in Asian families: summary of findings relevant to oral health. *British Dental Journal*, 188, 16–20.

WHO Expert Consultation (2004) Appropriate body-mass index for Asian populations and its implications for policy and intervention strategies. *The Lancet*, 363, 157–63.

Williams, S., Sahota, P. & Fairpoo, C.G. (1989) Infant feeding practices within white and Asian communities in inner city Leeds. *Journal of Human Nutrition and Dietetics*, 2, 325–38.

Winter, H., Cheng, K.K. *et al.* (1999) Cancer incidence in the south Asian population of England (1990–92). *Br J Cancer*, 79, 645–54.

World Health Organization (1998) *Obesity: Preventing and Managing the Global Epidemic. Report of WHO Consultation on Obesity*. World Health Organization, Geneva.

World Health Organization (2002) *The World Health Report: Reducing Risks to Health, Promoting Healthy Life*. World Health Organization, Geneva.

World Health Organization (2002) *Diet, Nutrition, and the Prevention of Chronic Disease: Report of a Joint WHO/ FAO Expert Consultation*. WHO Technical Report Series. World Health Organization/Food and Agriculture Organization, Geneva.

World Health Organization (2004) *Cancer: Diet and Physical Activity's Impact. Global Strategy on Diet, Physical Activity and Health*.

www.cdc.gov/tobacco/data_statistics/fact_sheets/smokeless/betel_quid.htm.

www.dh.gov.uk/en/PublicationsAndStatistics/PublishedSurvey/HealthSurveyForEngland/HealthSurveyResults/DH_4015530.

www.ic.nhs.uk/webfiles/publications/healthsur-vey2004ethnicfull/HealthSurveyforEngland210406_PDF.pdf.

www.statistics.gov.uk/pdfdir/meg1202.pdf.

www.who.int/dietphysicalactivity/publications/facts/cancer/en.

Bangladeshi Diet

Acheson, D. (1998) *Independent Inquiry into Inequalities in Health Report*. The Stationery Office, London.

Adams, C. (1994) *Across Seven Seas and Thirteen Rivers*. Eastside Books, London.

Aspinall, P.J. & Jacobson, B. (2004) *Ethnic Disparities in Health and Health Care: A Focused Review of the Evidence and Selected Examples of Good Practice*. www.lho.org.uk/Publications/Attachments/PDF_Files/Ethnic_Disparities_Report.pdf.

Balarajan, R., Bulusu, L., Adelstein, A.M. & Shukla, V. (1984) Patterns of mortality among migrants to England and Wales from the Indian Subcontinent. *British Medical Journal*, 289, 1185–7.

Balarajan, R. & Raleigh, V.S. (1995) *Ethnicity and Health in England*. HMSO, London.

Bose, K. (1992) NIDDM and obesity in Asians in the UK – scope for future studies. *Journal of the Royal Society of Health*, 112, 291–3.

Bose, K. (1995) A comparative study of generalised obesity and anatomical distribution of subcutaneous fat in adult White and Pakistani migrant males in Peterborough. *Journal of the Royal Society of Health*, 115, 90–5.

Bush, H.M., Anderson, A.S. et al. (1995) *Dietary Change in South Asian and Italian Women in the West of Scotland*. MRC Medical Sociology Unit Working Paper No. 54.

Cappuccio, F.P., Cook, D.G., Atkinson, R.W. & Strazullo, P. (1997) Prevalence, detection and management of cardiovascular risk factors in different ethnic groups in south London. *Heart*, 78, 555–63.

Census (2001) www.statistics.gov.uk/census2001/profiles/00bg.asp.

Erens, B., Primatesta, P. & Prior, G. (2001) *The Health Survey for England 1999. Volume 1: Findings. Volume 2: Methodology and Documentation*. The Stationery Office, London.

Fieldhouse, P. (1995) *Food and Nutrition. Customs and Culture*. Chapman and Hall, London.

Fox, C. (2004) Heart Disease and South Asians: Delivering the National Service Framework for Coronary Heart Disease. Department of Health and British Heart Foundation, London. www.dh.gov.uk/en/Healthcare/NationalServiceFrameworks/Coronaryheartdisease/DH_4098644.

Hamid, F. & Sarwar, T. (2004) *Global Nutrition: A Multicultural Pack*. DH, London.

Health Education Authority (1991) *Nutrition in the Ethnic Minority Groups: Asian and Afro-Caribbean in the UK*. Briefing papers. HEA, London.

Health Education Authority (1999) *The Health of Minority Ethnic Minority Ethnic Groups, Health Survey for England*. HEA, London.

Hillier, S. & Rahman, S. (1996) Childhood development: Bangladeshi parents in East London. In D. Kelleher & S. Hillier, *Researching Cultural Differences in Health*. Routledge, London.

Judd, P.A., Kassam-Khamis, T. & Thomas, J.E. (2000) *The Composition and Nutrient Content of Foods Commonly Consumed by South Asians in the UK*. Aga Khan Health Board.

Kassam-Khamis, T., Nanchahal, K. et al. (1999) Development of an interview administered food frequency questionnaire for use amongst women of South Asian ethnic origin in Britain. *Journal of Human Nutrition and Dietetics*, 12, 7–19.

Khan, G.B. (1982) *Al Dabh: Slaying Animals for Food the Islamic Way*. Islamic Medical Association, TaHa Publishers, London.

Knight, T.M., Smith, Z. et al. (1992) Insulin resistance, diabetes and risk markers for ischaemic heart disease in Asian men and non-Asian men in Bradford. *British Heart Journal*, 67, 343–50.

Landman, J. & Cruickshank, J.K. (2001) A review of ethnicity, health and nutrition-related diseases in relation to migration in the United Kingdom. *Public Health Nutrition*, 4(2B), 647–57.

Mather, H.M., Chaturvedi, N. & Kehely, A.M. (1995) Comparison of prevalence and risk factors for micro-albuminuria in South Asians and Europeans with type 2 diabetes mellitus. *Diabetic Medicine*, 15, 672–7.

McKeigue, P., Miller, G. & Marmot, M. (1989) Coronary heart disease in South Asians overseas: a review. *Journal of Clinical Epidemiology*, 42(7), 597–609.

McKeigue, P.M., Shah, B. & Marmot, H.G. (1991) Relation of central obesity and insulin resistance with high diabetes prevalence and cardiovascular risk in South Asians. *Lancet*, 337, 382–6.

Nazroo, J.Y. (1997) *The Health of Britain's Ethnic Minorities*. Policy Studies Institute, London.

Primatesta, P. & Brooks, M. (2001) Cardiovascular disease: prevalence and risk factors. In B. Erens, P. Primatesta & G. Prior, *Health Survey for England 1999. Volume 1: Findings*. The Stationery Office, London.

Raleigh, V.S. (1997) Diabetes and hypertension in Britain's ethnic minorities: implications for the future of renal services. *British Medical Journal*, 314, 209–13.

Rudat, K. (1994) *Black and Ethnic Groups in England: Health and Lifestyles*. Health Education Authority, London.

Smith, Z., Knight, T. *et al.* (1993) Dietary patterns in Asian and Caucasian men in Bradford: differences and implications in nutrition education. *Journal of Human Nutrition and Dietetics*, 6, 323–33.

The Tower Hamlets Partnership (2006) *Ward Data Report.* www.towerhamlets.gov.uk/data/discover/data/boroughprofile/downloads/ward-date-report/intro.pdf.

Thomas, B. (2001) *Manual of Dietetic Practice*. Blackwell, Oxford.

Thomas, J. (2002) Nutrition intervention in ethnic minority groups. *Proceedings of the Nutrition Society*, 61, 559–67.

Wild, S. & McKeigue, P. (1997) Cross-sectional analysis of mortality by country of birth in England and Wales, 1970–92. *British Medical Journal*, 314, 705–10.

Zannath, K. & Edholm, F. (2004) *Eating for a Healthy Life*. Camden Primary Care Trust, London.

Sri Lankan Diet

Abeywardena, M.Y. (2003) Dietary fats, carbohydrates and vascular disease: Sri Lankan perspectives. *Atherosclerosis*, 171(2), December, 157–61.

Amarasinghe, D.A.C.L., Fonseka, P., Fernando, D.J.S. & Dalpatadu, K.C.S. (2004) Risk factors for long-term complications in patients with type 2 diabetes in Sri Lanka. *Journal of the College of Community Physicians of Sri Lanka*, 9, 8–11.

Arambepola, C. & Fernando, D. (2005) Urban living and obesity. *Oxford Research Archive*, University of Oxford.

Census (2001) Office for National Statistics, London. www.ons.gov.uk/census/index.html.

Chowdhury, T. (2007) Type 2 Diabetes in People of South Asian Origin: Potential Strategies for Prevention. Department of Diabetic and Metabolic Medicine, Barts and London Centre for Diabetes.

FAO Nutrition Country Profiles (2004) *Sri Lanka*, 10 February. ftp.fao.org/es/esn/nutrition/ncp/SRLmap.pdf.

Fox, C. (2004) Heart Disease and South Asians: Delivering the National Service Framework for Coronary Heart Disease. Department of Health and British Heart Foundation, London. www.dh.gov.uk/en/Healthcare/NationalServiceFrameworks/Coronaryheartdisease/DH_4098644.

Glenday, K., Kumar, B.N., Tverdal, A. & Meyer, H.E. (2006) Cardiovascular disease risk factors among five major ethnic groups in Oslo, Norway: the Oslo Immigrant Health Study. *European Journal of Cardiovascular Prevention & Rehabilitation*, 13(3), June, 348–55.

Grulich, A.E., McCredie, M. & Coates, M. (1995) Cancer incidence in Asian migrants to New South Wales, Australia. *Br J Cancer*. 71(2), February, 400–8.

Hertzler, S., Washam, M. & Williams, J. (2007) Salacia oblonga extract reduces postprandial glycemia following a solid, high-starch meal. *The FASEB Journal*, 21, 832.

Hettiarachchi, P., Jiffry, M.T. *et al.* (2001) Glycaemic indices of different varieties of rice grown in Sri Lanka. *Ceylon Med J*, 46(1), March, 1–14.

www.who.int/ncd_surveillance/infobase/web/InfoBasePolicyMaker/reports/ReporterFullView.aspx?id=5.

Joshi, P., Islam, S. *et al.* (2007) Risk factors for early myocardial infarction in South Asians compared with individuals in other countries. *JAMA*, 297, 286–94.

Kumar, B.N., Meyer, H.E. *et al.* (2006) Ethnic differences in obesity among immigrants from developing countries, in Oslo, Norway. *International Journal of Obesity*, 30, 684–90.

Misra, A. & Vikram, N.K. (2002) Insulin resistance syndrome (metabolic syndrome) and Asian Indians. *Current Science*, 83(12), December.

Misra, A., Wasir, J.S. & Vikram, N.K. (2005) Waist circumference criteria for the diagnosis of abdominal obesity are not applicable uniformly to all populations and ethnic groups. *Nutrition*, 21(9), 969–76.

Perera, B., Fonseka, P., Ekanayake, R. & Lelwala E. (2005) Smoking in adults in Sri Lanka: prevalence and attitudes. *Asia Pac J Public Health*, 17(1), 40–5.

Pomerleau, J., McKeigue, P.M. & Chaturvedi, N. (1999) Factors associated with obesity in South Asian, Afro-Caribbean and European women. *International Journal of Obesity*, 23(1), January, 25–33.

Ramanujan, A. & Nestel, P. (2005) *Nutrition Country Profile: Sri Lanka*. FAO, UN, Geneva.

Rastogi, T., Vaz, M. *et al.* (2004) Physical activity and risk of coronary heart disease in India. *International Journal of Epidemiology*, 33(4), 759–67.

Smith, Z., Knight, T. *et al.* (1993) Dietary patterns in Asian and Caucasian men in Bradford; differences and implications for nutrition education. *Journal of Human Nutrition and Dietetics*, 6, 323–33.

Soysa, P. (1988) *The United Nations University Press Food and Nutrition Bulletin*, 10(1), March.

Sriskandarajah, D (2002) The migration–development nexus: Sri Lanka case study. *International Migration*, 40(5), 283–307.

Sriskantharajah, J. & Kai, J. (2007) Promoting physical activity among South Asian women with coronary heart disease and diabetes: what might help family practice. *Family Practitioner*, 24(1), 71–6.

Trivedy, C.R., Craig, G. & Warnakulasuriya, S. (2002) The oral health consequences of chewing areca nut. *Addict Biol*, 7(1), January, 115–25.

Vikram, N.K., Mohan, P.R., *et al.* (2003) Non-obese (body mass index $< 25\,kg/m^2$) Asian Indians with normal waist circumference have high cardiovascular risk. *Nutrition*, 19(6), 503–9.

Wandel, M., Gunawardena, P., Oshaug, A. & Wandel, N. (1984) Heating and cooling foods in relation to food habits in a southern Sri Lanka community. *Ecology of Food and Nutrition*, 14(2), 93–104.

Wickramasinghe, V.P., Cleghorn, G.J., Edmiston, K.A. & Davies, P.S.W. (2005) Impact of ethnicity upon body composition assessment in Sri Lankan Australian children. *Journal of Paediatrics and Child Health*, 41(3), March, 101–6.

Wijesuriya, M.A. (1997) Prevalence of diabetes in Sri Lanka. *International Journal of Diabetes in Developing Countries*, 17, 1–4.

2 West Indies

2.1 African-Caribbean Diet

Lorraine Bailey, Auline Cudjoe, Mandy Fraser,
Rose Jackson, Natalie Sutherland, Deborah Thompson

2.1.1 Introduction

African-Caribbean and Afro-Caribbean are inter-changeable terms used to describe people of African ancestry who are natives or inhabitants of the Caribbean (Lieback & Pollard, 2000). African-Caribbean people are primarily the descendants of West Africans. The Caribbean is situated in the region of the Americas, and incorporates the Caribbean Sea, its islands and the mainland surrounding it. The area consists of 30 countries, with an estimated population of 3 million distributed over 5,180 km^2 (Hamid & Sarwar, 2004) Figure 2.1.

History

The Arawak, Carib and Taino Indians were the first inhabitants of the Caribbean islands followed by approximately 10 million Africans. They were shipped by slave traders to work on the plantations of British, French, Spanish and Portuguese colonies during the 16th century. The main crops produced were sugar cane, bananas, cocoa, nutmeg, citrus fruits, cotton and rice (Hamid & Sarwar, 2004). European colonization caused the outbreak of war and consequently the depopulation of the natives (Bygott, 1996). Following the abolition of slavery in 1848 the Europeans sought indentured labour from India, China and Portugal.

Migration to the United Kingdom

There is some evidence of migration from the Caribbean to the UK as early as the 18th century. Small communities settled in the port cities of Cardiff, Liverpool and South Shields around the mid-19th century (Chambré-Hardman Archive, 2006). Migration from the Caribbean to Britain was rare prior to the Second World War, however owing to labour shortages after the war, the British government encouraged mass immigration from the British Empire and Commonwealth. The '*Windrush* generation' of 1948 marks the period when the first group of African-Caribbeans arrived in the UK (Grosvenor & Chapman, 1982). Most were recruited by British Rail, the National Health Service and London Transport (Philips & Philips, 1998).

Current UK population

In the UK census of 2001 approximately 566,600 individuals considered themselves to be black Caribbeans, equating to 1% of the total UK population.

Multicultural Handbook of Food, Nutrition and Dietetics, First Edition. Edited by Aruna Thaker, Arlene Barton.
© 2012 Blackwell Publishing Ltd. Published 2012 by Blackwell Publishing Ltd.

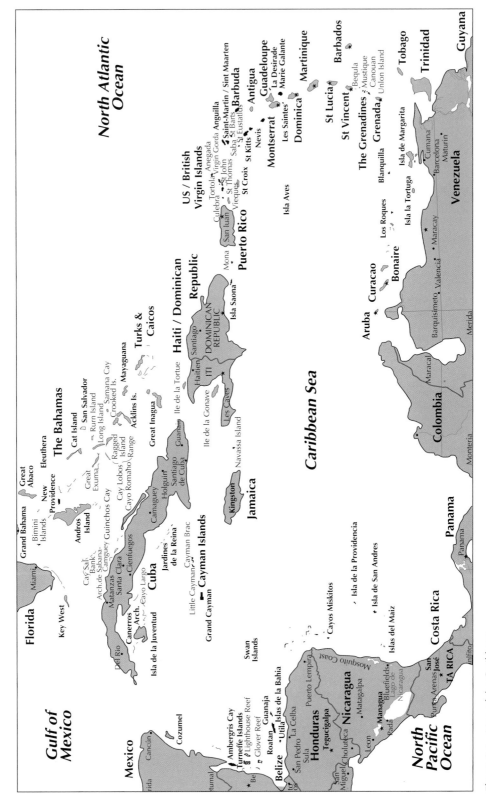

Figure 2.1   Map of the Caribbean

This does not take into account individuals who described themselves as mixed race, with one parent of African-Caribbean origin. The estimated figure in 2008 had risen to approximately 750,000, 1.3% of the British population (www.statistics.gov. uk). African-Caribbean communities exist throughout the UK, however the majority (61%) live in London with sizeable populations in the West Midlands – Birmingham, in particular. Smaller communities live in the South East, Yorkshire and Humberside.

2.1.2   Religion

Christianity is the main religion practised by African-Caribbeans, the largest denominations being Seventh Day Adventism and Pentecostalism.

Religious dietary restrictions

There does not appear to be any specific dietary practice associated with Christianity which impacts on nutritional status. However, some individuals may practise fasting.

Seventh Day Adventists and Pentecostals are encouraged to eat foods which are of natural origin (Bygott, 1996; Hamid & Sarwar, 2004). Eating habits are based on achieving optimum health. Some dietary restrictions exist, such as abstaining from pork and fish (without scales) as they are considered unclean. Alcohol and caffeine are prohibited and high intakes of sugar and salt are discouraged (Thomas & Bishop, 2007).

Within Rastafarianism a number of dietary practices are followed, foods described as *ital* (in their original state) are eaten. The degree of dietary restriction is dependent on the individual. Some are lacto-ovo-vegetarians, while others are vegans (Hamid & Sarwar, 2004). Individuals following a strict vegan diet are at risk of protein deficiency and possibly micronutrient deficiencies (Webster-Gandy et al., 2006).

2.1.3   Traditional diet and eating patterns

African-Caribbean diets have evolved through the influence of the original inhabitants and a combination of the dietary traditions and cuisines of migrant workers from Africa, India, China and Europe. The immigrant population combined their own traditional foods with those found on the islands. It has been suggested that the barbecue originated from the Arawaks, derived from the term *barbacoa*, a method for cooking meat slowly over of thin green wood strips. The Carib Indians flavoured their food with hot pepper and citrus juices and practised one-pot cooking. The Africans combined traditional foods with staples found on the islands. The arrival of Indian and Chinese labourers introduced curried meat and rice (Thompkins, 2008). The diet of older African-Caribbean tends to be more nutrient-dense as they usually to eat traditional foods (Sharma et al., 1999; Harding et al., 2007). This has resulted in a diet high in complex carbohydrates, fruit and vegetables and relatively low in fat, which meets current healthy eating guidelines.

There is a wide variety of dietary and food preparation practices among African-Caribbeans. However, in general, the basis of the Caribbean diet is starchy staples (rice, pasta) and starchy root vegetables (potatoes, plantain, yams), which are often used as a side dish, and various cuts of meat (fish, salt fish, chicken, pork, goat, lamb and salt beef), stewed, curried or grilled. Traditional drinks are also very popular, mostly natural or home-made, with sugar added to taste. These include mauby, sea moss, tamarind juice, mango juice, coconut milk, coconut water, ginger beer, soursop juice and guava juice. Flavoured beers and malt drinks are also popular with African-Caribbeans of all ages.

Fruits, vegetables and pulses are usually added to mixed and composite dishes. Fruits are often chopped or mixed with other ingredients or foods such as a mixed fruit salad, fruit-dense cake, 'Caribbean fruit cake', fruit pies and blended juices. Vegetables, lentils or pulses are usually added to composite dishes (i.e., pumpkin or callaloo soup), curries, sweet potato pie and side-dishes such as rice and peas. One-pot dishes in which starchy vegetables, such as cassava, dasheen, green bananas and breadfruit, are added to a highly flavoured soup base, are commonly consumed. The main features of the cuisine of African-Caribbean populations are summarized in (see Table 2.1).

Herbs and spices

Different types of seasonings are used in most dishes. The main seasonings are black and white

Table 2.1 Traditional African-Caribbean foods

	Encourage	Discourage
Bread, rice, potatoes, pasta and other starchy foods	Traditional foods: Rice, corn and cornmeal, oats and wheat-based foods (hard dough bread, dumpling), starchy fruits (green bananas, plantain, breadfruit), roots and tubers (cassava, yam, sweet potato), dasheen, coco yam (usually peeled and boiled like potatoes or mashed, creamed, baked, roasted or fried) Cooking tips: Preferred preparation methods include grilling, boiling, poaching, baking, braising, and stewing	Adding too much salt during preparation or at the table. Frying foods, keep to a minimum Adding butter, especially to wheat-based foods
Vegetables and fruits Eat at least five portions a day of a variety of vegetables and fruit each day. Fresh, frozen, tinned and dried fruit and vegetables	Traditional foods: Vegetables: callaloo (spinach), kale, peppers, karela and carrots (which are often used in soups, stews and one-pot meals) Other vegetables and fruit include sweetcorn, okra, cabbage, aubergine, pumpkin, tomato, ugu, chocho (christophene), green leaf, okazi, pineapple, guava, banana, pawpaw, mango, melon, strawberries, lime, apple, pear, orange	Caramelizing and adding sugar and cream to fruit preparations Adding salt and butter when cooking vegetables
Milk and dairy foods Dairy foods are nutrient rich and important for good health and at least three portions a day may be consumed	Traditional foods: Cheese, milk, yoghurt, fromage frais	Condensed and evaporated milks are usually high in sugar and fat. Choose reduced fat and sugar or lighter versions. Creamed coconut, as it is high in saturated fat so use it sparingly
Meat, fish, eggs, beans, nuts and seeds	Traditional foods: Snapper, red bream, red mullet, mackerel, herring, kippers, salmon and canned fish, as well as salted fish Egg, chicken, pork, lamb, Peas (black-eyed peas, gongo peas) and beans (kidney beans, butter beans) are commonly cooked with rice and coconut milk (rice 'n' peas) or added to stews and one-pot meals. Eat fish more often: grill, bake, steam or microwave rather than deep-frying Cooking tip: Use less salt in cooking and try not to add salt at the table. Eat fewer salty foods bacon, ham, cheese corned beef, crisps, salted nuts and packet soups	Salt fish, khobi, stockfish, salted mackerel, salt beef, salted pig's tail. If eaten they should be soaked before cooking to remove some salt. All-purpose seasonings as have salt in them Fatty meats. Visible fats from meat should be removed before cooking and after cooking some meats, excess fat should be drained off Skim the fat from the soups and stews after cooking
Fat- and sugar-rich foods	Fruit cakes, coconut-based sweets, biscuits, pastries Traditionally, rich beverages are served as drinks at meal times (e.g., *lassi*, sugary drinks) Cooking tip: Buy tinned fruit in natural juice rather than in syrup	Consumption in excess or find fruit or reduced-calorie cereal-based alternative
Other	Unsaturated oils (corn, sunflower, soya, rapeseed and olive oil) are better choices in small amounts Cooking tip: If using oil, measure the amount with a tablespoon and try to cut down gradually. Hot sauces or hot peppers may be used at the table instead of salt.	Palm and coconut oils which are high in saturated fats and should be used only occasionally

pepper, coriander, paprika, dried onions, chillies and garlic. These are usually a grounded pre-mix or all-purpose seasoning, which tends to be high in salt. Although these pre-mixes may be added sparingly, adding extra fresh or dried herbs and spices offers the flexibility not to add it at all or add it sparingly. Sweet dishes are often seasoned with vanilla essence, and nutmeg and mixed spices are added for flavour which allows for less sugar to be added.

Some foods are heavily salted as a means of preservation in hot climates, however salt added sparingly is perceived to reduce tastiness and unseasoned dishes or meals are viewed as poor cooking skills. Therefore traditional Caribbean dishes (e.g., ackee and saltfish) tend to be high in sodium.

Dietary supplements and natural remedies

More people are turning to alternative dietary therapies which often have little formal scientific basis and may be based on traditional folk medicine. Self-selected supplements or alternative therapies allow people to play a more active role in their health management. Historically, herbs and spices have enjoyed a rich tradition for their flavour enhancement characteristics and for their medicinal properties which present intriguing possibilities for health promotion due to their antioxidant content or laxative properties (Dragland, 2003; Kaefer & Milner, 2008).

Migration studies have identified some of the reasons for this change. First, African-Caribbean people appear to be altering their dietary habits and adopting the practices of the host country (Sharma et al., 1999). In recent decades a shift towards a less nutrient-dense diet has emerged (Sharma et al., 2008) (see Tables 2.2 and 2.3).

2.1.4   Healthy Eating

In recent years the proportion of African-Caribbean people with hyperglycaemia, hypertension and hyperlipidaemia has increased (DH, 2004). Migration, globalization and a complex interaction with the environment have resulted in changes in lifestyles, characterized by increased smoking, overweight and obesity, decreased exercise and changes in dietary habits to foods which are high in salt, fats and sugar, all of which may be contrib-

uting to the increase in chronic diseases such type 2 diabetes and cardiovascular diseases such as stroke and coronary heart disease (Aspinall & Jacobson, 2004). African-Caribbean people with hypertension have an increased risk of stroke and are at greater risk than their White counterparts (Cappuccio et al., 1997). While addressing healthier eating is essential in health promotion, it can be achieved by consuming a balance of traditional foods and dishes as well as healthy modern influences of the host country.

Most traditional African-Caribbean dishes and food choices are compatible with guidelines for healthy eating and many African-Caribbean people have maintained cultural food preferences. With the increased availability of popular Caribbean foods in some major supermarkets, the option to maintain a healthier traditional diet is possible. Nevertheless, second-generation African-Caribbean people tend to consume a westernized diet and fewer traditional foods (Millet et al., 2008).

The diet, whether micronutrient-dense, varied or unbalanced, may have an impact on health for better or worse, but cultural and lifestyle factors (i.e., physical inactivity, excess alcohol and poor preservation practices) may also play a role in the health outcomes of African-Caribbean people. Generally, the traditional African-Caribbean diet is higher in vegetables and fruit than the diet of the general population and as a result generally has less total and saturated fat compared with diet of younger UK-born African-Caribbean people (Sharma et al., 1999; DH, 2004) (See Figure 2.2). The diets of African-Caribbeans were also found to be higher in salt than those of the general population (DH, 2004) and African-Caribbean men were more likely to add more salt to foods during cooking than African-Caribbean women and Caucasian men and women (see Figure 2.3).

Cross-sectional and cohort studies suggest that diets rich in fruit and vegetables as well as starchy carbohydrates may protect against cardiovascular disease and some cancers (Steinmetz & Potter, 1991; Dauchet et al., 2006). For example, a cardio-protective ('Mediterranean') diet, characterized as a diet rich in vegetables, legumes, fruits, nuts, cereals and fish, has been long associated with good health (Knoops et al., 2004), however no single food group can be claimed to be responsible for the low rates of heart disease and cancers

Table 2.2　Traditional African-Caribbean eating pattern and dietary changes on migration

Meal	Traditional meal	Dietary changes on migration to the UK	Healthier alternatives
Breakfast	Saltfish with fried or baked dumplings Ackee and saltfish with fried or boiled banana Hard dough bread and tea Porridge: Cornmeal or porridge oats	Bread or toast Tea or coffee with (evaporated milk) Porridge: corn meal or oats, breakfast cereal with milk. Saltfish with fried or baked dumplings	Select high-fibre cereal and use semi- skimmed milk Try an artificial sweetener instead of sugar Baked dumpling instead of fried Low-fat dairy products
Lunch	Bulla cake, bun pattie or *roti* Rice with cabbage/saltfish Small version of main meal	Sandwiches Takeaways: chicken and chips, pizza, etc.	Select sandwiches or bread-based snacks Add fruit to very low-fat yoghurt
Evening meal (main meal)	Yam, sweet, potato Fish (steamed/fried) or curried meat Pea soup Gunga/red peas/oxtail soup with vegetables Rice and peas with chicken	Rice with chicken/meat curry/fish Vegetables Rice and peas with chicken Chicken/meat/fish Potatoes: boiled/roast/mashed Vegetables	Always include vegetables Select boiled potato, yam, green banana or jacket potato Measure oil and use sparingly
Puddings/ Desserts	Fruit, sweet potato pudding, banana fritters, baked custard	Cake, pudding	Fruit/low-calorie yoghurt
Snacks	Nuts, fruit	Nuts, crisps, biscuits, fruit, crackers and cheese, pattie, buns, cake, bread	Select fruit as the main snack Bread buns and plain cakes only occasionally Avoid eating nuts, crisp, biscuit regularly
Drinks	Lime juice, carrot juice, home-made lemonade Herbal teas, milk	Fizzy drinks, fruit juice Nutriment/Nourishment. Supermalt Punch, juice drinks, Ribena Horlicks, Milo, drinking chocolate	Unsweetened juices and diluted with water Sugar-free fizzy drinks or squashes Low-fat milks and artificial sweeteners for drinks such as Milo/drinking chocolate Avoid Nutriment/ Nourishment Punches can be made with low-fat milk and sweeteners

Table 2.3 Glossary of common African-Caribbean foods

Starchy foods

Bread fruit	Round fruit with green rough skin. Boiled or roasted. Can be sliced thinly and fried
Coo-Coo (Eddoe, Wangoo)	Caribbean equivalent to polenta, made exclusively from cornmeal which can be baked, fried or rolled into balls and poached in soups or stews
Cornmeal	Maize flour, used in many fried snacks or used in making dumplings
Dasheen (taro root)	Known as coco or taro, a starchy tuber usually served boiled or added to soups as a thickener
Dumplings	Made from flour and water and/or suet seasoned and poached separately or added to soup. Fried dumplings are made as above but with cornmeal added
Green banana	Fruit, usually boiled or steamed as too hard to be eaten raw
Plantain	Banana family fruit but generally regarded as a vegetable. Inedible raw, usually served as appetizer or starch dishes, boiled or fried
Bammy (cassava bread)	White flat and round, made from grated cassava. Mostly fried and served with fish
Farina	Porridge made from grated cassava
Yam	Similar in size and colour to potato but nuttier flavour. Served boiled, mashed or baked
Cassava	Long tuberous root, baked or boiled
Sweet potato	Starchy tubers, red or purple outer skin with a yellow or white centre. Boiled or baked
Tannia	A tuberous root vegetable similar to coco but larger
Hard dough bread	Made with enriched wholegrain flour
Foo-foo	Pounded plantain generally made into a savoury dish
Roti	Flat bread made from flour and split peas

Vegetables and fruit

Ackee	A bright red fruit of the Caribbean tree Blighia sapida
Christophene (*cho-cho*)	A small light-green or cream, pear-shaped vegetable
Avocado pear	Sometimes eaten with a sprinkling salt
Guava	Sweet fruit eaten fresh or made into jam
Jackfruit	Large oval fruit
Mango	Red or green smooth skin with sweet yellow flesh. Generally eaten whole, or made into jams, used in salads and added to fruit punch
Ortanique	Similar to tangerines in taste but much sweeter, larger and juicer
Paw-paw	Oblong, melon-like fruit. Thick yellow/orange flesh with black seeds. Green paw-paw is used as a vegetable
Callaloo (dasheen leaves)	Green vegetable like spinach but smaller leaves. Steamed with onions, garlic, peppers and butter. Served with salted cod and fried dumplings
Okra (ladies' fingers)	Green vegetable boiled and added to stews
Pakchoi	Dark-green leafy vegetable with a white stalk
Pumpkin	Boiled in soups, meat stews or served as a vegetable after steaming with butter
Sweetcorn	Boiled or roasted and often grated to make porridge, pudding or cakes

Meat, fish and offal

Conch	A shellfish usually fried or boiled
Escoveitched fish (fish with scales stripped off)	Mullet, bream, jack fish, red snapper fried and seasoned with spring onions, peppers, vinegar, salt and garlic
Cow's foot, goat, tripe, oxtail	Highly seasoned then, depending on the meat, roasted, fried, grilled boiled, braised or barbecued
Saltfish (salted dried cod)	Prepared by soaking in water to remove salt and soften then shredded and fried with onions, tomatoes and spices

(Continued)

Table 2.3 (*cont'd*)

Beans and pulses

Gungo (pigeon peas), black-eyed beans, cow-peas, adzuki and kidney beans	These are used in rice and peas or made into soups or stews
Broad beans, chickpeas (*channa*), lentils, mung beans and split peas	All used in meat stews

Dairy products

Evaporated milk and condensed milk	Used in hot and cold drinks, punches, puddings, cakes and cornmeal porridge
Coconut cream	High saturated fat used in the making of rice and peas
Corn oil	Used in frying and often reused
Hot beverages	
Bush tea (cerassee/carella)	Bitter-tasting infusion
Peppermint	Infused, added sugar is optional
Milo, Bournvita, Horlicks, Ovaltine, malted hot drinks	Made with evaporated, condensed or cow's milk with sugar

Cold beverages

Squash, cordials	Ribena, Vimto, Sarsaparilla mixed with water or used in punches
Nutriment/Nourishment	Used in punches and given to convalescents
Supermalt/Mighty Malt	Malt drink high in sugar and carbohydrate mixed with condensed milk. Light varieties now available
Egg punch	Made with raw eggs, Guinness, condensed milk and nutmeg, considered a very nutritious drink or tonic
Irish moss	Rich drink made from seaweed, linseed, condensed milk and sugar
Sorrel	Wine-coloured, sweet-tasting fruit, made into a drink with ginger, sugar, cinnamon and lime juice
Mauby	Bitter bark made into a drink and sweetened with sugar
Soursop	White flesh of this fruit is squeezed and blended into a punch with condensed milk, nutmeg, water and alcohol optional

Puddings and cakes

Bulla	Flat small circular cake made from flour, cinnamon, nutmeg, butter and milk, eaten with or without cheese
Bun	Sweet bread-like mixture with raisins and glacé cherries. Can be round or square, eaten with cheese throughout the day
Coconut grater cakes (sugar cakes/gizzarda)	Grated coconut, sugar and water boiled and allowed to harden and cut into squares. Eaten as a snack
Coconut drops	Dried coconut squares are boiled with ginger into a toffee-like mixture, allowed to harden and then eaten as a snack
Pone	Can be sweet or savoury. Made from cornmeal flour, sugar, butter, cow's or condensed milk, sultanas and spices. The sweet variety is made with an addition of coconut or ripe bananas or raisins, grated cassava or sweet potato is used in the savoury variety
Fritters	Self-raising dumpling mixture with either banana or flaked saltfish and onions and fried
Pattie	Oval-shaped savoury pastry filled with spicy minced beef. Vegetarian varieties are filled with or fish, ackee, callaloo

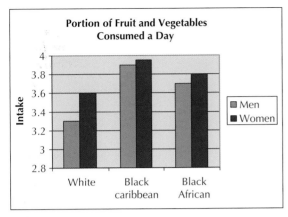

Figure 2.2   Comparison of portions of fruit and vegetables consumed by men and women (adapted from Department of Health, *Health Survey for England*, 2004, Health of Ethnic Minorities)

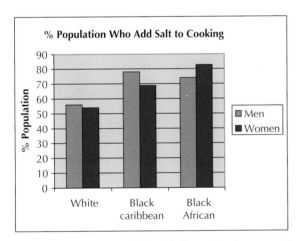

Figure 2.3   Comparison of salt added to cooking by men and women (adapted from Department of Health, *Health Survey for England*, 2004, Health of Ethnic Minorities)

or longer life expectancy observed among some populations.

Eight tips for healthier Choices

- Enjoy your food.
- Eat plenty fruit and vegetables.
- Eat a variety of foods.
- Don't eat too many foods containing a lot of fat.
- Eat the right amount to be a healthy weight.
- Don't have sugary food and drink too often.
- Eat plenty of foods rich in starch and fibre.
- If you drink alcohol, do so sensibly.

(FSA, 2005)

Dietary fibre

Eating a diet high in fibre may protect against risk factors associated with cardiovascular disease (CVD). Increasing the amount of wholegrain varieties of starchy foods (e.g., whole meal bread, wholegrain breakfast cereals, brown rice and wholegrain pasta) should be encouraged, as well as vegetables and fruit for sources of dietary fibre and health-promoting phytochemicals, essential vitamins and minerals and also antioxidants (Slavina, 2003).

Omega 3 fatty acids

Omega 3 fatty acids are now considered an important protective dietary measure against CVD, principally due to their anti-inflammatory and anti-thrombogenic properties. Major sources of omega 3 fatty acids are found in oily fish, rapeseed and linseed oil. Dietary recommendations are to consume 1–2 portions of oily fish a week for the general population and especially those at increased risk (0.2 g/day of omega 3 fatty acids) (ONS, 1991).

Evidence of good practice

Interventions to promote and encourage healthy eating need reliable baseline data on dietary habits, however this information is generally lacking for people in ethnic groups. Ethnic group participation rates are relatively small in national food consumption surveys, and analyses based on these surveys may not be reliable due to low subject participation. The overarching health promotion goal is to increase the quality and years of healthy life and eliminate health disparities between the Caucasian and minority populations.

Suggestions for the way forward

Lifestyle is a major factor in the development of disease and there is great potential to modify the environmental factors. Much of this is back to basics, with an emphasis on a balanced healthy diet which is low in sodium (salt), reducing the number of processed meals consumed and increasing the amount of wholegrain foods, cereals, fruit and vegetables in the diet. Other lifestyle measures include achieving a healthy weight, avoiding excessive alcohol intake and stopping smoking.

2.1.5   Obesity

Key points

- African-Caribbean women have higher levels of obesity than the general UK population.
- Encourage physical activity alongside dietary modifications.
- Promote traditional African-Caribbean foods such as fruit and vegetables, complex carbohydrates, fish and pulses, with modified cooking methods to reduce fat content.
- Weight-loss strategies specific to the African-Caribbean community need to be implemented.

Introduction

Research has identified that lower levels of chronic disease exist among indigenous populations compared to those of migrants (Harding *et al.*, 2008) and urbanization in the Caribbean may also be having a negative impact on the traditional diet and lifestyle patterns (Sharma *et al.*, 1999). Health surveys and cohort and comparison studies have repeatedly highlighted the increased risk of the chronic conditions of this ethnic group. The prevalence of chronic disease among individuals in the UK and the Caribbean exceeds that of Europeans (Abbotts *et al.*, 2004; Harding *et al.*, 2007; Sharma *et al.*, 2008) and this is an upward trend. Obesity, cardiovascular disease and diabetes are becoming the leading causes of death in the eastern Caribbean countries of St Vincent and the Grenadines, St Lucia, Grenada and Dominica (Albert, 2007). Other findings suggest that ethnic groups living in the UK are more likely to engage in poor dietary patterns and were also more susceptible to developing these conditions (Harding *et al.*, 2008). Modifiable factors such as smoking and inactivity are also contributing to the development of chronic disease (Pomerleau *et al.*, 1999).

High rates of obesity are also found in the Caribbean. In recent years there has been a marked increase among Caribbean populations (Sharma *et al.*, 2008). Approximately, 50% of the adult population are overweight, and 25% of adult Caribbean women are obese.

Prevalence

Levels of obesity are increasing throughout the world. It is a major problem in the Caribbean population. The findings of studies investigating the ethnic differences in overweight and obese adolescents are consistent with those in adults. Black girls in the UK, particularly those of Caribbean descent, were more likely to be overweight or obese than White UK girls. Contributory factors included being born in the UK and practising unhealthy dietary habits (DASH Study; Viner *et al.*, 2006; Harding *et al.*, 2007). This trend is also seen in the UK's Caribbean population with the Health Survey for England (2006) showing 32% of woman and 25% of men of Caribbean descent classified as obese as defined by the WHO classifications (BMI >30 kg/m^2) (see Tables 2.4 and 2.5). This compares to the national UK average for obesity of 24% for both men and women (HSE, 2004). As expected, the prevalence of obesity-related health disorders (e.g., CHD, type 2 diabetes and stroke) are also high among this population group.

Aetiology

The simplest description of obesity is an excess storage of fat in the body resulting from a positive

Table 2.4   The WHO classification for overweight and obesity

Classification	BMI (kg/m^2)	Risk of co-morbidity
Underweight	<18.5	Low
Healthy range	18.5–4.9	Average
Overweight	>25	
Pre-Obese	25–29	Increased
Obese class I	30–34.9	Moderate
Obese class II	35–39.9	Severe
Obese class III	>40	Very severe

(WHO 1998)

Table 2.5 Waist circumference cut-off points

	Increased risk	Substantially increased risk
Men	≥94 cm (≈37 inches)	≥102 cm (≈40 inches)
Women	≥80 cm (≈32 inches)	≥88 cm (≈35 inches)

(WHO 1998)

energy balance. While obesity can be the result of conditions such as Prader Willi or Bardet-Biedl syndrome, it is more likely to be caused by a combination of factors, including genetics, metabolic defects, behaviour and the environment.

Genetics and metabolic defects

The role of genetics in the development of obesity is much debated among all population groups. Numerous genes are involved in the control of appetite, satiety and energy expenditure and this is an ongoing area of research. At present the actual influence of genes on obesity is weak. A recent study looking specifically at the insulin-induced gene 2 transcriptions found that it had only a limited association with increased BMI (Smith et al., 2007).

Studies which specifically looked at defects in the *ob* gene and leptin found no differences in leptin levels between different ethnic groups even when adjusted for gender and BMI (Widjaja et al., 1997).

However, there is clearly a genetic susceptibility for excess weight gain in the African-Caribbean population, though whether this is a result of the exposure of this genetic profile to affluence and apathy is unclear and warrants further investigation.

Behaviour and environment

Inactivity and poor food choices will rapidly result in excess weight gain. In the West food intake is often governed by personal preference rather than a need to eat specific foods due to reduced availability. Traditional high-energy foods (e.g., sweetbreads, banana chips and sugary cakes), which in the past would have been made at home, are now mass-produced and easily available in shops, so

providing more opportunity for high energy input without the energy cost expended during food preparation.

Dietary modification in weight management

The first-line treatment for obesity is dietary and lifestyle change. Clients should be encouraged to reduce total fat, and sugary food and drink intakes. Particular emphasis should be placed on portion control of starchy foods, which are the main component of traditional West Indian diets.

Visual aids (e.g., pictures of portions), kitchen scales and household measures, should be used to help clients turn advice into practice. Reinforcement that traditional starchy foods such as plantain, rice, cassava, yam and breadfruit are healthy options should be given, with particular attention paid to cooking methods in order to maintain the lowest glycaemic factor of the starchy food. Clients should be encouraged to avoid frying and adding excess oil during cooking. Traditional herbs and spices should be promoted, and salt discouraged.

Physical activity

Regular exercise should be encouraged. The Department of Health recommendation of 30 minutes of moderate-intensity activity five days a week should be promoted along with all diet therapies (DH, 2004).

Anti-obesity drugs

Second-line treatments include anti-obesity drugs and bariatric surgery. As with the rest of the population, drug therapies should only be used when other dietary, exercise and behavioural methods have been explored (NICE CG43, 2006). There are currently two drugs licensed for the treatment of obesity in the UK: orlistat (Xenical) and sibutramine (Reductil). These are typically used separately, although there have been cases when they have been used in combination. This is not advocated by NICE.

2.1.6 Diabetes

Introduction

There are lower levels of type 2 diabetes and impaired glucose tolerance among Nigerians compared to Jamaicans and African-Caribbean migrants in the USA, suggesting that environmental or lifestyle changes rather than a genetic predisposition are the main contributory factors relating to the development chronic disease (Rotimi *et al.*, 1999).

Prevalence

A review of the prevalence of diabetes worldwide estimated it to be 2.8% of the total world population. It is projected that the number of people with diabetes will rise from 171 million in 2000 to 366 million in 2030 (Wild *et al.*, 2004). This is mainly due to more people living beyond 65 years. Asia and Africa are the regions with the greatest potential increase (Wild *et al.*, 2004). In the UK around 2.3 million people are affected (Diabetes UK, 2007).

The incidence of type 1 diabetes accounts for around 10% of all cases. It is more prevalent in temperate regions and declines progressively towards the equator (Amos *et al.*, 1997). Type 2 diabetes is much more common in the ethnic minority groups, in particular South Asian and African-Caribbean groups in the UK (Riste *et al.*, 2001). The prevalence of type 2 diabetes in adults is about three times greater in African-Caribbean people compared with the White European population. For men, it is 2.5 times as high and for women four times as high (DH, 2004). The Health Survey for England found that in African-Caribbean people aged 55 and over, 17.6% of men and 25.7% of women had type 2 diabetes (DH, 2004). There is a three-fold risk of death from diabetes in African-Caribbean men compared to Caucasian men and four-fold in African-Caribbean women compared to Caucasian women (The Stroke Association, 2006). Studies from the Caribbean are consistent with these findings, as they also illustrate a consistently high morbidity and mortality rate from diabetes among adults, particularly women (Sharma *et al.*, 2008).

Risk factors

Diabetes risk is primarily determined by increased genetic susceptibility as well as obesity and lifestyle factors, such as diet and exercise (Shai *et al.*, 2006). There is evidence that certain ethnic groups have a predisposition to type 2 diabetes in the presence of the same risk factors. In the African-Caribbean community there are higher rates of obesity – 33% in African-Caribbean women compared with 21% in the general population (DH, 2004). Although some studies have demonstrated a smaller amount of visceral adipose tissue in the Black population despite a larger amount of total body fat compared with the White population (Lovejoy *et al.*, 1996; Hill *et al.*, 1999), obese Black women are more likely to be insulin-resistant (Van der Merwe *et al.*, 2000).

A 20-year prospective study investigating the risk of type 2 diabetes found that a diet high in polyunsaturated fat and cereal fibre and low in trans fats and glycaemic load appears to have a stronger inverse association with diabetes risk among the minority ethnic groups compared with the White group. From this it was speculated that the ethnic differences observed in diabetes risk is likely to be due to an interaction between increased genetic susceptibility and diet and lifestyle (Shai *et al.*, 2006).

Complications

A UK cohort study showed that the prevalence of both macrovascular and microvascular disease was lower in African-Caribbean people compared with White Europeans; this includes a lower risk of heart disease (Chaturvedi *et al.*, 1996). African-Caribbean people with diabetes tend to have a lower incidence of cardiovascular disease, possibly due to lower triglyceride levels and higher HDL cholesterol levels compared with White people with diabetes. However, because diabetes is more prevalent in the African-Caribbean population, the net effect is still one of a high overall risk of mortality from coronary heart disease in this group.

A recent study comparing African-Caribbeans and Europeans with diabetes showed that they were five times more likely to die of stroke regardless of blood pressure (Tillin *et al.*, 2006). It was postulated that the regulation of cerebral blood vessels may be more adversely affected in African-Caribbeans compared with Europeans.

Diabetes is the main underlying cause of renal failure in African-Caribbean patients receiving renal replacement therapy – they have a relative risk 6.5 times greater compared with the White population.

The risk of amputation was found to be only one third that of Europeans in African-Caribbean men, and in African-Caribbean women the risk was no different compared with Europeans (Leggetter *et al.*, 2002).

Dietary modification

Management of diabetes includes lifestyle alterations in terms of dietary improvement and weight management, as well as including regular physical activity and compliance with medication (see Table 2.6).

Cultural beliefs may sometimes result in difficulty in compliance. Traditionally, in the African-Caribbean community big is seen as beautiful, and women were discouraged from reducing their weight. This is no longer true among younger generations; however, older people may still feel that it is better to be large than slim. Compliance with medication can also be an issue, due to the side-effects of the medication or the belief that if a person feels well, they do not need medication. Herbal remedies such as bush teas are increasingly common in the UK. They may be used with or instead of prescribed medication as they are often perceived to be more natural, as are some vitamin supplements and garlic.

The aim of lifestyle management of diabetes is to address the key risk factors (obesity, hypertension, dyslipidaemia) and lack of physical activity, as well as glycaemic control. The key dietary messages are to encourage healthy eating with regular meals, and a reduction in total fat, in particular saturated fat. An increase in fruit and vegetable intake is also encouraged, as well as a reduction in sugar and sugary foods and highly salted foods.

Several studies have shown that progression to type 2 diabetes in high-risk groups can be reduced.

Table 2.6 African-Caribbean dietary modification for diabetes

Food group	Examples of foods	Encourage
Starchy foods Root vegetables (tubers)	Sweet potato, yam, dasheen, coco, potato	Including a starchy food with each meal
	Bammy, breadfruit, cassava, oats, green banana, rice (easy cook), plantain, bread (wholegrain), breadfruit, dumplings	Lower GI foods
Vegetables and fruits	Pumpkin, callaloo, cho-cho, okra, sweetcorn, carrots, ackee, advocado	Add vegetables to soups and one- pot meals
	Mango, pineapple, grapefruit, melon, banana, paw-paw	Aim for at least five portions daily
		Have fruit as a snack or desert
		Tinned fruit in natural juice not syrup
Meat, fish and pulses	Beef, chicken, goat, mutton, pork, turkey	Remove skin before cooking
		Use less oil in cooking
		Reduce portion size
	Snapper, bream, mullet and jackfish.	Steam or bake fish rather than frying
	Mackerel, sardines and pilchards	Aim to have two portions of oily fish weekly
	Black-eyed beans, red kidney beans, gunga peas	Use more of these and less meat. Add to stews and soups
Milk and dairy foods	Fresh milk, condensed milk, Carnation milk, butter, cheese	Use lower fat milks and avoid sweetened condensed milk.
		Have low-fat yoghurt and reduced fat cheese
Sugary foods and drinks	Honey, molasses, brown sugar, ginger beer, fruit punch, carrot juice, sarsparilla Cakes, buns, biscuits, sweets, chocolate	Choose diet or no added sugar drinks Add less sugar to cereal and avoid in drinks Limit sweet snacks to small amounts

The American Diabetes Prevention Program included ethnic minority groups and showed that diabetes can be prevented through diet and exercise interventions (which resulted in weight loss) in people with impaired glucose tolerance (Knowler *et al.*, 2002).

Evidence of good practice

Diabetes UK is the first UK charity to create an Equality and Diversity team. This team is dedicated to helping diverse groups, including Black, Asian and minority ethnic communities. Their aim is to raise awareness of diabetes by working with healthcare professionals, link workers, social workers, community psychiatric nurses and staff from the voluntary sector as well as building relationships with organizations from diverse groups.

2.1.7   Coronary heart disease and stroke

Key points

- There is a higher risk and incidence of stroke among African-Caribbeans mainly due to a higher rate of hypertension.
- The traditional diet of African-Caribbeans is high in fruit and vegetables, complex carbohydrates, fish and pulses, and low in fat and processed foods.
- Promote diet as a natural way of preventing and treating hypertension in combination with medication.
- Health promotion strategies need to be specific to African-Caribbeans as cardiovascular risk factors differ from those in the general population.

Introduction

Cardiovascular disease is the collective term used to describe disorders of the cardiovascular system and includes coronary heart disease, hypertension and stroke.

African-Caribbean populations are prone to a range of chronic conditions such as obesity, diabetes, cardiovascular disease (mainly hypertension and stroke) and some cancers (Cruickshank & Landman, 2001; Abbotts *et al.*, 2004; Harding *et al.*, 2007). There is some evidence of migration as an

influential factor in the development of these conditions in this ethnic group.

The incidence and mortality for stroke is higher in black populations compared to other ethnic groups worldwide and they are more likely to suffer a stroke at an earlier age (Abbotts *et al.*, 2004; Wolfe *et al.*, 2005; Harding *et al.*, 2007). Multi-ethnic population studies have found that immigrants in the UK had the highest mortality rates and the occurrence of stroke was 10 years earlier in Blacks than in Whites (Wolfe *et al.*, 2005).

Trends for stroke and coronary heart disease mortality among migrants in England and Wales have also been observed. The findings consistently suggest that African-Caribbeans have the highest rates of stroke and hypertension (Balarajan, 1995). However, mortality from coronary heart disease was half that of the national rates compared to individuals born in England and Wales in the 1970s and 1980s (Chaturvedi *et al.*, 1996; Abbotts *et al.*, 2004).

Although rates of coronary heart disease among migrants have fallen, Jamaican women have higher rates than those born in England and Wales. It appears that smoking, obesity and minimal physical activity are key factors in relation to the risk of chronic disease (HSE, 2004; Harding *et al.*, 2008).

Hypertension is the most common chronic disease in the Caribbean and a major contributor to mortality, particularly hypertensive renal failure. The prevalence of hypertension is markedly high worldwide (Balarajan, 1995; Harding *et al.*, 2007). Approximately 30% of African-Caribbean men and 40% of African-Caribbean women have hypertension (The Stroke Association, 2006).

Furthermore, the risk of stroke is significantly higher in this population (Thomas & Bishop, 2007). There is a strong association with the increased risk of stroke and hypertension. A two-fold risk of stroke exists in African-Caribbeans compared to that of Caucasians. In addition, these individuals have a greater risk of having their first stroke at a younger age, primarily due to sickle cell disease (The Stroke Association, 2006). Stroke is a serious complication of the disorder. The strong association between these condition means that individuals may experience a stroke before the age of 16.

The evidence implies that people of African descent are at increased risk of chronic disorders, despite place of birth. The causes are multifactorial. To some extent there is a genetic predisposition, however the evidence also suggests that environmental and lifestyle changes are the primary cause. Individuals who have migrated to the West and second-generation African-Caribbeans appear to be at a greater risk.

Prevalence of coronary heart disease

The main manifestation of cardiovascular disease (CVD) among African-Caribbeans is stroke, which is largely attributable to small vessel disease. Both the risk and incidence of stroke is higher among African-Caribbeans living in the UK compared with national rates (Wolfe *et al.*, 2005), whereas coronary heart disease (CHD) occurs less commonly (Harding *et al.*, 2007). Cardiovascular mortality in people of Caribbean origin increases with increased duration of residence in the UK, mainly due to the effects of increased stroke mortality (Harding *et al.*, 2007), however compared with Caucasians African-Caribbeans experience better survival rates after stroke (Wolfe *et al.*, 2005).

Risk factors

The higher risk and incidence of stroke correlate to the higher prevalence of hypertension in this group, and is similar to the pattern observed in the Caribbean (Harding *et al.*, 2007). It is typically type 2 (low renin) hypertension and contributes to the high rates of end-stage renal disease found among African-Caribbeans (Lip *et al.*, 2007). The risk of

hypertension in African-Caribbeans is 3–4 times that of Caucasians (Lip *et al.*, 2007) and cannot be solely explained by environmental aspects, such as diet and lifestyle, although these appear to be major precipitating factors. Other potential causes independent of diet and lifestyle include lower renin activity with a further decrease with age, lower nephron mass and a genetic variant in the epithelial sodium channel (Browne, 2006). In addition, African-Caribbeans develop hypertension at an earlier age than Caucasians and the prevalence increases with age (Browne, 2006) (see Table 2.7).

Treatment

Hypertension detection rates are high among African-Caribbeans but blood pressures consistently remain above 140/85mmHg despite this (Harding *et al.*, 2007). This may be more a reflection of concordance with treatment than treatment efficacy and may be perpetuated by factors such as cultural and religious beliefs, use of traditional remedies, cultural differences that may affect communication with health professionals, and mistrust of doctors (Harding, 2004).

Based on the results of the Antihypertensive and Lipid-Lowering Treatment to Prevent Heart Attack randomized controlled trial (ALLHAT), NICE recommends first-line treatment with calcium-channel blockers or thiazide diuretics in African-Caribbean hypertensives (NICE, 2006). The latter have been found to be more effective at lowering and controlling blood pressure in African-Caribbeans (NICE,

Table 2.7 Cardiovascular risk factors

Higher prevalence		Lower prevalence	
Hypertension	More than double the risk of the UK general population	**Vascular risk factors**	Atrial fibrillation, transient ischemic attack
Diabetes mellitus	Higher risk of type 2 diabetes than the UK general population	**Smoking**	Lower population risk of stroke from smoking
Obesity and low activity	Greater morbid obesity among women and lower physical activity	**Dyslipidaemia**	Higher serum HDL concentrations
Sickle cell disorders	Stroke is more common in children aged 2–10 years than in adults	**High alcohol intake**	More likely to be non-drinkers and to drink less than the general population Lower rate of binge drinking

(Hajat *et al.*, 2004; Health Survey, 2004)

2006). In practice, most African-Caribbeans need two or more anti-hypertensive medications to reduce systolic blood pressure to <140 mmHg (Khan & Beavers, 2005).

Caribbean herbal remedies

Caribbean herbal remedies (bush teas) are the leaves of plants such as cerasee. They are widely used as adjunct therapy and are perceived to be more natural than prescribed medication, particularly among first-generation Caribbeans (Connell et al., 2005). For example, cod liver oil, evening primrose oil, green papaya and teas made from breadfruit leaf, garlic, leaf of life and soursop leaf are thought to lower blood pressure, while cerasee (karela) is believed to reduce the risk of both heart disease and hypertension. Some bush teas, such as rat ears (joy weed) boiled with mint, are also thought to purify the blood after it has been polluted by medication (Connell et al., 2005). Older African-Caribbeans often wait until they experience symptoms before they administer treatment and omit prescribed medication if asymptomatic or if their blood pressure is deemed normal (Connell et al., 2005). To increase compliance and efficacy of anti-hypertensive, there needs to be a greater emphasis on the prevention and treatment of hypertension irrespective of symptoms. Health professionals should describe blood pressure as 'controlled' rather than 'normal' to improve compliance with dietary advice and medication.

Dietary modification

Many older migrants from the Caribbean living in the UK continue to eat a traditional diet that is associated with a protective effect from CVD (Harding et al., 2007). This diet is high in fruit and vegetables, fish and pulses, and low in fat, with meals based on complex carbohydrates, with small meat portions and few processed foods. This was reflected in the results of the Health Survey (2004), which showed a lower fat intake among African-Caribbean people and a greater proportion of African-Caribbean men meeting the five-a-day fruit and vegetable recommendation than the general population However, in younger generations there has been a shift away from traditional diets and a greater intake of energy from fat compared to Caucasians (Harding et al., 2007). This pattern is likely to continue as future generations adopt more of the practices of the host nation and may give rise to the development of more atherogenic lipid profiles in African-Caribbeans.

The Dietary Approaches to Stop Hypertension (DASH) (Appel et al., 1997) study showed that a combination diet based on a high fruit and vegetable and wholegrain intake, and a low saturated and total fat intake lowered blood pressure in a sample that included 60% African-Americans (Appel et al., 1997). A later study showed that the combination of the eating plan and a reduced sodium intake gave the biggest benefit and may help prevent the development of hypertension (Sacks et al., 2001). This is significant because hypertension in African-Caribbeans is exacerbated by salt sensitivity and low salt excretion (Lip et al., 2007). In both studies the DASH diet was more successful in hypertensives than non-hypertensives, but all groups experienced a dramatic reduction in blood pressure. When giving dietary advice, dietitians should emphasize that diet can provide a natural method of both preventing and lowering high blood pressure and may facilitate a reduction in the amount of medications required to control blood pressure.

Increasing vegetable fruit and intake

It has been estimated that approximately 20% of strokes are due to fruit and vegetable intakes of below 600 g a day (DH, 2007). In line with both the Food Standards Agency (FSA) healthy eating guidelines and the DASH diet, intake of fruit and vegetables should be at least five portions a day. This will aid in both the prevention and management of hypertension and help to reduce the risk of CHD and stroke. Dietitians should particularly encourage the increased consumption of vegetables in salads, stews and soups in place of meat. (For further practical suggestions to increase fruit and vegetable intake (see Table 2.8.)

Reducing total fat and saturated fat intake

Reducing fat intake is important with regards to weight management and should be recommended, particularly as African-Caribbeans often have a higher mean BMI, waist/hip ratio and waist circumference than Caucasians (Health Survey, 2004). As well as the strategies listed, discourage the

Table 2.8   African-Caribbean dietary modification for cardiovascular disease

Foods	Encourage	Discourage
Increase vegetable and fruit intake	Vegetables: fresh, frozen or canned (drained to remove salt before consumption) Fruit juice (guava, passion fruit and soursop) Fruit: fresh dried or canned (in juice)	Ackee, particularly fried Avocado Coconut Fruit canned in syrup Fried plantain Vegetables canned in brine
Reduce saturated and total fat intake	Low-fat cheese Powdered skimmed milk Low-fat yoghurt	Cakes and biscuits (e.g., bulla, bun) Fried foods Convenience meat products Processed foods Foods containing coconut milk/cream High-fat dairy foods
Replace saturated and trans fats with mono- and polyunsaturated fats	Fish, particularly oily fish (anchovies, bloater, cacha, carp, eel, herring, hilsa, jackfish, katla, king fish (king mackerel), kipper, mackerel, orange roughy, pangas, pilchards, salmon, sardines, shad, sprats swordfish, tuna (fresh only), trout and whitebait) Rapeseed and olive oil Unsalted nuts	Fried fish Salted nuts
Whole grains/ high-fibre foods	Hard dough and hops bread made from whole meal flour Whole meal crackers Wholegrain breakfast cereal Cornmeal (e.g., savoury cornmeal dishes, such as turn cornmeal/coco) Brown rice Millet Legumes	West Indian bread with full-fat spread Cream crackers, particularly with cheese
Reduce salt intake	Soaking salted fish overnight to remove some salt Seasoning foods with herbs and spices, such as allspice (pimento), black or white pepper, cinnamon, coriander (cilantro), cumin (geera), garlic, ginger, nutmeg, scotch bonnet and thyme	Salty meat products and processed foods, e.g., beef jerky, bully beef (corned beef), luncheon meat, salted pigtail, salt beef, salt pork, trotters and oxtail Foods canned in brine Salted nuts Seasonings, such as all purpose seasoning, chicken, garlic salt, meat and fish seasoning, monosodium glutamate, packet soups, soy sauce and stock cubes

regular consumption of dishes that include coconut and coconut milk or cream, such as curries, cook-up rice/pilau (rice with pig's tail or salt beef fried in coconut milk and seasoned), rice and peas (rice with beans, such as red kidney beans or gungo peas), oil down/run down (pork trimmings/fried fish and breadfruit boiled in coconut milk and seasoned with herbs and spices) as coconut is high in cholesterol-raising saturated fatty acids, lauric and myristic acid. Saturated fats should be replaced

Table 2.9 Suggestions for reducing fat in the African-Caribbean diet

Foods	Examples	Suggestions
Root vegetables (tubers)	Coco (eddoe), dasheen (taro root/eddo), (Irish) potato, sweet potato, yam cassava	Boil Bake in foil rather than roasting or frying in oil
Other starchy foods	Breadfruit (bammy), cornmeal, dumplings/bake (droppers/spinners), festivals, green banana, rice, sweetbread (coconut bread), West Indian bread	Shallow fry Do not add butter/margarine to rice
Fruit and vegetables	Ackee, avocado, coconut (gizzada/coconut tart), fried plantain	Eat less
Caribbean soups **Stews**	Beef, chicken, goat, mutton, pork, turkey	Allow to cool slightly after cooking and skim off the fat Replace some meat with nuts, seeds and legumes (black-eyed peas, chickpeas (*channa*), lentils, lima beans, pigeon/gungo peas, red kidney beans, soy beans and split peas) Thicken sauces with cooked and puréed vegetables instead of coconut cream or milk
Curries **Jerky**		Try not to fry before using another cooking method Use lean cuts of meat Remove the skin on poultry before cooking
Fried and escoveitched (scaled) fish	Jackfish, mullet, parrot fish, porgies, red snapper, sprats	Steam Bake in foil
Meat products and snack foods	Bacon bits, bologna, fritters (accra, banana, saltfish and conch), hot dogs, patties, *rotis*, salami, sausages, souse (pickled pork trimmings), tails, tongue, tripe and trotters	Eat less

with mono- and polyunsaturated fats, particularly omega 3, and in line with current guidelines, African-Caribbeans should be encouraged to consume two portions of fish a week, including one portion of oily fish (Mead *et al.*, 2006) (see Table 2.9).

Reducing salt intake

Excess salt consumption is considered to be the greatest dietary risk factor for hypertension (DH, 2007). Although African-Caribbeans tend to add less salt at the table, often high quantities are used in cooking (Health Survey, 2004). Average salt intakes have been estimated at 8–9 g salt/day for African-Caribbean women and 10–12 g salt/day for African-Caribbean men, with marginally lower potassium intakes and a higher sodium/potassium

ratio than Caucasians (Cappuccio *et al.*, 1997). High intakes of salty foods and seasonings should therefore be discouraged and instead food can be flavoured with herbs and spices. In addition, salted fish, such as saltfish (salted cod) and salted mackerel, should be soaked overnight to remove some of the salt.

Increasing intake of low-fat dairy products

The DASH diet includes 2–3 portions of low-fat dairy foods a day, which is consistent with FSA guidelines. African-Caribbeans should be encouraged to consume low-fat dairy foods, such as low-fat cheese, fresh and powdered skimmed milk and low-fat yoghurt instead of evaporated milk, condensed milk and full-fat cheeses.

Increasing intake of wholegrain/high-fibre foods

Emphasis should be placed on the importance of basing meals on ground provisions (tubers) and complex carbohydrates; where possible high-fibre and wholegrain varieties should be consumed. Fibre intake can be increased by consuming West Indian breads made from whole meal flour, whole meal crackers, wholegrain breakfast cereals, brown rice and millet. In addition, some of the meat in dishes such as stews and soups can be replaced with legumes.

Evidence of good practice

The National Stroke Strategy (DH, 2007) and the regularly updated *National Clinical Guidelines for Stroke* (RCP, 2004) provide peer-reviewed, evidence-based guidelines for the secondary prevention of stroke. These guidelines recommend providing advice and information to anyone at risk of stroke on diet and achieving a satisfactory weight, reducing salt intake and avoiding excess alcohol (RCP, 2004; DH, 2007). In addition, individuals should be supported in possible strategies to modify their lifestyle and risk factors (DH, 2007). Since African-Caribbeans are considered to be a high-risk group, these guidelines are particularly pertinent to this population and their application could lead to a reduction in the number of strokes and recurrent strokes experienced.

Dietary guidelines for secondary prevention of CVD (specifically for secondary prevention following an MI) have been published (Joint WHO/FAO, 2003; Mead *et al.*, 2006; NICE, 2007). In summary, all the guidelines recommend that to reduce the risk of CVD individuals should be encouraged to increase their fruit and vegetable intake, reduce saturated and total fat intake and replace some saturated and trans fats with mono- and polyunsaturated fats (Joint WHO/FAO, 2003; Mead *et al.*, 2006). Wholegrain/high-fibre foods should be increased and intakes of sodium and alcohol should be reduced in line with current government recommendations (Joint WHO/FAO, 2003; Mead *et al.*, 2006). The guidelines also call for the identification of individual risk factors so that dietary information and advice can be individualized (NICE, 2007).

The traditional African-Caribbean diet has many influences, giving rise to a healthy foundation (The Stroke Association, 2006).

Suggestions for the way forward

The majority of research on CHD in people of African origin to date has involved African-Americans but these data are not necessarily transferable to first-generation African-Caribbeans due to differences in ancestry. More cohort studies need to be conducted with African-Caribbeans to establish which risk factors should be targeted to result in the optimum reduction of stroke and CHD risk in this group. Since the majority of African-Caribbeans living in the UK are UK-born, more epidemiological studies among second-generation descendants are warranted.

In general, there needs to be more health promotion strategies specific to African-Caribbeans as their cardiovascular risk factors clearly differ from the general population's. Namely, more resources should be focused on the prevention of risk factors such as hypertension, obesity and diabetes rather than smoking cessation, reducing alcohol intake and hyperlipidaemia, which are less significant. Strategies should be targeted at people of a younger age since strokes tend to occur approximately 10 years earlier in African-Caribbeans than in Caucasians (Wolfe *et al.*, 2005).

Websites

www.caricaon.com
www.statistics.gov.uk
www.diabetes.org.uk

Support groups

The Black Minority Ethnic Group Service
Email: cservices@stroke.org.uk
Web: www.stroke.org.uk

Black and Ethnic Minorities Diabetes Association (BEMDA)
St Pauls Church Centre
Rossmore Rd
London NW1 5DP
020 7723 5357

Sickle Cell & Young Stroke Survivors
801 Old Kent Road
London SE15 1NX
E-mail: info@scyss.org
Web: www.scyss.org
www.bmediabetes.org

Further reading

Appel, L.J., Moore T.J. *et al.* (1997) A clinical trial of the effects of dietary patterns on blood pressure. DASH Collaborative Research Group. *N Engl J Med*, 336(16), 1117–24.

Britain.tv (2006) www.Britain.tv/community_afro_demographis.shtml.

Department of Health (2004) *Health Surveys for England, Ethnic Minorities.* www.ic.nhs.uk/statistics-and-data-collections/health-and-lifestyles-related-surveys/health-survey-for-england/health-survey-for-england-2004:-health-of-ethnic-minorities–full-report

Department of Health (2006) *Health Survey for England.* National Centre for Social Research, London.

Erens, B., Primatesta, P. & Prior, G. (eds.) (2001) *Health Survey for England. The Health of Minority Ethnic Groups '99.* TSO, London.

Lane, D, Beevers, D.G. & Lip, G. (2002) Ethnic differences in blood pressure and the prevalence of hypertension in England. *Journal of Hypertension*, 16, 267–73.

NHS Global Nutrition (2004) *The Caribbean Diet.* Department of Health, London.

ONS (Office for National Statistics) (1991) *Census. Report for England, Regional Health Authorities.* ONS, London.

ONS (Office for National Statistics) (2003) *Regional Distributing: Minority Ethnic People.* ONS, London.

Ramdath, D.D., Isaacs, R.L., Teelucksingh, S. & Wolever, T.M. (2004) Glycaemic index of selected staples commonly eaten in the Caribbean and the effects of boiling v. crushing. *British Journal of Nutrition*, 91(6), 971–7.

Sacks, F.M., Svetkey, L.P. *et al.* (2001) Effects on blood pressure of reduced dietary sodium and the Dietary Approaches to Stop Hypertension (DASH) diet. DASH-Sodium Collaborative Research Group. *N Engl J Med*, 344, 3–10.

Wilks, R., Rotimi, C. *et al.* (1999) Diabetes in the Caribbean: results of a population survey from Spanish Town, Jamaica. *Diabetic Medicine*, 16, 875.

Wright, J.T., Dunn, J.K. *et al.* for the ALLHAT Collaborative Research Group (2005) Outcomes in hypertensive black and nonblack patients treated with chlorthalidone, amlodipine, and lisonopril. *JAMA*, 293, 1595–607.

References

Abbotts, J., Harding, S. & Cruickshank, K. (2004) Cardiovascular risk profiles in UK-born Caribbeans and Irish living in England. *Atherosclerosis*, 175(2), 295–303.

Albert J, (2007) Developing food-based dietary guidelines to promote healthy diets and lifestyles in the Eastern Caribbean. *Journal Nutrition Education Behaviour*, 39(6), 343–50.

Amos, A.F., McCarty, D.J. & Zimmet, P. (1997) The rising global burden of diabetes and its complications: estimates and projections to the year 2010. *Diabetic Med*, 14(Suppl. 5), S1–85.

Appel, L.J., Moore, T.J. *et al.* (1997) A clinical trial of the effects of dietary patterns on blood pressure. DASH Collaborative Research Group. *N Engl J Med*, 336(16), 1117–24.

Aspinall, P. & Jacobson, B. (2004) *Ethnic Disparities in Health and Health Care: A Focused Review of the Evidence and Selected Examples of Good Practice.* London Health Observatory, London.

Balarajan, R. (1995) Ethnicity and variations in the nation's health. *Health Trends*, 27(4), 114–19.

Browne, M.J. (2006) Hypertension and ethnic group. *British Medical Journal*, 332, 833–6.

Bygott, D. (1996) *Black and British.* Oxford University Press, Oxford.

Cappuccio, F., Cook, D., Atkinson, R. & Strazzulloc, P. (1997) Prevalence, detection, and management of cardiovascular risk factors in different ethnic groups in south London. *Heart.* 78, 555–63.

Chambré Hardman Archive (2006) *Culture and Ethnicity Differences in Liverpool – African and Caribbean Communities.* Liverpool.

Chaturvedi, N., Jarret, J. *et al.* (1996) Differences in mortality and morbidity in African-Caribbean and European people with type 2 diabetes: results of a 20-year follow-up of a London cohort of a multinational study. *British Medical Journal*, 313, 848–52.

Connell, P., McKevitt, C. & Wolfe, C. (2005) Strategies to manage hypertension: a qualitative study with black Caribbean patients. *British Journal of General Practice*, 55, 357–61.

Cruickshank, J.K. & Landman, J. (2001) A review of ethnicity and nutrition-related diseases in relation to migration in the United Kingdom. *Public Health Nutrition*, 4(2B), 647–57.

Dauchet, L., Amouye, P., Hercberg, S. & Dallongeville, J. (2006) Fruit and vegetable consumption and risk of coronary heart disease: a meta-analysis of cohort studies. *Journal of Nutrition.* 136, 2588–93.

DH (Department of Health) (2004) Anthropometric measures, overweight and obesity. *Health Survey for England Minority Ethnic Groups*, 6, 154–75.

DH (Department of Health) (2007) *National Stroke Strategy for England.* DH, London.

Diabetes UK (2007) *Reports and Statistics: Diabetes Prevalence.* www.diabetes.org.uk.

Dragland, S. (2003) Several culinary and medicinal herbs are important sources of dietary antioxidants. *Journal of Nutrition*, 133(5), 1286–90.

Food Standards Agency (2005) *Eat Well: Your Guide to Healthy Eating: 8 tips for Healthier Choices*. FSA, London.

Grosvenor, I. & Chapman, R. (1982) *West Indies and West Midlands*. Archives and Heritage, Birmingham City Council, Birmingham.

Hajat, C., Tilling, K. *et al*. (2004) Ethnic differences in risk factors for ischaemic stroke a European case-control study. *Stroke*, 35, 1562–7.

Hamid, F. & Sarwar, T. (2004) *The Caribbean Diet. NHS Global Nutrition – A Multicultural Resource Pack for Developing Dietary Competencies*. Brent NHS PCT and Westminster NHS PCT, London.

Harding, S. (2004) Mortality of migrants from the Caribbean to England and Wales: effect of duration of residence. *International Journal of Epidemiology*, 33, 382–6.

Harding, S., Rosato, M. & Teyhan, A. (2007) Trends for coronary heart disease and stroke mortality among migrants in England and Wales, 1979–2003: slow declines notable for groups. Heart. doi:10.1136/hrt 2007.122044.

Harding, S., Teyhan, A., Maynard, M.J. & Cruickshank, J.K. (2008) Ethnic differences in overweight and obesity in early adolescence in the MRC DASH study: the role of adolescent and parental lifestyle. *International Journal Epidemiology*, 37(1), 162–72.

Health Survey for England (2004) *The Health of Minorities – Full Report* [NS] 2006.

Hill, J.O., Sidney, S. *et al*. (1999) Racial differences in amounts of visceral adipose tissue in young adults: the CARDIA (Coronary Artery Risk Development in Young Adults) study. *Am J Clin Nut*, 69, 381–7.

Joint WHO/FAO Expert Consultation on Diet, Nutrition and the Prevention of Chronic Diseases (2003) *Diet, Nutrition and the Prevention of Chronic Diseases: Report of a Joint WHO/FAO Expert Consultation*. WHO, Geneva.

Kaefer, C. & Milner, J. (2008) The role of herbs and spices in cancer prevention. *Journal of Nutritional Biochemistry*, 19, 347–61.

Khan, J.M. & Beavers, D.G. (2005) Management of hypertension in ethnic minorities. *Heart*, 91, 1105–9.

Knoops, K., de Groot, L.C.P. *et al*. (2004) Mediterranean diet, lifestyle factors, and 10-year mortality in elderly European men and women: HALE project. *Journal of the American Medical Association*, 292, 1433–9.

Knowler, W.C., Barrett-Connor, E. & Fowler, S.E. (2002) Reduction in the incidence of type 2 diabetes with lifestyle intervention or metformin. *N Engl J Med*, 346, 393–403.

Leggetter, S., Chaturvedi, N. *et al*. (2002) Ethnicity and risk of diabetes-related lower extremity amputation: a population-based study of African-Caribbeans and Europeans in the UK. *Arch Intern Med*, 162, 73–8.

Lieback, H. & Pollard, E. (2000) *The Oxford Paperback Dictionary*. Oxford University Press, London.

Lip, G.Y.H., Barnett, A.H. *et al*. (2007) Ethnicity and cardiovascular disease prevention in the United Kingdom: a practical approach to management. *Journal of Human Hypertension*, 21, 183–211.

Lovejoy, J.C., De La Bretonne, J.A., Lemperer, M. & Tulley, R. (1996) Abdominal fat distribution and metabolic risk factors: effects of race. *Metabolism*, 45, 1119–24.

Mead, A., Atkinson, G. *et al*., on behalf of the UK Heart Health and Thoracic Dietitians Interest Group (Specialist Group of the British Dietetic Association) (2006) Dietetic guidelines on food and nutrition in the secondary prevention of cardiovascular disease – evidence from systematic reviews of randomized controlled trials (second update, January 2006). *J Hum Nutr Diet*, 19, 401–19.

Millet, C., Khunti, K. *et al*. (2008) Obesity and intermediate clinical outcomes in diabetes of a differential relationship across ethnic groups. *Diabetes Medicine*, 25(6), 685–91.

NICE (National Institute for Health and Clinical Excellence) (2006) *Obesity: The Prevention, Identification, Assessment and Management of Overweight and Obesity in Adults and Children*. www.nice.org.uk/CG43.

NICE (National Institute for Health and Clinical Excellence) (2006) *Hypertension: Management of Hypertension in Adults in Primary Care*. NICE, London.

National Institute for Health and Clinical Excellence (NICE) (2007) *MI: Secondary Prevention in Primary and Secondary Care for Patients Following a Myocardial Infarction*. NICE Guideline 44. NICE, London.

Philips, M. & Philips, T. (1998) *Windrush: The Irresistible Rise of Multiracial Britain*. HarperCollins, London.

Pomerleau, J., McKeigue, P. & Chaturvedi, N. (1999) Factors associated with obesity in South Asian, Afro-Caribbean and European women. *International Journal of Related Metabolic Disorders*, 1, 25–33.

Riste, L., Khan, F. & Cruickshank K (2001) High prevalence of type 2 diabetes in all ethnic groups, including Europeans, in a British inner city: relative poverty, history inactivity or 21st century Europe? *Diabetes Care*, 24, 1377–83.

Rotimi, C.N., Cooper, R.S. *et al*. (1999) Prevalence of diabetes and impaired glucose tolerance in Nigerians, Jamaicans and US blacks. *Ethnicity and Disease*, 9(2), 190–200.

Royal College of Physicians (RCP) (2004) National Clinical Guidelines for Stroke. 2nd edition. RCP, London.

Sacks, F.M., Svetkey, L.P. *et al*. (2001) Effects on blood pressure of reduced dietary sodium and the Dietary

Approaches to Stop Hypertension (DASH) diet. DASH-Sodium Collaborative Research Group. *N Engl J Med*, 344, 3–10.

Shai, I., Jiang, R. *et al.* (2006) Ethnicity, obesity and risk of type 2 diabetes in women: a 20-year follow-up study. *Diabetes Care*, 29, 1585–90.

Sharma, S., Cade, J., Riste, L. & Cruickshank, K. (1999) Nutrient intake trends among African-Caribbeans in Britain: a migrant population and its second generation. *Public. Health Nutrition*, 2, 469–76.

Sharma, S., Cao, X. *et al.* (2008) Assessing dietary patterns in Barbados highlights the need for nutritional intervention to reduce risk of chronic disease. *Journal of Nutrition and Dietetics*, 21(2), 150–8.

Slavina, J. (2003) Why whole grains are protective: biological mechanisms. *Proceedings of the Nutrition Society*, 62, 129–34.

Smith, A.J., Cooper, J.A., Li, L.K. & Humphries, S.E. (2007) INSIG2 gene polymorphism is not associated with obesity in Caucasian, Afro-Caribbean and Indian subjects. *International Journal of Obesity*, 31(11), 1753–5.

Steinmetz, K.A. & Potter, J.D. (1991) Vegetables, fruit, and cancer. I. Epidemiology. *Cancer Causes Control*, 2, 325–57.

The Stroke Association (2006) Stroke in Afro-Caribbean People. Factsheet 21. www.stroke.org.uk/document.rm?id=842.

Thomas, B. & Bishop, J. (2007) *The Manual of Dietetic Practice. People from Black and Minority Ethnic Groups.* Wiley-Blackwell, Oxford.

Thompkins, L. (2008) *Caribbean Food – A Little History.* ezinearticles.com.

Tillin, T., Forouhi, N., McKeigue, P. & Chaturvedi, N. (2006) The role of diabetes and components of the metabolic syndrome in stroke and CHD mortality in UK White and African-Caribbean populations. *Diabetes Care*, 29, 2127–9.

Van de Merwe, M.T., Crowther, N.J. *et al.* (2000) Evidence of insulin resistance in black women from South Africa. *International Journal of Obesity-Related Metabolic Disorders*, 24, 1340–6.

Viner, R.M., Haines, M.M. *et al.* (2006) Body mass, weight control behaviours, weight perception and emotional well-being in a multiethnic sample of early adolescents. *International Journal of Obesity*, 30(10), 1514–21.

Webster-Gandy, J., Madden, A. & Holdsworth, M. (2006) *Oxford Handbook of Nutrition and Dietetics.* Oxford University Press, Oxford.

WHO (1998) *Obesity: Preventing and Managing the Global Epidemic. Report of a WHO Consultation on Obesity.* WHO, Geneva

Widjaja, A., Stratton, I.M. *et al.* (1997) UKPDS 20: plasma leptin, obesity, and plasma insulin in type 2 diabetic subjects. *Journal of Clinical Endocrinology and Metabolism*, 82, 654–7.

Wild, S., Roglic, G. *et al.* (2004) Global prevalence of diabetes: estimates for the year 2000 and projections for 2030. *Diabetes Care*, 27, 1047–53.

Wolfe, C.D.A., Smeeton, N.C. *et al.* (2005) Survival differences after stroke in a multiethnic population: follow-up study with the South London Stroke Register. *British Medical Journal*, 331, 431–3.

3

East Asia

Heidi Chan, Keynes Chan, Wynnie Yuan Yee Chan, Mary Chong,
Emma Tsoi (China), Maclinh Duong (Vietnam), Fumi Fukuda (Japan)

The East Asian countries included in this part are China, Vietnam and Japan. China is a vast continent and the Chinese people who have migrated over the years have integrated into the many lifestyle aspects of the host country. During the Vietnam war many refugees came to United Kingdom as boat people and are now well settled. Japanese people mostly work in multinational companies in the United Kingdom. Many of the ingredients used in their diet are similar but the cooking style varies. Chinese food has become so popular that takeaway Chinese restaurants can be found in almost every town in the UK. As with other cultural groups, when migration occurs, the diet of the host nation may be adopted and diseases related to this can be seen. Within this chapter you will find information on migration, traditional diets, migration, religious influences and dietary considerations for healthy eating for each of the three countries discussed.

3.1 Chinese Diet

*Heidi Chan, Keynes Chan, Wynnie Yuan Yee Chan,
Mary Chong, Emma Tsoi*

3.1.1 Introduction

China is situated in the far east of Asia, on the west coast of the Pacific Ocean, bordering the Yellow Sea, Korea Bay, East China Sea and South China Sea, and lies between North Korea and Vietnam. Countries on its border include Russia, Mongolia, Afghanistan, Kazakhstan, Kirgizstan, Tajikistan, Pakistan, India, Nepal, Bhutan, Burma, Laos, Vietnam and North Korea. The land area consists of 9.6 million km^2, the fourth largest in the world after Russia, Canada and the United States. China is divided into 23 provinces, four municipalities, five autonomous regions and two special administration regions (Hong Kong and Macau). Beijing,

Multicultural Handbook of Food, Nutrition and Dietetics, First Edition. Edited by Aruna Thaker, Arlene Barton.
© 2012 Blackwell Publishing Ltd. Published 2012 by Blackwell Publishing Ltd.

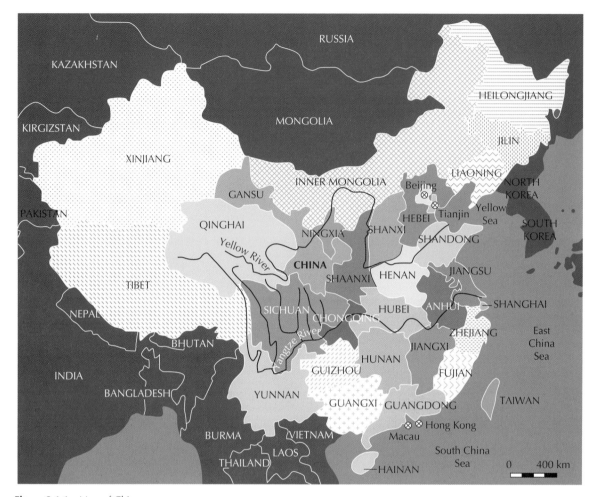

Figure 3.1.1   Map of China

Population

The total population of China is currently estimated at 1.3 billion, approximately 20% of the total world population (Central Intelligence Agency, 2010).

Language

As a result of the complex immigration pattern of the Chinese into the UK over the past 60 years there are many different dialects, countries of

the capital, is also the cultural and educational centre of China (see Figure 3.1.1).

origin as well as educational backgrounds and experiences. The two major dialects are Cantonese and Mandarin, although there are various local ones. The older generations are more likely to speak a local dialect in addition to Cantonese or Mandarin. The dialect spoken will vary depending on the part of China (including Hong Kong) they originated from. For example, many will speak Hakka if they are from that ethnic group of the southern provinces. There are also many different countries of origin (Hong Kong, mainland China, Taiwan, Vietnam, Malaysia, Singapore and the UK). Thus, the Chinese community is not a homogeneous entity.

A significant proportion of the Chinese in the UK, particularly the older the generation, do not speak English. If both parents speak a dialect, then it is possible the second generation will communicate with them and their grandparents in that language. However, we are witnessing the opening up of a generation gap as the younger generation pursue their own lives, develop career commitments and do not strictly adhere to the Chinese culture of 'family first'. This is exacerbated by the fact that younger family members, more so if they were born and raised in the UK, are often less able to speak the same language as their grandparents, or even their parents. The younger generation may understand what is said but are not able to speak the language. Many children attend Chinese school at the weekend where they are taught to read and write in Chinese (more specifically and commonly Cantonese due to communities largely originating from Hong Kong). The script is mostly interchangeable with Mandarin. However, modern Mandarin characters are simplified, whereas Cantonese people from Hong Kong will use traditional forms, but the component strokes of both types of characters are the same.

There are more likely to be language barriers with the first generation, but the majority are able at least to understand English if not converse in it. The second generation who have been born and brought up in the UK are less likely to experience any barriers and may be useful in acting as translators for their parents and/or grandparents. It is worth noting that these generational differences and the heterogeneity of the Chinese population have implications for health status and in particular nutritional status.

Migration to the United Kingdom

The Chinese are one of the several different groups of immigrants who have been continuously moving to the UK since the 1950s. In fact, the nation's first Chinese immigrants were 19th-century sailors who settled in Liverpool and London's Limehouse district. However, in the 1950s and 1960s a much larger influx followed. The chief reason for this migration, mainly of the Hong Kong Chinese, was economic. The industrialization of Hong Kong and the availability of cheap rice from South East Asia after the Second World War led to the declining use of the fields for rice production in the rural New Territories, thereby leaving the rice farmers unemployed.

There were two other notable factors for the postwar migration from Hong Kong to Britain. First, there was a demographic problem in Hong Kong caused by the arrival of refugees in the years immediately before and after the successful communist revolution in China. Since many Hong Kong Chinese had already been deprived of employment, the arrival of competitors for the limited job opportunities in conjunction with high land rental prices created a push factor. Then there was a pull factor generated by the demands in Britain. This largely consisted of a change in eating preferences, since at this time in Britain (and in other countries of Western Europe shortly afterward) there was a desire for more exotic and appealing food after the years of wartime austerity. Greek, Indian, Italian and other restaurants became popular, and Chinese food, long renowned as a high art, came into great demand both for its cheapness and for its fascinating, different ingredients, taste and presentation. Demographic and economic factors in Britain, such as the increased labour force participation of women, the growing number of single households and the dispersion of the population to the suburbs and council estates, also played a significant role in creating a market for ready-made foods. This was easily catered for by the incoming Chinese migrants.

For all these reasons, and the fact that they were guaranteed freedom of access to the UK as they were Commonwealth citizens, the Chinese contributed to a significant population flow from Hong Kong during the 1950s and 1960s. Similar to the early immigrants from the Indian subcontinent, male Chinese farmers initially saw themselves as temporary sojourners, hoping to raise enough money to support their families back home, before eventually returning. Ethnic Chinese also arrived from all over South East Asia, including from Malaysia, Singapore and Vietnam. Thus, Chinese communities were established in Britain, initially in Manchester and the Greater London area.

Current UK population

The percentage of ethnic Chinese living in the UK rose from 0.3% in 1991 to 0.4% in 2001. This equates to a population of 247,403, of whom approximately three-quarters are migrants and the rest born in the UK (British-born Chinese or BBC – a term often used by the Chinese when referring to those born in the UK). That figure is likely to be significantly higher now due to the arrival of new migrants and students, particularly from mainland China, over the last two decades. When compared with the UK general population, the UK Chinese population in 2001 is much younger, with 78% aged 16–64 compared with 64% in the general UK population. The Chinese make up 5.3% of the non-White population in the UK. Chinese people are found in greatest numbers in Cambridge, Westminster, the City of London and the London borough of Barnet. They form more than 2% of the population in these areas. They make up the third largest ethnic group in the UK (Census, 2001).

3.1.2   Religion

Buddhism, Confucianism and Taoism are the most common religions of the Chinese, however most Chinese in the UK are non-religious and so religion does not place any specific restrictions as such on dietary habits. However, there is a strong cultural element to the Chinese diet, which stems from Taoist teachings and in particular its philosophy on health and illness.

Cultural dietary influences

Balance and harmony are central to representations of health and illness in the Chinese. The healthy working of the body is thought to depend on a harmonious balance between elements and forces within the body, and between the body and the social, natural and supernatural environment (Jovchelovitch & Gervais, 1999). Balance and harmony provide structure and meaning to the understanding of the complementary, yet antagonistic forces by which everything that exists is formed. This system of thought is underlined by the well-known principles of Yin and Yang. The Chinese see the human body, the natural environment, the social relations that organize society and the supernatural world as elements linked and regulated by the adequate management of opposites and similarities. Thus, the binaries hot/cold, wet/dry and Yin/Yang, to name but a few, operate

within and across each domain. The principle of similarity – the idea that 'like helps like' or 'like fights like' – also organizes the internal structure of each domain and its relations to other domains. For the Chinese, balance and harmony are fundamental to health, not only within the body, but also within social relations, in relations with the landscape and nature, and in relations with the supernatural. The human organism is seen as a microcosm mapping onto and mirroring the structure of society, the image of nature and the macrocosm of the universe (Anderson, 1987).

Food is paramount in Chinese culture and is closely intertwined with concepts of health and illness. Since health is conceived as the product of a sufficient and adequate flow of energy (*ch'i*) through the body, and since food is an important source of energy, the careful selection of food and drinks, as well as the disciplined timing of meals, are thought to be integral to good health. Manipulation of nutrition remains the first and major recourse of almost all Chinese families in order to maintain good health and to prevent or cure illness (Anderson, 1987). It has been suggested that dietary prescriptions and proscriptions articulate the complex interactions between the individual, social and natural conditions. They link each individual to the family and to Chinese culture as a whole. Together with language, food is probably the most important vehicle for the transmission of traditional health beliefs. The Chinese have a long history of using food, herbs, animal parts and insects to maintain health and to treat illness (Jovchelovitch & Gervais, 1999). Traditional Chinese medicine (TCM) is widely used. Not only is food fundamental to the maintenance of health, as a whole it comprises the objectification of a number of concepts and rituals that keep the cultural system of the Chinese community alive and provide for each of its individual members a clear sense of identity and belonging. It is exceptionally important not only in relation to what one eats (the properties of the food itself), but also in relation to how one eats, in other words, the rituals of preparing, timing and socially organizing food intake.

The notion of balance between the forces of Yin and Yang guide the classification and use of food for medicinal purposes. Thus the categories of hot/cold, warm/cool, dry/wet and tonic/ poisonous are ascribed to different foods on the

Table 3.1.1   Classification of Yin and Yang foods

	Yin: Cold/Cool/Wet	Neutral	Yang: Hot/Warm/Dry
Foods	Most fruits and vegetables, e.g.:	Rice	Meat
	Chinese cabbage	Wheat noodles	Wine
	Watercress	Pork	Ginger
	Water chestnuts	Chicken	Garlic
	Spinach	Fish	Peanuts
	Melon		Oils
	Banana		Spices
	Honey		Chillies
	Chrysanthemum tea		Pepper
	Herbs		Brown sugar
Characteristics	Bland		Spicy
	Low-calorie		High-calorie
	Crisp		Protein-rich
			Oily
Flavour	Watery		Sharp
	Fresh		Intense
Colour	Green		Red
	White		Orange
			Yellow
Cooking method	Raw	Stir-fried	Deep-fried
	Refrigerated	Steamed	Baked
	Frozen		Grilled
	Boiled		Roasted

basis of the effects they have on the human body (see Table 3.1.1).

Hot, dry and tonic foods stimulate health and are used to increase energy in the body, while cold and wet substances are used when the opposite is required to restore balance. For example, in hot weather, people drink cooling teas and eat more cold and cooling foods, while in cold weather they consume hot or warming foods, thus the balance of Yin and Yang is maintained (Gould-Martin & Ngin, 1981). Poisonous foods are so called on the basis of the observation that scaly animals such as snakes and scorpions are known to be poisonous. Some seafood and shellfish are termed 'poisonous' as they are believed to affect one's skin although they are known to be safe to eat by most.

It is important to note that the cooking method can modify or enhance the properties of food. For example, deep-fried food can add more Yang, and so it is said that having too much deep-fried food can give you *yeet hay*, perceived as a negative state of being, characterized by a sore throat – a manifestation that the body is out of equilibrium. Therefore, in order to balance out with Yin, one would consume more vegetables, soup, fish and chrysanthemum tea, while cutting down on greasy, deep-fried foods and meat.

Traditional Chinese medicine

The Chinese are able to integrate different systems of knowledge and incorporate new information originating from different traditions. The idea of complementarity between opposites allows for the simultaneous use of different resources; it empowers the Chinese to cope in an alien environment.

The Chinese will take on new information and either anchor it to their system of thinking regarding health and illness or allow it to exist alongside their prior knowledge. This is made possible because, according to the Chinese way of thinking, Chinese and western health beliefs belong to different realms and therefore do not compete. One believes and trusts in Chinese medicine. western medical knowledge, by contrast, is grounded in science: it is open to proof and challenge and, by its very logic, challenges beliefs. Rather than turning these systems into mutually exclusive domains, the Chinese reconcile them to suit their purposes and needs.

Chinese medicine is therefore ingrained in the culture of Chinese people, with the older generations making more use of it than of conventional western medicine. It is a traditional medical system which has a holistic approach to diagnosing, preventing and treating diseases by identifying patterns and then applying the individual or combined therapies of acupuncture, Chinese herbal medicine, *tuina* (therapeutic massage) as well as other techniques. According to the Association of Traditional Chinese Medicine its unique characteristics which distinguish it from western medicine are rooted in the concept of holism and treatment according to syndrome differentiation. TCM has grown in popularity in the UK over recent years, with Chinese pharmacies now being a common sight on the high street due to the rising demand from people other than the Chinese.

3.1.3   Traditional diet and regional variations

China is a vast country and as a result, different regions lend themselves to extensive variations of cuisine and food choice due to crop production and the resultant locally produced foods, influenced by their climatic and geographical situations. Broadly speaking, dietary habits can be divided into those of the rice-growing areas of the south and central regions of the country, and those of the wheat and mixed grain-producing regions in the north. Within this division, five distinctive cuisines can be identified, although many minor variants exist.

Northern China

This large area includes the provinces of Inner Mongolia, Henan, Shandong, Shaanxi, Shanxi and Hebei. Beijing (formerly Peking) is located in Hebei and is central to one of the country's best-known cuisines. The agriculture in these areas is dominated by wheat, maize, sorghum, rice, cotton and sesame. The main vegetables found here are cucumbers, celery and Chinese cabbage. As it is the main wheat-growing area, wheat-based foods are a major source of carbohydrate. Wheat flour dumplings are a common dietary feature. They may be steamed or stuffed with a sweet or savoury filling and boiled or shallow-fried. Other wheat-based items such as bread and noodles are also widespread. A sandwich is made by filling pockets of wheat flour bread (similar to pitta) with thinly sliced and flavoured barbecued meat (Thomas & Bishop, 2007).

There are two predominant cooking traditions in the north: the imperial food of Peking and the food of Shandong and Inner Mongolia. The imperial cooking of Peking evolved over centuries and through the succession of great dynasties. It is elaborate, characterized by lavish banquets and complex, rich dishes, such as Peking duck, and refined recipes including the more pungent flavours of peppers, ginger, coriander, garlic and leeks. The foods of Shandong and Inner Mongolia revolve around lamb and mutton dishes, whereas pork and chicken are favoured elsewhere in the country (Shulman, 2002).

Eastern China

This area covers the lower Yangtze valley and the Yangtze delta area and includes the coastal provinces of Jiangsu, Anhui and Zhejiang. Rich agricultural products are grown here such as wheat and rice, as well as abundant seafood. Eastern China has a rich, decorative and slightly sweet style of cuisine, and in contrast to Peking, garlic is rarely used, whereas oil is used generously, as is sugar, sweet bean paste and rice wine.

The eastern school of cooking is focused on Shanghai, but there are other culinary centres in this region, such as Hangzhou, Yangzhou, Suzhou and Wuhsi. The red-braising method of cooking (*hung-shao*) originated in the East and involves the slow cooking of ingredients in a mixture of thick, dark soy sauce and rice wine, which is then reduced and poured over the main ingredient. Seasonings are used to accentuate natural flavours. Delicate vegetables are paired with delicate fish or meat, such as baby cabbage hearts with crabmeat or prawns, which brings out their natural sweetness. There is great emphasis on soups, stews and rich meaty stocks and various *congee* (rice porridge). Soup bases are commonly made from fish balls, turtle meat, small clams or fungi. Pork, coagulated pig and poultry blood, and soya beans are also frequent features. Noodles are more common than rice and often added to soups and other dishes.

There was a strong European presence in Shanghai which left its gastronomic mark in the form of breads, cakes, pies, sweets, as well as sumptuous cold appetizer platters – a legacy of the Russians (Shulman, 2002). As a result, Shanghai's cuisine is the most eclectic of all in China, incorporating ingredients from East and West.

Central China

This region is known as the 'spicy zone' of China's culinary repertoire, and encompasses Sichuan, Hunan and Yunnan provinces. Garlic, chilli, cassia, black and brown pepper, star anise, five spice, coriander, pepper oil and dried citrus are key ingredients. Some dishes here are delicately spiced, however those cooked 'village style' are fiery. The cuisines of the central areas were influenced during the medieval era of the Silk Route by the cuisines of China's trading partners to the west. Broad beans and walnuts were brought in from Iran, and halva-type desserts became popular. Salting, smoking, drying and pickling are common means of food preservation in the central region.

Of the central provinces, the cuisine of Sichuan is the most distinctive and has greatly influenced those of its surrounding regions. Main crops include wheat, rice, maize, bamboo shoots, rapeseed and citrus fruits, particularly tangerines. Sichuan cooking is not just hot, but includes various flavours such as sweet, salty and vinegary. Specialities of this kind include hot and sour soup, fragrant and crispy duck, twice-cooked pork, beef

with dried tangerine peel, camphor and tea-smoked duck, many fish dishes, bean curd (*ma po*) and an oily walnut paste and sugar dessert. Pickled vegetables, bamboo shoots, broad beans and pastes made from them are important in Sichuan cooking, and a strong Buddhist influence has resulted in many vegetarian dishes.

Smoking and barbecuing are common cooking methods in the region, especially for spare ribs. Splash-frying is another technique used here, as well as in Beijing: ingredients are hung over a pot of boiling oil and are cooked in the continuous splashes of oil (Shulman, 2002).

Hunan cooking is focused on rice, noodles, pork, chicken, cabbage, white radish, freshwater fish and mountain products such as fungi, game, bamboo shoots, wild roots and herbs. Maize, sweet potatoes and chilli peppers found their way to this region as New World foods, along with maize cakes and white potatoes, which were introduced by French missionaries in the 18th and 19th centuries. A wide range of fruit is consumed here, as well as nuts, particularly pine nuts and gingko nuts.

The cooking of Yunnan is less spicy than Sichuan's and is influenced by local minorities, in particular by the Tibetan and quasi-Tibetan peoples who live there, and by its proximity to India. As a result, unlike in most other regions of China, there is extensive use of dairy products such as yoghurt, cheese and fried milk curd. Noodles and steamed bread are eaten in preference to rice. China's finest hams originate from Yunnan, which also produces sausages, bacon, brawn and other cured pork products (Shulman, 2002).

Western China

The Xinjiang province of western China has a large Urghurs population. Consequently the food of this region bears more resemblance to the food of Central Asia than with the food of the rest of China.

Wheat is the main crop within this region, and as a staple it is eaten largely in the form of flat breads, noodles and dumplings. Flatbreads (*uighur naan*) are baked in tandoor ovens and flavoured with onion and cumin seeds, garlic and sesame seeds. Grilled kebabs (known as *shashlik* in Central Asia) are made with lamb and mutton. Spiced kebabs are the most popular street food in the oasis towns of the Takla Makan Desert. Cumin, black peppercorns and cayenne are rubbed into the skewered pieces of meat, which are quickly grilled. These are served with mint-flavoured yoghurt, stir-fried peppers and naans. In contrast to the rest of China, pork does not feature often in Xinjiang due to a significant Muslim influence.

Southern China

Cooking in the south is centred on the coastal provinces of Fujian and Guangdong and includes Cantonese cuisine. Rice is the region's staple food, so much so that a meal without rice is not considered a meal at all. Maize, sweet potatoes, taro, wheat and leafy green vegetables are also cultivated, as are oranges, peaches, tropical fruits and tea. Fish and shellfish, especially prawns, crabs, crayfish, clams and scallops, are bountiful. Bread and other baked products have become increasingly popular in areas exposed to western influence from Hong Kong.

This region's cooking is the most refined, varied and indeed renowned in China. Cantonese cuisine is not highly seasoned. For example, steamed fish, boiled prawns, steamed or stir-fried vegetables, fried oysters, boiled chicken and consommé are at their best when they are simple. The key is in the harmonious blending of different fresh and delicate flavours. Dipping sauces and seasonings most often found at the Cantonese table include soy sauce, oyster sauce, chilli sauce, vinegars, sesame oil, white pepper and black beans.

The Cantonese use the full range of Chinese cooking techniques and have an enormous variety of dishes. However, they are especially renowned for the quality and aromas of their stir-fries, prepared using a wok with a little oil. They are also known for the quality and variety of their dim sum, an umbrella term to describe small dishes of chopped meat, seafood or vegetables wrapped in a wafer-thin coating of pastry or dough, eaten as a late breakfast, lunch or snack. The Chinese love of snacks and light bites is most evident in this part of the country (Shulman, 2002).

In addition to the Cantonese, the Hakka have a cuisine that is simple and straightforward and demonstrates the Chinese appreciation of the many textures of offal. The Hakka are known for their skill with liver, kidney and tripe, stir-fried with vegetables. Hakka specialities include beef balls, chillies, salt-baked chicken, aubergine, bitter melon and a fish paste seasoned with onion and ginger stuffed in fried bean curd.

In the province of Fujian, there is a great emphasis on soups and one-dish preparations ranging from consommés to thick stews and rice *congees*. Noodles are common, and the region is also known for a type of thin pastry or dough skin (*yen pi*), which consists of pounded and finely chopped meat mixed with flour or corn flour. Shark's fin and bird's nest is cooked at its best here. Lard is commonly used as a cooking fat, and deep-frying is popular, as well as slow simmering and long steaming.

The majority of Chinese immigrants and subsequent generations in the UK originate from Hong Kong, and so the focus of this chapter will be based largely on those dietary habits and culinary styles. There is, however, a notable steady influx of asylum seekers from mainland China, which has been occurring more recently over the past 20 years and consists largely of Mandarin speakers from Fujian province.

Typical meal pattern

Breakfast

A traditional Chinese breakfast consists of *congee*, noodles, rice and steamed buns. *Congee* can be plain, or may include meat, fish, dried scallops, dried mussels, small dried shrimps, preserved eggs or peanuts and is usually accompanied by fried dough (*yow ja gwai*) to balance the textures of smooth and crispy. However this is time-consuming to prepare and most Chinese, including the first and second generations, will have a western-style breakfast consisting of bread, toast or breakfast cereal with milk. A cup of 'English' tea with milk is usually drunk with or without sugar, depending on personal preference.

Lunch and dinner

The midday and evening meals can be quite similar. They will include rice, noodles, buns or dim sum. Dim sum is eaten mid-morning (traditionally as breakfast) or in the afternoon. Among UK immigrant Chinese populations, its consumption tends to be confined to weekends, often with family and friends in restaurants for lunch or during the afternoon. However, they can now be purchased ready-made and chilled or frozen and so may also be eaten at home at the weekend.

Examples of dim sum include:

- Steamed dumplings filled with beef (*nau yuk yuen*), prawns (*har kau*), or pork, shrimp and mushroom (*siu mai*).
- Steamed or baked buns with barbecued pork (*char siu bau*), chicken and vegetables (*gai choi bau*).
- Rice noodle roll (*cheung fun*) filled with prawns, pork, beef, vegetables or fried dough stick (*yow ja gwai*).
- Taro paste with minced Chinese sausage (*wu tao go*).
- Egg custard tart (*dan tart*).
- Sweet lotus seed buns (*ling yong bau*).
- Sticky glutinous rice parcels filled with dried shrimp, chicken, Chinese sausage, spring onions and Chinese mushrooms steamed in dried lotus leaves (*lo mai gai*).
- Steamed shredded white radish (*daikon*) mixed with glutinous rice flour.
- Spare ribs.
- Chickens' feet.
- Tripe and other types of offal.

A typical midday or evening meal revolves primarily around a staple such as rice or noodles (*fan* – the most substantial part of the meal) with several main dishes containing meat, poultry, fish, tofu or bean curd (*choi* – the complementary dish). A clear soup is generally served, both as a beverage and as a palate cleanser. One or two vegetable dishes are likely to be included. There are usually fewer dishes served at lunch than at dinner, particularly as dinner is considered to be the main meal of the day and is the one most likely to be eaten at home with the family.

The Chinese style of eating is a communal affair involving the whole family sitting down together and sharing the dishes. There is no specific order in which to eat unlike the three-course meal of western cultures. The Chinese table is usually round, which facilitates the sharing of dishes. Each place setting has a rice bowl, a saucer and a pair of chopsticks. Each diner receives a full bowl of rice (*fan*) and uses their chopsticks to pick small portions of the dishes (*choi*) at a time from the table throughout the meal.

This traditional way of eating is usually only carried out for the evening meal as Chinese people in the UK adopt a more convenient western-style of eating for lunch. However, this is dependent on their degree of acculturation, so the older Chinese tend to follow the more traditional approach of communal eating. The second generation are less likely to have a Chinese meal in the evening every day, particularly if they do not live at home with their first-generation parents. A variety of cuisines are cooked, such as Italian pastas and pizzas (usually ready-made), or traditional English foods such as sausages and mash (although the mash might be substituted with rice), roast dinners or fast food such as burgers and chips. Simple Chinese stir fries or instant noodles are also a popular and easy way to make a meal. Single portions may be eaten more so than the traditional communal sharing of dishes at dinner.

Dessert
Desserts are not commonly consumed, although fresh fruit, particularly oranges, may be served after a meal. Sweet mango or coconut and red bean puddings or custard cream buns may be eaten, but usually as part of *yum cha*, as here a variety of savoury and sweet dim sum items is consumed throughout the meal. The second generation are more likely to consume desserts such as cake, pudding, ice cream or chocolate after a meal, but more often than not as snacks between meals.

Snacks
The Chinese are well known for their array of snacks. In the past, dried cuttlefish, pork or beef jerky were the most popular Chinese snacks alongside dried mango slices and sweet pickled plums. Nowadays, the average household will also have dried nori seaweed sheets, sesame crackers or plain with nori flavouring, shelled peanuts, yam or almond cookies, dried haw flakes, wasabi or chilli-flavoured nuts, potato and rice crackers. Fresh or dried fruit is also eaten between meals, as well as cakes, pastries, biscuits, and in the second generation crisps, chocolate and sweets.

Beverages
The most commonly consumed drinks, particularly among the older generation, are hot boiled water (*gwan sui*) and tea (green, white, blue or

flower teas). Black 'English' teas are consumed by both generations with the addition of milk and perhaps sugar.

Chinese people traditionally drink many chilled sweetened drinks rather than squash or fruit juice. Examples include flavoured soya milk (chocolate, yam, strawberry or coconut), lychee, chrysanthemum tea, green tea, raw sugar cane drinks, coconut milk and iced coffee or tea. In cold weather, hot milky tea or honey and lemon are consumed. In traditional cafés, tea and coffee are mixed and served as one drink with plenty of evaporated or condensed milk and sugar.

Globalization has introduced western coffee shops, therefore the consumption of latte, mocha and traditional Italian coffees has increased. This is certainly true of the second generation. Carbonated drinks and fruit squashes are also more popular with children and young adults.

3.1.4   Festivals and special occasions

New Year or Spring Festival

This celebrated in late January/early February according to the lunar calendar. In ancient China (and many areas of present-day China), life revolved around farming. Hence the New Year was celebrated as the planting of a new season of crops. After all, a successful planting is the best guarantee for a successful and delicious year to come. Further to the main feast dishes, foods traditionally associated with New Year include sweet soya bean soup, glutinous rice cakes and fruit and seeds, which symbolize renewal. The Chinese will also expect their children to eat as many cakes, oranges and orange-inspired dishes as they can stomach, so they are prepared for the sweetness that the New Year will bring. Oranges symbolize good fortune because they are sweet and one of China's most abundant fruits.

On the first day of the New Year it is traditional for adults to give their children and younger relatives *hong bao* or *lai see* (small red envelopes) filled with money. The envelopes symbolize good luck and wealth. Visiting, feasting and exchanging gifts of food, money and items may continue for three days.

The Dragon Boat Festival

This takes place in mid-summer. Glutinous rice dumplings, sweet or savoury and sometimes stuffed with meat are traditionally consumed. They are served wrapped in lotus leaves and then steamed.

Moon or Mid-Autumn Festival

This usually takes place in late September/early October, depending on the lunar calendar, and coincides with the end of the harvest year. It involves moon cakes being bought and exchanged as gifts. Moon cakes are sweetened, mashed lotus nuts encased in a thin, sweet pastry which usually contains duck egg yolk. There is a traditional custom that family and friends meet to dine under the bright mid-autumn harvest moon. Pomelos (yellow-green citrus fruit) may also be eaten.

Feasting demands the preparation and consumption of highly calorific foods that people at other times may not be able to afford. Throughout the year as well as at the traditional festivals, each family holds its own round of feasts to which other families are invited.

Dietary changes on migration

Immigrant Chinese have made adaptations to their diet since living and settling in the West. Although rice remains the staple of their diet, many western foods are consumed. These include bread, breakfast cereals, milk, dairy products and soft drinks. The older generation consider it important to consume a low-fat diet, high in fruit and vegetables (Satia-Abouta *et al.*, 2002). However, the younger generation, being relatively more accustomed to the western diet, are less likely to adhere to the traditional Chinese diet, except perhaps for the evening meal, as they believe cooking such meals is inconvenient (see Table 3.1.2 and Table 3.1.3).

Herbs and spices

The Chinese in the UK largely use ginger, garlic, five spice, spring onion and coriander in their cooking. Meats are traditionally marinated in herbs and spices prior to cooking. It is not uncommon to marinate with salt, sugar, soy sauce, rice wine and sesame seed oil too. Dried mandarin skin is added to casseroles or stews in addition to the above ingredients. Shreds of ginger and sliced garlic are

Table 3.1.2   Traditional Chinese eating pattern and dietary changes on migration

Meal	Traditional meal	Dietary changes on migration to UK	Healthier alternatives
Breakfast	*Congee*, steamed buns, rice/noodles	White bread/toast with butter, sugary cereal with whole milk	Whole meal bread/toast with low-fat spread, wholegrain cereal with skimmed milk
Lunch	Rice/noodles with barbecued/stir-fried meat, buns, dim sum	Instant/pot noodles, fast food/ takeaway, sandwich with fried egg and pork luncheon meat, meat pie/pasty, sausage roll	Boiled/steamed dim sum, whole meal sandwich/jacket potato with low-fat filling or boiled/poached egg and lean ham with salad
Evening meal	Clear soup, rice/noodles, meat, poultry, fish, tofu or bean curd, vegetables	Fast food/takeaway, pasta, pizza, roast dinner, sausages and rice, stir fry	Boiled/steamed brown rice or whole wheat noodles/ pasta, meat, poultry, fish, tofu or bean curd, vegetables (use less oil, salt, soy sauce)
Desserts	Oranges	Cake, pudding, ice cream, chocolate	Fruit, low-fat yoghurt, low-fat mousse/desserts
Snacks	Dried cuttlefish, pork or beef jerky, dried mango slices, sweet pickled plums, peanut/walnut/almond paste	Dried nori seaweed sheets, sesame crackers or plain with nori flavouring, shelled peanuts, yam/almond cookies, dried haw flakes, wasabi/chilli-flavoured nuts, potato/rice crackers, cakes, pastries, biscuits, crisps, chocolate, sweets	Fresh/dried/tinned fruit, low-fat yoghurt, crisp bread, rye bread, rice crackers, baked wholegrain snacks
Beverages	Flavoured soya milk (chocolate, yam, strawberry or coconut), lychee juice, chrysanthemum tea, green tea, raw sugar cane drinks, coconut milk, honey and lemon tea, iced coffee, hot/ iced tea with evaporated or condensed milk and sugar	Whole milk, flavoured milk, milkshakes, fizzy soft drinks, fruit squash, coffee/tea with whole milk and sugar	Diet soft drinks, low sugar squash, fruit juice, smoothies, hot boiled water (*gwan sui*), tea (green, white, blue or flower teas), unflavoured soya milk, tea/ coffee with skimmed milk and sweetener

commonly used in stir-fries. Dried herbs and vegetables are added to Cantonese soups, which are boiled for several hours to produce a rich broth. There are various combinations of dried herbs, vegetables and meat or fish selected for their functions in balancing Yin and Yang. A traditional saying is that 'to perfect a good pot of soup is the way to win a man's heart'.

Alcohol

Only 3% of Chinese men in the UK consume more than the recommended 21 units of alcohol a week (DH, 2001) and only 4% of Chinese women compared to 16% of women in the general population.

As part of a large (2,000) telephone survey conducted in Hong Kong, men and women were asked: 'On how many days per week during the past 30 days, on average, did you drink at least one alcoholic drink?' In response 74% of women and 49% of men reported they had none. The survey also found 67 men answered that they drank alcohol every day but only 10 women reported this (Department of Health Hong Kong Centre for Health Protection, 2009). There appears to be a slight upward trend in these figures as the telephone survey is conducted annually.

Table 3.1.3   Glossary of Chinese foods

Name of foods	Description of foods
Abalone	White-fleshed shellfish with a firm texture and a delicate, scallop-like flavour. Available tinned, dried or fresh, these are delicacies served on special occasions.
Bamboo shoots	Fibrous, cream-coloured shoots with a firm, crunchy texture – one of the most widely used vegetables in stir fries or available as pickles or in chilli oil.
Bean curd/tofu *ma po*	Made from puréed yellow soya beans. Traditionally in areas of China where meat was scarce or expensive, bean curd/tofu was a vital source of protein and as a result there are many different varieties available.
Bean sprouts	The young sprouts of mung beans. Popular in stir fries due to their fresh flavour and crunchy texture.
Bitter gourd/bitter melon	Mostly light green to white in colour with a bumpy skin containing rosy-red seeds. It has a rather bitter taste as the name suggests and usually complements rich pork dishes. If not available, marrow or courgette can be used.
Char siu	Barbecued pork, usually red-brown in colour. *Char siu bau* – steamed or baked bun containing *char siu*.
Chinese buns	Steamed/baked/fried bread buns made of dough containing sugar, water, yeast, flour and corn oil.
Chinese cabbage/ Chinese leaves/ Chinese celery	A wide variety of cabbages are used in all sorts of dishes as well as in chutneys and pickles. They usually have succulent, broad white stems with dark green leaves, e.g., *choi sum, pak choi, gai lan*.
Chinese mushrooms/fungi	Both fresh and dried forms are popular since they add a particular texture to a dish, and so are rarely served alone. There are many varieties, e.g., shiitake, oyster, cloud ears.
Chinese sausage	Thin dried sausage made of pork, beef or pork liver and duck. Generally have a sweet-salty flavour.
Chinese five spice powder	Very pungent, combination spice powder consisting of star anise, cinnamon, clove, fennel and Sichuan pepper. Often used in the batter of fried vegetables or meat or in meat marinades. The combination of five spices may stem from the ancient Chinese belief that the universe is composed of five elements – wood, metal, water, fire and earth – a system which is ingrained in many aspects of daily life.
Congee	Rice cooked with plenty of water until the rice grains split releasing the starch to form a thick, white, porridge-like soup. This can be served on its own but is most popular with peanuts, meat or fish. Traditionally, these were served in poor families where rice was scarce. It is also the preferred food during illness as it is considered easy to digest.
Corn starch	Powdery flour, nearly all starch obtained from the endosperm of corn. Mixed with water to form a paste. Often added to stir fries as a thickening agent.
Daikon	Mild-flavoured, large white radish.
Dim sum	An umbrella term to describe steamed, baked, braised, boiled or fried dumplings or other small dishes served traditionally for breakfast, lunch or afternoon tea. The customary event of going out to eat dim sum is called *yum cha* which literally means to 'drink tea' as tea is always served with dim sum and forms part of the meal as a whole.
Fan	The staple, most substantial part of the meal, e.g. rice, noodles, millet or steamed breads. Literally means 'cooked grain' or 'cooked rice', but is also used to denote food in general. *Choi* is the complementary dish, e.g. the stew, or meat, fish or vegetable preparation, though literally means 'vegetables'. In day-to-day eating, there is always more *fan* and less *choi*, whereas festive meals emphasize, and so include more, *choi*. In dim sum foods, the *fan* and *choi* are combined into one dish. These are the two elements that essentially make up the Chinese meal.

Table 3.1.3 (Con'd)

Name of foods	Description of foods
Gwan sui	Hot boiled water – commonly consumed particularly during illness as it is believed to flush out toxins and aid digestion.
Hoisin sauce	Thick sauce valued for its unique combination of sweet and spicy flavours. Made from soya bean paste and flavoured with garlic, sugar, chillies and other spices and ingredients. Used in cooking as a dipping sauce and in barbecue sauce recipes.
Noodles	Egg noodles (*chow mein*) – soft yellow noodles made from wheat flour and egg.
	Rice noodles (*ho fun*) – flat, opaque noodles made from rice flour.
	Vermicelli – glass-like, opaque white threads made from mung bean flour.
	Buckwheat noodles – beige-coloured noodle strips made from buckwheat flour.
	Noodles symbolize longevity and are often served at birthdays and weddings.
Oyster sauce	Made from oysters and soya beans, this thick salty sauce is used to flavour beef and vegetable dishes.
Salted eggs	Whole boiled eggs in their shells are preserved in salty solution and accompanied with rice. Traditionally, this was eaten by poorer families who could not afford meat.
Seaweed	Popular for both their flavours and textures and are generally used in soups or stews.
Soy sauce	Used in savoury dishes, made from fermented soya beans with a rich, salty taste. There are two main types: dark which is used with strong-flavoured dishes such as beef or pork, and light, which is used for more delicate food, like seafood, poultry and vegetables.
Taro	A dark-red-brown root vegetable with a flavour similar to sweet potato.
Water chestnut	Small round root plants commonly added to stir fries and casseroles to give a crisp, crunchy texture and a light sweet flavour.

Smoking

The marketing of smoking in East Asia has intensified – hence the prevalence is around 50% for men and 10% for women there (Lopez, 1998). A community-based study in Seattle also found smoking rates were significantly higher in men (21%) than in women (1%) out of a sample of 395 immigrant Chinese (Taylor *et al.*, 2007). In a three-year longitudinal study of over 2,000 Hong Kong Chinese subjects aged 70 years and older, mortality risks were observed to be elevated in both sexes: 80% of deaths arose from cancer, cardiovascular and respiratory diseases for which smoking is an established risk factor (Woo *et al.*, 1998). However, only 17% of Chinese men and 9% of Chinese women smoke cigarettes according to the Health Survey for England (DH, 2001) (see Figure 3.1.2).

3.1.5   Healthy eating

Key points

- Yin and Yang elements play a major role in conventional Chinese cuisine.
- With immigration and subsequent generations within the UK, some of these perspectives may have been lost. What was once a diet consisting of rice with vegetables and low-fat, high-value protein has been replaced by high-calorie 'western' convenience foods.
- The lack of nutritional awareness in this population group may have contributed to chronic diseases typical of western citizens.

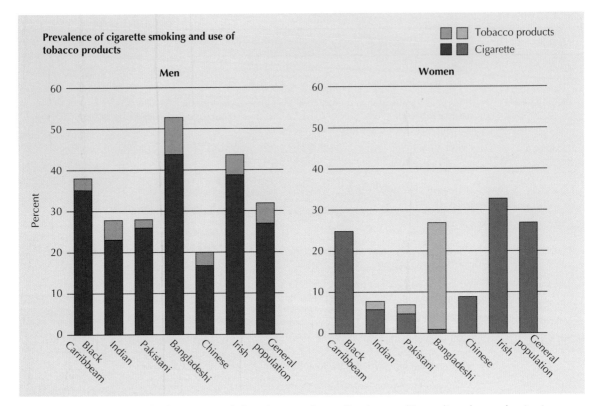

Figure 3.1.2   Prevalence of all tobacco use including cigarette, pipe and/or cigar smoking and/or tobacco chewing in a range of ethnic populations (DH, 2001)

Traditional eating patterns among the Chinese consist of four main food groups on which the Chinese healthy eating pyramid (see Figure 3.1.3) is based (similar to the UK Food Standards Agency's eatwell plate). They include:

- Grains and cereals.
- Fruits and vegetables.
- Meat, poultry, eggs, fish, beans and dairy products.
- Fat, oil, salt and sugar.

Grains and cereals

Rice and noodles
These are the staples of a Chinese diet; they are the equivalent of bread and potatoes in a typical UK diet and represent the core carbohydrates. Rice is the mainstay of every meal in the south of China and wheat products more so in the north. In a typical western diet, bread and potatoes may be served as a side-dish, whereas rice is always the central focus of a Chinese meal.

Rice
Rice dishes at midday or in the evening are typically served with vegetables and meat. Types of rice include long grain, short grain, jasmine, brown, red and glutinous. These are prepared by various methods (e.g., steamed, *congee*, fried, boiled or cooking all the ingredients in one pot). Each grain of rice is treated with respect in China. An old wives' tale that one will end up marrying an ugly, pimple-faced person if every single grain of rice in the bowl is not eaten can still be heard in Chinese households today.

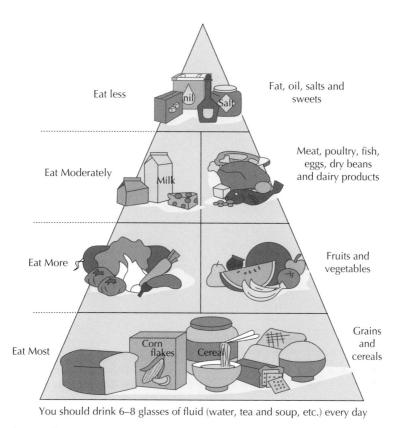

Eat less — Fat, oil, salts and sweets

Eat Moderately — Meat, poultry, fish, eggs, dry beans and dairy products

Eat More — Fruits and vegetables

Eat Most — Grains and cereals

You should drink 6–8 glasses of fluid (water, tea and soup, etc.) every day

Figure 3.1.3   The food pyramid
Department of Health. The Government of the Hong Kong Special Administrative Region (2008)

Noodles

Noodles are available in various shapes and sizes. They are comparable to different types of pasta. If they are made from wheat flour they are slightly coarse in texture. Mung bean flour is used to make vermicelli (thin white noodles) or rice flour for *ho fun* (flat, wide, slippery noodles). Because noodles are so versatile, they can be served at any time of day and can be stir-fried or boiled and served in soup. Noodles symbolize longevity and so are traditionally served on birthdays and weddings.

Buns

Particularly the sweet glazed variety are typically eaten 'on the go' at breakfast and also as a snack. Fluffy white buns with savoury fillings may be eaten instead of rice in northern China.

Fruits and vegetables

The recommendations of the healthy eating pyramid specify eating 2–3 portions of fruit and vegetables a day, fewer than UK the guideline of five-a-day. Fresh fruit tends to be served as an after-dinner snack or dessert. These are typically orange or apple segments, melon slices or bunches of grapes. However, fruit is also consumed dried, salted and pickled. Vegetables are served with the midday and evening meal, either cooked with meat or fish, or as a dish on its own. These provide colour and crunchiness to the meal and include fresh pak choi, gai lan, choi sum and other Chinese leaves and gourds. Japanese mushrooms (e.g., shiitake, enoki) are commonly used to flavour a dish but are never served as a dish in their own right. Other vegetables (e.g., broccoli, peppers, tomato, cucumber, pumpkin, courgette and aubergine) are always cooked as a mixed vegetable dish or to accompany meat. Families may serve traditional preserved or pickled vegetables (e.g., bamboo shoots).

Meat, poultry, eggs, fish, beans and pulses, dairy foods

Meat, poultry and eggs

Traditionally, slivers or dices of meat and/or poultry were served with vegetables and rice or noodles. As capitalism has amplified, fast-food cafés are now offering whole pork chops, numerous sausages and chicken wings at low cost to entice customers. Thus protein portions have increased and a meal is never complete without either a portion of meat, poultry, fish or eggs. Eggs are a common household food in the Chinese kitchen. If noodles were served with vegetables and there was no meat in the house, a fried egg would be cooked to accompany the meal. If an extra guest arrived unexpectedly for dinner, they will have brought an extra dish with them (e.g., barbecued pork (*char siu*), roast belly pork or duck). The host will then add an extra side-dish using eggs from the kitchen and a tinned meat such as luncheon meat. Thus eggs and tinned meat are common additions to a Chinese meal.

Fish and seafood

These feature widely in the Hong Kong Chinese (Cantonese) menu due to its coastal location. Fresh fish, crab, lobsters, king prawns, mussels can be hand-picked at the market or local restaurant. Fish are usually steamed whole with spring onion and ginger to bring out its fresh flavour. White fish made into fish balls are also popular. Crab and lobster tend to be fried in the wok with other ingredients. In addition to the fresh produce, dried versions of shrimp, scallops and mussels are used to enhance the flavour of a dish.

Beans and pulses

The Chinese use a huge variety of beans and pulses. These include soya and mung beans (both largely used to make tofu or bean curd), red beans such as adzuki, kidney beans and rice which are boiled and used as constituents in soups. Fresh green beans, often long ones, are commonly sliced and added to stir fries.

Tofu and soya products

These feature widely in Chinese cuisine. There is a perception among many Chinese families that these products are 'vegetables', but they are in fact a high-protein food and can be used as a meat substitute. Tofu of varying textures dictate how they should be cooked – softer types of tofu are steamed and firmer ones fried. Textured vegetable protein or soya products are eaten in Buddhist temples or specialist vegan/vegetarian restaurants.

Milk and dairy products

These do not feature widely in the diets of the majority of Chinese people and are only common among the minority peoples of the central and west. Traditionally, dairy products such as cheese, cow's milk and yoghurt are less frequently consumed as they are believed to be difficult to digest. Cheese in particular can have a strong flavour and pungent aroma which disturbs the balance of Yin and Yang and thus adversely affects health. Cheese is not always included in Chinese healthy eating advice due to this belief. Lactose intolerance or 'maldigestion' in this population group often results in a reduced dairy intake.

Fats, oil, salt and sugar

Vegetable oil (derived from rapeseed), sesame oil and peanut oil are frequently used in Chinese cooking. Less oil is used in domestic cooking than in commercial cooking (i.e., when eating out). The typical Chinese kitchen is small and does not facilitate the sort of cooking appliances one finds in a fast-food café or restaurant. Chinese chefs will prepare most of their foods by frying in the wok and re-heating it when ordered. Lard is rarely used for cooking at home, but remains an ingredient in many Chinese buns, cakes and pastries bought commercially (see Table 3.1.3).

Dried, salted or preserved snacks are popular. Soy sauce, fish sauce, oyster sauce, hoisin sauce and monosodium glutamate (MSG) also contribute to Chinese people's sodium intake. MSG is used less often now in domestic cooking, and MSG-free alternatives are available. There is also a growing availability of reduced salt products, such as soy sauce.

Chinese buns, pastries or fruit are eaten as snacks or desserts. With the recent trend towards slimming, local bakeries are selling reduced sugar and lower fat cakes and pastries. These are often garnished with fresh fruit such as mangoes and strawberries, or have flavourings of green tea or yam/taro giving them a distinct green or deep-purple colour. Occasionally sweet soup (*tong sui*) is prepared as an afternoon snack or served at the end of a meal. There are many varieties of this sweet soup which consist of a range of ingredients sweetened with unrefined rock or cane sugar. They are cooked in a similar way to the savoury soups. They can be served chilled and sold in cans in convenience stores. Combinations include:

- Dried soya curd sheets and nuts.
- Taro, sago and coconut cream.
- Mango, grapefruit and tapioca.
- Red or green mung beans and dried citrus peel.
- Sweet potato chunks and a little root ginger.
- White lotus seed and poached egg.

Other chilled sweetened drinks are traditionally consumed such as flavoured soya milk, fruit drinks and teas.

Traditional Chinese food and drink can be high in fat, oil, salt and sugar. Cooking methods are different in the home from the commercial setting and the former is often perceived as healthier. However, Chinese people use convenience food and drink extensively as part of their current lifestyle.

- Incorporating starchy food and vegetables in the midday and evening meal should be encouraged as part of healthy eating.
- Reducing the amount of soy sauce, preserved snacks, sweetened buns and commercial drinks is recommended to cut down the intake of salt and sugar.

- Consuming fried food or snacks less frequently and advising on the use of vegetable oil (derived from rapeseed), peanut, canola, corn, sesame or olive oils will have positive impact on general health.

Chinese who have not migrated but who have adopted a western diet are experiencing a rise in chronic conditions. A news item concluded that Chinese women who consume more western foods are at increased risk of cancer. A study of 1,500 Chinese women found those that consumed a diet high in meat, fish, sweets, white bread, milk and puddings were twice as likely to develop breast cancer as those consuming a vegetable-based diet (BBC, 2007). Women with a BMI > 25 kg/m^2 were at most risk as were postmenopausal women. Another example of health implications after adopting a western diet and lifestyle is discussed in an editorial in the *British Medical Journal* (BBC, 2007). Meat intake has increased among the Chinese from 8% to 25% from 1982 to 2002. China experienced an astonishing 28-fold increase in obesity between 1985 and 2000. With such changes to their diet, it will not be surprising if there is a concurrent rise in prevalence of other 'western' diseases such as diabetes and cardiovascular disease.

3.1.6   Recent evidence of good practice to promote healthy eating

At present there are few national public health projects promoting healthy eating among Chinese inhabitants of the UK. The national recommendations (e.g., five-a-day and Change4Life) are not specifically aimed at the Chinese population. The eatwell plate does not encompass the food groups of a typical Chinese diet for those not following a western diet. As it is not tailored to this population, dietetic advice to these patients with or predisposed to chronic disease is a challenge. Where Chinese populations are found in the UK, Primary Care Trusts or community groups may have set up health promotion projects – for example, the Healthy Chinese Takeaway Menus project currently being conducted by the Chinese National Healthy Living Centre in London. This is a pilot project supporting Chinese takeaways to develop, display and maintain a Healthy Choice Menu in terms of nutritional balance so as to reinforce the value of traditional Chinese good cooking practices (Chinese National Healthy Living Centre, 2010).

Suggestions for the way forward

As eating practices among immigrants and the older generation have changed in the past decade or more, it has become apparent that this is contributing to major chronic diseases. It would be appropriate to address such trends. Whether Chinese immigrants adopt a westernized diet or continue to consume traditional foods, it would be beneficial to make recommendations for healthy eating. Reducing salt consumption, increasing calcium intake and increasing dietary fibre would all help to reduce the risk of hypertension, osteoporosis and bowel cancer. It would be valuable for the Chinese population to become more aware of the benefits of dietary fibre in relation to chronic disease prevention (Woo *et al.*, 1998). Smoking is also one of the main lifestyle factors that need to be tackled since it has a direct link with premature mortality. Clear, concise and appropriately tailored messages are necessary in the campaign to promote healthy eating and lifestyle by healthcare professionals, advertising companies and in schools.

3.1.7   Obesity

Key points

- Overweight and obesity are defined as abnormal or excessive fat accumulation that may impair health and are usually measured using the body mass index (BMI).
- The prevalence of overweight and obesity is increasing globally in both adults and children.
- Overweight and obesity are associated with an increased risk of developing chronic diseases such as cancer, cardiovascular disease and type 2 diabetes.
- The combination of a weight-reducing diet and increased physical activity are recommended for overweight or obese adults.

Introduction

Obesity is a global concern not only in adults but also among children and adolescents (WHO, 2000;

International Obesity Taskforce, 2006). There is international consensus on the negative impact of obesity on the social, mental and physical functions in children (Swallen *et al.*, 2005; Reilly & Wilson, 2006). Furthermore, the majority of obese children remain obese in their adulthood (Vanhala *et al.*, 1998), with possible increased risk of adult mortality and morbidity (Rudolf *et al.*, 2001; Burke, 2006).

Comparisons between rural and urban Chinese populations show a direct association between rising household income and a higher percentage of energy intake from fat. Daily consumption of grains decreased as intake of animal foods and edible oils rose. 38% of men and 34% of women in Hong Kong are overweight and have a BMI > 25 kg/m^2. The prevalence of obesity (BMI >30 kg/m^2) is 5% for men, 7% for women and alarmingly 8% for children. As obesity is linked with metabolic syndrome which leads to increased mortality and morbidity, these figures are of great concern. The prevalence of diabetes has increased from 10% to 20–30% from 1985 to 1995 among the Hong Kong Chinese older generation (Woo, 1998).

The estimated hospitalization costs in Hong Kong in 2002 were US$0.43 billion, accounting for 8.2–9.8% of total public expenditure on health in Hong Kong (Ko, 2008). In China, the total medical cost was estimated by Zhao *et al.* (2008) to be US$2.74 billion, or 3.7% of national total medical costs in 2003.

BMI is an index of weight-for-height and is commonly used to classify underweight, overweight and obesity in adult populations. BMI is measured by dividing a person's weight (in kg) by their height (in m)^2. The correlation between the BMI and body fatness is fairly strong, however correlation varies by sex, race and age. These variations (Gallagher *et al.*, 1996; Prentice & Jebb, 2001) include:

- At the same BMI, women tend to have more body fat than men.
- At the same BMI, older people tend to have more body fat than younger adults.
- Trained athletes may have a high BMI because of increased muscle rather than increased body fat.

Since abdominal fat is a predictor for risk of obesity-related diseases, an individual's waist

Table 3.1.4   Classification of weight by BMI in adult Asians

Classification	Asian BMI (kg/m^2)
Underweight	<18.5
Normal range	18.5–22.9
Overweight	>23
Overweight: At risk	23–24.9
Overweight: Obese I	25–29.9
Overweight: Obese II	>30

(WHO, 2000)

circumference should be assessed in addition to their BMI (International Diabetes Federation, 2003):

- Men > 94 cm; and
- Women (not pregnant) > 80 cm = increased risk

People who are overweight or obese are more likely to suffer from types of cancer, cardiovascular disease, type 2 diabetes, gallstones, osteoarthritis (especially in the knees) and hypertension.

In general, BMI is classified in four categories according to level of body weight; cut-off points vary for Europeans and Asians (see Table 3.1.4). The WHO Child Growth Standards (2006) include BMI charts for infants and children up to five years. However, measuring overweight and obesity in children aged 5–14 years is challenging because there is currently no standard worldwide definition of childhood obesity. The US Centers for Disease Control and Prevention (CDCP) recommend first calculating a child's BMI and then plotting it onto their BMI-for-age growth charts. This will take into account the changes in the amount of body fat with age and difference in the amount of body fat between girls and boys (CDCP, 2000).

Prevalence

It has been estimated that 1.6 billion adults (age 15+) are overweight, at least 400 million adults are obese and more than 20 million children over the age of five are overweight (WHO, 2007). The WHO project that by 2015 approximately 2.3 billion adults will be overweight and more than 700 million will be obese.

The Hong Kong Population Health Survey (2003/4) estimates that 17.8% of the population aged 15 and above are overweight and 21.1% are obese.

According to data from the Chinese National Surveys on Students' Constitution and Health conducted in 2000, the prevalence of overweight and obesity in children from urban areas increased from 1% to 25% between 1985 and 2000 (Zhou, 2002), and among adolescents, the prevalence is estimated to be 16% using the International Obesity Task Force BMI cut-offs (Li et al., 2006). The prevalence rates are comparable to those in the USA and Australia where one in four children are overweight or obese.

Urban and rural differences in the prevalence of obesity are also evident in Malaysia where 5.6% of urban men are obese compared to 1.8% of rural men and 8.8% of urban women compared to 2.6% of rural women.

The Hong Kong Student Health Service recorded a rising trend of obesity (defined as age- and sex-specific weight more than 120% times the median weight for height) among primary school students (10–13 years) from 16.4% in 1997/8 to 18.7% in 2004/5.

In the UK, data from the Health Survey for England (DH, 2001) reported the prevalence of obesity (using >30 kg/m^2 as a cut-off) among Chinese as low: 6.2% of men and 4.5% of women.

Risk factors

Global increases in overweight and obesity are attributable to a western diet characterized by an increased intake of energy-dense foods high in fat and sugar but low in vitamins, minerals and other micronutrients; a trend towards decreased physical activity due to the increasingly sedentary nature of many types of work, changing modes of transportation and increasing urbanization. James et al. (2002) estimated that with urbanization China has reduced daily energy expenditure by about 200–400 kcal a day. Furthermore, with the introduction of mechanization, TV, media and computerized changes, energy demands have dropped by a further 400–800 kcal/day.

In China, dietary patterns characterized by a low intake of fruit and vegetables and a high intake of fatty meat have been identified as a risk factor for obesity (Li *et al.*, 2006). The increase from about 15% to 20% in the proportion of calories from fat is sufficient to explain some of the weight gain in the population (Paeratakul *et al.*, 1998).

According to the Hong Kong Nutritional Survey, varieties of grain and meat are negatively correlated, whereas snacks are positively correlated with obesity indices in Hong Kong adults (Sea *et al.*, 2004).

Lam *et al.* (2004) examined the relationship between leisure-time physical activity (LTPA) and mortality in Hong Kong. When compared with an exercise frequency of less than one episode/month, one or more episodes of LTPA a month was inversely related with all causes of mortality for both men and women (multivariable OR (95% CI) = 0.63 (0.59, 0.69) for men; 0.75 (0.70, 0.80) for women after adjusting for education, age, smoking, alcohol intake and physical demands at work). A 2001 survey found that 80% of children watched TV during leisure-time, while only 33% chose to exercise; moreover 45% of children watched more than three hours of TV a day. In 2001, Hong Kong adults spent 2.4 hours a day watching TV and only 55% of adults had exercised in the past month, much less than those in other developed countries (Lam *et al.*, 2002).

The relationship between sleeping hours and obesity in 4,793 Hong Kong subjects aged 17–83 years found that increasing BMI was associated with fewer sleeping hours and more working hours. Those who slept six hours or less a night and worked more than nine hours a day had the highest BMI compared with those who slept longer and worked shorter hours.

Prevention

Chronic diseases such as overweight and obesity are largely preventable by:

- Achieving energy balance and maintaining a healthy weight.
- Limiting energy intake from total fats.
- Shifting from saturated fats to unsaturated fats.
- Increasing consumption of fruit and vegetables, legumes and whole grains.
- Limiting the intake of sugars.
- Increasing physical activity.

The Chief Medical Officer's report on physical activity (DH, 2004) emphasizes the beneficial relationship between physical activity and health. It recommends a minimum of 30 minutes of at least moderate-intensity physical activity five or more days a week for weight management. However, in the absence of a reduction in energy intake, many individuals will need to participate in 45–60 minutes of moderate intensity physical activity each day to prevent obesity. People who were obese and who have lost weight may need 60–90 minutes of activity a day to maintain weight loss.

Nutrition and lifestyle interventions in the workplace, schools and health settings have shown significant changes in BMI in intervention groups in addition to sustained modifications in dietary and exercise behaviour (Li *et al.*, 2008; Liu *et al.*, 2008; Togami 2008).

Sustained commitment from governments, international agencies, NGOs, public and private stakeholders are needed to help shape healthy environments in order to make healthy diet options accessible and affordable. Food industry involvement is essential to initiating a policy to reduce the portion sizes, fat, sugar and salt content of processed foods, which are being consumed increasingly by the Chinese population in the UK.

Dietary modification

A low-calorie, low-fat, high-fibre diet combined with an emphasis on short-term, realistic goals is warranted. A deficit of 500–1,000 kcal a day below energy requirements will lead to a weight loss of 0.5–1 kg per week.

Development of long-term maintenance of a healthy diet is also essential. Retrospective studies suggest that long-term, low-fat, high complex-carbohydrate diets are the most effective for weight loss and weight maintenance (Klem *et al.*, 1997; Kennedy *et al.*, 2001) (see Table 3.1.5).

3.1.8 Diabetes

Introduction

Diabetes mellitus is reaching epidemic proportions worldwide, with the past two decades witnessing a increase in its incidence (Amos *et al.*, 1997;

Table 3.1.5 Chinese Dietary modification for weight reduction

	Discourage	Encourage
Energy	High-energy foods and drinks, e.g., chocolate, confectionery, crisps, chips, egg custard tart (*dan tart*), spring rolls and other deep-fried dim sum, sweet soup (*tong sui*), sugarcane drink, sweetened soya milk, sweetened lemon tea, soft drinks	Lower-energy foods and drinks, e.g., vegetables, fruit, legumes (e.g., red beans, black-eyed peas, mung beans), plain biscuits, steamed buns, *congee*, tofu, water, tea, diet/sugar-free drinks.
Fat	Deep-fried foods and dim sum, fried rice or noodles, Chinese sausage, roast belly pork, roast duck, chicken wings, hamburgers, luncheon meat e.g. spam, cream-filled buns, lard, whole milk, full-fat yoghurt, hard cheese	Boiled/steamed/baked/grilled foods and dim sum, plain rice, boiled noodles, lean cuts of meat, e.g., chicken breast, pork leg and meat trimmed of fat before cooking, fruit, monounsaturated oil (but sparingly), skimmed milk, low-fat yoghurt, soft/cottage cheese.
Fibre	White rice, white bread, cornflakes, white pasta, instant noodles and other processed foods	Brown or red rice, whole meal or wholegrain bread/breakfast cereals, whole wheat pasta, whole wheat/buckwheat noodles, fruit and vegetables.
Alcohol	Limit wherever possible	When drinking alcohol use low-calorie mixers (e.g., diet tonic, diet coke) or choose 'light' beers

---

Key points

- Diabetes is approaching epidemic proportions. The WHO estimates that there will be 300 million adults with diagnosed diabetes by 2025.
- Eating a healthy balanced diet, maintaining regular physical activity and maintaining a healthy body weight can help to prevent or delay the onset of type 2 diabetes.
- People with diabetes need to maintain a healthy weight by eating a low-fat, low-salt diet, which includes whole grains, fruit and vegetables.

Zimmet, 2000). This is largely of type 2 diabetes and associated conditions of diabetes and metabolic syndrome (Shafrir, 1997). Diabetes is associated with significant morbidity and mortality. People with diabetes have increased rates of death from heart disease, stroke and renal disease, as well as blindness (Stamler *et al.*, 1993).

Prevalence

The prevalence of diabetes is increasing rapidly in both developed and developing countries. WHO

estimated that the number of adults with diabetes increased from 110 million in 1994 to around 240 million in 2010. It is projected that the number will reach 300 million by 2025 (King *et al.*, 1998).

In the UK, there are 1.4 million people with diagnosed diabetes of whom around one million have type 2 diabetes. Many more people may have undiagnosed diabetes.

In China over the past two decades, the number of people with diabetes or impaired glucose tolerance has increased rapidly (Leung & Lam, 2000, Chan *et al.*, 2001, Chowdhury & Lasker, 2002). Data from the National Diabetes Survey of 1996 (Pan *et al.*, 1997) showed the overall prevalence of type 2 diabetes and impaired fasting glucose among 25–64 year olds in China to be 2.5% and 3.2% respectively. It is estimated that prevalence in rural areas is around half that of urban areas, the differences being related to urbanization, diet, lifestyle and income. The 2008 Inter-ASIA study (Hu *et al.*, 2008) estimates the prevalence of type 2 diabetes and impaired fasting glucose to be 5.49% and 7.33%. Tests conducted on a representative sample of 46,000 adults aged 20 and over from 14 provinces in China suggest that more than 92 million adults have diabetes and nearly 150 million more have pre-diabetes, pushing the prevalence figure to 10%, much higher than previous estimates (Yang *et al.*, 2010).

The Hong Kong Cardiovascular Risk Factor Prevalence Study (Janus *et al.*, 2000) estimates the prevalence of diabetes and impaired fasting glucose to be 9.8% and 6.2%. It has been estimated from epidemiological studies that up to 60% of Hong Kong Chinese with diabetes were previously undiagnosed (Cockram *et al.*, 1993). The International Diabetes Federation estimates the number of sufferers will increase to more than 1 million in Hong Kong by 2025.

WHO estimates that mortality from diabetes, heart disease and stroke will cost China US$555.7 billion in lost national income over the next 10 years.

Although type 1 diabetes remains the main form of the disease in children, it is likely that type 2 diabetes will be the prevalent form within 10 years in many ethnic groups (Zimmet *et al.*, 2001). In Japan, type 2 diabetes accounts for 80% of childhood diabetes (Kitagawa *et al.*, 1998).

Risk factors

Age, BMI, a family history of diabetes and dyslipidemia in men and age, BMI, hypertension, dyslipidemia, total cholesterol and history of gestational diabetes in women (Cockram *et al.*, 1993; Lau *et al.*, 1993; Ko *et al.*, 2000) are associated with an increased likelihood of developing diabetes in Hong Kong Chinese. These risk factors are associated with increasing age and have additive effects on the risk of developing diabetes.

Metabolic syndrome

Metabolic syndrome is a cluster of major risk factors which substantially increase the risk of premature cardiovascular diseases (CVD) and type 2 diabetes (Hu *et al.*, 2004; Malik *et al.*, 2004). Up to 80% of the almost 200 million adults with diabetes worldwide will die as a result of cardiovascular disease. People with metabolic syndrome are also at increased risk, being twice as likely to die from a heart attack and three times as likely to die from a stroke compared to people without the syndrome (Isomaa *et al.*, 2001; International Diabetes Federation, 2003).

Prevalence of metabolic syndrome in adolescents is relatively low in China – 3.7% compared with 10% in US adults – however, prevalence of the metabolic syndrome among overweight Chinese adolescents is similar to those living in the USA (Li *et al.*, 2008). Using data from the 2002 China National Nutrition and Health Survey (Li *et al.*, 2008), it is estimated that the prevalence of the metabolic syndrome is 35.2%, 23.4% and 2.3% among adolescents who were overweight (BMI ≥ 95th percentile), at risk of overweight (BMI 85th–95th percentile) and normal weight (BMI < 85th percentile), respectively. Based on these figures, it is estimated that more than 3 million Chinese adolescents have the metabolic syndrome.

Using International Diabetes Federation criteria (Kong *et al.*, 2008), it is estimated that 1.2% of Chinese adolescents in Hong Kong have metabolic syndrome and among the working Chinese population in Hong Kong (Ko *et al.*, 2006), estimates equate to a prevalence of 7.3% in men and 8.8% in women for metabolic syndrome.

Prevention

Recent studies have demonstrated the efficacy of lifestyle intervention in people with impaired glucose tolerance to progression to type 2 diabetes. The Diabetes Prevention Program in the USA demonstrated that diet and exercise delay the progression from impaired glucose tolerance to diabetes by 58% (Larkin, 2001). Similar results have been shown in the Da Qing IGT and Diabetes study in China (Pan *et al.*, 1997) and in the Finnish Diabetes Prevention Study Group trial (Tuomilehto *et al.*, 2001).

Diet modification (see Table 3.1.6) and physical activity are the two key approaches in the treatment of type 2 diabetes. The aim is for patients to control their blood glucose levels and to aid overweight patients in losing weight. Usually it is possible to control type 2 diabetes by diet and activity, however complex patients may require medication (oral hypoglycaemic agents) and/or insulin injection.

The use of plants and herbs (e.g., ginseng, ivy gourd (coccinia indica), garlic and aloe vera) for glycaemic control is common, particularly among the Chinese. There is relatively little known regarding the efficacy, safety and drug interactions of herbs, plants, vitamins or other dietary supple-

Table 3.1.6 Chinese Dietary modification for diabetes

	Discourage	Encourage
Fats	Frying, coconut cream/milk, fried dim sum, duck, belly pork, Chinese sausage, luncheon meat (spam), prawn crackers, fried rice or noodles	Boiling/steaming/baking/grilling, stir fry (monounsaturated oil), steamed dim sum, pork leg, skinless chicken breast, lean meat, plain boiled/steamed rice or noodles
Sugar	Lychee drink, sweetened soya/sugar cane drink, sweet fried/steamed bun, egg custard tart (*dan tart*), moon cake, sweet soup (*tong sui*)	Fruit juice, smoothies, water, diet/sugar-free drinks, sweetener, tea cake, rice cakes, rye/crisp bread, plain biscuits or crackers
Salt	Salt added at table and in cooking, corned beef, luncheon meat, black bean sauce, soy/hoisin sauce, salted duck eggs, monosodium glutamate, stock cubes	Herbs (coriander), spices (ginger, star anise, five spice powder, pepper), garlic, spring onion, lean, unsalted meats, plain boiled egg, lower/reduced salt soy sauce and stock cubes
Fibre	White bread, white rice, white rice noodles, white pasta, cornflakes, and other processed foods	Granary/multi-grain bread, brown or red rice, whole wheat/buckwheat noodles, whole wheat pasta, wholegrain breakfast cereals, adzuki beans, black eyed peas, lentils, potatoes, taro

ments for diabetes. The American Diabetes Association (2001) encourages healthcare providers to question patients on their use of alternative therapies and practices and be cognizant of any potential harm to patients.

3.1.9   Coronary heart disease and stroke

Key points

- The coronary heart disease (CHD) mortality rates in western countries are higher than in East Asian countries, while those for stroke are higher in East Asian than in western countries. This differential pattern is related to the contrasting dietary patterns between East Asian and western countries.
- The higher total and saturated fat intake in western countries appear to give rise to increased rates of dyslipidaemia, resulting in CHD.
- The greater intake of salt and higher dietary sodium/potassium ratio in East Asians are likely to be major contributors to hypertension, which increases the risk of stroke.
- Young East Asian immigrants are found to have adopted a diet in which the positive aspects of their traditional diets are replaced by the negative aspects of western diets, which are rela-

tively high in fat and cholesterol, but low in fibre.
- It is of concern if immigrants retain some of their unfavourable native eating habits which when combined with some of the unfavourable eating habits of their host country, will multiply their risk of CHD.
- To lower the risk of CVD, less salt and fats (particularly saturated fats) and a greater variety of fruit and vegetables are encouraged.

Introduction

The prevalence of coronary heart disease is lower in the Chinese compared to Caucasians. This may be attributed to the lower percentage fat in the traditional Chinese diet. In addition, the Chinese population in China consume mainly fish, seafood, vegetables but few dairy products, therefore the nutritional profile of these foods may be cardio-protective. These include antioxidants, omega 3 fatty acids, folic acid and phytoestrogens and are significantly higher than in western diets (Heaney, 1999).

Prevalence

Mortality rates for coronary heart disease in the UK and USA have always been higher than in East

Table 3.1.7 CHD and stroke mortality rate, age-standardized, 1970, 1994–98, men and women aged 35–74 years by country

Year	1970			1994–98			
Cause of death	Japan	UK	US	Japan	PR China	UK	US
Men							
Coronary heart disease	94[a]	509[b]	652	57	100[c]	267	202
Stroke	385	141	120	79	251	57	42
Women							
Coronary heart disease	47	164	252	20	69	96	84
Stroke	225	113	90	41	170	44	33

a. Age-standardized rate per 100,000 population.
b. England and Wales.
c. Urban. (WHO American Heart Association, 2001)

Asian countries such as Japan. In contrast, East Asian countries have higher mortality rates for stroke compared to their western counterparts. This trend has long been recognized (see Table 3.1.7).

There is increasing evidence from large epidemiological studies (Kuulasmaa *et al.*, 2000; Ueshima *et al.*, 2003; Zhou *et al.*, 2003) to show that this differential pattern is related to the dietary patterns in East Asian and western countries.

Dietary patterns in East Asian and western populations

Macro- and micronutrient intakes have been found to differ markedly in East Asian and western populations. The western diet is higher in total fat, saturated fat, trans fatty acids and sugar, but lower in total carbohydrate and starch. In contrast, the East Asian diet is lower in calcium, phosphorus, selenium and vitamin A. Dietary sodium is higher and potassium lower, hence the sodium/potassium ratio is higher in the Asian diet, particularly in the Chinese. The Japanese diet contains a higher intake of omega 3 polyunsaturated fatty acids, almost certainly reflecting a greater fish intake; a higher intake of cholesterol, probably due to greater egg consumption; and for Japanese men greater average intake of alcohol (Ueshima *et al.*, 2003).

These findings indicate that despite economic development, globalization (including of the food supply), national and international public health

recommendations for CHD/CVD prevention and control, which may have influenced dietary trends in recent decades (Worth *et al.*, 1975; Robertson *et al.*, 1977), important differences remain, albeit blunted, across East Asian and western populations.

Risk factors and treatment

It is well known that the underlying pathology leading to most clinical CHD is severe coronary atherosclerosis. The aetiology of the modern epidemic of severe atherosclerotic disease is adverse lifestyles, especially with regard to eating pattern – diets high in total fat, saturated fat, trans fat, cholesterol, calories (for level of energy expenditure) and salt, and often inadequate in protective micronutrients and fibre, and excessive in alcohol. Excess dietary lipid is of major importance, primarily because it causes a rise in population average serum cholesterol and its atherogenic fractions from youth through to middle age, with resultant high population average levels and high rates of dyslipidaemia (Zhou *et al.*, 2003).

It has been inferred that the key factor accounting for persistent low CHD rates in China and Japan is the low average serum cholesterol that has prevailed throughout adulthood for both men and women (Kuulasmaa *et al.*, 2000).

On the other hand, the underlying pathology of stroke is more variegated and complex compared to CHD. A small percentage of stroke is due to atherothrombotic disease of the large arteries supplying the brain. Other types of stroke include cerebral haemorrhage, cerebral ischaemia and embolism to the brain. For all these types of stroke, high blood pressure is a prime risk factor. Cigarette smoking also enhances risk markedly (Zhou *et al.* 2003).

In this context, the greater East Asian intake of salt and higher dietary sodium/potassium ratio (Na/K), especially for China, are likely to be major contributors to hypertension in adulthood. Thus, there is high average systolic blood pressure to diastolic blood pressure ratio (SBP/DBP) for the population from middle age onwards and high prevalence rates of adverse SBP/DBP levels, despite low average body mass index (BMI). For the Chinese in China, comparatively low intakes of total protein, especially animal protein, and of calcium may also be factors playing a role in the development of adverse SBP/DBP levels and high risk of stroke (Zhou *et al.*, 2003).

Dietary pattern in immigrant East Asians

It is well known that with increasing acculturation, immigrants adopt the dietary patterns in their host country. More dramatic changes in dietary patterns can be found in the younger generation of Asians since they assimilate western culture to a greater extent than their parents. Young Asians living in the USA have been found to have a higher fat diet and consume more cholesterol than their older counterparts. They also ate out three times more and ate less ethnic foods than the older Asians. Young Asians' diets were more Americanized in that they ate more fast foods and drank more juices. This process of acculturation has led to young Asians acquiring a diet in which the positive aspects of their traditional diets are replaced by the negative aspects of the western diets, which are relatively high in fat and cholesterol, but low in fibre (Wu-Tso *et al.*, 1995). These findings indicate that the degree of acculturation of immigrants certainly affects dietary intakes in ways that may alter risks of several chronic diseases.

It is of concern if immigrants retain some of their unfavourable eating habits (e.g., a high salt diet) as, when combined with some of the unfavourable

eating habits of their host country, their risk of CHD will be multiplied. Recent studies have indicated that average serum cholesterol levels of middle-aged Chinese rose during the 1990s, as diets became 'richer' and BMI increased (serial data from the PRC-USA collaborative study, 1992). Similarly, data from the Japanese–Hawaii INTERLIPID study indicate that the decades-long favourable serum lipid levels of Japanese middle-aged populations (Keys *et al.*, 1984) no longer exist. This, plus the extraordinarily high smoking rates of Chinese and Japanese men, along with high average blood pressures, indicates that the East Asian serum lipid trend is to be regarded as a warning signal.

There is a positive association between salt intake and hypertension which is well documented for the older Chinese. The recommended daily intake of sodium is 6 g. Astonishingly, the northern Chinese diet consists of preserved vegetables contributing to approximately 15 g of salt daily (Woo *et al.*, 2002). A reduction in the population's hypertension will have positive effects on stroke and multi-infarct dementia prevention.

Dietary modification

Reduce and replace salt intake:

- Balance salt intake by having one flavourful dish, accompanied by a less salted dish at each meal.
- Flavour the dish with vinegar, lemon juice or juice from other citrus fruits, or adding tomatoes (and less salt) to give it a tangy twang.
- Use herbs (e.g., coriander), spices (e.g., ginger, star anise, five spice, pepper), and garlic to flavour dishes instead of salt.
- Garnish the dish with celery, spring onions and chilli to enhance the flavour of the dish.
- Use Chinese mushrooms, dried scallops or white fungus, together with chicken or pork bones, to create a tasty stock for soups. No or little salt is thus needed.
- Reduce intake of preserved and salted products like salted eggs, salted fish, preserved vegetables, fruit and snacks and tinned products.
- High salt products include soy sauce, monosodium glutamate (MSG), seasoning, fish sauce,

therefore limit use of these during cooking and at the table or use lower/reduced salt versions.

Reduce saturated fats, trans fats and foods high in cholesterol:

- These include fatty meat such as duck, pork belly, spare ribs, luncheon meat, chicken's feet, tripe and other types of offal.
- Traditional cakes and pastries may be rich in lard or butter. Make use of monounsaturated oils and spreads (e.g., vegetable oil derived from rapeseed, peanut oil, canola oil or olive oil) in cooking.
- Have steamed fish or lean meat, instead of fried.

Emphasize fish, soya and bean products to increase protein and calcium intake:

- When steamed and in soups, these provide the more beneficial fats (mono- and polyunsaturates).
- Take moderate amounts of dairy products if tolerated (e.g., milk, yoghurt, low-fat cheese).

Increase fruit and vegetable intake:

- The WHO recommended daily intake is 400 g.
- Consume a variety to maximize intake of the range of nutrients fruit and vegetables to provide vitamin C, potassium, folate, fibre, carotenoids and flavonoids. These have been shown to help reduce CVD risk (see Table 3.1.8).

3.1.10   Cancer

Key points

- Approximately 6.7 million people worldwide die each year as a result of cancer (Cancer Research UK). The most common cancers are lung, breast, bowel, stomach and prostate.
- Cancer has become the major leading cause of death in China, accounting for 22% of all deaths. Nasopharyngeal, lung, stomach and oesophageal cancer are most prevalent (He *et al.*, 2005).
- Increased physical activity, smoking cessation and adopting a healthier diet are important lifestyle changes for reducing risk of cancer.

Introduction

For many Chinese people, cancer is a taboo subject and there remain various misconceptions surrounding the disease. There is a lack of knowledge and understanding, but many Chinese acknowledge that the disease is serious and life-threatening (Papadopoulos *et al.*, 2007). Western medicines and treatments are well known and available to the Chinese but many seek alternative or complementary therapy while they are undergoing such treatments (Chui *et al.*, 2005). Traditional Chinese medicines are acknowledged for their holistic

Table 3.1.8   Chinese Dietary modification for treatment of coronary heart disease

	Discourage	Encourage
Food products	Preserved and salted products, e.g., preserved vegetables/fruit/snacks, salted eggs, salted fish, tinned products	Fresh produce, e.g., fresh fruit and vegetables, fish, soya and bean products
Flavourings	Salt, soy sauce, monosodium glutamate, seasoning, fish sauce	Lower/reduced salt, soy sauce/seasoning/fish sauce, vinegar, lemon juice, citrus fruits, tomatoes, herbs (coriander), spices (ginger, star anise, five spice powder, pepper), garlic, celery, spring onion, chilli
Types of fat	Fatty meat, e.g., duck, pork belly, spare ribs, luncheon meat, chicken's feet, tripe, offal, cakes & pastries rich in lard and butter (saturated fat)	Lean, skinless meat, monounsaturated cooking oils and spreads, e.g., vegetable oil (rapeseed), peanut oil, canola oil, olive oil, sesame oil, corn oil
Cooking methods	Deep frying	Steaming, boiling, grilling, stir frying

properties and are often viewed as an important element in the treatment of cancer.

Nationwide campaigns for smoking cessation continue to play a major part in health promotion in China, as there are around 303 million smokers and 530 million passive smokers in the country (Yang *et al.*, 2008). Educating the population on the health risks associated with both smoking and passive smoking are therefore vital to reduce the high prevalence of lung cancer in the country (Parkin *et al.*, 2005).

Traditional Chinese medicine (TCM) is renowned for its holistic approach to health treatments, including cancer care, and plays a key role in treatment for many Chinese patients. Individuals may choose to use western medicines as well as TCM for their treatment of cancer. TCM may be used as an adjunct to aggressive cancer treatments or as a palliative to ease pain or other symptoms (Chui *et al.*, 2005).

Prevalence

It has been estimated that 10 million cases of cancer are diagnosed worldwide each year with 2.2 million new cases diagnosed in China in comparison to 1.6 million cases in North America (Parkin *et al.*, 2005). Around 24.6 million people are living with cancer worldwide and China has 3.1 million with the disease (Parkin *et al.*, 2005) (see Table 3.1.9).

Approximately 6.7 million deaths result from cancer worldwide each year with around 1.6 million in China. The global deaths from stomach cancer stand at around 700,000 cases and 45% of these are from China alone. The incidence of stomach cancer is highest in Japan, and China is the second highest worldwide (Parkin *et al.*, 2005). This type of cancer is the most commonly diagnosed in Chinese women and the second most commonly diagnosed cancer in men (Table 3.1.9).

The incidence of lung cancer is high in China; in fact, the number of cases in Chinese women is the third highest in the world and the cases seen in Chinese men are the sixth highest in the world (Parkin *et al.*, 2005). It is the leading cancer diagnosis for Chinese men and the second highest for Chinese women.

The third most common diagnosis for Chinese males is liver cancer. The number of total cases in China represents 55% of all cases seen worldwide. For females in China, the third highest incidence of cancer is of the breast. However, the incidence of breast cancer is relatively low when compared to North America, where it is more than five times of that found in China (Parkin *et al.*, 2005).

There is a lack of information on the incidence of cancer in Chinese people living in the UK. However, it has been observed that Chinese people who migrate to western countries tend to be at increased risk of cancers which are more prevalent there, such as colorectal and breast (McCracken *et al.*, 2007).

A study found that the attitude to cancer screening, such as the use of flexi-sigmoidoscopy for colorectal cancer, can differ between ethnic minorities in the UK. Many British Chinese interviewed were able to suggest a cause of colorectal cancer but stated they would not undergo such screening due to embarrassment and shame (Robb *et al.*, 2008). It has also been found that the low uptake of screening in ethnic groups may be due to cultural differences, language and accessibility to healthcare (McCracken *et al.*, 2007).

Risk factors and treatments

A number of factors may increase the risk of developing cancer. These include obesity, an insufficient intake of fruit and vegetables, high intake of meat and meat products and poor dietary fibre intake (World Cancer Research Fund, 2007). Rice and

Table 3.1.9 Cancer incidence per 100,000

Site of Cancer	Male	Female
Lung	42.4	19.0
Breast	N/A	18.7
Colorectal	13.6	9.2
Stomach	41.4	19.2
Prostate	1.6	N/A
Liver	37.9	14.2
Cervical	N/A	6.8
Oesophageal	27.4	12.0
Bladder	3.8	1.4
Non-Hodgkin's lymphoma	3.0	1.6
Leukaemia	0.2	0.2

(Parkin *et al.*, 2005)

wheat are the staples of the Chinese diet as well as products made from these ingredients, such as noodles, rice cakes, bread and dumplings. The traditional Chinese diet can therefore be low in wholegrain cereal products but high in fruit and vegetables (Thomas & Bishop, 2007). Cases of bowel cancer are rising in parts of Asia including Hong Kong and Japan, which could be a result of low consumption of cereal fibre in the diet as well as physical inactivity and smoking (Parkin *et al.*, 2005; McCracken *et al.*, 2007).

Nasopharyngeal cancer is rare but is more commonly diagnosed in China. Both environment and lifestyle factors have been shown to be the main risk factors for the high incidences of nasopharyngeal cancers especially in southern China (Chang & Adami, 2006). It is well documented that the risk of head and neck cancers increases with smoking and alcohol consumption (Blot *et al.*, 1988).

The use of salt and monosodium glutamate in Chinese cooking is common for both flavouring and preservation. Cured meats and salted fish are frequently used in Chinese dishes and considered a delicacy. It is suspected that the high levels of nitrosamine and bacterial mutagens present are the key risk factors for nasopharyngeal carcinoma (Zou *et al.*, 2000; Jiang *et al.*, 2004). The high prevalence of Epstein-Barr virus also contributes to the high incidence of this type of head and neck cancer. As there are different methods for producing salted fish in various areas of China, incidences of nasopharyngeal cancer also vary between the different provinces (Zou *et al.*, 2000).

One of the main health problems in China is hepatitis B infection. It has been estimated that around 10% of the population are affected by it (Zhao *et al.*, 2000). As the hepatitis B virus has been shown to increase the risk of hepatocellular carcinoma, patients should be monitored closely to assess for any development of cancer (Yang *et al.*, 2002). Awareness of the disease needs to be improved as well as access to appropriate treatments to prevent the spread of hepatitis B within the Chinese population.

The high incidence of stomach cancer is linked with tobacco smoking and *Helicobacter pylori* infection as well as high intake of salted and preserved products (Tsugane & Sasazuki, 2007). In developing countries and areas with overcrowding and

low income, *H. pylori* infection is widespread and its prevalence has also been found to be high in areas where gastric cancer is common. Other factors, such as a large number of young children in the family and lower educational status, have also been suggested as factors for cases of the infection (Shi *et al.*, 2008). More studies are needed to establish a link between diet and this type of infectious disease.

The use of TCM is common in Chinese culture. Herbal remedies are concocted by mixing ingredients derived from plants with the aim of restoring the balance of Yin and Yang in the body (Lee *et al.*, 2000). Acupuncture may also be used to ease the flow of energy (*ch'i*) in the body. Some patients may choose to follow conventional treatments such as chemotherapy and radiotherapy but will use Chinese medicine to counter any effects these treatments may have on their energy balance. There is no doubt that TCM is effective for conditions such as eczema and malaria, however, more randomized controlled trials are needed to establish the clinical effectiveness of such remedies for the treatment of cancer (Tang & Wong, 1998; Pu *et al.*, 2008).

Dietary modification

The traditional Chinese diet is high in carbohydrates, grains, fruits and vegetables, and low in red meat and dairy products (see Table 3.1.10). The dietary pattern of western countries historically has differed from that of East Asia as the populations consume more red meat, animal fats and sugar and fewer grains and vegetables. These differences are one of the explanatory factors of the variation in the prevalence of cancer between the countries.

As the Chinese diet becomes increasingly westernized, with it come the health implications of a diet higher in fat and sugar, such as breast cancer, coronary heart disease and obesity (Cui *et al.*, 2007; McCracken *et al.*, 2007; Thomas & Bishop, 2007). The number of cases of breast cancer witnessed in China has steadily increased due to the changes in dietary pattern. More red meat, dairy products and sugary foods are consumed on a regular basis by the Chinese, particularly the younger generation. The availability of such foods has vastly increased due to the growth in the economy.

Table 3.1.10 Chinese Dietary modification for treatment of cancer

Food	Discourage	Encourage
Carbohydrates	Fried white rice or noodles	Boiled/steamed rice – brown or red
		Boiled noodles – buckwheat, whole wheat
Proteins	Fatty, salted or preserved meat	Lean meat (with skin or fat removed)
	Large amounts of meat	Fish
	Deep-fried	Soya (tofu) and other bean curd
		Steamed, boiled or stir-fried
Milk and dairy foods	Condensed/evaporated milk	Milk – skimmed
	Cream	Low-fat dairy products – yoghurt, soft/cottage cheese
Fruit and vegetables	Salted or preserved fruit and vegetables	Fresh fruit and vegetables
	Added sugar	Steamed or stir-fried vegetables
	Deep-fried	
Fats and oils	Lard	Use less oil and use monounsaturated oil:
	Butter	Olive oil
		Rapeseed oil
		Sesame oil
		Canola oil
		Peanut oil
		Corn oil
		Low-fat spread made from these oils
Herbs, spices and flavourings	Monosodium glutamate	Ginger
	Salt	Garlic
	Soy sauce	Coriander
	Sugar	Pepper
		Chilli
		Star anise
		Chinese five spice
		Spring onion
		Lemon juice
		Celery
Drinks	Alcohol	Water
	Sugary/sweetened drinks	Chinese tea
		Fruit juice/smoothies
		Diet/no added sugar drinks

The Chinese diet is traditionally high in soya but there is conflicting evidence demonstrating whether these products can increase risk or offer a protective effect against breast cancer. Isoflavones found in soya have similar chemical structures as oestrogen. It is thought that isoflavones may be of benefit to those with oestrogen-receptive breast cancer as the compound competes with oestrogen to bind with the receptors (Messina & Wood, 2008). A recent study showed no increased risk of breast cancer with higher intake of soya but there was increased risk with higher meat consumption (Cui et al., 2007). While more studies are needed to substantiate the effect of soya on cancer, such food items should be included in the diet in reasonable quantities if any.

Due to the identified risk factors for various cancers in the Chinese population, the key dietary recommendations are:

- Avoidance of salted eggs, salted fish and preserved meat as well as following the traditional Chinese diet, which is low in fat.
- Alcohol should be limited to recommended levels (21 units/week for men, 14 units/week for women) due to the increased risk of oesophageal and oral cancer with higher intakes (World Cancer Research Fund, 2007).
- The use of wholegrain products should be encouraged.
- Increase the amount of fruit and vegetables consumed. A higher intake of vitamin C has been shown to have a protective effect against gastric cancer, which is especially prevalent in the Chinese (Tsugane & Sasazuki, 2007).
- Traditional cooking methods, such as steaming and stir-frying, should continue, as less fat is used compared with methods such as deep frying and roasting.

As well as reducing dietary intake of preserved and salted food products to reduce cancer risk, lifestyle factors should be taken into consideration as these can also impact health. Cessation of smoking and the prevention of viral infections should be recommended to help reduce the risk of cancer in the Chinese population. An increase in physical activity levels would also help to improve the health of many Chinese across the world. Raising awareness and improving understanding of the impact of both dietary and lifestyle factors on the risk of cancer should result in a reduction on the number of cancer diagnoses seen in Chinese people.

Evidence of best practice

Having a basic understanding of the concept of Yin and Yang and the Chinese holistic approach to treatment would be of significant benefit when providing dietetic advice for a Chinese patient (see Introduction). Foods are classed as 'hot' or 'cold' for the balance of Yin and Yang in the body. For example, a patient may increase their intake of 'cold' food to counter any effect from their

body being in a 'hot' state such as when receiving radiotherapy (Chui et al., 2005). It is therefore important to consider these practices when advising patients from this ethnic group. Patients should be advised to consult their doctor or dietitian before taking any complementary treatments, including TCM.

Suggestions for the way forward

Health professionals often have little or no knowledge of the use of TCM. Since it is such an integral part of Chinese culture, there is a real need for more quality studies to demonstrate its clinical effectiveness in the treatment of cancer (Tang & Wong, 1998). When undertaking a dietary consultation with a patient of Chinese origin, it may be of benefit to ascertain whether any herbal remedies are taken, or indeed whether other complementary therapies are being used.

3.1.11   Nutrition support

Introduction

Food plays an integral part in Chinese culture with diverse cooking styles found in the various provinces of China (see Introduction). During illness, food is usually viewed as an essential part of the healing process and family members are often keen to support patients.

Many Chinese patients may choose to use TCM when they are ill, either on its own or as a complementary treatment to conventional medicines (Chui et al., 2005). TCM may use herbal remedies derived from various types of plants boiled together in water or treatments such as acupuncture (Lee et al., 2000).

Dietary needs

Oral nutrition support may be required for patients who are unable to meet their nutritional requirements with their usual food intake due to various clinical conditions and stages of their conditions. Or they may not be able to consume their usual food intake due to physical, social, psychological and behavioural factors. The use of ordinary foods and drinks should be considered first for all patients requiring nutrition support prior to the introduction of nutritional sip feeds (Thomas & Bishop, 2007). Patients requiring nutrition support should be provided with first-line information on food fortification and practical ideas on adding nutritional value to their diet. Advice on ethnic foods should be given to patients of Chinese origin, as familiar foods may be more acceptable to this group, particularly in the older generation.

Dietary advice

The Chinese diet usually consists of three meals a day, with the evening meal constituting the main meal of the day. The staple foods include rice and wheat and their products, such as noodles, bread and dumplings.

Advice should include increasing the frequency of oral intake as well as the addition of nutrient-dense foods and beverages. Dietary advice for a high-energy diet largely includes adding milk-based drinks, meat, dairy products and sugary food and drinks to the diet. For many Chinese living in Britain, it is important to advise on these foods as well as typical Chinese foods readily available in stores and supermarkets. The younger generation of Chinese will most likely be familiar with both western and Chinese foods, hence the importance of providing dietary information on both diets (Thomas & Bishop, 2007) (see Table 3.1.11).

Poor appetite

Patients may experience loss of appetite (anorexia) due to the physical effects of their illness or disease, such as pain, nausea, vomiting, diarrhoea or a sore mouth. Psychological effects may also occur as a result of their illness or disease progression, which may include anxiety, depression, general malaise, lethargy and lack of motivation to eat and drink. Nutrition support is vital to prevent malnutrition. Below are examples of high-energy and high-protein Chinese foods and fluids (Cancer Equality, 2008).

Early satiety

Gastric resection, abdominal tumours or radiotherapy to the upper abdominal area, and the resultant psychological effects, may lead to patients feeling full much earlier than usual. It is therefore essential

Table 3.1.11 Chinese Dietary modification for Nutritional support

Meals	Foods
Main and light meals	Rice *congee* with pork, chicken, egg or fish and/or with grains, beans, nuts and seeds
	Scrambled egg with ham and spring onion
	Fried noodles or rice with meat and vegetables
	Thick soup with pork, black-eyed peas, almonds, mushrooms and dried dates
	Selection of dim sum (fried ideally)
Desserts	Sweet soup (*tong sui*) made with egg, coconut, milk, sugar and nuts
	Peanut or sesame glutinous rice dumplings
	Bean curd pudding with sugar
	Red bean soup pudding
	Sweet peanut soup
	Jelly and ice cream
High-energy and protein snacks	Twisted or spicy doughnuts
	Ox tongue crisps
	Dumplings
	Tea leaf eggs
	Toast/bread with peanut butter and butter or fried egg and ham
	Green or red bean cakes
	Sweets and biscuits
	Fried cashew or peanuts
	Peanut brittle
Nourishing drinks	Soya milk with sugar
	Peanut and rice drink
	Lemon and honey tea
	Red bean and cream drink
	Raw sugar cane drink
	Mango and milk bubble tea

for these patients to consume energy-dense foods and drinks to augment the nutritional content of their intake. Patients should also be advised to eat little and often by including regular snacks and drinks throughout the day. Avoid drinking fluids with meals or for an hour beforehand.

Nausea and vomiting

These symptoms may occur as a result of illness, exacerbation of a condition or a side-effect of treatment such as medication or chemotherapy. Anti-emetics may be needed to mitigate the symptoms of nausea and vomiting.

Patients should be advised to eat small meals more frequently throughout the day with nourishing drinks in between their meals. Patients may find cooking smells exacerbate their symptoms; therefore, it may be advisable to ask other members of the family to help prepare their meals.

Ginger has been found to have anti-emetic properties; the use of foods and drinks containing this plant may be of benefit to patients suffering nausea and vomiting (Ernst & Pittler, 2000). The use of ginger is common in stir-fry dishes, and it can also be consumed in ginger tea, ginger beer and ginger sweets and desserts. Chinese patients may find it useful to add ginger when they are cooking their rice or main dishes with meat and vegetables.

Taste changes (dysgeusia)

Treatments such as chemotherapy and radiotherapy can often lead to a change in taste for patients. Foods and beverages may taste blander than usual or metallic.

Patients should be encouraged to choose foods that are strong in flavour such as sweet and sour, hot and sour, lemon or pineapple sauce, black bean sauce, black pepper and the use of herbs. Other sharp-tasting foods such as mints, sweets, preserved fruits and ginger-containing products may be useful when a patient is experiencing taste changes.

The use of different sauces, seasonings and spices may also be useful in helping foods to taste less metallic. Soy sauce, sweet chilli sauce, hoisin sauce, rice wine vinegar, five spice, honey, sugar, chilli oil and sesame oil are just a few of the many sauces and spices that can be used in Chinese cooking. Marinating food with these may help to enhance the flavour. Patients may find certain foods too sweet, in which case the use of lemon, bitter melon and wine vinegar may help to neutralize the sweetness.

Sore mouth

Certain treatments, such as chemotherapy and radiotherapy, may cause a sore and painful mouth (stomatitis and mucositis). Other factors, such as infection, inflammation, ulceration of the oral areas or oral thrush, may also cause this unpleasant side-effect. As well as dietary advice, oral hygiene and appropriate pain control should be offered to patients.

Dietary advice for patients suffering from a sore mouth should focus on eating soft, moist foods as well as using plenty of sauces. Examples of soft, moist foods include *congee*, soup, stew and porridge. Foods that are very dry or rough in texture (e.g., crackers, biscuits and crisps) should be avoided. Patients should also avoid very salty, spicy and acidic foods and sauces.

Cold drinks, such as iced tea or coffee, red bean and cream drink or even ice cubes, ice cream and ice lollies, may be soothing and could be beneficial to patients.

Dry mouth (xerostomia)

This unpleasant damage to the salivary gland can be caused by surgery or radiotherapy to the head and neck region, but can also be a side-effect of medications, poorly controlled diabetes or dehydration. The use of an artificial saliva product may be useful for patients with damage to the salivary gland.

Patients should be encouraged to have a soft, moist diet, using plenty of sauces. Any food items that are extremely dry (e.g., nuts, crackers and toast) should be avoided. Fluids should be taken throughout the day to help keep the oral cavity moist and avoid dehydration. Adding honey or slices of lemon to water if the mouth is not sore are both sharp tasting and refreshing. As well as cold fluids, sucking ice cubes, ice lollies, boiled sweets or slices of chilled melon may be soothing.

This advice is likely to be welcomed by the Chinese patient as it is aligned with the principles of Yin and Yang, whereby xerostomia would be perceived as being in a hot/dry state similar to *yeet hay* and so must be counterbalanced with cold/wet food and drink.

Food fortification

Energy and protein can be added to the diet using everyday foods to boost nutritional intake when appetite is poor. Practical ideas on food fortification using energy-dense foods should be provided to patients who require oral nutrition support as first-line advice.

The following foods are high in energy and protein and can be added to fortify meals and drinks:

- Milk powder added to whole/full-fat milk (4 tablespoons of milk powder/1 pint milk). This mixture can then be used in food and drinks such as breakfast cereal, porridge, milk puddings, tea or coffee.
- Butter or oil added to vegetables, sauces, pasta, rice and during cooking.
- Butter or spread thickly spread on in sandwiches or on toast.
- Cream, cheese and/or milk added to soup, sauces, pasta and mashed potato.
- Sugar, jam, syrup or honey added to breakfast cereals, milk puddings, fruit smoothies, milkshakes or other drinks and desserts.
- Evaporated/condensed milk added to tea, coffee and desserts.
- Ice cream, double cream, full-fat yoghurt or custard added to desserts such as brownies, apple pie or waffles.
- Full-fat foods and drinks, e.g., whole/full-fat milk, thick and creamy/full-fat yoghurt, rather than low-fat, low-calorie, 'light' or 'diet' food and drinks.
- Fried food (e.g., vegetables, meat, fish, tofu, rice, noodles), using plenty of oil, butter or sauces.
- Dips (e.g., hoisin sauce, plum sauce, oyster sauce, sweet chilli sauce).
- Shredded meat, beans, egg, fried onions or noodles added to soup, stew and *congee*.
- Snacks and light meals (e.g., dim sum, pork pies, scotch eggs, nuts, sweets, jellies, milk puddings, cakes, biscuits, bean curd pudding, red bean pudding, coconut cream buns, egg custard tarts (*dan tart*), peanut glutinous rice dumpling)

eaten throughout the day if a main meal cannot be managed.
- Glucose powder or over-the-counter nutritional supplements such as Complan or Build Up powder added to food and drink. Milkshakes and soup versions are available in a variety of flavours and can be bought in pharmacies and larger supermarkets.

Nutritional supplements

If ordinary foods and drinks are insufficient to improve a patient's nutritional status, the use of nutritional supplements may be necessary to prevent weight loss and malnutrition. Oral nutritional supplements are high in energy and protein and are available in a variety of forms including sip feeds, powders, puddings and energy-dense liquid supplements. The use of ordinary foods and drinks should always be considered first, prior to the introduction of proprietary supplements. Details of both oral nutritional supplements and enteral feeds, including types of feeds and their appropriate use, are well documented in *The Manual of Dietetics* (Thomas & Bishop, 2007).

If a Chinese patient needs to introduce nutritional supplements into their diet, clear instructions and an explanation should be given to ensure compliance. Although dairy intake is relatively low in East Asia, it is not uncommon for Chinese patients to include milk and other dairy products in their diet (Lau *et al.*, 1988). The introduction of proprietary supplements or enteral feeds should therefore be relatively well received.

Suggestions for the way forward

Traditional Chinese medicines may be used by patients to enhance their health and well-being (Lee *et al.*, 2000). As there could be a reaction between conventional treatments and Chinese medicines, patients should always seek medical advice before introducing any of these medicines into their healthcare plan.

3.1.12   Nutritional deficiencies

Calcium

The exclusion or lower consumption of dairy products in the Chinese diet can lead to a low intake of calcium, however this is likely to be offset by the higher intake of non-dairy, calcium-rich foods such as soya milk, tofu, bean curd and green, leafy vegetables. However, reported calcium intakes in some Chinese Americans have been as low as 400 mg/day in comparison to Caucasians' > 1,000 mg/day (Jackson & Savaiano, 2001). Mean calcium intakes in a sample population of 142 Chinese, Japanese and Korean women showed low calcium intakes in the younger population as well as the older women. These figures mirror calcium consumption of other ethnic minorities, which is much lower than the recommended daily intake.

Low dairy product consumption in the Chinese population and a high salt intake causes urinary calcium secretion, which predisposes to osteoporotic fractures. This is particularly true of the older generation of Chinese, who are more likely to follow a traditional diet. The calcium intake across China ranges from 300 mg to 800 mg per day which is low in comparison to 1,200 mg in North Americans. Vegetables and soy products provide 41% of calcium intake in the Chinese population and absorption from some of these foodstuffs is higher than that of milk.

Fibre

Fibre intake, particularly of insoluble fibre, may be low in the Chinese diet as wholegrain cereals are infrequently consumed. White rice is the staple and dumplings, noodles and bread are largely made from white rice or refined wheat flour. Fruit and vegetable, and hence soluble fibre, consumption is higher, as these foods are seen to impart 'cooling' properties and thus feature in every meal as they balance the 'heating' properties of meat and spices. An overall lack of insoluble fibre may predispose the Chinese population to a higher risk of constipation.

Anaemia

Anaemia is common among women of Chinese ethnic origin in the UK, occurring much more frequently than in women of European origin (Fischbacher *et al.*, 2001). It is predominantly microcytic and may be related to iron deficiency secondary to a low consumption of red meat.

Another type of anaemia prevalent in the Chinese population is alpha-zero-thalassaemia. It is an important genetic risk for those originating from Hong Kong, South China, Vietnam, Singapore, Malaysia, Thailand and the Philippines.

Haemoglobin H disease is a sub-type of alpha-thalassaemia. Patients present with chronic haemolytic anaemia of variable severity. Though a less prevalent form of anaemia in the Chinese population, for those with elevated ferritin levels, the diet should be low in iron. If the reticulocyte count is elevated, the diet should be supplemented with folic acid (Cheerva & Ashok, 2009).

3.2 Vietnamese Diet
Maclinh Duong

Key points

- The traditional Vietnamese diet can be low in fat, high in starchy carbohydrates and abundant in fruit and vegetables – especially eaten raw.
- Low-fat cooking methods are common. This should be encouraged as part of healthy eating messages.
- Fish sauce is commonly used in cooking rather than salt.
- As in Chinese culture, the concept of Yin and Yang is often followed in terms of its application to diet, nutrition and well-being.
- Vietnamese who have migrated to the UK or are UK-born .readily adopt UK dietary practices, especially a western-style breakfast and midday meal.
- In the UK a traditional Vietnamese meal is often consumed in the evening when more time is available and all family members are present.

3.2.1 Introduction

Long periods of domination and interaction with its northern neighbour, China, have resulted in Vietnam's historical inclusion as part of the East Asian cultural sphere known widely as the Chinese cultural sphere. Following independence from China in the 10th century, Vietnam began a southward expansion which saw the annexation of territories formerly belonging to the Champa civilization (now central Vietnam) and parts of the Khmer

French introduced Roman Catholicism and the Latin alphabet (Vietnam is the only non-island nation of Indochina which uses the Latin alphabet). The vast majority of the first Vietnamese immigrants to the UK spoke no English at all, but second-generation Vietnamese British people, as well as more recent immigrants, have a better understanding of English (Sims, 2007). It is unknown how many of the 55,000 Vietnamese people presently in the UK speak English as their first or second language, and Vietnamese is the main language of some 22,000 Vietnamese people in the UK.

Migration to the United Kingdom

Mass migration to the UK started after the end of the Vietnam War in 1975, with the UK being one of only six countries accepting refugees. Early immigrants were the so-called boat people fleeing persecution by the victorious communists, as well as students, academics and business people. Vietnamese refugees found it difficult to adapt to the British way of life, and as the established Vietnamese British community was very small, the new wave of immigrants found it much harder to settle in compared with those who migrated to, say, France or the USA. Many came to the major cities, including the capital, London (33,000), with around approximately a third of all Vietnamese Londoners settling in the boroughs of Lewisham (where Vietnamese is now the second most common language), Southwark and Hackney (Sims, 2007). A significant (>4,000) Vietnamese community lives in Birmingham, and over 2,500 are in Leeds and Manchester (Burrell, 2000).

Current UK population

The 2001 census recorded 23,347 Vietnamese-born people of whom 65% originate from northern Vietnam. According to most recent estimates there are at least 55,000 people of Vietnamese origin living in England and Wales (0.01% of the UK's population), of these around 20,000 are thought to be undocumented migrants and 5,000 students on temporary visas (Sims, 2007).

3.2.2   Religion

The most common religions for Vietnamese people in the UK are Mahayana Buddhism and Roman

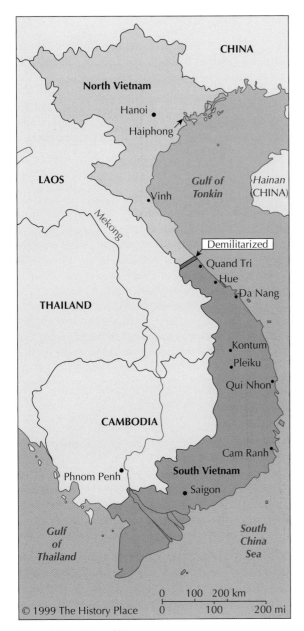

Figure 3.2.1   Map of Vietnam

empire (now southern Vietnam) which explain minor regional variances in Vietnam's culture due to contact with these different groups (Figure 3.2.1).

Language

During the French colonial period (1874–1954), Vietnam was influenced by European culture. The

Catholicism, followed by approximately 80% and 20% respectively of the community's total population. This is different from the religious breakdown in Vietnam, where 85% of the population are Buddhist/Confucian and 6.8% are Roman Catholic. (Cheney, 2005). Besides the 'triple religion', Vietnamese life is profoundly influenced by ancestor worship as well as animism. Most Vietnamese people, regardless of religious denomination, practise ancestor worship and have an ancestor altar in their home or business alongside a statue of Buddha – a testament to the emphasis Vietnamese culture places on filial duty.

3.2.3 Traditional eating pattern in Vietnam

The Chinese concept of Yin and Yang (see Table 3.1.1 page 139, Chinese Diet) also plays a major part in Vietnamese life in terms of health maintenance and treating illness.

There are, however, major differences between Chinese and Vietnamese cuisine. In part this is the result of French colonial rule, which has resulted in the use of making consommé, braising techniques and French bread and coffee being a ubiquitous part of the Vietnamese diet.

The main differences lie in the seasonings used, the cooking methods employed and the emphasis on the use of fresh and plentiful amounts of herbs and vegetables either cooked mixed in the dish itself or served raw with a dipping sauce. Vietnamese cuisine also has regional variations, with notable differences in the spices used and how hot (chilli heat) the food is cooked.

Northern Vietnam

Vietnamese cuisine can be divided into three categories, each pertaining to a specific region. With northern Vietnam being the cradle of Vietnamese civilization, many of Vietnam's most famous dishes, such as *phở* (noodle soup) and *bánh cuốn* (literally rolled cake) originated in the north. The north's cuisine is more traditional and conservative in its use of spices and other ingredients. It is also lighter and fresher in taste. Seafood, particularly on the east coast, is popular and stir-fried dishes appear more frequently as a result of Chinese influence.

Central Vietnam

The cuisine of central Vietnam is quite different from the cuisines of both the northern and southern regions in its use of many small side-dishes (similar to tapas in Spanish cuisine) and its highly decorative presentation. Its cuisine is also spicier due to the liberal use of hot chilli peppers and shrimp paste, which gives piquancy to the dishes.

Southern Vietnam

The cuisine of south Vietnam has been influenced historically by the cuisines of southern Chinese immigrants and French colonists, such as the use of fondues. Southern Vietnamese prefer sweet/ tangy flavours in many dishes, using pineapple, tamarind and galangal. There is also more use of vegetables such as potatoes and asparagus than the green leafy vegetables used in the rest of the country. As a region of more diversity, the south's cuisine uses a wider variety of the herbs and spices often used in neighbouring Thailand and India.

Bread, rice, potatoes, noodles and other starchy foods

White rice is the main staple food in Vietnam and is usually served boiled and occasionally fried. Rice is a useful source of iron and calcium. A variety of noodles made from rice, wheat or green beans are stir-fried or served with salads or cooked as noodle soups and are very common in Vietnam. Other less common starchy foods eaten are green bananas, cassava, maize, sweet potatoes and tapioca.

- *Bun thit nuong*: Thin rice vermicelli served cold with grilled marinated pork chops and *nước nước chấm* (fish sauce, served with julienned kohlrabi and carrot). A similar northern version is *bún chả* (see below) with grilled pork meatballs in place of grilled pork chops.
- *Bún chả*: One of the more popular and simple Vietnamese dishes, a combination vermicelli, grilled pork meat balls or belly pork (often shredded) and served on a bed of greens (salad and sliced cucumber), herbs and bean sprouts. Often includes a few chopped Vietnamese spring rolls and a small bowl of *nước chấm* to drizzle over.

- *Bún bò huế*: Spicy beef noodle soup originated in the royal city of Hue in central Vietnam. Beef bones, fermented shrimp paste, lemongrass and dried chilies give the broth its distinctive flavour. Often served with mint leaves, bean sprouts, lime wedges, shredded banana blossoms and shredded herbs.
- *Bún riêu*: Noodle soup made of thin rice noodles and topped with crab and shrimp paste, served in a tomato-based broth and garnished with bean sprouts, prawn paste, herb leaves, water spinach and chunks of tomato.
- *Phở*: Beef noodle soup with a rich, clear broth/consommé achieved from slow boiling meat and bones, roasted ginger, onion and herbs. There are many varieties of *phở* made from different types of meat (most commonly beef and chicken) along with beef balls. *Phở* is typically served with spring onions and coriander and slices of cooked beef or chicken and broth. Wedges of limes or lemon are squeezed over the top and fresh chilli or chilli sauce is added for those who like heat. In *phở tai* slices of raw beef are placed on top of the noodles and boiling hot *phở* stock is poured over the slices to cook them. In the south, bean sprouts, hoisin sauce and various herbs such as mint and holy basil are also added.
- *Chao*: Rice *congee*. There is also a variety of different broths and meats, including duck, chicken, salted egg, offal, fish, etc.
- *Bánh chưng*: Sticky rice wrapped in banana leaves and stuffed with mung bean paste, lean and fatty pork and black pepper, traditionally eaten during the lunar New Year (*Tet*). *Bánh chưng* is popular in the north, while a similar version, *bánh tét*, is more popular in the south. (*Bánh tét* is cylindrical in shape and includes no fatty pork.)
- *Banh xeo*: Vietnamese pancake made from rice flour with turmeric, shrimps, slivers of fat pork, sliced onions, and sometimes button mushrooms, fried in oil (usually coconut oil). It is eaten with lettuce and various local herbs and dipped in *nước chấm* (sweet fermented yellow bean sauce). Rice papers are sometimes used as wrappers to contain *banh xeo* and the accompanying vegetables.
- *Bánh cuốn*: Rice flour rolls stuffed with minced pork, prawns and wood ear mushroom. They are eaten in a variety of ways with many side-dishes including *chả* (Vietnamese sausage).
- *Gỏi cuốn*: Salad rolls (also known as Vietnamese fresh rolls or summer rolls). They are rice paper rolls stuffed with prawns, herbs, pork, rice vermicelli and other ingredients and dipped in *nước chấm*. Spring rolls constitute almost an entire category of foods, as there are many different kinds with different ingredients.
- *Bánh mi thit*: A Vietnamese baguette containing paté, Vietnamese mayonnaise, various selections of cold cuts (of which there is a large variety, most commonly ham and a Vietnamese bologna), pickled daikon, pickled carrot and cucumber slices. The sandwich is often garnished with coriander and black pepper. This food is common throughout Vietnam as a favourite with factory workers and students, and eaten for any meal of the day, most commonly breakfast and lunch.

Vegetables

Leafy green vegetables similar to spinach or watercress in the UK, such as Morning Glory, *pak choi* and *choi sum*, are lightly boiled (with the water used to boil them turned into *canh*, a thin soup with various ingredients added, such as vegetables, ginger, prawns/meat, etc., and poured over boiled rice, or stir-fried or added to noodle soup dishes. Fresh, uncooked vegetables and salads are an integral part of many Vietnamese meals and lettuce, cucumber, coriander and mint (of which there are many varieties) are almost always included (see Table 3.2.1) lists vegetables commonly used with their Vietnamese name and English translation.

Fruit

Fruit is commonly eaten between meals as a snack and at the end of the main meal instead of a dessert course. Fruit is rarely cooked; however, banana or pineapple fritters are made for special occasions (see Table 3.2.2).

Meat, fish, eggs, beans and other non-dairy sources of protein

Pork is the most widely used animal protein in Vietnam, followed by chicken and beef.

Table 3.2.1 Vegetables commonly used in Vietnamese diet

Vietnamese name	English name	Vietnamese name	English name
Cà rốt	Carrot	Mồng tơi	Ceylon spinach
Cà tím	Aubergine	Ớt	Chilli pepper
Cải bắp	Cabbage	Rau dền đỏ	Joseph's coat
Cải bó xôi	Pak choi	Rau muống	Water morning glory
Cải xoong	Watercress	Rau cần ta	Hemlock water dropwort
Cải cúc or tần ô	Crown daisy	Rau ngót	Katuk
Củ cải trắng	Daikon	Su su	Chow chow
Dưa leo/chuot	Cucumber	Súp lơ or Bông cải	Cauliflower
Muop dang/Khổ qua	Bitter melon		

Table 3.2.2 Fruit commonly used in Vietnamese diet

Vietnamese name	English name	Vietnamese name	English name
Na/Mãng cầu	Custard apple	Mít	Jackfruit
Bòn bon	Langsat	Mãng cầu tây	Cherimoya
Bưởi	Pomelo	Na or Mãng cầu ta	Sweetsop
Cà chua	Tomato	Ổi	Guava
Chôm chôm	Rambutan	Phật thủ	Buddha's head
Chùm ruột	Gooseberry	Roi/Mận Đà Lạt	Rose apple
Du đủ	Papaya	Roi in the north, Mận in the south	Water apple
Dưa hấu	Watermelon	Sầu riêng	Durian
Hồng xiêm or Xa-pô-chê	Sapodilla	Táo tàu	Chinese date
Hồng	Persimmon	Thanh long	Pitaya – dragon fruit
Khế	Star fruit	Trái trứng gà	Canistel
Nhan	Longan	Vải	Lychee
Mận	Plum	Vú sữa11	Green star apple
Mãng cầu Xiêm	Soursop	Xê-ri	Acerola
Măng cụt	Mangosteen	Xoài	Mango

Fish and seafood are widely consumed also, especially in the coastal regions.

Tofu (bean curd) is common, especially among strict Buddhists or those on a low income as it is cheap.

Beans, lentils and nuts are not used in dishes on a daily basis but commonly used in desserts, as snacks and as a garnish such as on *xôi* (sticky glutinous rice).

Meat or fish is typically grilled, stir-fried, braised, roasted or boiled in Vietnam and often fat and skin from meat and poultry are not removed.

- *Bo kho/Bo sot vang*: Beef and vegetable stew often cooked with warm, spicy herbs and served very hot with baguettes for dipping.
- *Gio lua/Cha lua*: Sausage made with ground lean pork and potato starch. Also available fried when it is known as *chả chiên*. There are various kinds of *chả* (sausage): ground chicken (*chả gà*), ground beef (*chả bò*), fish (*chả cá*) or tofu (*chả chay*, or vegetarian sausage).
- *Ca kho to*: Caramelized fish cooked in a clay pot.
- *Nom du du/Gỏi đu đủ*: Vietnamese papaya salad typically made from shredded papaya, herbs, various meats (shrimp, slices of pork, liver or meat jerky) and herbs, and with a more vinegar-based rendition of *nước chấm*.
- Curry is popular, especially in the south. Curried chicken can be similar to the Thai curries (i.e., thin and fragrant with coconut milk) or like Caribbean curries (i.e., stir-fried with no coconut milk). It is usually served with rice.

As pork and beef are the main red meats consumed in Vietnam, encouraging clients to choose leaner cuts and smaller portions will help reduce the overall saturated fat intake. Likewise, encouraging skinned poultry, fish, tofu and seafood will help reduce the overall saturated fat and total fat intake.

Milk and dairy foods

The one food group that is a concern in the Vietnamese diet is the dairy group as cheese, milk and yoghurts are not commonly eaten although some use is made of evaporated and sweetened condensed milk in hot drinks and desserts. Most Vietnamese people will not be achieving the recommended three servings of dairy foods a day to obtain the 700 mg of calcium required in the adult diet. Calcium intake in the diets of Vietnamese people living in the UK may be low because:

- Milk and cheese are consumed in small quantities, if at all.
- Rice grown in Vietnam contains much more calcium than the rice imported into the UK.
- Fruit and vegetables commonly found in the UK contain less calcium than some tropical varieties.

Lack of dietary vitamin D is also a concern as a low vitamin D intake has been identified in some Vietnamese children. In Vietnam, the main source of vitamin D is from sunlight and oral supplements may be necessary for those living in the UK, particularly for the housebound.

Fats and oils

Vegetable/coconut oils or lard are used in stir-fry cooking in Vietnam. In the UK the main oil of choice is sunflower or corn oil. Olive oil is rarely used, except in salads. Butter and margarines are used sparingly but used more often by the Vietnamese people who eat more bread. Coconut milk/cream is mainly used for desserts or in drinks or curries.

It is important to educate Vietnamese clients on the importance of choosing healthier fats/oils as coconut oil and lard, which are high in saturated fat, are the preferred choice in Vietnam. Encouraging low-fat cooking methods (e.g., steaming, poaching, braising, grilling or stir-frying) in place of shallow- or deep-fat frying is advantageous.

Desserts and beverages

Desserts are not eaten on a daily basis but generally limited to social occasions or festivals such as the New Year (*Tết*) or Moon Festival or weddings/anniversaries, etc. They are generally consumed in small quantities after the main meal. Various cakes and confectionery are made with any combination of sweet beans, tropical fruit and glutinous rice.

Beverages can often be high in sugar from the use of sugar cane and fat from sweetened condensed milk or coconut milk. Below are some examples of well-known Vietnamese desserts and beverages.

- *Chè*: A sweet dessert beverage or pudding usually made from beans and sticky rice. Many varieties are available, each with different fruits, beans (e.g., mung beans or kidney beans), and other ingredients. *Chè* can be served hot or cold – such as *sâm bổ lường*, which includes dried jujube, longan, fresh seaweed, barley, lotus seeds and crushed ice cubes.
- *Deep-fried banana*: Banana fried in batter and often served hot with ice cream, usually vanilla or coconut flavour.
- *Sinh tố*: A fruit smoothie made with a few tea-spoons of sweetened condensed milk, crushed ice and fresh local fruits. The smoothies come in many varieties including custard apple, sugar apple, avocado, jackfruit and durian.
- *Yoghurt*: Made with condensed milk it has a sweet, tart flavour. It can be eaten in its chilled soft form or frozen. In Vietnam, it can be seen served frozen in small, clear bags.
- *Cafe sua da*: Strong iced coffee, most often served with sweetened condensed milk. The beverage is very popular among the Vietnamese.
- *Nước mía*: Sugar cane juice, served with ice.
- *Sữa đậu nành*: A soybean drink served hot or cold, sweetened or unsweetened.
- Slushes and tropical sorbets.

Herbs and spices

The use of soya sauce is due to Chinese influence, as well as pickled foods, particularly pickled vegetables (e.g. pickled mustard greens or pickled leeks similar to those eaten in China) (see Table 3.2.3).

Many Vietnamese people use monosodium glutamate (MSG) as a flavour enhancer in cooking. It can be purchased from Asian supermarkets. MSG as a food ingredient has been the subject of scientifically unsubstantiated health concerns. A report from the Federation of American Societies for Experimental Biology (FASEB) compiled in 1995 on behalf of the US Food and Drug Administration (FDA) concluded that MSG was safe for most people when 'eaten at customary levels'. However, it also said that, based on anecdotal reports, some people may have an MSG intolerance which causes 'MSG symptom complex'

Table 3.2.3 Herbs and spices used in Vietnamese diet

Vietnamese name	English name
Rau thơm	Herbs
Giấp cá or diếp cá	Houttuynia cordata
Húng cây or rau bac hà	Peppermint
Húng lủi	Spearmint
Kinh giới	Elsholtzia ciliata
Ngò gai/Mui tau	Long coriander/cilantro
Ngò om	Rice paddy herb
Rau đắng	Bacopa monnieri
Rau ngò or ngò rí	Coriander
Rau quế, húng quế, or rau húng quế	Thai basil (sometimes substituted with sweet basil in the United States)
Rau mui/ngo	Vietnamese coriander
Thì là	Dill
Tía tô	Perilla
Xả or sả	Lemon grass

(commonly referred to as Chinese restaurant syndrome) and/or a worsening of asthmatic symptoms (Geha *et al.*, 2000). Subsequent research found that while large doses of MSG given without food may elicit more symptoms than a placebo in individuals who believe that they react adversely to MSG, the frequency of the responses was low and the responses reported were inconsistent, not reproducible, and were not observed when MSG was given with food (Tarasoff & Kelly, 1993). While many people believe that MSG is the cause of these symptoms, a statistical association has never been demonstrated under controlled conditions, even in studies with people who were convinced that they were sensitive to it (Tarasoff & Kelly, 1993; Walker, 1999; Freeman, 2006).

Condiments and sauces

- *Nước mắm* (fish sauce): This can be used alone or mixed with water, lemon/lime juice, garlic, vinegar, sugar, salt and chili for the classic

Vietnamese fish sauce dip. Sodium intake can be high due to the use of fish sauce which is used in cooking and for dipping.

- *Mắm tôm* (shrimp paste): Used for sauces, soups and curries.
- Hoisin sauce: Mostly used for *phở* in south Vietnam or served with roasted duck or barbecued pork.
- Hot chilli sauce: Such as *sriracha* used in noodle soups, stir fries or as a dip for spring rolls, etc.

Typical meal pattern

Given the strong Chinese influence, many Vietnamese eating practices and cuisine are similar to those of southern China (e.g., stir-fry cooking, use of soya sauce, chopsticks, rice bowls and communal eating). All dishes, apart from the individual bowls of rice, are communal. Each individual has chopsticks, a spoon and a rice bowl. Each protein course, vegetable course and soup/broth will be served with a serving spoon.

Breakfast

Often bought away from home, as there is an abundance of cheap, high quality stalls selling nutritious and quick meals. Vietnamese people traditionally eat beef/chicken noodle soup (*phở*) or sticky rice (*xôi*), or *bánh cuốn* (rolled filled rice pancake). *Bún riêu*, a tomato-based noodle soup with fresh crab paste, coriander and chillies with thin rice stick noodles and eaten with fresh salad and more fresh herbs is another favourite. *Mien gà*, another classic noodle soup consumed particularly in the north, is a green bean thread noodle in chicken soup with chicken, spring onions and Chinese mushrooms and can be eaten for breakfast. The French influence can be seen in French bread filled with paté or a fried egg or cold meat/sausage made from pork known as *gio lua* or *chả* and given a Vietnamese twist by being served with fresh coriander and mint and seasoned with salt, pepper and fish sauce. Fried rice is another breakfast favourite utilizing leftovers from the previous night's meal. French-style coffee served with condensed milk is commonly taken at breakfast or a variety of Chinese teas without milk.

Lunch

Most Vietnamese people come home from work or school to have *cơm* (rice) or the lunch meal (similar to the example provided above but with fewer dishes) with the family. If it is too far to travel, lunch will often be bought from one of the many pavement stalls that sell *phở*, various stir-fried noodle dishes such as *mien* or *xôi*, a sticky glutinous rice cooked with peanuts or green or black beans, or *bánh cuốn*, a crêpe-like roll made from a thin sheet of rice flour filled with ground pork, minced wood ear mushroom and other ingredients and served with a dipping sauce and consumed at the stall. A packed lunch can also be bought to take back to the workplace with rice and meat (chicken, pork, beef, fish, prawn, egg or tofu) and vegetables. The containers are similar to the takeaway containers used in the UK but the container is bigger, with a separate compartment for rice and other food to eat with the rice. Fried rice with leftovers from the previous night's meal may be consumed for lunch. Some schools prepare lunches for pupils which the parents pay for.

Evening meal

The evening meal is eaten with the whole family and is considered to be the main meal of the day. Plain boiled rice is always served along with one or two protein dishes – beef or fish either stir-fried or steamed, one or two vegetable dishes either raw or lightly stir-fried, a bowl of *canh* (thin broth) with vegetables and meat or prawns or tofu to ladle over the rice and various small dishes of dipping sauces. The evening meal is more elaborate and has more dishes than lunch (see Table 3.2.4).

3.2.4   Traditional pattern in the UK

For second-generation Vietnamese, particularly for those living in western countries such as the UK, the foods consumed at breakfast and lunch are typically western owing to lack of time to prepare traditional dishes and lack of availability of certain ingredients unique to Vietnamese cooking. Continental-style breakfast foods such as cereals, particularly the low-fibre or sugary varieties (e.g., Cornflakes or Frosties) served with milk or bread/toast with butter/margarine and jam or peanut butter or processed cheese slices are common

Table 3.2.4 Common Vietnamese food and how it is prepared and served

Food	Vietnamese name	Food description and how it is consumed
Rice	*Cơm*	Plain boiled short grain or Thai jasmine rice cooked in a rice cooker. Leftover rice is fried for breakfast or lunch. Served in individual bowls. The number of bowls consumed varies depending on the individual, usually 1–2 for women, 2–3 for men.
Vegetables	*Rau luộc* (boiled vegetables) *Khuấy rau xào* (stir-fried vegetables) *Rau tươi* (fresh vegetables)	Mainly green leafy variety, although some western-style vegetables (carrots, cauliflower and aubergine) are consumed. Vegetables can be boiled/steamed or raw especially salads/bean sprouts or stir-fried with garlic/ginger/onion and herbs with fish sauce, salt and stock powder.
Red meat, poultry, fish, tofu, eggs, shellfish	*Thịt đỏ* (red meat) *Cá* (fish) *Dậu phu/hu* (tofu) *Trứng* (eggs) Trai (shellfish) *Thịt gia câm* (poultry)	Protein foods are usually grilled, poached, steamed, braised, fried or stir-fried with a sauce and herbs and seasoning (e.g., fish sauce or soya sauce).
Broth/Soup	*Canh*	A clear broth made from the liquid from boiled vegetables and bones and often has vegetables, meat or seafood and fresh herbs (dill, coriander, holy basil). The soup is poured over the rice in the rice bowl at the end of the meal or consumed on its own.
Sauces/Dips	*Nước sốt* (sauces) *Nước mắm* (fish sauce)	Little dipping plates filled with fish sauce made with limes, garlic, vinegar, salt, chillies and sugar and/or soy sauce with ginger, spring onions and sesame oil or chilli sauce or chilli oil. Used to dip protein foods or raw/boiled vegetables/salads for extra flavour

examples. Alternatively, instant noodle packets (*mì ăn liền*) with fried or boiled eggs are another favourite. Tea or coffee served with milk and sugar is commonly drunk at breakfast along with fruit juice. The practice of coming home to have lunch with the family for second-generation Vietnamese is impractical owing to distance and the short lunch break. Therefore, sandwiches either brought from home or shop-bought are common. If sandwiches are not brought and the place of work has kitchen facilities, instant noodle packets served in disposable polystyrene bowls are a common alternative. Leftovers from the previous night's evening meal brought are commonly eaten for lunch. Fried rice is a useful way to use up leftover rice, protein foods and vegetables (see Table 3.2.5).

3.2.5 Healthy eating

The typical Vietnamese diet can be healthy and similar in benefits but equally in terms of negatives like its Chinese counterparts.

● The Vietnamese diet is generally high in carbohydrates as rice, noodles and other starchy foods form the basis of meals.

- Low in overall fat and sugar due to the cooking methods used and the relatively low intake of foods/drinks high in fat and sugar.
- High in soluble fibre due to abundance of fruit, vegetables and pulses/lentils.
- Low in insoluble fibre as intake of wholegrain starchy carbohydrates are not readily available in Vietnam, with white rice and noodles are favoured over brown rice and whole wheat noodles.
- Saturated fat sources are prevalent due to coconut oil/lard often used in cooking, fatty meats and skin on poultry often left on and the use of coconut milk/cream used in desserts and sweet drinks.

Encouraging Vietnamese clients to eat plenty of fruit, vegetables, beans and lentils will help to increase their overall fibre intake and to choose healthier types of fats/oils, leaner cuts of meat and remove skin from poultry will help improve lipid profiles and reduce risk of heart disease (see Table 3.2.6).

Table 3.2.5   Health benefits of traditional Vietnamese foods

Foods	Health benefits
Noodle soups	Nutritionally balanced meal containing carbohydrate, protein and vegetables.
	Low in fat, moderate in calories and good source of fluid
Encourage consumption of raw vegetables/salads and fresh herbs or lightly cooked	Helps to increase fibre intake
Liquid used to boil vegetables made into soup (*canh*)	Increases micronutrients, antioxidants and phytochemicals
	No wastage of nutrients that may be leached out during the boiling process
Encourage soya milk (unsweetened) and tofu/bean curd in dishes and desserts	Helps to increase soya protein which may help control cholesterol levels and aid heart health. Soya isoflavones may help with menopausal symptoms and bone health
Encourage fresh fruit/fruit smoothies eaten as snacks and after meals	Helps to increase fibre intake
	Increase micronutrients and antioxidants
Encourage use of beans/lentils/nuts in drinks or desserts made with less sugar or on sticky rice	Helps to increase soluble fibre intake to aid bowel regulation and help to lower cholesterol levels and regulate blood sugar levels
Encourage low-fat cooking methods for grilling, stir-frying, braising, roasting, more noodle soup dishes	Helps to lower total fat intake and aid with weight maintenance

Table 3.2.6   Foods to encourage and discourage in the Vietnamese diet

	Encourage	Discourage
Fibre	Granary/multi-grain bread, brown rice/pasta, taro/yam Whole wheat/buckwheat noodles, green bean vermicelli, adzuki beans, black-eyed peas, lentils, green split peas, potatoes with skins	White bread, low-fibre breakfast cereals, white rice, white noodles
Fats	Boiling/steaming/baking/grilling/barbecue/stir fry (with small amount of monounsaturated oil) Steamed dim sum, *banh cuon*, summer rolls, pork leg, lean meat, skinless poultry/duck, fish, seafood, steamed bean curd/tofu, plain boiled rice	Frying, using coconut cream/milk/oil, fried spring rolls, fried dim sum, fried doughnuts, duck/poultry with skin, belly pork, fatty cuts of meat, Chinese/Vietnamese sausages, prawn crackers, fried rice, banana/pineapple fritters
Sugar	Fruit juice (limit to 1 small glass and avoid adding extra sugar to sweeten), water, diet/sugar-free drinks, plain Chinese/Vietnamese tea with no sugar or use sweetener, tea cake, plain biscuits/sponge cake	Sugar cane, sugar, sweetened condensed milk in drinks/desserts, honey, lychee drink, fizzy drinks, other soft drinks/teas made with sugar, sweetened soya drink, sweet steamed bun, egg tart, moon cake, sweet soup (*chè*)
Salt	Use herbs (coriander, mint, sweet holy basil, etc.), spices (ginger, star anise, five spice powder, pepper), lean, unsalted meats, lower sodium soy sauce/stock cubes/powder if available	Salt added at table and in cooking, instant stock powder/cubes, monosodium glutamate, corned beef, spam, black bean sauce, soy/hoisin sauce, salted ducks' eggs, fish sauce, pickled leeks/mustard greens/cabbage

3.3   Japanese Diet

Fumi Fukuda

Key points

- Japanese emigrants who settled abroad, and their descendants, are called Nikkei. Worldwide there are more than 2.5 million Nikkei living in their adopted countries.
- The primary religions of Japanese are Shintoism (83%) and Buddhism (70%). Many Japanese practise aspects of both religions and do not see themselves as adhering exclusively to either.
- Life expectancy in Japan is one of the highest in the world at 82 years of age (world average is 66 years). This may be due to a lower rate of deaths from cancer, cardiovascular disease and coronary heart disease.
- Japanese in Japan eat approximately 100g of fish or other seafood a day, which is their second largest source of protein.
- Soybean (*daizu, Glycine max*) is one of the most important ingredients in the Japanese diet. It is referred to as 'meat in the field' in Japanese as

its high protein content (30–50%) is comparable to that of meat.
- A decrease in the production of lactase is found in 85% of the adult Japanese population and is genetically determined. This is not a problem because small amounts of lactose can be tolerated even by people suffering from lactose malabsorption.
- The traditional Japanese diet consists of a bowl of rice, a bowl of miso soup, a source of protein and vegetables.
- It is important to follow a traditional Japanese diet and minimize use of fat and salt to minimize risk of developing diseases such as cardiovascular disease.
- Finding traditional ingredients can be challenging and expensive for Japanese living abroad.

3.3.1   Introduction

Japan (Nippon or Nihon in Japanese) is one of the East Asian island nations located in the northwestern part of the Pacific Ocean. It consists of four

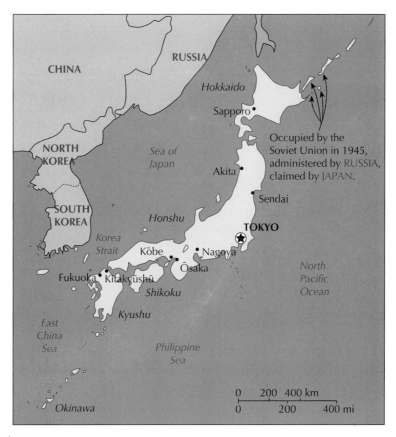

Figure 3.3.1   Map of Japan

large islands (Hokkaido, Honshu, Shikoku and Kyushu) and more than 3,000 small islands. It is divided into eight regions (Hokkaido, Tohoku, Kanto, Chubu, Kinki, Chugoku, Shikoku and Kyushu) (see Figure 3.3.1). In January 2010, the population was estimated as 126,804,433, making it the 10th most populated country in the world (CIA, 2010).

Japan began to import Chinese culture from the 4th century onwards and adapted it to its own customs and traditions, which resulted in today's unique culture. In the middle of the 16th century, European culture began to gain a foothold in Japan, but this was limited to certain areas, and in the 17th century, the country was closed to foreign influence for 200 years. After the Meiji Restoration in the mid-19th century, Japan opened up again and began a process of orientation towards Western Europe in order to modernize the country and increase its international competitiveness – a process interrupted by the Second World War. After 1945, the American way of life began to exert an increasing influence on Japanese culture.

Language

More than 99% of the population speak Japanese as their first language (CIA, 2010) and Japanese is the sixth most spoken language in the world (Web-Japan, 2009). English is not widely understood. The Japanese writing system consists of three character sets: Kanji (several thousand Chinese characters) and Hiragana and Katakana (two syllabics of 48 characters each; together called Kana). Japanese texts can be written in the western style, in horizontal rows from the top to the bottom of the page, or in the traditional Japanese style, in vertical columns from right to the left across the page. The two styles coexist.

Migration to the United Kingdom

Japanese emigrants who settle abroad, and their descendants, are called Nikkei. Worldwide there are more than 2.5 million Nikkei living in their adopted countries, mainly in the USA (1,200,000) and Brazil (1,400,000) (Association of Nikkei & Japanese Abroad, 2010). In the 19th and early 20th centuries agricultural labourers moved to those two countries as economic migrants. Among the Japanese who live abroad (semi-)permanently are diplomatic staff and representatives of Japanese companies who are seconded to overseas branches. There are also university students who study abroad to further their professional qualifications.

Current UK population

In 1884, 264 Japanese people migrated to the UK. Most were government officials or students. Their number increased to 500 within 10 years (Itoh, 2001). According to the Ministry of Foreign Affairs (2009), 59,431 Japanese are residents in the UK, most of whom live in London. They comprise the fifth largest Japanese population living abroad.

3.3.2   Religion

The primary religions of Japanese are Shintoism (83%) and Buddhism (70%) (MEXT, 2007). The total exceeds 100% as many Japanese observe both. Generally speaking, most Japanese do not see themselves as an adherent of just one of these religions but practise aspects of both Shintoism and Buddhism in a syncretic way. Dietary restrictions and influences from Shintoism and Buddhism in the modern Japanese diet are not commonly seen.

3.3.3   Traditional diet and eating pattern

The Japanese put great emphasis on seasonal foods, the quality of ingredients and on presentation. Agricultural land is limited, therefore, the focus is on quality rather than quantity. A traditional Japanese meal consists of a bowl of rice, a bowl of miso (a paste made from fermented and salted soy beans), soup and dish of seafood (mostly fish) or meat. This is called *ichijyu-issai*, which means one bowl of soup and one dish of seafood or meat. In addition, pickled vegetables (*tsuke-*

mono), stir-fried or stewed vegetables and/or tofu (soybean curd)-based dishes are often served together. According to Nakamura and colleagues (2001) native Japanese refer to tofu, fish and *tsuke-mono* as traditional Japanese foods. In former times, *ichijyu-issai* meant a simple meal. However, due to the westernization of the diet in modern Japanese society, this term is generally used to describe a healthy balanced diet.

In terms of serving methods, each member of the family has his or her own bowl for rice and soup and a pair of chopsticks. Seafood or meat are served on individual plates, while dishes such as cooked and pickled vegetables are often served on a common plate and shared.

Rice, bread, potatoes, pasta and other starchy foods

Rice is Japan's most important crop. It has been cultivated for over 2,000 years. Its fundamental importance to the country and its culture are reflected in the fact that rice was once used as a currency – in some remote villages up to the Second World War (Allen, 2009) – and that the Japanese word for cooked rice (*gohan*) also has the general meaning of meal. The literal meaning of breakfast (*asagohan*), for example, is morning rice. However, for the last 50 years, Japanese per capita rice consumption has declined steadily – a phenomenon also observed in Taiwan and Korea (see Figure 3.3.2).

The rice produced in Japan is almost exclusively the subspecies *Oryza sativa japonica*. Compared to the other major subspecies, *O. sativa indica*, which is mainly cultivated in India (patna rice, basmati rice), it is shorter grained and, owing to its higher amylopectin content, it becomes sticky when cooked. In the UK, it is sold as sushi rice.

Since unpolished or brown rice (*gemmai*) is generally considered less tasty, the rice is mainly *hakumai* (white rice), where the outer layers (*nuka*) of the grain which contain most of the thiamine (vitamin B_1) have been removed. Vitamin B_1 deficiency (beriberi) is avoided through consumption of foods rich in thiamine, such as pulses and pork, and food supplements. Recently, in order to stem declining rice consumption in Japan, efforts have been made to promote germinated brown rice as a healthier alternative to *hakumai* as it is believed to

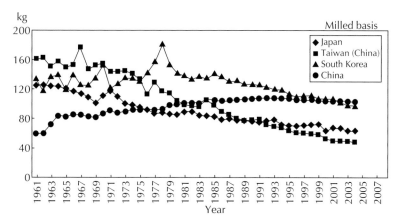

Figure 3.3.2 Development of per capita rice consumption in selected East Asian countries (Ito & Ishikawa, 2004)

have a wide range of health benefits (Ito & Ishikawa, 2004), in addition to a high thiamine content.

Rice is usually boiled, but can also be served fried, as porridge (*kayu*) or *congee* (*zousui*).

Sushi and *onigiri* are unique to Japan. *Sushi* is made from rice mixed with vinegar, sugar and salt, boiled and left to cool. For *nigiri-zushi*, it is formed into small cubes and topped with fish or seafood; for *maki-zushi*, it is formed into rolls and filled with fish, seafood, egg or vegetables. *Onigiri* is typical Japanese fast food, available in supermarkets and corner shops where it is sold as rice balls, mostly triangular in shape weighing around 100–120 g. Either plain, seasoned or with a filling of seafood, vegetables, egg or meat, they are usually covered in an edible wrapper of *nori*, which makes it ideal as takeaway food, to be consumed on the way to or from work.

A special variety of japonica rice is *mochi gome*, a short-grained glutinous rice with a particularly high amylopectin content making it stickier than conventional Japanese rice. It is used for some ceremonial dishes, cooked and served with red beans, and eaten to celebrate special events such as graduation or weddings. Rice cakes (*mochi*) made from pounded and cooked glutinous rice were traditionally eaten at New Year, grilled and served wrapped in seaweed or in a soup. They are now available throughout the year. *Mochi gome* is also the base material for rice crackers (*sembei*) and prepared with sugar for sweets.

Various Japanese sweets (*wagashi*) are made from rice flour, as are savoury or sweet rice crackers (*sembei*). Given the increasing popularity of *pan*, attempts have been made to introduce bread based on 80% rice flour enriched with 20% gluten (rice does not contain gluten, which is necessary to make bread dough rise) (Ito & Ishikawa, 2004).

The Japanese also consume various types of noodles (*udon*, *somen* and *ramen*) which mainly differ in dimension and the way they are served, are made from wheat, and *soba* from buckwheat. They are served either in hot or cold soup with or without a variety of toppings such as vegetables, herbs, meat, seafood and egg. The majority of Japanese noodle restaurants specialize in one of these types of noodles, which they then offer in many varieties. It is not an uncommon in Japan to see customers queuing outside popular noodle restaurants, and then have only a few minutes to enjoy their lunch. However, instant pot noodles are becoming increasingly popular, and many corner shops provide customers with boiling water so they can prepare them themselves. As in Japan, in the UK these noodles are available either dried or fresh, or as complete instant meals. In recent years, Italian-style pasta has become popular in Japan, particularly among the younger generation. However, the Japanese prefer to serve it with their own sauces, based on soy sauce.

Bread was introduced to Japan by Portuguese traders in the middle of the 16th century, and

Table 3.3.1 Vegetables used in Japanese diet that are available in the UK

English name	Japanese name	English name	Japanese name
Bamboo shoots	Takenoko	Japanese radish	Daikon
Bean sprouts	Moyashi	Leek	Negi
Broad beans	Soramame	Lotus root	Renkon
Broccoli	Burokkori	Mizuna	Mizuna
Burdock	Gobo	Okra	Okura
Cabbage	Kyabetsu	Onion	Tamanegi
Carrots	Ninjin	Pepper	Piman
Cauliflower	Karifurawa	Pumpkin	Kabocha
Celery	Serori	Snap beans	Snap endou
Chinese cabbage	Hakusai	Sweet corn	Toumorokoshi
Chinese chives	Nira	Spinach	Horensou
Cucumber	Kyuri	Taro	Satoimo
Elephant foot	Konnyaku	Tomato	Tomato
Fine beans	Ingenmame	Turnips	Kabu
French beans	Sayaingen		

termed *pan* (from the Portuguese *pão*). However, until the end of the 19th century, it was mostly consumed by western visitors. Baked products from wheat dough then became more widely known through a bun filled with sweetened red bean paste (*an*), invented in 1874 (Otani, 2006). More than 100 years later, *an-pan* is still hugely popular among adults and, even more so, children. Today, buns with a wide range of fillings are available, such as melon *pan*, choc *pan* or the savoury curry *pan*. White wheat bread similar to that marketed in the UK is also called *pan*. Rye-based sourdough bread is virtually unknown in Japan. The per capita consumption of *pan* is slowly increasing, but is negligible compared to the consumption of rice.

Potatoes (*Solanum tuberosum*) and sweet potatoes (*Ipomoea batatas*) are seldom served as a main source of starchy carbohydrate, but small amounts are cooked with vegetables and meat and served as a side-dish. A common sight in winter are street vendors who sell freshly roasted sweet potatoes (*yaki-imo*). Puréed sweet potato is an ingredient of various types of sweets.

Vegetables, mushrooms, seaweeds and fruits

The Japanese diet includes a wide range of vegetables. Most are also commonly consumed in the UK (see Table 3.3.1).

An exception is *gobo* (Arctium lappa). In the UK, where it was once a popular root vegetable, it is today better known as an ingredient of dandelion and burdock beverages and health potions, but is not easy to find as a vegetable. In Japan, it is either stewed or fried, and commonly served with chicken dishes. Despite having an English name, devil's tongue or elephant foot (*Amorphophallus konjac*) is virtually unknown in the UK. *Konnyaku* is widely used in the Japanese diet and either boiled, fried or stewed. It is a healthy food as it is very low in calories and high in fibre. However, when younger children or the elderly consume *konnyaku*, supervision may be necessary due to the sticky consistency which poses a risk of choking. Lotus (*Nelumbo nucifera*) root is mostly stewed with shiitake mushrooms and chicken, but also served battered and deep fried or pickled. It is traditionally eaten on New Year's Day. It is claimed that the future can be seen through the large vessels which in the sliced root appear as holes.

Several types of mushrooms are commonly consumed in Japan. Those available in the UK are shiitake (*Lentinula edodes*, also known as Chinese black mushroom), enoki (*Flammulina velutipes*, golden needle mushroom), buna-shimeji (*Hypsizygus tessellatus*, marketed in the UK as brown clamshell mushroom) and maitake (*Grifola fron-*

dosa, known as hen-of-the-woods in the UK). Mushrooms are low in calories and prepared in the same way as vegetables. Maitake is also used in traditional Japanese and Chinese medicine to boost the immune system. Pharmaceutical research has confirmed the medicinal properties of maitake, which has a hypoglycaemic effect (Kubo *et al.*, 1994) and also inhibits some types of cancer cell (Nanba & Kubo, 1997; Konno, 2007).

Seaweeds (*kaiso*) have been an important part of the diet for centuries. They are not only low in calories but also nutritious. Various types of seaweed are used extensively as soup stock, seasonings and other forms in daily Japanese cooking. The three most commonly used are *nori* (dried paper seaweed, produced from the red alga *Porphyra sp.*), *kombu* (edible kelp from the *Laminariaceae* family) and *wakame* (*Undaria pinnatifida*). *Nori* is used to wrap rice (e.g., to make *onigiri* and *sushi*). *Wakame* can be used in many dishes such as soup and salad. *Kombu* is considered the king of the seaweed and has been a key ingredient in Japanese cooking for over 1,000 years. It is an essential ingredient of *dashi* (soup stock), because of its natural content of the flavour enhancer glutamic acid. Furthermore, it offers a range of health benefits for weight control because it is low in fat (less than 2 g per 100 g) and rich in vitamins especially vitamins B_1 and A, minerals such as calcium and potassium, and fibre (Japanese Science and Technology Agency, 2010).

Many of the vegetables, mushrooms and seaweeds in the Japanese diet are also known and consumed in the UK. Most of those that can be grown here are widely available. Some growers in the UK have specialized in lesser known Japanese vegetables, but their products are not available everywhere. It is possible to grow many Japanese herbs or vegetables in the garden or even as container plants. However, it should be noted that the import of some seeds to the UK is prohibited, and for others, a phytosanitary certificate may be required (FERA, 2008). Many other vegetables that have become popular as ingredients of the Asian cuisine are imported, depending on the demand and their shelf-life either as preserves or fresh. Only those that, like *konnyaku*, are virtually unknown in the UK and can only be kept fresh for a limited time, are difficult to find in UK shops.

The range of fruits consumed in Japan is similar to that in the UK. In general, they are eaten fresh or dried as a snack, as well as dessert. Lesser known in the UK, but occasionally available in larger supermarkets, are *nashi* (Japanese pear, *Pyrus pyrifolia*) and *kaki* (Japanese persimmon, *Diospyros kaki*). Japan is home to a wide range of citrus fruits (e.g., *iyokan, ponkan* and *yuzu*), which are rich in vitamin C and appreciated for their rich flavour and refreshing acidity. They are not marketed in the UK.

Fish, meat, legumes, eggs and nuts

Japanese in Japan eat approximately 100 g of fish and other seafood every day; it is their second largest source of protein (MAFF, 2010). According to MAFF (2010), the top 10 types of fish consumed are salmon (*sake*), tuna (*maguro*), saury (*sanma*), yellowtail (*buri*), horse mackerel (*aji*), mackerel (*saba*), plaice (*karei*), bonito (*katuo*), sardine (*iwashi*) and sea bream (*tai*). Although available in Japan, whale meat consumption is insignificant.

A Japanese specialty is *fuku* (various species of the *Tetraodontidae* family, known in English as puffers or blowfish). What makes *fuku* unique is the presence of a lethal toxin in some organs. In order to avoid fatalities, only licensed restaurants with specially qualified chefs are allowed to serve *fuku* dishes. In the EU, the sale of puffers is prohibited.

Other seafoods, such as prawn (*ebi*), shellfish (*kai*), squid (*ika*), octopus (*tako*) and cod roe (*tarako*), are also regularly eaten in Japan. A delicacy is sea urchin (*uni*), of which the ovaries are eaten, usually as *sushi*. A product (mainly) based on seafood is *surimi*, developed in Japan in the 1960es and now known worldwide. The English name, crab sticks, is misleading because any animal protein – minced, rinsed, puréed and then flavoured and pressed into various shapes – can be processed as *surimi*. A special form of *surimi* is *kamaboko*, made exclusively from white fish and known in Japan since the 14th century. Prepared in the auspicious colours red and white, it is served for festive meals.

Fish dishes are prepared in the same way as in other countries, grilled, stewed or fried. Unique to Japan is the consumption of raw seafood. It is essential that the ingredients are absolutely fresh. Served on top of small balls of vinegared rice, it is known as *nigiri-sushi*. As *sashimi*, it is eaten on its own, arranged and served on top of shredded *daikon and/or shiso* leaves (see below). Depending on the kind of *sashimi*, *wasabi* (ground ginger) is used as a condiment. Both *nigiri-sushi* and *sashimi* are dipped into a mixture of soy sauce and *wasabi*.

Compared to Japan, the availability of fresh fish and seafood in the UK is limited. Therefore, Japanese living in the UK predominantly stew, grill or fry fish, rather than preparing it as *sashimi*. Boiled fish paste (e.g., *kamaboko* and *chikuwa*) is commonly eaten in Japan and is available in the UK as a frozen food in Asian supermarkets.

Meat has been eaten in Japan in larger quantities only since the second half of the 20th century – the annual per capita consumption of meat and poultry increased from 3.1 kg in 1950 to 23.4 kg in 1975 (Kagawa, 1978). After meat and poultry consumption peaked in the early 1990s (27.7 kg per capita in 1992), it steadily decreased in the following years, to around 23.3 kg in 2002 (Statistics Bureau, 2008). Japanese know a variety of meat dishes. The main types of meat consumed are chicken, pork and beef. Lamb and mutton are not commonly eaten except in Hokkaido. Specialist restaurants serve horse meat (*sakuraniku*).

Soybean (*daizu*, *Glycine max*) is one of the most important ingredients in the Japanese diet. It is referred to as 'meat in the field' as its high protein content – 30–50% – is comparable to that of meat. Soybeans are used in a wide range of preparations, for example like pulses, bean sprouts or boiled green soybean in a pod (*edamame*). Toasted soybeans ground into flour (*kinako*) are used to flavour *mochi* and prevent it from sticking, but also to prepare a kind of milkshake. Bean curd (*tofu*) is produced from coagulated soy milk and widely used in a large range of preparations in the traditional Japanese diet. *Natto* (fermented soy beans) are eaten as a topping for rice, either on their own or mixed with a raw egg. Soybean products are widely available in Asian supermarkets in the UK.

While soya has been subjected to many unsubstantiated health claims, a study conducted for the American Heart Association came to the conclusion that 'many soy products should be beneficial to cardiovascular and overall health because of their high content of polyunsaturated fats, fiber, vitamins, and minerals and low content of saturated fat' (Sacks *et al.*, 2006).

The second most popular legume in Japan is the adzuki bean (*Vigna angularis*). Prepared with *mochi*, it is known as *sekihan* and served for celebrations, the red colour symbolizing good luck and happiness. Like soy beans, adzuki beans are used for bean sprouts. Red bean paste (*an*), the key ingredient of many popular Japanese sweets (see below), is produced by boiling adzuki beans with sugar. In its liquid form, this preparation is known as *shiruko* (red bean soup). As already mentioned, many more legumes are consumed in Japan as vegetables.

Eggs are another commonly consumed food high in protein – mainly chicken but also quail eggs. Seven per cent of total protein consumed comes from eggs in Japan (MAFF, 2010). Eggs are eaten boiled (e.g., on their own), *as sushi*, as a component of egg tofu or raw with soya sauce on top of rice or noodles.

With the exception of *kuri* (chestnuts, *Castanea sativa*), which are predominantly sold by street vendors during winter, nuts are not widely consumed in Japan.

Milk and dairy foods

Milk and dairy products were relatively unknown in Japan until they were promoted on a large scale after 1945: in 1950, the per capita consumption in Japan was 2.5 kg, which rose to 53.3 kg in 1975 (Kagawa, 1978). The most recent official figures (Statistics Bureau, 2008) are available for 2002 and give a domestic per capita consumption of (cow's) milk of 32 l. In a survey conducted by the National Milk Promotion Association of Japan, 60% of the respondents claimed they drink between 100 ml and 200 ml of milk a day, and 11% that they do not consume any milk. Yoghurt is eaten as part of a western-style breakfast or as dessert, but only occasionally. Cheese is available, but (apart from in delicatessens) usually as processed cheese of domestic production, and consumption is negligible (see Figure 3.3.3).

In 85% of the adult Japanese population, the ability to digest lactose is reduced to a lesser or greater degree (hypolactasia) (Vesa *et al.*, 2000) due to a genetically determined decrease in the production of lactase, the enzyme that breaks down

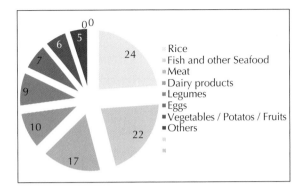

Figure 3.3.3   Sources of protein in the Japanese diet (MAFF, 2010)

lactose, soon after weaning. This does not pose a problem for most Japanese, because a daily intake of 10–15 g of lactose, provided it is consumed in small quantities, can be tolerated even by people suffering from lactose malabsorption (Garrow *et al.*, 2000). Given that the average lactose content of cow's milk is 4.6%, this would enable Japanese to consume 220–330 ml milk per day without suffering from the symptoms of lactose intolerance (diarrhoea and abdominal pain and distension).

Fats and oils

According to the Japanese Ministry of Health, Labour and Welfare, the average Japanese daily calorie intake is 1,867 kcal, of which 24.9% come from fat; this meets the official recommendations for 30–69 year olds who should meet 20–25% of their energy requirements from fat (MHLW, 2009). Of the daily fat consumption of 52.1 g, an average of 25.9 g is from animal sources. Between 1980 and 2002, the average annual per capita consumption of butter (excluding that in processed food) was 150 g (± 10%), which is approximately a third of the margarine consumption (USDA, 2007).

With regard to vegetable oil, rapeseed oil is consumed most (approximately 40%) followed by soya oil. This does not only include home consumption as cooking oil but also its use in processed foods such as margarine and mayonnaise, and in restaurants (JOPA, 2008). It is reported that the annual Japanese per capita consumption of vegetable oil is 13 kg (MAFF, 2010).

Desserts, sweets and beverages

The dessert that concludes a typical Japanese meal usually consists of seasonal fruits. Sweets are eaten as snacks, known as *oyatsu* or *sanji* (literally, 3 o'clock as it is often eaten midway between lunch and dinner). Sweets snacks are known as *wagashi*, which are mainly based on cooked and sweetened adzuki beans, e.g., *yokan* (made from bean paste, sugar and agar), *monaka* (crackers filled with sweet bean paste) or daifuku (*an* wrapped in rice flour dough). *Kushi-dango* are rice flour balls on skewers, dipped in a sweet soy sauce. Western-style sweets (e.g., those based on cocoa) are a recent introduction. Savoury snacks (*sembei*, rice crackers) are also consumed.

The most typical and traditional Japanese beverage is unfermented green tea, of which 18.5 l are consumed per person per year (MAFF, 2004); The World Green Tea Association (n.d.) estimates an annual per capita consumption of 760 g. It is not only consumed as a refreshing or stimulating beverage, but also for ceremonial purposes (*chado*) and always taken unsweetened. To a lesser extent, Japanese drink fermented 'English-style' tea, either plain, or with milk or lemon and/or sugar. Coffee consumption in Japan has increased from 1.1 kg per capita in 1975 to 3.3 kg in 2007 (AJCA, 2009), and is thus considerably higher than that of tea.

Caffeine-free beverages typical for Japan are prepared from buckwheat (*soba cha*) or from roasted wheat (*mugi cha*). Other beverages such as fruit juice and sparkling juice are also consumed.

Most (non-alcoholic) beverages are available round the clock from the omnipresent vending machines.

Herbs and spices

The traditional Japanese cuisine only knows a limited number of herbs and spices, and these are used sparingly.

Myoga (Japanese ginger, *Zingiber myoga*) is an essential ingredient for pickles, but also commonly used in the preparation of noodle soup. *Sansho* (*Zanthoxylum piperitum*), despite its English name, Szechuan pepper, is not related to black or white pepper but to citrus fruits; while the leaves serve as a garnish (e.g., for soups), a paste prepared from the seeds together with *miso* is used to reduce the smell of some fish dishes. The aromatic leaves of *shiso* (beefsteak plant, *Perilla frutescens*) are not only used to garnish *sashimi*, but also to add flavour to *somen* and *udon* dishes. Unlike Japanese radish (*daikon, Raphanus sativus*), Japanese horseradish (*wasabi, Eutrema japonica*) is not eaten as a vegetable, but ground into a paste that has a strong, hot flavour. Mixed with soy sauce, it is used to flavour *sushi*, *sashimi* and *soba* noodles. Due to its long shelf-life, *wasabi* paste is easily available in UK supermarkets. In Isu Hanto, a region south-west of Tokyo where much of the *wasabi* is produced, even *wasabi*-flavoured ice cream is marketed.

The use of herbs and spices such as basil, coriander, curry powder, dill, garlic and others, is a relatively recent phenomenon; in the traditional way of Japanese cooking, they were not known.

Herbs and spices are particularly useful to reduce the use of soy sauce/salt which is contributing to the high intake of salt.

Condiments and sauces

Among the various products derived from fermented soy beans, soy sauce (*shoyu*) is the most important for Japanese cuisine. *Shoyu* owes its popularity to its glutamic acid content, which acts as a flavour enhancer. On the Japanese dining table, a bottle of *shoyu* is as essential as salt and pepper are in northern Europe. In Japan, the current annual per capita consumption of *shoyu* is approximately 7 l, but statistics show a decreasing trend over recent decades (SOYIC, 2010), possibly due to the westernization of Japanese cuisine.

Miso is a thick paste, prepared by fermenting varying proportions of soy beans, cereals (e.g., rice, wheat and barley) and various other ingredients. It is used as a base for soups, as an ingredient for pickling vegetables, to prepare a glaze for *mochi*-based sweets and for various other purposes.

Compared to other soy-based products, soy sauce is lower in isoflavones than other soy products, and its high NaCl content of 14–18% makes it problematic for a low sodium diet. However, low sodium soy sauce is available, containing up to 50% less sodium. Since wheat is a common (though not essential) ingredient, soy sauce and

miso are not generally suitable for coeliac disease sufferers; however, gluten-free soy sauce (*tarami*) is available.

A popular condiment for use with rice is *furikake*, a mixture of one or all of sesame seed, seaweed, fish flakes, egg powder and various other ingredients. Some preparations contain industrially produced monosodium glutamate (see Table 3.3.2).

3.3.4 Food preservation and cooking methods

The traditional Japanese methods used to preserve food are drying, pickling and curing.

The most common method, drying, was used predominantly for all types of fish, seaweed, *shiitake*, *daikon*, *tofu* and noodles. For pickling, various ingredients are used, in particular vinegar, soy sauce and *miso*. *Nuka-doko* is a method in which a preparation of rice bran (*nuka*) chilli and *kombu* is fermented together with the vegetables to be pickled – mostly carrots, aubergines and cucumber. Although *tsukemono* (the generic term for pickled vegetables) is sold in supermarkets, many Japanese households still prepare their own. Only salmon and pork are preserved by curing.

Of the various cooking methods, boiling is predominatly used for rice, noodles and vegetables. One of the most common ways to prepare fish is grilling, and most Japanese kitchens have a grill designed specifically for fish. Fish is also fried, as for meat and vegetables. The technique of stir-frying was imported from China. A traditional method for preparing fresh vegetables, *tofu*, seafood and meat is *nabemono*. A special broth is heated on a rechaud, and the diners add the food they have selected. *Nabemono* is typically prepared during winter, and the social aspect is as important as the nutritional. Similar to *nabemono* is *oden*, for which mainly processed seafood and preserved vegetables are used.

Deep-fried food is known as *agemono* and can be prepared with batter (*tempura*) or without (*suage*). The batter is usually based on wheat flour. Not only fish, meat and *tofu* but also vegetables can be deep-fried and are often served with dips made from soy sauce. Thus, *agemono* dishes can be high in both fat and salt.

Table 3.3.2 Condiments and sauces used in the Japanese diet

English name	Japanese name	Food description and how it is consumed	Notes and suggestions
Soy sauce	*Shoyu*	Used on its own as well as with other seasonings, e.g., sugar for cooking. It may be used as 'table soy sauce' to add to dishes or used as a dip.	High in salt. Reduced salt versions are more expensive and the availability in the UK is limited. Use of soy sauce should be limited and substituted with herbs.
Sugar	*Satou*	Used together with soy sauce to stew meat and fish, or with other spices to season vegetable dishes.	Can be replaced by artificial sweetener.
Sweet sake	*Mirin*	Made from sugar and fermented rice. Used to enhance flavour.	High in sugar. Should be used in small quantities only.
Salt	*Shio*	Added to dishes already seasoned with soy sauce. Used to pickle vegetables.	Minimize or, where possible, avoid use and replace with herbs.
Vinegar	*Su*	Mainly prepared from rice, but also from fruits such as *ume* (Japanese plum). Mixed with sugar, sweet sake and soy sauce and used as a Japanese-style dressing.	Can be used on its own to replace soy sauce.
Miso	*Miso*	Fermented and salted soy bean paste. As important as soy sauce in Japanese cuisine since it is used in wide variety of dishes. There is huge range of varieties.	High in salt. Reduced salt version is available but more expensive and the availability in the UK is limited. Use should be minimized. Eat toppings in miso soup but avoid drinking all miso soup.

3.3.5 Alcohol

Of all the alcoholic beverages consumed in Japan, sake is probably the most typical. The first known written records of sake date back to the 8th century, but it is assumed it was produced much earlier than that (Antoni, 1988). The English name, rice wine, is misleading, because the sugar which is fermented to alcohol first has to be obtained by hydrolysis of rice starch. Sake – which is also the general term for alcohol – contains 15–20% alcohol. It is mainly consumed on social occasions – cold in summer or warmed in winter. Per capita consumption in 2004 was 7.31 (Brewers Association of Japan, 2006) (see Figure 3.3.4).

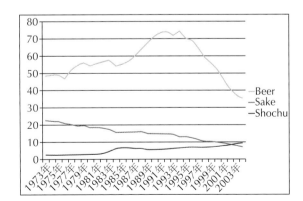

Figure 3.3.4 Annual per capita consumption (litres) of selected alcoholic beverages in Japan (Brewers Association of Japan, 2006)

Although beer first began to be brewed in Japan in 1853, it was marketed only to foreigners and upper-class Japanese. The first brewery that sold beer to the general public was established in 1872. In 1883, the production of beer in Japan was 208,000l and the imports 450,000l. By 1887, the domestic production – 3,151,000l – exceeded imports of 1,630,000l. Production continued to rise and with 11,829,000l in 1897 dwarfed the 154,000l of imported beer (Brewers Association of Japan, 2004). Due to its lower alcohol content than sake, it is also consumed as refreshing beverage – 35.4l per capita in 2004 (Brewers Association of Japan, 2006).

Another alcoholic beverage typical for Japan is *shochu*. With regard to production process and alcohol content, it is best compared to vodka. Produced by fermentation of various starchy base materials – most commonly cereals such as rice or barley, but also sweet potatoes or sugar cane – an alcohol content of up to 40% is obtained through subsequent distillation. Average per capita consumption in 2004 was 9.6l (Brewers Association of Japan, 2006). In the same year, 14.5l of various other alcoholic beverages (whisky, wine, etc.) were consumed per capita (Brewers Association of Japan, 2006).

For Japanese, consumption of alcohol can be more problematic than for people of European descent. It is estimated (Fukui & Wakasugi, 1972) that some 90% of the Japanese carry a less efficient variant of the gene that regulates the production of alcohol dehydrogenase, the enzyme responsible for breaking down alcohol. Thus, the effects of alcohol intoxication appear after ingestion of smaller amounts of alcohol than in westerners, and hangover symptoms persist for longer.

In their survey of 2,547 adult Japanese (aged 20+ years; the legal age for drinking alcohol and smoking is 20 in Japan), carried out in 2003, Osaki *et al.* (2005) found that 28.9% of males and 7.6% of females drank 4 or more units of alcohol (1 unit = 10 g) daily, and 12.7% of males and 3.4% of females 6 units or more; 0.9 % of the respondents met the ICD-10 criteria for alcohol dependence; and 2.5 % engaged in hazardous alcohol use. With regard to age groups, MHLW (2004) reported that most at risk from alcohol abuse were females aged 20–29 years and males aged 20–29 and 40–49 years.

3.3.6 Smoking

A survey conducted in 2008 by the Ministry of Health, Labour and Welfare (2009) revealed that 36.8% of Japanese males and 9.1% of females are regular smokers, almost exclusively cigarettes. These figures have decreased for both genders and in all age groups compared to a survey conducted in 2003. The number of people who smoke more than 21 cigarettes per day has decreased from 32.7% in 2003 to 25.3% in 2008 for males and 9.6% in 2003 to 9.2% in 2008 for females. In addition, the number of smokers who expressed a desire to give up smoking has increased from 24.6% to 28.5% of males and 32.7% to 37.4% of females. This could be due to an increasing awareness of the consequences of smoking for health, as the same survey revealed.

3.3.7 Typical meal pattern and the changing eating patterns of second-generation Japanese

While studies on the changing eating pattern of Japanese in the UK are limited, more research has been carried out in the USA and Brazil. A study in the USA showed that Japanese-Americans were consuming a diet high in fat, sugar, sodium and calories (Kudo *et al.*, 2000). Japanese-Americans were also consuming more simple carbohydrates and animal protein than native Japanese (Nakanishi *et al.*, 2004). A study in Hawaii revealed that expatriate Japanese women consumed more grains and meat but less seaweed, fish, vegetables and soy products than Japanese women in Japan (Takata *et al.*, 2003).

There was a significant difference between native Japanese and Brazilians of Japanese origin in terms of percentage energy gained from fat despite the similar total energy intake (Freire *et al.*, 2003). In Japan, the total energy intake is 1,902 kcal, made up of 15% protein, 25.3% fat and 59.7% carbohydrates (MHLW, 2004). However, Japanese-Brazilian intake is as follows: 13–14% protein, 31–33% fat and 52–54% carbohydrates (Freire *et al.*, 2003). The other study showed that the figure is close to an estimated value of non-Japanese-Brazilians in metropolitan areas which is 30% (Cardoso *et al.*, 1997,

2000). Similar results were obtained by a study of Japanese women in Hawaii who consume 2,032 kcal, as 14.2% protein, 29.7% fat and 55.2% carbohydrates (Takata *et al.*, 2003).

From these observations, it may be necessary to suggest choosing complex carbohydrates, consuming traditional a Japanese diet of seaweed, fish and soy products but less meat, as a source of protein.

To reduce the total energy intake, foods which are low in calories, such as *konnyaku*, seaweed and mushroom, are useful. However, sourcing these traditional ingredients can be challenging, especially for Japanese who live in small towns and villages. With regard to cooking methods, it is important to minimize the use of fat and to avoid deep-fried foods (see Table 3.3.3).

Table 3.3.3   Typical Japanese meal pattern

	Encourage	Discourage
Breakfast Japanese-style		
Rice, miso soup, protein-rich food (e.g., grilled fish or egg or *natto*), pickled vegetable, *nori*	Most calories from carbohydrates Traditional and low-calorie foods such as fish, tofu, seaweed, mushrooms and *konnyaku*	Use of soy sauce and salt Drinking all miso soup Use of fat for cooking, i.e., deep frying such as tempura (battered seafood/meat/vegetables)
Western-style		
Bread, salad, egg, bacon, yoghurt or breakfast cereals	Low-fat dairy products Complex carbohydrates Low-sugar breakfast cereals	Use of fat for cooking High saturated fat products, e.g., butter and bacon Sugary breakfast cereals
Lunch Japanese-style		
A dish of noodles or fried rice or leftovers from the night before prepared in a lunch box (*obentou*)	Include most calories from carbohydrates Increase intake of mushrooms, vegetables and seaweed	Drinking all soup from noodles
Western-style		
Sandwich with a packet of crisps, juice	Choose complex carbohydrates Low-calorie fillings	Fatty and sugary foods High-fat fillings
Dinner Japanese-style		
Ichijyu-Issai plus some vegetable-based dish	Include most calories from carbohydrates Use more mushrooms, vegetables and seaweed.	Use of soy sauce and salt. Herbs can be alternatives Avoid table soy sauce and salt Drinking all miso soup Use of fat, i.e., deep-fat frying such as tempura
Western-style		
Meat or fish, vegetables (salad or cooked) with potatoes or rice	Complex carbohydrates Low-fat cooking methods Fish	Use of fat Simple carbohydrates Animal protein

3.3.8 Health and life expectancy in Japan

Worldwide, the average life expectancy at birth is 66 years (UN, 2007). In Japan, according to WHO (2009), life expectancy at birth is 83 years (or 82.6 years; UN 2007; or 82.17 years; CIA, 2010). According to CIA (2010) the life expectancy in Japan is fifth highest in the world. There is a difference between males (78.87 years) and females (85.66 years).

In terms of the infant mortality rate (infant deaths per 1,000 live births) it is 3.2 in Japan and 53.9 in the world (UN, 2007) (or 2.79; CIA, 2010). According to CIA (2010), this is the fifth lowest in the world.

The possible reason Japan has one of the highest life expectancy in the world is that the three major causes of death (cancer, cardiovascular disease and coronary heart disease) have decreased (MHLW, 2010).

According to MHWL (2010), the current dietary reference intakes for Japanese in terms of salt is 9 g/day for males and 7.5 g/day for females. It has decreased by 10 g/day for males and 8 g/day for female from the previous recommendation as the average intake of salt has decreased in Japan. This is one of the possible reasons why the death rates from these diseases have decreased. In addition, the high fish consumption in the Japanese diet may be a protective factor against heart disease (Ueshima et al., 2003).

Support groups

Chinese Diet

Cancer Equality
Riverside House
27–29 Vauxhall Grove
London, SW8 1SY
Telephone: 020 7735 7888

Macmillan Cancer Support
89 Albert Embankment
London SE1 7UQ
Telephone: 0808 808 0121

South East Scotland Cancer Support Group
50 Pentland Drive,
Edinburgh EH10 6PX
Telephone: 07904 362 854

Provides practical help and emotional support to Chinese people living with cancer through meetings, visits and social activities. Provides culturally competent information and resources in the Chinese language.

Further reading

Chinese Diet

The Association of Traditional Chinese Medicine (2007) *About Traditional Chinese Medicine*. www.atcm.co.uk/medicine.htm.

The Boys' and Girls' Clubs Association of Hong Kong (2003) *Taipei, Hong Kong and Shanghai Children's Living Survey*. Department of Health, Hong Kong.

Cancer Equality (2008) *Coping with Eating Difficulties When you have Cancer: A Guide for Chinese Patients*. Cancer Equality, London.

Group of China Obesity Task Force (2004) Body mass index reference norm for screening overweight and obesity in Chinese children and adolescents. *Chinese Journal of Epidemiology*, 25(2), 97–102.

Kim, S.M., Lee, J.S. *et al.* (2006) Prevalence of diabetes and impaired fasting glucose in Korea: Korean National Health and Nutrition Survey 2001. *Diabetes Care*, 29(2), 226–31.

Payne-James, J., Grimble, G. & Silk, D. (1995) *Artificial Nutrition Support in Clinical Practice*. Edward Arnold, London.

People's Republic of China–United States Cardiovascular and Cardiopulmonary Epidemiology Research Group (1992) An epidemiological study of cardiovascular and cardiopulmonary disease risk factors in four populations in the People's Republic of China: baseline report from the P.R.C.–U.S.A. Collaborative Study. *Circulation*, 85, 1083–96.

WHO/IASO/IOTF (2000) *The Asia-Pacific Perspective: Redefining Obesity and its Treatment*. Health Communications Australia, Melbourne.

Woo, J., Ho, S.C. *et al.* (2003) Diet and glucose tolerance in a Chinese population. *European Journal of Clinical Nutrition*, 57, 523–30.

Vietnamese Diet

Lewis, M.P. (ed.) (2009) *Ethnologue: Languages of the World*. 16th edition. SIL International, Dallas, TX. www.ethnologue.com.

Japanese Diet

Eng, M.Y., Luczak, S.E. & Wall, T.L. (2007) ALDH2, ADH1B, and ADH1C genotypes in Asians: a literature review. *Alcohol Research & Health*, 30(1), 22–7.

International Coffee Organization (2008) *Historical Coffee Statistics*. ICO, London. www.ico.org/historical.asp.

MAFF (Ministry of Agriculture, Forestry and Fisheries) (2008). Food Supply in 2008. www.maff.go.jp/j/zyukyu/fbs/index.html.

Toriyama, K., Heong, K.L. & Hardy, B. (eds.) (2005) *Rice is Life: Scientific Perspectives for the 21st Century*. International Rice Research Institute, Los Baños, Philippines.

Watanabe, Y. & Suzuki, N. (2006) Is Japan's milk consumption saturated? *J Fac Agr*, 51(1), 165–71. Kyushu University, Japan.

References

Chinese Diet

American Diabetes Association (2001) Clinical practice recommendations. *Diabetes Care*, 24(Suppl 1), S1–133.

American Heart Association (2001) *Heart and Stroke Statistical Update*. American Heart Association, Dallas, TX.

Amos, A., McCarty, D. & Zimmet, P. (1997) The rising global burden of diabetes and its complications: estimates and projections to the year 2010. *Diabetic Medicine*, 14, S1–S85.

Anderson, J.M. (1987) Migration and health: perspectives on immigrant women. *Sociology of Health and Illness*, 9(4), 410–38.

BBC (2007) *Western Diet Risk to Asian Women*. news.bbc.co.uk/1/hi/health/6284830.stm.

Blot, W.J., McLaughlin, J.K. *et al.* (1988) Smoking and drinking in relation to oral and pharyngeal cancer. *Cancer Research*, 48(11), 3282–7.

Burke, V. (2006) Obesity in childhood and cardiovascular risk. *Clinical & Experimental Pharmacology & Physiology*, 33(9), 831–7.

Cancer Equality (2008) *Coping with Eating Difficulties When You Have Cancer. A Guide for Chinese Patients*. Cancer Equality, London.

Centers for Disease Control and Prevention (2000) *CDC Growth Charts for the United States: Methods and Development*. Series Report 11, No. 246. Washington, DC.

Central Intelligence Agency (2010) *The World Factbook*. www.cia.gov/library/publications/the-world-factbook/geos/ch.html.

Chan, J., Ng, J. *et al.* (2001) Diabetes mellitus – a special medical challenge from a Chinese perspective. *Diabetes Research & Clinical Practice*, 54, S19–S27.

Chang, E.T. & Adami, H.O. (2006) The enigmatic epidemiology of nasopharyngeal carcinoma. *Cancer Epidemiology, Biomarkers and Prevention*, 15(10), 1765–77.

Cheerva, A.C. & Ashok, B.R. (2009) *Hemoglobin H Disease: Treatment & Medication*. emedicine.medscape.com/article/955496-treatment.

Chinese National Healthy Living Centre (2010) *Healthy Chinese Takeaway Menus Project*. www.cnhlc.org.uk/english.html.

Chowdhury, T. & Lasker, S. (2002) Complications and cardiovascular risk factors in South Asians and Europeans with early onset type 2 diabetes. *Quarterly Journal of Medicine*, 95, 241–6.

Chui, Y.Y., Donoghue, J. & Chenoweth, L. (2005) Responses to advanced cancer: Chinese-Australians. *Journal of Advanced Nursing*, 52(5), 498–507.

Cockram, C.S., Woo, J. *et al.* (1993) The prevalence of diabetes mellitus and impaired glucose tolerance among Hong Kong Chinese adults of working age. *Diabetes Research & Clinical Practice*, 21, 67–73.

Cui, X., Dai, Q. *et al.* (2007) Dietary patterns and breast cancer risk in the Shanghai breast cancer study. *Cancer Epidemiology, Biomarkers & Prevention*, 16(7), 1443–8.

DH (2001) *Health Survey for England 1999: The Health of Minority Ethnic Groups*. Series HS, no.9. Department of Health, London.

DH (2004) *At Least Five a Week. Evidence on the Impact of Physical Activity and its Relationship to Health. A Report from the Chief Medical Officer*. Department of Health, London.

Department of Health. The Government of the Hong Kong Special Administrative Region. (2008) *Health Zone – Central Health Education Unit*. www.cheu.gov.hk/eng/info/exercise_04.htm.

Department of Health. The Government of the Hong Kong Special Administrative Region. Centre for Health Protection (2009) *Statistics on Behavioural Risk Factors*. www.chp.gov.hk/en/data/4/10/280/390.html.

Ernst, E. & Pittler, M.H. (2000) Efficacy of ginger for nausea and vomiting: a systematic review of randomized clinical trials. *British Journal of Anaesthesia*, 84(3), 367–71.

Fischbacher, C., Bhopal, R. *et al.* (2001) Anaemia in Chinese, South Asian, and European Populations in Newcastle upon Tyne: cross-sectional study. *British Medical Journal*, 322, 958–9.

Gallagher, D., Visser, M. *et al.* (1996) How useful is BMI for comparison of body fatness across age, sex and ethnic groups? *American Journal of Epidemiology*, 143(3), 228–39.

Gould-Martin, K. & Ngin, C. (1981) Chinese Americans. In A. Harwood (ed.) *Ethnicity and Medical Care*. Harvard University Press, Cambridge, MA and London.

He, J., Gu, D. *et al.* (2005) Major causes of death among men and women in China. *The New England Journal of Medicine*, 353, 1124–34.

Heaney, R.P. (1999) Age-related osteoporosis in Chinese women. *American Journal of Clinical Nutrition*, 69(6), 1291–2.

Hu, D., Fu, P. *et al.* (2008) Increasing prevalence and low awareness, treatment and control of diabetes mellitus among Chinese adults: The InterASIA study. *Diabetes Research & Clinical Practice*, 81, 250–7.

Hu, G., Qia, J. *et al.* (2004) DECODE Study Group. Prevalence of the metabolic syndrome and its relation to all cause and cardiovascular mortality and its relation to all cause and cardiovascular mortality in nondiabetic European men and women. *Archives of Internal Medicine*, 164, 1066–76.

International Diabetes Federation (2003) *Diabetes Atlas*. 2nd edition. IDF, Brussels.

International Obesity Task Force (2006) www.iotf.org/database/GlobalAdultsAugust2005.asp.

Isomaa, B., Almgren, P. *et al.* (2001) Cardiovascular morbidity and mortality associated with the metabolic syndrome. *Diabetes Care*, 24(4), 683–9.

Jackson, B.S. & Savaiano, D. (2001) Lactose maldigestion, calcium intake and osteoporosis in African-, Asian-, and Hispanic-Americans. *Journal of the American College of Nutrition*, 20, 198S–207S.

James, W.P.T., Chen, C. & Inoue, S. (2002) Appropriate Asian body mass indices? *Obesity Reviews*, 3, 139.

Janus, E.D., Wat, N.M.S. *et al.* (2000) The prevalence of diabetes, association with cardiovascular risk factors and implications of diagnostic criteria (ADA 1997 and WHO 1998) in a 1996 community based population study in Hong Kong Chinese. *Diabetic Medicine*, 17(10), 741–5.

Jiang, J.H., Jia, W.H. *et al.* (2004) Genetic polymorphisms of CYP2A13 and its relationship to nasopharyngeal carcinoma in the Cantonese population. *Journal of Translational Medicine*, 2(1), 24.

Jovchelovitch, S. & Gervais, M.C. (1999) Social representations of health and illness: the case of the Chinese community in England. *Journal of Community & Applied Social Psychology*, 9, 247–60.

Kennedy, E.T., Bowman, S.A. *et al.* (2001) Popular diets: correlation to health, nutrition and obesity. *Journal of the American Dietetic Association*, 101, 411–20.

Keys, A., Menotti, A. *et al.* (1984) The seven countries study: 2,289 deaths in 15 years. *Preventive Medicine*, 13(2), 141–54.

King, H., Aubert, R.E. & Herman, W.H. (1998) Global burden of diabetes 1995–2025: prevalence, numerical estimates and projections. *Diabetes Care*, 21(9), 1414–31.

Kitagawa, T., Owada, M., Urakami, T. & Yamanchi, K. (1998) Increased incidence of noninsulin dependent diabetes mellitus among Japanese school children correlates with an increased intake of animal protein and fat. *Clinical Pediatrics*, 37, 111–16.

Klem, M.L., Wing, R.R. *et al.* (1997) A descriptive study of individuals successful at long term maintenance of substantial weight loss. *American Journal of Clinical Nutrition*, 66, 239–46.

Ko, G.T.C. (2008) The cost of obesity in Hong Kong. *Obesity Reviews*, 9(Suppl. 1), 74–7.

Ko, G.T.C., Chan, J.C.N. *et al.* (2000) Outcomes of screening for diabetes in high risk Hong Kong Chinese subjects. *Diabetes Care*, 23, 1290–4.

Ko, G.T.C., Cockram, C.S. *et al.* (2006) Metabolic syndrome by the International Diabetes Federation definition in Hong Kong Chinese. *Diabetes Research & Clinical Practice*, 73, 58–64.

Kong, A.P.S., Ko, G.T.C. *et al.* (2008) Metabolic syndrome by the new IDF criteria in Hong Kong Chinese adolescents and its prediction by using body mass index. *Acta Pædiatrica*, 97(12), 1738–42.

Kuulasmaa, K., Tunstall-Pedoe, H. *et al.* (2000) Estimation of contribution of changes in classic risk factors to trends in coronary-event rates across the WHO MONICA Project populations. The WHO MONICA Project. *The Lancet*, 355, 675–87.

Lam, T.H., Chan, B. & Ho, S.Y. (2002) *A Report on the Healthy Living Follow-up Survey 2001*. Department of Health, Hong Kong.

Lam, T.H., Ho, S.Y. *et al.* (2004) Leisure time physical activity and mortality in Hong Kong: case control study of adult deaths in 1998. *Annals of Epidemiology*, 14, 391–8.

Larkin M. (2001) Diet and exercise delay onset of type 2 diabetes, say US experts. *Lancet*, 358(9281), 565.

Lau, E., Donnan, S., Barker, D.J. & Cooper, C. (1988) Physical activity and calcium intake in fracture of the proximal femur in Hong Kong. *British Medical Journal*, 297(6661), 1441–3.

Lau, E., Woo, J. *et al.* (1993) Serum lipid profile and its association with some cardiovascular risk factors in an urban Chinese population. *Pathology*, 25, 344–50.

Lee, M.M., Lin, S.S. *et al.* (2000) Alternative therapies used by women with breast cancer in four ethnic populations. *Journal of the National Cancer Institute*, 92(1), 42–7.

Leung, G. & Lam, K. (2000) Diabetic complications and their implications on health care in Asia. *Hong Kong Medical Journal*, 6, 61–8.

Li, M., Dibley, M., Sibbritt, D. & Yan, H. (2006) An assessment of adolescent overweight and obesity in Xi'an City, China. *International Journal of Pediatric Obesity*, 1, 50–8.

Li, M., Li, S., Baur, L.A. & Huxley, R.R. (2008) A systematic review of school based intervention studies for the prevention or reduction of overweight among Chinese children and adolescents. *Obesity Reviews*, 9, 548–59.

Li, Y., Yang, X. *et al.* (2008) Prevalence of the metabolic syndrome in Chinese adolescents. *British Journal of Nutrition*, 99(3), 565–70.

Liu, A., Hu, X. *et al.* (2008) Evaluations of a classroom based physical activity promoting programme. *Obesity Reviews*, 9(Suppl. 1), 130–4.

Lopez, A.D. (1998) Counting the dead in China. *British Medical Journal*, 317, 1399–400.

Malik, S., Wong, N.D. *et al.* (2004) Impact of the metabolic syndrome on mortality from coronary heart disease, cardiovascular disease and all causes in United States adults. *Circulation*, 110(10), 1245–50.

McCracken, M., Olsen, M. *et al.* (2007) Cancer incidence, mortality, and associated risk factors among Asian Americans of Chinese, Filipino, Vietnamese, Korean, and Japanese ethnicities. *CA: A Cancer Journal for Clinicians*, 57(4), 190–205.

Messina, M.J. & Wood, C.E. (2008) Soy isoflavones, estrogen therapy, and breast cancer risk: analysis and commentary. *Nutrition Journal*, 7, 17.

Muztagh Travel Service (2010) *Map of China: At a Glance.* www.muztagh.com/map-of-china.

Office for National Statistics (1991 and 2001) *Census.* ONS, London.

Paeratakul, S., Popkin, B.M. *et al.* (1998) Changes in diet and physical activity affect the body mass index of Chinese adults. *International Journal of Obesity*, 22, 424–31.

Pan, X., Yang, W., Li, G. & Liu, J. (1997) Prevalence of diabetes and its risk factors in China 1994 – National Diabetes Prevention and Control Cooperative Group. *Diabetes Care*, 2, 1664–9.

Pan, X.R., Li, G.W. *et al.* (1997) Diet and exercise in preventing NIDDM in people with impaired glucose tolerance. The Da Qing IGT and Diabetes Study. *Diabetes Care*, 20(4), 537–44.

Papadopoulos, I., Guo, F., Lees, S. & Ridge, M. (2007) An exploration of the meanings and experiences of cancer of Chinese people living and working in London. *European Journal of Cancer Care*, 16(5), 424–32.

Parkin, M., Bray, F., Ferlay, J. & Pisani, P. (2005) Global cancer statistics. *CA: A Cancer Journal for Clinicians*, 55, 74–108.

Prentice, A.M. & Jebb, S.A. (2001) Beyond body mass index. *Obesity Reviews*, 2(3), 141–7.

Pu, C.Y., Lan, V.M., Lan, C.F. & Lang, H.C. (2008) The determinants of traditional Chinese medicine and acupuncture utilization for cancer patients with simultaneous conventional treatment. *European Journal of Cancer Care*, 17(4), 340–9.

Reilly, J.J. & Wilson, D. (2006) ABC of obesity: childhood obesity. *British Medical Journal*, 333, 1207–10.

Robb, K.A., Power, E., Atkin. W. & Wardle, J. (2008) Ethnic differences in participation in flexible sigmoidoscopy screening in the UK. *Journal of Medical Screening*, 15(3), 130–6.

Robertson, T.L., Kato, H. *et al.* (1977) Epidemiologic studies of coronary heart disease and stroke in Japanese men living in Japan, Hawaii and California. Coronary heart disease risk factors in Japan and Hawaii. *American Journal of Cardiology*, 39, 244–9.

Rudolf, M.C., Sahota, P., Barth, J.H. & Walker, J. (2001) Increasing prevalence of obesity in primary school children: cohort study. *British Medical Journal*, 322, 1094–5.

Satia-Abouta, A.J., Patterson, R.E. *et al.* (2002) Psychosocial predictors of diet and acculturation in Chinese American and Chinese Canadian women. *Ethnicity & Health*, 7(1), 21–39.

Sea, M.M., Woo, J. *et al.* (2004) Associations between food variety and body fatness in Hong Kong Chinese adults. *Journal of the American College of Nutrition*, 23, 404–13.

Shafrir, E. (1997) Development and consequences of insulin resistance: lessons from animals and hyperinsulinaemia. *Diabetes & Metabolism*, 22, 131–48.

Shi, R., Xu, S. *et al.* (2008) Prevalence and risk factors for helicobacter pylori infection in Chinese populations. *Helicobacter*, 13(2), 157–65.

Shulman, M.R. (2002) *The World on Your Plate.* Carroll & Brown Publishers, London.

Stamler, J., Vaccaro, O., Neaton, J.D. & Wentworth, D. (1993) Diabetes, other risk factors and 12 year cardiovascular mortality for men screened in the Multiple Risk Factors Intervention Trial (MRFIR). *Diabetes Care*, 16, 434–44.

Swallen, K.C., Reither, E.N., Haas, S.A. & Meier, A.M. (2005) Overweight, obesity, and health-related quality of life among adolescents: the National Longitudinal Study of Adolescent Health. *Pediatrics*, 115, 340–7.

Tang, J.L. &Wong, T.W. (1998) The need to evaluate the clinical effectiveness of traditional Chinese medicine. *Hong Kong Medical Journal*, 4(2), 208–10.

Taylor, V.M., Yasui, Y. *et al.* (2007) Heart disease prevention among Chinese immigrants. *Journal of Community Health*, 32(5), 299–310.

Thomas, B. & Bishop, J. (2007) *Manual of Dietetic Practice.* 4th edition. Blackwell, Oxford.

Togami, T. (2008) Interventions in local communities and worksite through physical activity and nutrition programme. *Obesity Reviews*, 9(Suppl. 1), 127–9.

Tsugane, S. & Sasazuki, S. (2007) Diet and the risk of gastric cancer: review of epidemiological evidence. *Gastric Cancer*, 10(2), 75–83.

Tuomilehto, J., Lindstrom, J. *et al.* (Finnish Diabetes Prevention Study Group) (2001) Prevention of type 2 diabetes mellitus by changes in lifestyle among subjects with impaired glucose tolerance. *The New England Journal of Medicine*, 344(18), 1343–50.

Ueshima, H., Okayama, A. *et al.* (2003) Differences in cardiovascular disease risk factors between Japanese in Japan and Japanese-Americans in Hawaii: the INTERLIPID study. *Journal of Human Hypertension*, 17, 631–9.

Vanhala, M., Vanhala, P. *et al.* (1998) Relation between obesity from childhood to adulthood and the metabolic syndrome: population-based study. *British Medical Journal*, 317, 319–20.

WHO Expert Consultation (2004) Appropriate body mass index for Asian populations and its implications for policy and intervention strategies. *The Lancet*, 363(9403), 157–63.

Woo, J. (1998) Nutrition and health issues in the general Hong Kong population. *Hong Kong Medical Journal*, 4(4), 383–8.

Woo, J., Ho, S.C. & Yu, A.L.M. (2002) Lifestyle factors and health outcomes in elderly Hong Kong Chinese aged 70 years and over. *Gerontology*, 48, 234–40.

Woo, J., Ho, S.C. *et al.* (1998) Impact of chronic diseases on functional limitations in elderly Chinese aged 70 years and over: a cross sectional and longitudinal survey. *Journal of Gerontology: Medical Sciences*, 35A, 102–6.

Woo, J., Leung, S.S. *et al.* (1998) Dietary intake and practices in the Hong Kong Chinese population. *Journal of Epidemiology & Community Health*, 52(10), 631–7.

World Cancer Research Fund (WCRF) (2007) *Food, Nutrition, Physical Activity, and the Prevention of Cancer: A Global Perspective*. American Institute for Cancer Research, Washington, DC.

World Health Organization (2000) *Obesity: Preventing and Managing the Global Epidemic. Report of a WHO Consultation*. WHO Technical Report Series 894. WHO, Geneva.

World Health Organization (2006) *WHO Child Growth Standards: Methods and Development: Length/Height-for-Age, Weight-for-Age, Weight-for-Length, Weight-for-Height and Body Mass Index-for-Age*. WHO, Geneva.

World Health Organization (2007) *The World Health Report 2007 – A Safer Future: Global Public Health Security in the 21st Century*. WHO, Geneva.

Worth, R.M., Kato, H. *et al.* (1975) Epidemiologic studies of coronary heart disease and stroke in Japanese men living in Japan, Hawaii and California: mortality. *American Journal of Epidemiology*, 102, 481–90.

Wu-Tso, P., Yeh, I. & Tam, C.F. (1995) Comparisons of dietary intake in young and old Asian Americans: a two generation study. *Nutrition Research*, 15(10), 1445–62.

Yang, G., Kong, L. *et al.* (2008) Emergence of chronic non-communicable diseases in China. *The Lancet*, 372(9650), 1697–705.

Yang, H.I., Lu, S.N. *et al.* (2002) Hepatitis B antigen and the risk of hepatocellular carcinoma. *The New England Journal of Medicine*, 347, 168–74.

Yang, W., Lu, J. *et al.* (2010) The China National Diabetes and Metabolic Disorders Study Group. 2010. Prevalence of diabetes among men and women in China. *The New England Journal of Medicine*, 362, 1090–101.

Zhao, S., Xu, Z. & Lu, Y. (2000) A mathematical model of hepatitis B virus transmission and its application for vaccination strategy in China. *International Journal of Epidemiology*, 29, 744–52.

Zhao, W., Zhai, Y. *et al.* (2008) Economic burden of obesity-related chronic diseases in Mainland China. *Obesity Reviews*, 9(Suppl. 1), 62–7.

Zhou, B.F. (2002) Predictive values of body mass index and waist circumference for risk factors of certain related diseases in Chinese adults – study on optimal cut-off points of body mass index and waist circumference in Chinese adults. Cooperative Meta-Analysis Group of the Working Group on Obesity in China. *Biomedical & Environmental Sciences*, 15(1), 83–96.

Zhou, B.F., Stamler, J. *et al.* (2003) Nutrient intakes of middle-aged men and women in China, Japan, United Kingdom, and United States in the late 1990s: The INTERMAP Study. *Journal of Human Hypertension*, 17, 623–30.

Zimmet, P. (2000) Globalisation, coca-colonisation and the chronic disease epidemic: can the doomsday scenario be averted? *Journal of Internal Medicine*, 247(3), 301–10.

Zimmet, P., Alberti, K.G.M.M. & Shaw, J. (2001) Global and societal implications of the diabetes epidemic. *Nature*, 414, 782–7.

Zou, J., Sun, Q. *et al.* (2000) A case-control study of nasopharyngeal carcinoma in the high background radiation areas of Yangjiang, China. *Journal of Radiation Research*, 41(suppl.), 53–62.

Vietnamese Diet

Burrell, I. (2000) Vietnamese boat people came to Britain for a new life. They found unemployment and despair. *The Independent News*, 22 January. www.independent.co.uk/news/uk/this-britain/vietnamese-boat-people-came-to-britain-for-a-new-life-they-found-unemployment-and-despair-727739.html.

Cheney, D.M. (November 2005) *Statistics by Country by Catholic Population*. www.catholichierarchy.org/country/sc1.html.

FDA and Monosodium Glutamate (MSG) (31 August 1995). vm.cfsan.fda.gov/~lrd/msg.html.

Freeman, M. (October 2006) Reconsidering the effects of monosodium glutamate: a literature review. *J Am Acad Nurse Pract*, 18(10), 482–6. www3.interscience.wiley.com/journal/118565688/abstract.

Geha, R.S., Beiser, A. *et al.* (April 2000) Review of alleged reaction to monosodium glutamate and outcome of a multicenter double-blind placebo-controlled study. *J Nutr*, 130(Suppl 4S), 1058S–62S.

Sims, J.M. (January 2007) *The Vietnamese Community in Great Britain – Thirty Years On.* Runnymede Trust, London.

Tarasoff, L. & Kelly, M.F. (1993). Monosodium L-glutamate: a double-blind study and review. *Food Chem Toxicol*, 31(12), 1019–35.

Walker R. (October 1999) The significance of excursions above the ADI. Case study: monosodium glutamate. *Regul Toxicol Pharmacol*, 30(2 Pt 2), S119–S121.

Japanese Diet

Allen, L. (2009) *The Encyclopedia of Money.* ABC-CLIO, Santa Barbara, CA.

AJCA (All Japan Coffee Assciation) (2009) *The Consumption of Coffee in Japan.* coffee.ajca.or.jp/data/data04.html.

Antoni, K. (1988) *Miwa – The Sacred Beverage.* Franz Steiner Verlag, Stuttgart.

Association of Nikkei & Japanese Abroad (2010) *Who are 'Nikkei & Japanese Abroad'?* www.jadesas.or.jp/EN/aboutnikkei/index.html.

Brewers Association of Japan (2004) *The History of Beer.* www.brewers.or.jp/100ka/history/mokuji.htm.

Brewers Association of Japan (2006) *Consumption of Different Types of Alcohol in Japan.* www.brewers.or.jp/data/t07-seijin.html.

Cardoso, M.A. *et al.* (December 1997) Dietary patterns in Japanese migrants to southeastern Brazil and their descendants. *J Epidemiolo*, 7(4), 198–204.

Cardoso, M.A. *et al.* (2000) Secular changes in dietary patterns in the metropolitan areas of Brazil (1988–1996). *Rev. Saúde Pública*, 34(3), 251.

Central Intelligence Agency (CIA) (June 2010) *The World Fact Book.* www.cia.gov/library/publications/the-world-factbook/geos/ja.html.

FERA (Food and Environment Research Agency) (2008) *Plant Health Guide for Importers.* www.fera.defra.gov.uk/plants/publications/documents/importersGuide0909.pdf.

Freire, R.D., Cardoso, M.A. *et al.* (2003) Nutritional status of Japanese-Brazilian subjects: comparison across gender and generation. *British Journal of Nutrition*, 89, 705–12.

Fukui, M. & Wakasugi, C. (1972) Liver alcohol dehydrogenase in a Japanese population. *Japanese Journal of Legal Medicine*, 26, 46–51.

Garrow, J.S., James, W.P.T. & Ralph, A. (2000) *Human Nutrition and Dietetics.* 10th edition. Churchill Livingstone, Edinburgh.

Ito, S. & Ishikawa, Y. (2004) *Marketing of Value-Added Rice Products in Japan: Germinated Brown Rice and Rice Bread.* FAO International Rice Year, 2004 Symposium. Rome, 12 February.

Itoh, K. (2001) *The Japanese Community in Pre-War Britain.* Routledge/Curzon, London.

JOPA (Japan Oilseeds Processors Association) (2008) *The Supply of Rapeseed Oil.* www.oil.or.jp/topNews/bn20021002.html.

Japanese Science and Technology Agency (March 2010) *Food Composition Database.* fooddb.jp.

Kagawa, Y. (1978) Impact of westernization on the nutrition of Japanese: changes in physique, cancer, longevity and centenarians. *Preventive Medicine*, 7(2), 205–17.

Konno, S. (March 2007) Effect of various natural products on growth of bladder cancer cells: two promising mushroom extracts. *Alternative Medicine Review*, 12(1), 63–8.

Kubo, K., Aoki, H. & Nanba, H. (August 1994) Anti-diabetic activity present in the fruit body of *Grifola frondosa* (maitake). I. *Biological & Pharmaceutical Bulletin*, 17(8), 1106–10.

Kudo, Y., Falciglia, C.A. *et al.* (August 2000) Evolution of meal patterns and food choices of Japanese-American females in the United States. *European Journal of Clinical Nutrition*, 54(8), 665–70.

MAFF (Ministry of Agriculture, Forestry and Fisheries) (2004) www.maff.go.jp/www/counsil/counsil_cont/sougou_syokuryou/recycle/6/siryou06.pdf.

MAFF (Ministry of Agriculture, Forestry and Fisheries) (2010) *Characteristics of Consumption of Fish and Seafoods in Japan.* www.maff.go.jp/j/syouan/tikusui/gyokai/g_kenko/tokucyo.

MEXT (Ministry of Education, Culture, Sports, Science and Technology) (2007) *Statistical Report on Religion in 2008.* www.estat.go.jp/SG1/estat/OtherList.do?bid=000001024763&cycode=8.

Ministry of Foreign Affairs (2009) *Annual Report of Statistics on Japanese Nationals Overseas.* www.mofa.go.jp/mofaj/toko/tokei/hojin/10/pdfs/1.pdf.

MHLW (Ministry of Health, Labour and Welfare) (2004) *Annual Report on Diet.* www.mhlw.go.jp/houdou/2006/05/h0508-la.html.

MHLW (Ministry of Health, Labour and Welfare) (2004) *Facts and Associated Problems due to Alcohol in Adults.* www.mhlw.go.jp/topics/tobacco/houkoku/061122b.html.

MHLW (Ministry of Health, Labour and Welfare) (2009). Summary of the 2008 National Health Survey. http://www.mhlw.go.jp/houdou/2009/11/dl/h1109-1b.pdf.

MHLW (Ministry of Health, Labour and Welfare) (2009) Dietary Reference Intake for Japanese. www.mhlw.go.jp/houdou/2009/05/h0529-1.html.

MHLW (Ministry of Health, Labour and Welfare) (2010) *Cause of Death.* www.mhlw.go.jp/toukei/saikin/hw/life/life09/04.html.

MHLW (Ministry of Health, Labour and Welfare) (2010) *International Comparison of Life Expectancy.* www.mhlw.go.jp/toukei/saikin/hw/life/life09/03.html.

Nakamura, M., Whitlock, G. *et al.* (2001) Japanese and western diet and risk of idiopathic sudden deafness: a case-control study using pooled controls. *International Journal of Epidemiology*, 30, 608–15.

Nakanishi, S. *et al.* (2004) A comparison between Japanese-Americans living in Hawaii and Los Angeles and native Japanese: the impact of lifestyle westernization on diabetic mellitus. *Biomedicine & Pharmacotherapy*, 58, 571–7.

Nanba, H. & Kubo, K. (1997) Effect of maitake D-fraction on cancer prevention. *Annals of the New York Academy of Sciences*, 833, 204–7.

Osaki, Y., Matsushita, S. *et al.* (2005). Nationwide survey of alcohol drinking and alcoholism among Japanese adults. *Japanese Journal of Alcohol Studies & Drug Dependence*, 40(5), 455–70.

Otani, H. (2006) Bon appetit! *NIPPONIA*, 38. web-japan.org/nipponia/nipponia38/en/appetit/index.html.

Sacks, F.M., Lichtenstein, A. *et al.* (2006) Soy protein, isoflavones, and cardiovascular health. *Circulation*, 113(7), 1034–44.

SOYIC (Soy Sauce Information Center) (2010) Production and Consumption of Soy Sauce. www.soysauce.or.jp/arekore/index.html.

Statistics Bureau (2008) *Economic and Financial Data for Japan.* www.stat.go.jp/data/kakei/2002np/02nh.htm.

Takata, Y., Maskarinec, G. *et al.* (2003) A comparison of dietary habits among women in Japan and Hawaii. *Public Health Nutrition*, 7(2), 319–26.

Ueshima, H., Okayama, A. *et al.* (2003) Differences in cardiovascular disease risk factors between Japanese in Japan and Japanese-Americans in Hawaii. The INTERLIPID study. *Journal of Human Hypertension*, 17, 631–9.

United Nations (2007) *World Population Prospects: The 2006 Revision.* www.un.org/esa/population/publications/wpp2006/WPP2006_Highlights_rev.pdf.

USDA (United States Department of Agriculture) (2007) *Japan Dairy Products Semiannual Report 2007.* GAIN Report JA7067. www.fas.usda.gov/gainfiles/200711/146293059.pdf.

Vesa, T., Marteau, P. & Korpela, R. (2000) Lactose intolerance. *Journal of the American College of Nutrition*, 19(2), 165–75.

Web-Japan (2009) *Japan Fact Sheet. Japanese Language: A Rich Blend of Outside Influence and Internal Innovation.* web-japan.org/factsheet/en/pdf/e19_language.pdf.

WHO (World Health Organization) (2009) *Global Health Observatory.* apps.who.int/ghodata/?vid=720#.

World Green Tea Association (n.d.) *Production and Consumption of Tea in the World.* www.o-cha.net/english/cup/pdf/6.pdf.

4 Israel

4.1 Jewish Diet

Ruth Kander

4.1.1 Introduction

The state of Israel is officially the homeland of the Jewish people, however there are many Jewish communities to be found all around the world. Sephardic Jews originated in the Iberian Peninsula (Spain and Portugal), whereas Ashkenazi Jews (German Jews) are those who migrated to the east, thus 'Ashkenaz' Jews came from Hungary, Poland, Belarus, Lithuania, Russia, Ukraine and Eastern Europe whereas Mizrahi Jews came from India, North Africa, Iran and Yemen.

This chapter focuses on the eating patterns of British Jews living in the UK.

Israel is located in the Middle East on the eastern shore of the Mediterranean Sea (Figure 4.1.1). It has borders with Lebanon in the north, Syria in the north-east, Jordan and the West Bank in the east, and the Gaza Strip and Egypt in the south-west, and within its relatively small area is geographically diverse. Israel is the world's only predominantly Jewish state, with a population of 7.5 million people, of whom 5.7 million are Jewish. Arabs form the country's second largest ethnic group, and include Muslims, Christians, Druze and Samaritans.

The modern state of Israel derives its historical and religious roots from the biblical land of Israel, also known as Zion, a concept central to Judaism since ancient times. Political Zionism took shape in the late 19th century, and the Balfour Declaration of 1917 formalized by British policy established the Jewish state. Following the First World War, the League of Nations had granted Great Britain the Mandate for Palestine and the responsibility to establish 'the Jewish national home' within it.

In November 1947, the United Nations voted in favour of the partition of Palestine, proposing the creation of a Jewish state, an Arab state and a UN-

Multicultural Handbook of Food, Nutrition and Dietetics, First Edition. Edited by Aruna Thaker, Arlene Barton.
© 2012 Blackwell Publishing Ltd. Published 2012 by Blackwell Publishing Ltd.

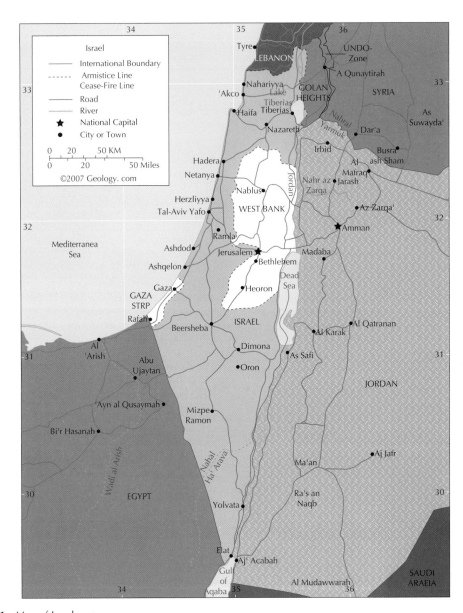

Figure 4.1.1 Map of Israel

administered Jerusalem. Partition was accepted by the Zionist leaders but rejected by Arab leaders, resulting in civil war. Israel declared independence on 14 May 1948 and neighbouring Arab states attacked the next day. Since then, Israel has successfully fought a series of wars with its neighbours, and in consequence occupies territories, including the West Bank and Gaza Strip, beyond those delineated in the 1949 Armistice Agreements. Israel has signed peace treaties with Egypt and Jordan, but efforts to resolve the conflict with the Palestinians have met with limited success and some of Israel's international borders remain disputed (en.wikipedia.org/wiki/Israel).

Language

The majority of Jews in the UK speak English but some speak Yiddish (a High German language of Ashkenazi origin). Hebrew (also called *Ivrit*) is spoken in Israel and by some Israelis living in the UK. Children in Jewish orthodox schools in the UK learn to read and write Hebrew from the age of five.

Migration to the United Kingdom

There is evidence that Jews first settled in the UK during the Roman occupation and were expelled during the reign of Edward I in 1206. In 1664 Oliver Cromwell officially readmitted the Jews to England, mainly because of their worldwide commercial connections and the wealth they would bring with them. Until the 17th century the Jews who settled in England were mainly of Sephardic origin (i.e., from Spain and Portugal) and had their own customs and backgrounds. In the late 19th century and again in 1930s and after the Second World War there was more immigration of European Jews, many of whom settled in the East End of London.

In the postwar years these groups have been added to by the arrival of more Sephardic groups. These are Jews who define themselves in terms of the Jewish customs and traditions which originated in the Iberian Peninsula before the expulsion of Jews from that area in the late 15th century (after Islam was replaced by Christianity as the governing religion), and usually defined in contrast to Ashkenazi and Mizrahi Jews.

Ashkenazi Jews are literally 'German Jews'. Later, Jews from Western and Central Europe came to be called 'Ashkenaz' because the main centres of Jewish learning were located in Germany. Many Ashkenazi Jews later migrated, mostly eastward, forming communities in non-German-speaking areas, including Hungary, Poland, Belarus, Lithuania, Russia, Ukraine and Eastern Europe. The Jewish population at the turn of the 20th century lived principally in the East End of London, a large, impoverished, industrial area. As their situation improved they moved into other areas, such as Hackney, Stamford Hill and Clapton. The majority (56%) of Jews now live in north and north-west London. Jewish communities are also found in Manchester, Leeds, Gateshead, Sunderland and Glasgow.

Current UK population

There are approximately 12 million Jews worldwide, the majority living in Israel and the United States. According to the 2001 census, the UK population was estimated at 270,499 (0.5% of the total population) and the majority (83%) were born in the UK; 96.7% live in England, 2.5% in Scotland, 0.8% in Wales. Jews have the oldest age profile of all communities in the UK, with 22% over the age of 65. Only 7% of Jews have no qualifications and about 44% of Jews have a university education. Jews are most likely to be self-employed and one third of Jewish men work in banking, finance or insurance. There were 33,000 children compared with 13,000 places in Jewish schools. In the UK 2001 census 97% of Jews registered themselves as White (www.statistics.gov.uk).

4.1.2   Religion

In Judaism it is believed that everything in the universe is under the direct control of one God. All aspects of the Jewish religion are taken from the Torah (i.e., the Old Testament) – the written law. Rabbis throughout the ages have interpreted the Bible and this is called the oral law. The practice of Judaism requires the observance of the 613 commandments, and Judaism as a way of life involves all these commandments. However, there are different types of Judaism.

Orthodox/ultra orthodox Judaism

It is important to understand that Jewish people have very different levels of observance, The ultra orthodox adhere very strictly to both Jewish written or oral law. An individual who is born Jewish but doesn't follow any of the laws will have a similar way of life to the average British/Caucasian citizen. Observant Jews live within their own communities and have support systems and make friends through their local synagogues and schools. As patients, they will strictly follow the dietary laws, including those applying to the Sabbath and all the Jewish festivals.

Reform Judaism

This form of Judaism grew out of the 18th-century Enlightenment. Reform Jews follow some traditions but do not feel obliged to follow customs which in their view are not adapted to modern times. A reform Jew is unlikely to follow strict dietary laws and they are also unlikely to observe a strict Sabbath and festival laws.

Liberal Judaism

This is a progressive form of Judaism which aims to bring Judaism and modernity together. Liberal Jews apply Judaism's religious and cultural tradition within a framework of modern thinking and morality. They seek to live to do justice, love and kindness and to walk humbly. There is no obligation on them to obey the dietary laws, but can if they wish to do so. Liberal Jews believes that all festivals and days of celebration or mourning should be upheld in tandem with traditional beliefs (www.bbc.co.uk/religion/religions/judaism).

Kashrut

Kashrut is the term given to the dietary laws regarding what can and cannot be eaten, and how food should be prepared and consumed. The word kosher is used to describe foods prepared in accordance with the Jewish dietary laws. Rabbis and other rabbinical authorities do not bless food to make it kosher; rather they supervise its production to ensure it is in accordance with Jewish dietary laws, which are derived from the Bible. Thus food can be intrinsically kosher without any rabbinical authority being involved. For instance, vegetables and fruit are undoubtedly kosher as long as they have no insects on them. Keeping kosher is a way of Jewish life. It is important to understand that people will observe different standards when following a kosher diet. The strictest people will eat only food that has an orthodox certification, including all packaged products, meat, fish and bakery products. In addition, they will only eat in restaurants with a kosher certification from an orthodox rabbi. Others will be more flexible; some will eat any product that is vegetarian or vegan, and will read ingredients to ensure that they do not contain obviously non-kosher ingredients. Some will eat vegetarian dishes in restaurants or a non-kosher home, and some will only eat meat that comes from a kosher animal (see Table 4.1.1).

Table 4.1.1 Jewish dietary restriction

- All meat eaten must be from animals that chew the cud and have cloven hooves (e.g., cow and sheep).
- The Torah lists 24 forbidden birds. Poultry allowed includes chicken, duck, goose, Cornish game hen, turkey.
- Forbidden animals include all insects, rodents, reptiles and amphibians. The Torah prohibits eating game, hyrax (rock badger), hare and pig.
- There are some parts of meat/poultry that must not be eaten. Kosher cuts of meat are taken from the front up to the 12th rib of the animal.
- A qualified person (shochet), in accordance with Jewish law, must slaughter all meat/poultry. In the Torah the way the meat is slaughtered is called shechita. There are special abattoirs and kosher butchers.
- After the animal has been slaughtered it must be made kosher by draining all the blood. This is done by a complex method but will involve covering the meat in salt, which can make kosher meat higher in salt than non kosher meat.
- Kosher fish must have fins and scales (e.g., cod, trout, mackerel, salmon, tuna). Shellfish and scavengers (e.g., catfish, monkfish) are forbidden as they don't have fins and scales.
- Meat and milk must not be eaten together. In a kosher home all utensils, pots, pans, crockery and cutlery must be separated (i.e., one set for milk and another for meat).
- Meat and milk foods should be stored separately on different shelves; some people keep separate fridges or freezers (but this is not common).
- Products with grape juice should not be eaten without kosher supervision.
- All fresh fruits and vegetables are permitted but they must not contain any insects. Even eating the tiniest insect can be a major transgression.

4.1.3   Food production and cooking methods

Separation of meat and milk

The Torah states that meat and milk must not be consumed at the same time. Separate dish cloths, sponges, sinks and draining boards should be used for these foods. It is also a requirement to wait between the consumption of eating meat and milk. This varies from 3 to 6 hours.

Milk

Rabbinic law requires that there be supervision during the milking process to ensure that the source of the milk is from a kosher animal. The UK Department for Environment, Food and Rural Affairs' regulations and controls are sufficiently stringent to ensure that only cow's milk is sold commercially. It is therefore accepted by some that milk sold in the UK is suitable for consumption. However, some individuals are more stringent and only consume milk produced with full-time supervision.

Parev (neutral)

Parev food is neither milk nor meat. *Parev* foods include fruits, vegetables, nuts, crisps, raw potatoes, raw pasta, raw rice, raw eggs, soft drinks, tea bags/granules, pure coffee powder and sweets/biscuits/chocolate. Packaged foods that have a kosher certification will specify if they are *parev* or not. *Parev* food can be served with either meat or milk. A kosher kitchen will usually have *parev* pots, utensils and cutlery. These are always washed separately from meat/milk. A *parev* food will become meat or milk depending on what it is cooked in or what is added to it. For example, pasta cooked in a *parev* pot is neutral until either meat or cheese is added.

Grape products

Wine represents the holiness and separateness of the Jewish people. Wine or grape juice is used for the sanctification of the Sabbath and at festivals. In addition, wine was poured on the altar of sacrifices in the days of the temple. For this reason Jews must produce and handle wine or grape juice. This can affect a number of food products: fruit juices made with grapes, tinned fruits in grape juice, wine vinegar, foods with grape flavourings (e.g., yoghurts, jams, all wine and alcoholic drinks made with grapes) and some mustards. Spirits (e.g., whisky and vodka) are permitted. All these foods should only be used if they have a kosher certification.

4.1.4   The Sabbath

Upon completing the creation God rested on the seventh day and gave the Sabbath as a gift. The central theme of the Sabbath is being with family and friends. On the Sabbath all forms of work are prohibited. Work is seen as most things associated with the developed world – using electricity, cooking, shopping, driving, watching TV, drawing, etc. The Sabbath starts at sundown on Friday (in the winter months this can be as early as 3.30 pm and in the summer often communities bring in the Sabbath at 7.30 pm) and ends after nightfall on Saturday. The Sabbath is typically a day of rest. The head of the house and families will go to the synagogue for prayers on Friday evening, Saturday morning and afternoon.

On the Sabbath three meals are taken. Meals can start with the sanctification of the wine/grape juice and then a blessing over bread (*challa*, people generally like this and will eat a number of slices or a whole roll, it may be homemade) (see Table 4.1.2).

Healthy foods for the Sabbath meals

- Starters: Salad, fruit (e.g., melon, grapefruit, pineapple) or fish.
- Soup: Chicken soup with vegetables, the fat removed and no vermicelli (pasta).
- Main course: Grilled meat or chicken with rice or baked potato with salad or steamed/roasted vegetables, freshly cooked meat salad (e.g., chicken or beef).
- Desserts: Fruit, meringue, fruit fool, mousse, small amount of ice cream.

4.1.5   The Jewish calendar

The dates of the Jewish festivals are determined by their position in the Hebrew calendar. The Hebrew

Table 4.1.2   Foods eaten on the Sabbath

Meal	Food eaten	Nutritional implications for healthy eating
Friday night	Meat in pastry or chopped liver	High in fat
Traditional examples but it will vary according to families	Chicken soup with vermicelli	Need to ensure fat is skimmed off soup and watch portion of vermicelli
The meal is high in carbohydrates; as they are at every course need to strike a balance.	Roast chicken	Ensure no oil/fat used; check for high-fat sauces poured over. Recommend using spray oil or cooking in water.
	Roast potatoes	Can be high in fat. Have rice instead.
	Vegetables or salad	Make sure no high-fat dressings are used or that vegetables have been cooked in too much oil.
	Dessert	Encourage a small portion or just fruit. Could compromise and tell patient to have dessert either on Friday night or on the Sabbath.
Sabbath breakfast (*kiddish*) Snack after prayers in synagogue before lunch	Crackers	Encourage not to have too many 1–3 crackers with pickled herring (as others have mayo/oil added).
	Herrings pickled, in oil (*shmultz*), chopped, tuna, egg or avocado dips (all will have mayonnaise)	Should limit cakes/biscuits.
	Cakes (yeast cake)	It could be recommended that the first course at lunch be avoided if *kiddish* has been eaten.
	Biscuits	
	Whisky is often drunk by the men, about 1–3 shots	
Sabbath lunch	Egg mayonnaise	High in fat. Recommend using less and a lower-fat variety.
	Cholent (meat stew)	Encourage lean meat. Plenty of vegetables and pulses and small amounts of potatoes. Could recommend the use of sweet potatoes.
	Kegul (potato pie) traditionally made with a lot of oil, but this can be modified	Advise to find lower-fat recipes.
	Chopped liver	High fat content. Encourage small portion.
	Schnitzel (fried chicken breast)	Encourage baking in the oven.
	Cold meats	Encourage freshly made meat cold rather than the high-fat processed meats.
Sabbath day supper (called the third meal)	Salads containing mayonnaise (i.e., egg mayo, tuna, coleslaw, potato salad)	All high in fat due to mayonnaise. Encourage smaller portions and use of less mayonnaise.

Table 4.1.3 Dates for Jewish festivals

Festival	Jewish month	English month
Rosh Hashanah	1–2 Tishrai	September/October
Fast of Gedaliah	3 Tishrai	September/October
Yom Kippur (fast)	10 Tishrai	September/October
Sukkot	15–20 Tishrai	September/October
Hoshanna Rabba	21 Tishrai	September/October
Shemini Atzeret	22 Tishrai	September/October
Simchat torah	23 Tishrai	September/October
Channuka	25–30 Kislev, 1–2 Tevet	December
10th Tevet (fast)	10 Tevet	December/January
Tu B'ishvat new year trees	15 Shevat	January/February
Fast of Esther	13 Adar	February/March
Purim	14 Adar	February/March
Pesach	15–22 Nissan	March /April
Shavvuot	6–7 Sivan	May/June
Shiva Asar B'Tammuz (fast)	17 Tammuz	June/July
Tisha B'Av (fast)	9 Av	July/August

calendar is based on the lunar/solar cycle. Each Hebrew month consists of 29 or 30 days. The length of the days and hours varies by seasons, and controlled by times of sunset, nightfall, dawn and sunrise (see Table 4.1.3).

4.1.6   Religious festivals and foods

Rosh Hashannah

This festival marks the beginning of the New Year (the first month, Tishrai, is usually in September). The theme of the New Year is sweetness and a sweet new year. Many sweet foods are eaten at this time. Rosh Hashannah is also a time of reflection on the past year, to contemplate the future and to pray that we are inscribed into the book of life. Rosh Hashannah is celebrated over two days unless it links in with the Sabbath, in which case it can last three days, which would mean consuming

six large meals. The pattern of the meals is similar to the Sabbath in that a blessing over wine is said and then a blessing over the *challa*. On Rosh Hashannah the *challot* (plural of *challa*) are round, symbolizing the continuity of life. Instead of putting salt on the *challa*, it is dipped in honey, to express a wish for a sweet new year. On the first night of Rosh Hashannah and generally over the festival there are a number of foods that are eaten as symbols for a good new year ahead.

Honey is one of the most common symbolic foods taken on the first night, by dipping apple in honey Jews are asking for a sweet new year. Other traditional symbolic foods include pomegranate, fenugreek, head of fish, cake, *tzimmes*; stewed carrots with honey and dried fruits, especially dates. Some main dishes are also cooked with honey/sugar.

Yom Kippur

This comes 10 days after Rosh Hashannah; it marks the end of 10 days of repentance and is the most important day of the year. On this day adults and children over the age 12/13 years fast, confess all their sins and ask God for forgiveness and to be written and sealed into the book of life.

Fasting is a fundamental aspect of the day and the fast lasts for 25 hours from sunset to sundown the following day. During this time no food or drink can be taken. A festive meal is taken before the fast. This is usually quite similar to the Sabbath meal and a light meal is taken after the fast.

Allowances can be made for people with chronic medical conditions (e.g., diabetics, oncology patients or pregnant/breastfeeding women).

Sukkot

This comes four days after Yom Kippur and is a celebratory festival. Sukkot lasts for eight days. During this time there are many family and social gatherings. The last two days are a celebration of the end the yearly cycle of the Torah readings. Traditionally, sweets and chocolates are given to the children in the synagogue.

Channuka

This festival lasts for eight days and is in the Jewish month of Kislev, which generally occurs in

December. During this time it is customary to eat foods made with oil, in particular doughnuts and *latkes* (fried potato cakes).

This can have implications for weight reducers and heart disease and diabetic patients.

Tu Beshvat (New Year for the Tree)

It is customary to eat 15 different fruits that all grow from trees, including the seven fruits species for which the Land of Israel is praised, a land of wheat, barley, (grape) vines, figs, pomegranates, olives palms and honey. Some families will have a celebratory meal and the fruits as dessert.

Diabetics may experience high blood sugar levels if they take too many dried fruits or fresh fruits.

Purim

Purim is on the 14th of Adar, which is usually the month of March. The main event is reading the Book of Esther. People give each other sweetmeats, and family and friends will gather together for a celebratory meal. Hamentashen (a puff pastry, triangular in shape, with a poppy seed/date/chocolate or jam filling) is traditionally eaten.

Patients should be encouraged to limit high-calorie foods during the day and to eat moderately at the main meal.

Passover

This festival usually falls in the spring and coincides with Easter. It lasts for eight days with the first two and last two being similar to the Sabbath. During this time it is forbidden to eat any foods made from the five types of grain (wheat, barley, oats, rye and spelt) that have been leavened. The orthodox communities will go to great lengths to ensure that the entire house, garage, cars are clean from *chametz* (anything made from the five types of grain). The kitchen is also thoroughly cleaned and a completely different set of dishes, pots, pans, utensils and cutlery is used for these seven days. The staple foods for the week are matzos which are made from unleavened bread (wheat that has only been in contact with water for a short amount of time; special types permitted by the rabbis). There are different levels of observance.

Some will simply avoid bread for the week; others will buy kosher food and have matzos. The ultra orthodox will be more stringent and eat only matzos, potatoes, eggs, chicken, fruits and vegetables. The modern orthodox will buy all foods with a kosher stamp marked 'kosher for Passover' and buy meat or fish from kosher-certified stores. On the first and second night of Passover the family will gather together for the Seder, this is the reading from the Haggadah of the exodus from Egypt. During the Seder symbolic foods are eaten and four cups of wine are taken. Symbolic foods include egg, lettuce, radish, horseradish and *charoset* (a paste made of apples, wine, hazelnuts and ground almonds) (see Table 4.1.4).

In hospital a patient who is orthodox will require kosher meals with a special stamp that states 'kosher for Passover'; in addition they will probably prefer not to take any nutritional supplements that week unless they have discussed this with their local rabbi.

Shavuot

This festival comes exactly seven weeks after Passover starts. It lasts for two days and is similar to rules to the Sabbath. It commemorates the time when Moses received the Torah on Mount Sinai. During this festival it is customary to eat dairy foods such as cheesecake and pastry with cheese (cheese blintz). The milky meal will often include vegetable soups, salmon, potatoes, salads and cheesecake for dessert.

As many high-fat products will be eaten at this time this will have implications for weight reducers and lipid-lowering patients.

Fasting

There are six fast days in the Jewish year. All boys over the age of 13 years and girls over the age of 12 years are expected to fast. Pregnant and breast-feeding women, the elderly and the sick should seek guidance from their local rabbi. A fast will start at sunrise and end at sunset. There are two fasts that start at sundown the day before and end at one hour after sunset the next day and so last 25 hours.

During a fast it is prohibited to have any foods or drinks.

Table 4.1.4 Jewish foods eaten during Passover

Food group	Foods	Nutritional considerations
Carbohydrates	Matza	Low fat about 80 kcal a slice as bread but not filling can eat too many.
	Potatoes Encourage diabetics to have sweet potato as lower GI	Ensure appropriate portion sizes and that margarine is not added if advising diabetes/weight reduction.
	Rice (the Sephardim eat rice but not Askenazim)	Watch portion sizes if advising for diabetes/weight reduction
Protein	Meat, fish, poultry	Can easily have too much as many large meals, encourage meat twice daily but only at one course in a meal.
Fruit and vegetables	Most acceptable. Many will avoid legumes (sweet corn, peas, beans)	Discourage oil dressings, mayonnaise.
Cakes and biscuits	Often home-made with many eggs used	Quite high protein/fat. Need to control portion size.
Nuts	Many cake and biscuit/dessert recipes contain a large proportion of groundnuts	

Health in the Jewish religion

It is mentioned in the Bible that people must look after themselves both physically and spiritually. The Talmud (the basis for all rabbinic laws) advises wise men not to live in a town without a doctor. Maimonides, a famous Spanish Jewish philosopher and Torah scholar, who lived in the 12th century, wrote a classic code which stresses that saving a life should take precedence over the sanctity of the Sabbath. There is a principle that life is supremely important (Spitzer, 1998). Although good health is highly regarded, it is somewhat paradoxical that orthodox and Hassidic Jews have high levels of obesity and heart disease and engage in low levels of physical activity (Spitzer, 1998).

4.1.7 Typical eating pattern

Eating patterns depend on level of observance, interest in eating healthily and life and social circumstance, just like any others in the UK. On Sabbath and Jewish festivals kosher food is available. It is also important to remember the concept of the Jewish mother, who will often give large helpings of food. Many Jews in UK have generally adopted the British eating habits into the kosher lifestyle.

4.1.8 Healthy eating

Key points

- Healthy eating can be difficult as families get together for big meals and many of the traditional foods at the time of festivals are high in fat.
- Encourage healthier versions of high-fat products; give examples and negotiate a reasonable compromise, for example having fried foods no more than once a week, on the Sabbath or festivals.

Healthy eating should generally be encouraged as one of the commandments in the Torah is to look after ourselves. In the UK the eatwell plate model (FSA 2007) can be encouraged as it is for the general population. (See Table 4.1.5) for a description of Jewish foods.

Dietary modification for an orthodox patient who keeps a strictly kosher home

- They are not allowed to eat meat and milk together, for example they would not be allowed to have a meat sandwich for lunch followed by a yoghurt.

Table 4.1.5   Description of Jewish foods

Food group	Kosher availability	Retail shops
Breads	Granary, wholemeal, rye, white. Wholegrain varieties are limited and not GI tested.	Bought from strictly kosher bakeries/shops.
Breakfast cereals	Most commercial cereals are acceptable, some contain milk (e.g., Special K) which is unsupervised and therefore will not be taken by some groups.	Can buy in supermarkets or any grocery store.
Rice and pasta	All plain dried varieties are acceptable	Can buy in supermarkets or any grocery store.
Cheese and yoghurt	There is a very limited variety of low-calorie/low-fat yoghurts/cheese. Encourage smaller portions of regular and low-fat varieties if possible (can be expensive).	Kosher shops, some local supermarkets in north-west London, Stanford Hill area may have a kosher section.
Milk	All ultra orthodox will buy kosher milk which is available as full, semi-skimmed and skimmed	Kosher shops.
Butter and margarine	These must be kosher and there are no low-fat varieties. All polyunsaturated	Kosher shops.
Meat and poultry	Encourage patients to buy lean meat. Encourage chicken and fish	Kosher butcher/shops.
Fish	The main fish taken is salmon, mackerel, cod, sea bass, trout, tuna, herrings	Kosher fish shop.
Beans and lentils	All acceptable	Can be bought from any shop.

- Unlikely to have a cooked breakfast (as this would make them meaty for hours).
- Will nearly always have large meals on Friday night and Saturday/festival days. Try to reach a compromise on cutting down/calorie modification as many foods are traditional and would be difficult to avoid (e.g., *kegul*).
- Foods that can be purchased from a supermarkets; fruits, vegetables, drinks, pasta, rice, oil, tea, coffee, sugar, flours, breakfast cereals.
- Some ultra orthodox will buy all food and drink from a strictly kosher shop. These can be sourced online or contact the Beth Din (rabbinical court).

Kosher bakeries sell many types of cakes, biscuits, pastries and croissants; these are useful when advising on increasing calories. In general they will all be *parev* (neutral). Some will have a range of milky cakes. Kosher sweets and chocolates are widely available, as is ice cream. Ice cream can be *parev* or dairy (in north-west London there is even a kosher ice cream van!)

Herbs and spices

Cumin, cilantro and turmeric are very common in Sephardi cooking. Caraway and capers were brought to Spain by the Muslims and feature in the cuisine. Cardamom (*hel*) is used to flavour coffee. Chopped fresh cilantro and parsley are popular garnishes. Chopped mint is added to salads and cooked dishes, and fresh mint leaves (*nana*) are served in tea. Cinnamon is sometimes used as a meat seasoning, especially in dishes made with ground meat. Saffron, which is grown in Spain, is used in many varieties of Sephardic cooking, as well as spices found in the areas where Jews have settled (en.wikipedia.org/wiki/Cuisine_of_the_Sephardic_Jews).

Sephardic Jews tend to eat foods that have more flavour than Ashkenazi Jews. The latter are more likely to use salt, pepper, garlic and paprika as seasonings rather than those described above. Their food is not spicy (www.inmamaskitchen.com/FOOD_IS_ART_II/food_history_and_facts/Jewish_Cooking.html).

Table 4.1.6 Jewish Dietary modification for weight reduction

Food group	Example of foods	Dietary advice
Starchy foods	Breads, pitta bread, rolls, French stick	Choose grainy breads. e.g., granary or rye or wholemeal pitta/rolls. Advise on portion sizes.
	Rice	Basmati or long grain. Advise on portion size.
	Pasta	Any type. Advise on portion sizes.
	Potatoes	Avoid with large amounts of oil e.g., *kegul, latkas*, chips. Recommend sweet potato. Advise on portion size.
Meat, fish, eggs and beans	Meat, chicken, duck	Avoid frying. Try lean cuts. Have smaller portions. Remove skin before cooking,
	Fish	Bake in oven with no added fats. Avoid fried fish.
Vegetables	Any fresh, frozen, tinned	Avoid cooking with oil, use low-calorie sprays or steam them. Plate model with half-plate with vegetables (should be encouraged).
Fruits	Any fresh, frozen, tinned	Have three fruits daily (any type). Have fruits spread across the day not in one sitting. Avoid compote with added sugar – use sweetener or nothing.
Drinks		Diet fizzy drinks. No added sugar squash.
Cakes, biscuits, sweets and chocolate		Eat less; maybe treat yourself on the Sabbath.
Large meals		Encourage smaller portions and fill up on vegetables.
Physical activity		Encourage to incorporate into daily lifestyle

4.1.9   Obesity

There are no data in the UK on rates/prevalence of obesity in the Jewish population but in view of the religious cultural lifestyle there are many overweight men, women and children who are obese.

As an ultra orthodox man will prefer not to have his waist and hips measured by a female dietitian, if possible find a male to measure males and a female to measure females.

Suggestions for the way forward

Patterns of obesity could be looked at in the ultra orthodox and development of weight-reducing programmes developed for their lifestyle and culture (see Table 4.1.6).

4.1.10   Coronary heart disease, stroke

There are no data in the UK on rates/prevalence of coronary heart disease (CHD) in the Jewish population as there is very little research on CHD, stroke and hypertension in this group. In the ultra orthodox communities exercise is often not undertaken by adult men and women. If this is to be encouraged, then they would require separate facilities as men and women do not mix together. There are separate gyms in Stamford Hill area of north London.

Dietary modification for Jewish orthodox patient (weight management for coronary heart disease)

- Regular meals.
- Increase fruits and vegetables.
- Pulses/lentils instead of red meat.
- Reduce oil in cooking.
- Lower-fat dairy products where available.
- Avoid high-fat foods (e.g., pastry products) and *kegul*.
- Reduce fried foods; grill, boil or bake instead.
- Eat more oily fish (available in kosher fish shops and kosher stores).
- Use poly- or monounsaturated fat in cooking, and use sparingly.
- Increase activity by general lifestyle modifications, e.g., more walking, using stairs instead of a lift, joining exercise classes.
- Portion control (important as it is traditional for mothers to give large portions).
- Avoid snacking.
- Take care during festivals. They should be encouraged not to overindulge.

The advice is mainly the same as that for any Caucasian. It is important to remember that there are many family gatherings on the Sabbath and during festivals when many calories consumed.

Blood pressure

There are no data on hypertension rates in the UK Jewish population. Offer the same advice as for the general population:

- Reduce salt in cooking.
- Avoid packet soups.
- Reduce ready-made sauces.
- Reduce the use of stock cubes.
- Reduce fast/convenience foods.
- Flavour food with herbs and spices.

The process by which meat from kosher animals is made kosher involves using a large amount of salt. Although the salt is thoroughly rinsed off much is absorbed. Therefore all kosher meat (even if it is fresh and not processed) will contain salt, but there are no data on how much. It is important to consider this when assessing the salt intake of someone who follows a strict kosher diet. Encourage patients to wash meat thoroughly before cooking.

Stroke

Texture-modified diets

- A puréed diet can be ordered from companies that provides kosher meals. In the event that the hospital cannot provide the appropriate texture in a kosher meal the family should be asked if they are able to bring in meals.
- Thickeners or thickened drinks should be checked for suitability (this can be checked with the manufacturers or the Beth Din).

4.1.11 Type 1 and type 2 diabetes

There are no data on the prevalence of diabetes in the Jewish populations in the UK. Dietary treatment for an orthodox Jew would be the similar to advice given to a non-Jewish patient. There are no known herbal remedies used for the treatment of diabetes. Diabetics should consult their local rabbi with regard to fasting. A regular diabetes diet sheet is appropriate (see Table 4.1.7).

Complications associated with diabetes, such of renal failure, can involve modification of the diet. All advice will be similar to that for a non-Jewish patient.

Chronic kidney disease stages 1–3

Reduce protein in the diet only if intake is excessive, such as on the Sabbath and festivals when two meat courses may be consumed in one meal: suggest that only one is taken.

- Reduce salt as per general population.
- Strict diabetic control.
- Lose weight.
- A patient with ESRF (stage 4/5) and on dialysis may need potassium and/or phosphate restriction. Traditional foods high in potassium include *kegul* eaten on Sabbath and festivals, *cholent* (meat stew) eaten on the Sabbath which may include potatoes and vegetables that have not been pre-boiled, and *boraka* (potato or spinach pasty).

There is no known literature on diet and diabetes for the Jewish population in the UK, or known support groups.

Table 4.1.7 Jewish dietary modification for diabetes

Food group	Example of foods	Dietary advice
Starchy foods	Breads, pitta bread, rolls, French stick	Choose grainy breads, e.g., granary, rye or whole meal pitta or rolls.
	Rice	Basmati or long grain.
	Pasta	Any type. Watch portion sizes.
	Potatoes	Avoid with large amounts of oil e.g., *kegul*, *latkas*, chips, sweet potato.
Meat, fish, eggs and beans	Meat, chicken, duck	Avoid frying. Have lean cuts. Have smaller portions. Remove skin before cooking.
	Fish	Bake in oven with no added fat. Avoid fried fish.
Vegetables		Avoid cooking with oil, use low-calorie sprays or steam them.
Fruits		Have three fruits daily (any type). Have fruits spread across the day not in one sitting. Avoid compote with added sugar – use sweetener or nothing.
Drinks		Diet fizzy drinks. No added sugar squash.
Cakes, biscuits, sweets, and chocolates		Eat less – maybe a treat on the Sabbath.

4.1.12   Cancer

The risk for cancers differs between the various ethnic groups. There are no data on cancer rates among Jews in the UK. Care for a cancer patient who is orthodox will be similar to that for a non-Jewish British patient.

4.1.13   Nutritional support

Modification of the diet to improve oral intakes must consider keeping milk and meat separate. For example, it would not be acceptable to fortify chicken soup with cream or have milk/cheese with a meaty meal.

- Margarine (e.g., Tomor, which is dairy-free) could be added to potatoes and vegetables.
- Have more fried foods. Traditional Jewish fried foods include *schnitzel* (fried chicken breasts) and *latkas* (fried potato cakes).

- If having a dairy meal, then fortify soup/mashed potato with cream and cheese.
- In a meat meal encourage pastry foods (e.g., *borakas*) or the use of non-dairy margarine.
- Add extra oil or margarine to rice and pasta.
- Encourage desserts such as pies/crumble (these can be *parev* and therefore eaten after a meat meal), high-calorie dairy yoghurts and milk puddings (only after milk meals).
- Snacks between meals. After a meat meal patients must wait 3–6 hours before eating a dairy snack: non-dairy snacks include croissants, pastries, biscuits, cake, non-dairy (*parev*) chocolate, toast with peanut butter/jam/soya cream cheese with Tomor margarine, fruit with non-dairy ice cream and soya ice cream.

Sip feeds

Many sip feeds are acceptable and are considered dairy. This needs to be considered when advising on numbers to take and what else the patient is eating (i.e. meat meals). Some supplements will be non-dairy (i.e., non-milk-based, e.g., Calogen, Maxijul). Some sip feeds contain gelatin and if from animal origin are not acceptable. Flavours such as strawberry, raspberry and forest fruits maybe not accepted as they may contain a red colourant (E120) from a non-kosher source.

The manufacturers or Beth Din can advise on which sip feeds are suitable.

Enteral feeding

The dietician should check if the standard feed used in the hospital is kosher; if not the family should be consulted and they will make the decision. The family may or may not want to contact their rabbi.

4.1.14   Maternal and child nutrition

In Jewish culture families and children play a major role. Jewish tradition values childbearing, from the biblical commandment 'be fruitful and multiply'. The Jewish lifecycle begins at birth.

A Jewish boy (considered Jewish only if his mother is Jewish) will have been circumcised when he is eight days old. This is a commandment from God first given to Abraham and is an accepted law. The circumcision ceremony is very important and a celebratory occasion. At this time the baby boy is named (often after a male member in the families that has passed away) and a special meal is taken afterwards, where the name of the newborn is traditionally discussed. When a boy reaches 13 years he celebrates his Bar Mitzva, which literally means a boy is responsible for observing the 613 commandments. This is a celebratory occasion and the boy will read the chapter in the Torah, which is called a portion. The family will often host a party and festivities for family and friends.

A girl is named in the synagogue at any time and traditionally a party is given for her within the first year known as a *kiddish* to welcome her into the world and celebrate the beginning of life, either on the Sabbath or on any day of the week. A girl becomes of age when she reaches 12 years. She is then considered a woman and is expected to take on all the 613 commandments just like boys do at the age of 13. Traditionally, she will have a party

to celebrate this coming of age with her parents, friends and family. This could have implications if a child is overweight as 12–13 year olds may be going to parties on a weekly basis. A compromise needs to be sought by a dietitian giving advice.

The issues surrounding Jewish children are no different from those outside the Jewish faith. Requirements for pregnant mothers and young children are the same, and advice given to pregnant or breastfeeding Jewish women are the same as for anyone else. However, one would need to consider kosher dietary restrictions.

Key points to consider for pregnant and breastfeeding Jewish women
Fast days
Out of the six fast days held during the year, two are generally considered more important, and the most important is Yom Kippur. This is the 25-hour fast, during which time no food or drink may be consumed, not even sips of water. However, since the health of the mother and baby is of paramount importance, some pregnant or breastfeeding women do not fast and there are those who choose to fast for just a few hours and then break the fast.

Key points to consider in infant and child nutrition
Infant feeding
Many Jewish mothers choose to breastfeed, and due to ultra orthodox restrictions on contraception use, some mothers adopt breastfeeding as a method of contraception. The reliability of this method is controversial, but still widely practised in ultra orthodox circles.

Formula feeds
If a baby cannot tolerate breast milk, or if there are problems establishing breastfeeding or expressing breast milk, formula feeding is an option. Most commercial baby formulas are kosher; however, they do not have kosher certification for the milk content, including soy-based formula. If a special formula is required, then the Beth Din should be consulted. If they don't know, there is usually a pharmacist attached to them who will know or who will be able to make enquiries.

Websites

www.aish.org.uk
www.chabad.org.uk
www.jewishcare.org
www.statistics.gov.uk/cci/nugget.asp?id=293
www.bbc.co.uk/religion/religions/judaism/living/
    communitysurvey.shtml

Support groups

Chai Cancer Care: available to all cancer patients in the
    Jewish community.
www.chaicancercare.org
Camp Simcha: a support organization for Jewish chil-
    dren with cancer and other life-threatening diseases.
www.campsimcha.org.uk

Resources

The London Beth Din Kashrut Division
735 High Road
London N12 0US
Telephone: 020 8343 6255, Kashrut enquiries: 020 8343
    6247
email: info@kosher.org.uk
www.kosher.org.uk/intro.htm

References

Spitzer, J. (1998) *A Guide for the Orthodox Way of Life for
    Healthcare Professionals*. The Department of General
    Practice and Primary Care, St Bartholomew's and the
    Royal London School of Medicine and Dentistry and
    the East London and The City Health Authority.

5

Eastern Mediterranean Region

Christina Merryfield (Arab League), Zelalem Debebe (Somalia)

This is the region around the Mediterranean Sea and its Arabic-speaking peoples are mostly adherents of Islam. This chapter focuses on the Arabic diet as well as the diet of Somalia. Arab migrants make up a significant minority of the UK population, particularly as a result of the wars in Iraq and civil war in Somalia, which has resulted in an increase in the number of refugees seeking asylum in the UK. Somalis are the most recent arrivals. Some of the Arabic people have settled but many also come for medical treatment. As most of the Arabic-speaking countries are Muslim, this chapter has extensive information on the religious and dietary needs of this religious group. Religion dictates which foods are allowed or permissible (*halal*) and which are forbidden (*haram*). There is information on migration, traditional diets and changes in migration, religious influences and on dietary considerations for specific disease conditions such as obesity, diabetes and cardiovascular disease.

5.1 Arabic Diet

Christina Merryfield

5.1.1 Introduction

Arab countries

Since 1945 most Arab countries have joined the Arab League, which aims to strengthen ties among member states, coordinate policies and consider matters of common interest. The Arab League has 22 members which can be grouped into the African-Arab countries (Egypt, Libya, Tunisia, Algeria, Morocco, Mauritania, Sudan, Comoros, Djibouti and Somalia) and the Asian-Arab countries (Bahrain, Kuwait, Syria, Lebanon, Jordan, Iraq, Oman, Palestine [Gaza and the West Bank], Qatar, Saudi Arabia, Yemen and the United Arab Emirates). The World Health Organization (2005) often refers countries in

Multicultural Handbook of Food, Nutrition and Dietetics, First Edition. Edited by Aruna Thaker, Arlene Barton.
© 2012 Blackwell Publishing Ltd. Published 2012 by Blackwell Publishing Ltd.

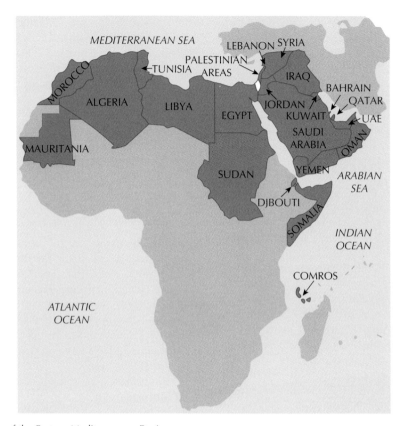

Figure 5.1.1   Map of the Eastern Mediterranean Region

the Arab League collectively as the eastern Mediterranean region (Figure 5.1.1).

Current population in the Arab region

The total population of the Arab region was estimated at 300 million in 2002 or 4.8% of the world's population. By 2025 this figure is projected to reach 395 million or 5.5% of the world's population, with Egypt by far the most populous country (United Nations, 2002).

Language

Arabic belongs to the Semitic language group which can be divided into classical or Qur'anic Arabic (mainly used for reading and religious text); colloquial Arabic, of which there are many spoken dialects; and modern Arabic, which provides a lingua franca. Arabic dialects are spoken by

approximately 100 million people. The main difficulty in classifying the dialects arises from basing the classification on both sociological and geographical criteria, although these overlap. According to geographical criteria, seven divisions emerge:

1. Saudi Arabia, Syria–Iraqi–Jordanian Gulf.
2. South Arabic (Yemen, Oman and Zanzibar).
3. Iraq.
4. Syria–Lebanon–Israel–Jordan.
5. Egypt (some parts excluded as they belong to the Maghrebine dialect).
6. Sudan and Central Africa.
7. Maghrebine dialects, including Malta.

Arab is the name originally applied to the Semitic peoples of the Arabian peninsula; it is now used also for populations of countries whose primary language is Arabic, and includes Algeria, Egypt, Iraq, Jordan, Lebanon, Libya, Morocco,

Syria and Yemen. Socially, Arabs are divided into the settled *fellahin* (villagers) and the nomadic Bedouin (Moussa *et al.*, 2008).

Migration to the United Kingdom

The UK is home to a multiracial, multicultural and multi-faith community and the added feature of inter-ethnic marriage makes racial classification progressively more complex. It is known that the Romans brought Arab archers with them and established a town called 'Arabiya', present-day South Shields (Al-Jalili, 2004).

In the 19th century, Yemeni seamen, called Lascars, worked on British ships and many stayed to take employment in the docks and related industries, or the expanding rail network. London's East End, Tyneside, Liverpool and Cardiff became centres of small Arab communities. By 1948 there were nearly 1,000 Arabs in Tyneside, some marrying local women, thus giving rise to the British-Arab identity that many native-born British-Arabs, especially those of mixed ancestry, are now establishing. In the 1950s, many of these relocated to Birmingham and Sheffield. A number of Somalis from what was British Somaliland also settled in these areas as a result of serving on British ships. Frequently overlooked, but vitally important, the traditional trading skills of Syrians and Lebanese brought them to 'Cottonopolis' – Manchester. Large-scale Arab immigration began after 1945, with the Palestinians, followed by Egyptians and Sudanese, and the 1960s saw people coming from Morocco. Political repression in some home countries has partly contributed to Arab immigration, particularly in the 1960s to the 1990s from countries such as Iraq, Egypt, Sudan, Algeria and Somalia (McCoy, 2003).

Current UK population

Arab migrants make up a significant minority of the UK population, particularly as a result of war in Iraq and Somalia from where there has been an increase in the number of Arab asylum seekers; therefore this population group is expected to increase (Goenka *et al.*, 2007). According to the 2001 census, there were 106,833 people from the Arab League living in London, the largest group

being aged 25–44 years (Greater London Authority, 2005). Greater London is the main centre for British Arabs, with an estimated 300,000 in the capital. There are also traditional areas of Arab settlement such as Sheffield, where many Yemenis moved to work in the steel industry. Britain's main Arab population originate primarily from Iraq, Lebanon, Egypt and Morocco. The numbers place people from these countries among one of the largest non-Commonwealth immigrant groups in Britain (Census, 1991).

5.1.2   Religion

Among the Arab League countries most of the population are practising Muslims, divided mainly into Sunnis and Shia. There is also a minority of Christians, including Eastern Orthodox, Copt, Catholic and Assyrian in some countries (e.g., Jordan, Lebanon, Djibouti and Sudan). The UK has a documented Muslim population of around 1.2 million and 7% have an Arab background (UK Census (ONS, 2001)).

Although the basic beliefs and practices of Islam are universal, there are different branches and denominations, each of which has its own traditions and practices. The two main branches are Sunni and Shia.

Most practising Muslims follow five main duties or pillars of Islam:

- Faith in one God.
- Prayer at five set times every day.
- Giving a required amount to charity each year.
- Fasting during the holy month of Ramadan.
- Making a pilgrimage (*hajj*) once in their lives to the sacred city of Mecca if they can.

Religious dietary restrictions

Restrictions on what Muslims can eat are laid down in the Qur'an and are regarded as the direct command of Allah. Most practising Muslims do not eat pork or anything made from pork or from pork products. All other meat and meat products are eaten provided they are *halal* (permitted – that is, killed according to Islamic law). Seafood is allowed as fish is considered to have died naturally when taken out of the water, so the question of a specific method of killing does not arise. Alcohol is forbidden (Henley & Schott, 2004).

Guidelines for halal products

The Muslim Food Board (UK) advises that food products must be free from the following:

- Any product or by-product derived from pig or dog.
- Blood.
- Carnivorous animals (except fish).
- Birds with talons or birds that feed by snatching and tearing (e.g., birds of prey).
- Reptiles and insects.
- Any marine animals, except fish.
- Animals that live on land and in water (amphibians, e.g., frogs, crocodiles).
- Animals that have died by any means other than slaughtering according to the Islamic law.
- Animals that are generally considered repulsive (e.g., lice, maggots, mice, rats, spiders).
- The bodies of animals permitted under the Islamic law (cattle, sheep, lamb, goat, deer, poultry) but not slaughtered according to Islamic law. Most animals in the UK are not slaughtered according to Islamic law.
- Wine, ethyl alcohol or spirits, where these remain in their original chemical form.
- Any product or by-product (including any product used temporarily as a substitute) which contains, or is derived from, any one or more of the above products, in however minute a quantity, whether as an ingredient or sub-ingredient, as a processing aid, as a releasing agent, as a glazing agent, as an additive, as a colour or in any other form, is *haram* (unlawful).
- The preparation, processing and the manufacturing equipment must be free from all of the above.
- Packaging material that comes into contact with the food product must be free from all of the above.

Fasting during Ramadan

Ramadan occurs in the ninth lunar month of the Islamic calendar year, the dates changing each year. Abstaining from eating and drinking occurs from dawn (*sahur*) to dusk (*iftar*), with the length of fasting varying with geographical location and season. For example, the fasting period can be about 13 hours in Jordan while in London it can be as short as 9 hours in the winter months or as long as 18 hours in the summer months (Khatib & Shafagoj, 2004).

Most healthy practising Muslims over the age of 12 will fast during Ramadan, however some Muslims are exempt; they include the elderly, pregnant and breastfeeding women and people who suffer from an illness that could be adversely affected by fasting. Ramadan is intended to teach self-discipline, self-restraint and remind Muslims of the plights of the impoverished.

5.1.3   Traditional diet and eating patterns

Traditional eating patterns vary across the Arab countries depending on various influences from neighbouring regions and food supply. Originally Arab food was the food of the desert nomads and therefore was simple and portable. Nomads stopped at oases and in settled farming areas to get some of their food, such as flour for bread, dates, vegetable, spices and some fruits. They brought animals with them to provide meat and milk (e.g., goats and camels) and often would have cooked over campfires (see Tables 5.1.1, 5.1.2 5.1.3 & 5.1.4).

Food consumption patterns have dramatically changed in some Arab countries as a result of the sudden increase in income from oil revenue. Mass media, especially televised food advertisements, play an important role in altering eating habits. Migration, particularly during the 1970s, has had a great impact on the food practices in many Arab countries (Musaiger, 2002).

Typical meal pattern

A typical, simple meal, commonly served as *mezzeh* (a selection of dishes), may consist if the following foods:

- Wheat: a staple of Arabic cooking and used in bread (often served with a main meal) and pastries.

- Rice: the basis of most main dishes cooked with vegetables, chicken, lamb or beef.
- Vegetables and beans, particularly aubergine, cauliflower, courgettes and spinach: chickpeas and broad beans are often used in dips such as hummus or eaten as *fool*. Salads are commonly taken as a side-dish with meals; the basic dressing consists of olive oil, garlic and lemon.
- Desserts: filo pastries stuffed with dates or nuts, spices and butter and covered in a honey or sugar syrup.

Table 5.1.1 Foods commonly consumed in Arabic diets

Bread, rice, potatoes, pasta and other starchy foods	Milk and dairy foods	Vegetables and fruits	Meat, fish, eggs beans and other non-dairy sources of protein	Foods and drinks high in fat and or/sugar
Rice	Cow's milk/cheese/yoghurt	Aubergine	Lamb/mutton	Olive oil
Couscous	Sheep's milk/cheese/yoghurt	Courgettes	Beef	Peanut oil
Bread	Goat's milk/cheese/yoghurt	Okra	Chicken	Corn oil
Macaroni	Camel's milk/cheese	Artichokes	Quail	Sesame oil
Potatoes		Spinach	Offal	Ghee
Cassava		Carrots	Goat	Butter
Yam		Asparagus	Camel	Sugar cane
Millet		Onion	Sardines	Honey
		Green beans	Mullet	Pastries (often with nuts, honey and dried fruit)
		Cauliflower	Bream	Cakes (often with nuts and honey)
		Beetroot	Salmon	
		Salad leaves	Monkfish	
		Cucumber	Mackerel	
		Tomato	Trevally	
		Bananas	Shrimp	
		Grapes	Shellfish	
		Plums	Eggs	
		Apricots	Chickpeas	
		Melon	Broad beans	
		Pineapple	Lentils	
		Pomegranate	Sesame seeds	
		Lemons	Pistachio	
		Oranges	Almonds	
		Dried fruit	Walnuts	
		Apples	Hazelnuts	
			Pine nuts	

Table 5.1.2 Description of typical Arabic foods

Name of food	Description
Baklava	A sweet dessert made from chopped walnuts or pistachios, cinnamon and orange blossom wrapped in a thin pastry shell and drenched in syrup
Bean/lentil salad	Based on the ingredients of beans or lentils (usually boiled), chopped onion, garlic, lemon and tomatoes. Dressings usually parsley or coriander
Cheese *fatayer*	Cream cheese, parsley, mint wrapped in bread dough and oven-baked
Fattoush	Bread salad – cucumber, tomatoes, pepper, lettuce, mint and parsley with lemon juice mixed with toasted chopped bread
Falafel	Fried, made from ground chickpeas, onion, potato and flour
Fool	Broad beans, garlic, lemon and olive oil
Hummus	Ground chickpeas with sesame seed paste, lemon, garlic and sometimes olive oil
Kibbeh	Minced meat (or potato) fritters mixed with cracked wheat, onion, cinnamon and allspice. Usually fried, but can be baked
Labneh	Yoghurt – often with olives and mint
Mahalabia	Milk pudding – often with rice, cream, rose water, sugar and salt
Shawarma	Cuts of lamb, chicken or beef, wrapped in pitta bread. Sometimes *taboula* (sesame seed)-based sauce added
Taboula	Finely chopped salad of tomatoes, parsley, fresh mint and crushed wheat
Taboulleh	Cracked wheat with chopped parsley, mint spring onions, garlic, lemon and tomatoes
Tzaziki	Dip consisting of chopped cucumber, garlic, mint in yoghurt
Umm Ali	Pastry with milk, nuts and raisins

Table 5.1.3 Herbs and spices used in Arabic diet

English name	Arabic name (pronunciation may vary from country to country)	Use in cooking
Allspice	*Bahar heloo*	Often in sweets and dessert and to flavour stews
Cardamom	*Hail*	Used to flavour Arabic coffee
Cinnamon	*Qurfa*	Usually in a mixture of spices – the blend differs in each country. This mixture is referred to as *baharat*
Coriander	*Kuzbara*	Usually ground; added to most vegetable-based dishes
Black pepper	*Filfil aswad*	Added to most main dishes
Nutmeg	*Basbasa*	Often use in meat-based dishes
Paprika	*Paprika*	Sprinkled to taste
Chilli	*Filfil har*	Often added to curry-type dishes
Turmeric	*Kurkum*	Usually ground and added to most main dishes
Cumin	*Kamoon*	Strong, used sparingly in main dishes and rice
Samak	*Samak*	Dark-red berries, sour, often used as a substitute for lemons
Mint	*Nana*	Mainly used in salads and dips, often with parsley and yoghurt
Salt	*Mileh*	Added to most dishes
Parsley	*Badoonis*	Used widely in salad and vegetable dishes

Table 5.1.4　Glossary of Arabic foods

Arabic pronunciation (this may vary from country to country)	Food/dish
Baba Ghannouj	Puréed aubergine with sesame butter
Baamieh	Okra
Baydh	Eggs
Dajaaj	Chicken
Haleeb	Milk
Loubeih	Green beans
Lahm	Meat
Murabba	Jam
Qarnabeet	Cauliflower
Roz	Rice
Shurba	Soup
Smaiskeh	Lamb
Samak	Fish
Taheeni	Sesame oil
Teen	Figs
Tamour	Dates
Yakhnie	Stew
Zayt	Oil

Table 5.1.5　Average energy from macronutrients in the UK

Energy supply	Major food groups
Carbohydrate 48% Protein 16% Fat 35%	Cereals and cereal products 31%
	Milk and milk products 10%
	Egg and egg dishes 2%
	Fruit and nuts 2%
	Meat and meat products 15%
	Vegetables 4%

(HMSO, 2003)

5.1.4　Healthy eating

Key points

- Traditional patterns of the eastern Mediterranean region have changed to become more westernized.
- Nomadic people may well keep their traditional eating pattern, which is simple and portable.

Introduction

Traditional eating patterns of those native to the eastern Mediterranean region have changed to become more westernized. Those from this region living in the UK have shown similar trends, but often to a greater degree. In some Arab countries, such as Sudan and Saudi Arabia, protein availability has doubled and fat has increased three-fold; rice and wheat availability has increased five- and eight-fold respectively. At the same time, there has been no comparable increase in vegetable consumption and even a general decrease in some countries (Alwan, 1997).

There have been rapid changes in diets and lifestyle resulting from urbanization. These are causing a rise in diet-related diseases, including obesity, diabetes, cardiovascular disease, hypertension, stroke and various forms of cancer, which are taking over traditional public health concerns like undernutrition and infectious diseases (WHO, 2010).

Many of these changes are reflected in UK eating patterns, along with an increase in fast-food consumption. Chronic diseases, as a result of a change to a more westernized diet, has increased the incidence of obesity, cardiovascular disease, diabetes and some forms of cancer in Middle East countries (Musaiger, 2002).

The percentage of energy from macronutrients varies in the Arab League countries; Table 5.1.5 shows the average UK intake and the following sections the comparison with other Arab countries.

Sudan

The main food supply is from cereals, vegetables and milk (see Table 5.1.6). Sudan is an example of an Arab country with large inequalities and malnutrition. In rural areas the main staples are millet and sorghum. Cassava, yam and sweet potatoes are also consumed, whilst in urban areas wheat (bread) is the main staple.

Table 5.1.6 Average percentage energy from macronutrients in Sudan

Energy supply (2000–2)	Major food groups
Carbohydrates 61%	Cereals 53%
Protein 13%	Milk and eggs 13%
Lipids 26%	Vegetable oil 7%
	Pulses, nuts and oils 6%
	Meat and offal 6%
	Fruit and vegetables 4%
	Animal fats 1%

(Food and Agriculture Organisation of the United Nations FAO 2005)

Table 5.1.8 Average percentage energy from macronutrients in Kuwait

Energy supply (2000–2)	Major food groups
Carbohydrates 58%	Cereals 58%
Protein 11%	Milk and eggs 6%
Lipids 31%	Vegetable oil 17%
	Pulses, nuts and oils 3%
	Meat and offal 10%
	Fruit and vegetables 3%
	Animal fats 2%

(FAO, 2006)

Table 5.1.7 Average percentage energy from macronutrients in Lebanon

Energy supply (2000–2)	Major food groups
Carbohydrates 58%	Cereals 33%
Protein 11%	Milk and eggs 13%
Lipids 31%	Vegetable oil 11%
	Pulses, nuts and oils 10%
	Meat and offal 8%
	Fruit and vegetables 11%
	Animal fats 2%

(FAO, 2007)

Lebanon

Lebanon is a middle-income country where wheat (bread) is the main staple accompanied by lamb or chicken with rice, or fish with vegetables. Ghee is used more compared with North African-Arab countries (see Table 5.1.7).

Kuwait

Kuwait lies on the coast of the Persian Gulf; one third of the population compromises Kuwaiti nationals and two-thirds are immigrants (34% Arabs, 61% non-Arab Asians and 5% stateless nomads), hence the influence of Asian foods. It is also situated near the coast and fish and other seafoods are consumed more frequently (see Table 5.1.8). Staple foods are rice, wheat (bread, but along with many of the Gulf State countries, sizeable amounts of processed foods are consumed).

Over the past four decades changes in socioeconomic status, lifestyle and dietary habits have occurred, along with an increase in chronic diseases often associated with western diets and high-income countries. The traditional diet, which consisted of dates, milk, fresh vegetables and fruit, wholewheat bread, rice and fish or meat, has changed to a more mixed diet, with often an excess of energy-dense foods rich in fat and refined sugars and low in complex carbohydrates. Although sugar consumption is already relatively high, it continues to rise. The same trend applies to fat consumption. This is shown particularly in high-income Arab countries such as in the Arab Gulf. Larger cities in low-income Arab countries, such as Djibouti, Somalia, Sudan and Yemen, have similar dietary intakes to their counterparts in the intermediate and high-income Arab countries (Musaiger, 2002).

Changes in dietary habits and lifestyle in the Arab states from traditional lifestyles to a more westernized diet, characterized by high-fat, salt and low-fibre intakes along with sedentary lifestyles are widely reported in these countries (Musaiger, 2002). In the UK, these foods are more freely available, hence the incidence of these chronic diseases potentially increasing.

The Department of Health eatwell plate model (DH 2011) is relevant to this ethnic group and healthy eating tips are shown in Tables 5.1.9–5.1.11 compared with traditional eating patterns.

Recent evidence of good practice to promote healthy eating

An unhealthy diet is a modifiable risk factor that can contribute to chronic diseases prevalent in many of the eastern Mediterranean countries. Primary prevention based on comprehensive population-based programmes has been identified to help in containing an emerging epidemic of these chronic diseases. The WHO Regional Office has established a comprehensive integrated approach, 'Eastern Mediterranean Approach to Noncommunicable Diseases Network' (EMAN), to control chronic diseases such as diabetes, cardiovascular disease and cancer by promoting for example, healthy eating and physical activity and discouraging smoking. EMAN aims to link eastern Mediterranean countries through community-based programmes and raising community awareness in the region (WHO EMAN 2010).

Alcohol

Few studies have been undertaken to assess the intake of alcohol in the Arab countries. In most there is zero tolerance and abstinence is consequently usually high. A report on alcohol consumption in 12 of the 21 member states of the eastern Mediterranean region in 2004 showed a lower association of disease related to alcohol in the Middle East (1.3%) than in West and North Europe (6.8%), the protective role of local religious and cultural factors having a major influence on Arab Muslims (WHO, 2006).

However, with the adoption of a more westernized lifestyle, particularly in the UK, where alcohol is freely available and there is peer pressure from social events that offer alcohol, this is likely to have some impact in consumption.

Among the UK population, the average number of units of alcohol consumed per week in 2005 was 6.5 for women and 14.9 for men. Although these figures show the average intake is below the recommended maximum limits (14 units for women and 21 units for men), 24% of men and 13% of women over the age of 16 years exceeded that limit (IAS, 2008).

Smoking

In the UK (2005) 24% of adults over 16 years in Great Britain smoke, a slight fall since the late 1990s.

In Arab countries, particularly in the Middle East, the *shisha* (hookah, water-pipe or hubble-bubble) is taken instead of cigarettes (see Figure 5.1.2).

The *shisha* is mixed with certain flavours and aromatic herbs (e.g., apple, mango, strawberry, mint or other additives). Among women, who rarely smoke cigarettes, less stigma is attached to smoking the *shisha* and it is often seen as fashionable.

Shisha smoking in general is less frequent than cigarette smoking but has more concentrated exposure, that is, 15–90 minutes which is the equivalent of 2–12 cigarettes per portion of tobacco used. However the *shisha* produces more smoke and it is estimated that smoke exposure is equivalent to 100–200 cigarettes a session, therefore the health magnitude is different from cigarette smoking.

Prevalence of smoking overall in adult males in Egypt, in 2002, was 34% cigarette only and 10% *shisha*. Adult females were less than 1%. Data suggest that prevalence is increasing in Egypt and similar trends are occurring in nearby countries, including Syria and Kuwait, consequently adding to the burden of smoking-related diseases. Smoking aggravates the complications of diabetes; causes hypertension which is prevalent in many of the Arab countries; and can increase the risk of cancers. Another health issue of the *shisha* is the lead piping and other heavy metals, which pose a risk to toxic substances on the lips, oral cavity and hands (skin). There is very little literature to date on the health consequences of these heavy metals (WHO, 2006).

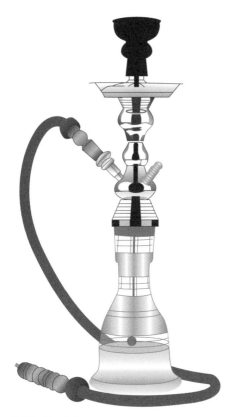

Figure 5.1.2   Hookah

5.1.5   Obesity

Key points

- An increase in energy and fat consumption has been shown in the Arab League countries over the last three decades.
- Barriers to physical activity need to be addressed and options provided, particularly for women who wear the *hijab*.
- The transition from traditional to more western diets and lifestyle has influenced the increased rates of obesity.
- Plumpness may often be perceived as a sign of affluence and fertility (in women in particular).

Table 5.1.9   Traditional Arabic eating patterns

Healthy eating tips (eatwell plate)	Traditional Arabic eating patterns
Base meals on starchy foods	Meals are usually based on refined starchy foods, particularly in more urban areas and rapidly developing countries
Eat lots of vegetables and fruit	Vegetable and fruit consumption is often associated with economic status and availability. Surveys of intakes have shown that the recommended five portions are often not achieved
Eat more fish, including one portion of oily fish	Intake of fish varies greatly; those near the sea (e.g., the Gulf States) will have a higher consumption. Oily fish is available as in UK (e.g., mackerel, sardines)
Reduce saturated fats and sugar	Higher income countries (e.g., Saudi Arabia and Kuwait) tend to have a higher fat and sugar consumption; the intake increasing over the last decade, this relationship has also shown an increase rate of obesity. Saturated fat is particularly high in areas where ghee and butter is used rather than vegetable oils
Try to eat less salt – no more than 6 g a day	Many of the Arab countries are hot and an increased intake of salt may be required. However salt is commonly added to traditional cooking so intake is likely to be more than necessary
Get active and try to maintain a healthy weight	Populations particularly in urban areas will often undertake little physical activity. In rural areas activity (walking) is essential for survival
Drink plenty of water	Water is usually consumed frequently; in addition, sugary drinks are commonly taken
Don't skip breakfast	In most cases three meals, which includes breakfast, are consumed

(Bashour, 2004; Dehghan, 2005)

Table 5.1.10 Traditional meal pattern foods to encourage in Arab diet

	Traditional foods to encourage	Reason to encourage
Breakfast		
	Breakfast cereals – high-fibre	Source of fibre
	Flatbread – wholemeal varieties	Source of fibre
	Fool (broad beans, garlic, lemon and olive oil)	Source of fibre, but limit use of oil
	Labneh – with low-fat yoghurt	Source of calcium
	Low-fat milk	Source of calcium
Snacks		
	Dried fruit (but limited quantity)	Source of fibre and vitamins
	Fresh fruit	
Lunch		
	Couscous/rice (long-grain/high-fibre)	Usually steamed/boiled
	Taboulleh (cracked wheat and parsley salad)	Source of fibre and vitamins
	Kibbeh (potato variety and oven-baked)	Lower in fat than meat version especially if oven-baked. Can be used in soups or in a tomato sauce or yoghurt, providing a good basis for a meal
	Bean or lentil salad	Low in fat, source of fibre
	Vegetables and pulses in main meals	Low in fat, good source of fibre
	Fish, poultry (without skin)	Lower in saturated fat than lamb/mutton, beef
	Dressings based on tomato sauces, lemon, pepper and crushed garlic	Low-fat dressing variety
	Olive oil (limited quantities)	Source of MUFAs
Evening meal or lighter meal		
	Soup, e.g., lentils, vegetables, vermicelli	Low in fat, source of fibre

Introduction

Obesity has become epidemic worldwide and in the eastern Mediterranean region overweight has reached alarming levels although the proportion varies from country to country and between geographical areas. It is well documented that morbidity and mortality rates rise with increase in body weight and are associated with chronic non-communicable diseases such as type 2 diabetes, hypertension, cardiovascular disease and some cancers. Changes in lifestyle, dietary habits, physical activity and the social and cultural environment are associated with obesity. Migration from countries where manual labour was a significant part of daily life to those, such as the UK, where

labour-saving jobs and the popularity of consuming convenience foods, including increased availability of these foods, is more common, will inevitability have a detrimental effect on health.

Definition

The most widely used classification of obesity in adults is based on body mass index (BMI) (see Table 5.1.12), the values being the same for men and women. BMI may not correspond to the same degree of fatness across different populations, due in part to different body proportions. It can therefore be considered a useful tool and used to estimate obesity. Waist circumference is a good measure

Table 5.1.11 Dietary modifications of the Arabic diet to promote healthier eating

Meal	Traditional foods	Changes to make a healthier option
Breakfast		
	Labneh – often not low-fat varieties used	Low-fat yoghurt variety, omit salt
	Fool – usually with a large amount of olive oil	Reduce oil
	Flat bread – commonly based on white flour	Wholemeal/grain variety – check quantity taken
	Cereal – various, but often low-fibre varieties	Choose high-fibre variety taken with low-fat milk
Snacks		
	Dates (often stuffed)/figs/Baklava/cakes – various (e.g., date or semolina). Consumed in large quantities	Limit number of dates, fresh fruit. Avoid ghee and butter when making cakes
Lunch (often the main meal)		
	Potatoes	Potatoes are usually taken fried or in a stew, therefore encourage use in a stew than fried
	Dips, e.g., *tzaziki* (often not low-fat yoghurt), hummus (presented with a lot of oil)	Use low-fat yoghurt for *tzaziki*, limit sesame seed paste, oil and salt for hummus
	Starters: Cheese *fatayer* (made with cheese cream)	Use cottage cheese or low-fat soft cheese
	Rice – boiled with water or from chicken/meat extract	Use stock cube rather than meat extract
	Flat bread	Check quantity especially if rice also consumed, chose wholemeal variety. Limit or omit spreads
	Dressings (olive oil)	Use oil sparingly
	Stew or dish combined with vegetables, red meat, poultry or fish	Use plenty of vegetables and pulses and skim fat from surface before adding vegetables. Limit oil. Use poultry/fish more often than fish or pulses as an alternative
	Desserts; fruit, *mahalabia* (milk pudding), dates, baklava	Encourage fruit. *Mahalabia* – use low-fat milk, avoid cream and reduce sugar (or use sweetener) and salt. Limit baklava to special occasions
	Fats often used: butter, ghee	Avoid butter and ghee. Use fats sparingly
Evening meal		
	Sandwich	Use wholegrain bread and low-fat cheese, bulk with salad
	Meat *kibbeh*	Use potato instead of meat to prepare and oven-bake instead of frying
	Shawarma (bread with red meat or chicken, often with salad (*tabouli*) and/or sauce (sesame-based)	Use wholegrain bread. Avoid energy-dense sauces, fill with salad, less meat/chicken
Drinks		
	Water, tea, coffee, fruit juices and fizzy drinks	Use low-fat milk. Limit fruit juices to one small glass a day, unsweetened. Diet/light fizzy drinks. Encourage water
Other		
	Honey	High in sugar

Table 5.1.12 Classification of body mass index

	BMI (kg/m^2)
Underweight	≤18.5
Healthy/normal weight	18.5–24.9
Overweight	25–29.9
Obese moderate (class1)	30–34.9
Severe (class 2)	35–39.9
Morbid (class 3)	≥40

(WHO, 1998)

of central obesity; it is unrelated to height and correlates closely with BMI and waist/hip ratio. Central obesity is associated with raised plasma triglycerides and reduced high-density lipoproteins which can be responsible for negative health consequences, such as cardiovascular disease.

Prevalence

The WHO estimates there will be 2.3 billion overweight adults in the world by 2015 and more than 700 million will be obese (see Table 5.1.13 for eastern Mediterranean region predictions). Obesity particularly exists among women in this region and will vary between rural and urban populations. In North Africa, approximately half of all women are overweight (BMI > 25) with rates of 50.9% in Tunisia and 51.3% in Morocco (Mokhtar *et al.*, 2001).

There have been few prevalence studies of obesity to date in the UK Arab population; however, it is interesting to note that the first UK cases of type 2 diabetes in children were in girls of Arab or South Asian origin. Studies of Arab-American migrants have a greater incidence of obesity and diabetes compared to the overall US population. It is likely that a similar trend exists in the UK Arab population. While UK Arabs share the increase in diabetes and cardiovascular risk that is seen in South Asian migrants, they are distinct in terms of customs and traditions (Goenka, 2007).

BMI and waist circumference

It is useful to use BMI along with waist circumference, as this provides a better measure of intra-abdominal fat. Different ethnic groups have different cut-off values for waist circumference. In the UK the classification to measure waist circumference is shown in Table 5.1.14.

Table 5.1.13 The percentage of obesity in adults (BMI > 30 kg/m^2), 15+ years (UK 16+ years) by gender in the eastern Mediterranean region in 2002 and predicted percentage in 2010

Country	2002 Female	2002 Male	2010 Male	2010 Female
Algeria	11.9	4.5	6.4	16.2
Bahrain	33.5	21.2	21.2	37.9
Comoros	5.8	0.9	1.9	9.6
Djibouti	5	1.2	1.8	7.4
Iraq	15.5	6.6	8.3	19.1
Jordan	40.2	19.6	19.6	37.9
Kuwait	49.2	29.6	29.6	55.2
Lebanon	23.9	14.9	14.9	27.4
Libya	21.1	10.7	12.7	24.9
Mauritania	20.6	2.9	5.3	26.9
Morocco	19	3.7	3.7	23.1
Oman	13.5	7.7	7.7	17
Qatar	27.9	16.6	18.7	31.6
Saudi Arabia	32.8	22.3	23	36.4
Somalia	2.1	0.3	0.6	3.4
Sudan	4.3	1	1.5	6.5
Syria	20.8	10.5	12.4	24.6
United Arab Emirates	37.9	24.5	24.5	42
Tunisia	28.8	7.7	7.7	32.6
United Kingdom	21.3	18.7	23.7	26.3

(WHO, 2005)

A few studies have attempted to suggest the optimal cut-off values for waist circumference and BMI in the Arab population. A BMI of >22.9 for women and >22.6 for men has been suggested and waist circumference measurement has varied from >84.5 cm to >99 cm for women and >78.5 cm to 97 cm for men (Mansour *et al*, 2007; Al Lawati *et al.*, 2008).

It is interesting to note the variation among studies; however, the International Diabetes Federation currently recommends the use of

Table 5.1.14   Waist circumference

Men	
Increased risk	94–102 cm
Substantially increased risk	>102 cm
Women	
Increased risk	80–88 cm
Substantially increased risk	88 cm

(WHO, 1998)

European data until more specific information becomes available.

Dietary modifications for weight reduction diet

In the Near East and North Africa energy consumption has been increasing steadily from 2,290 kcal per capita per day in 1964–6 to 3,006 kcal per capita per day in 1997–9 with a predicted increase to 3,170 kcal per capita per day by 2030. Similarly trends are shown in dietary fat intake such that the supply of fat has increased by 20 g per capita per day between 1967–9 and 1997–9 in North Africa. Similar trends are reported in other Arab League countries (WHO FAOSTAT, 2003). It is therefore not surprising that the prevalence of obesity has increased along with adopting more of a western-style diet and lifestyle.

The energy content of the diet can be reduced by:

- Restricting fast foods eaten out and providing suitable alternatives.
- Reducing the amount of fat in cooking and introducing alternative low-fat methods, such as boiling, baking and grilling.
- Avoiding extras at mealtimes, such as bread in addition to rice, dips and energy-dense side-dishes.
- Avoiding energy-dense desserts/snacks such as baklava and cakes and limiting the amount, e.g., of dates consumed (these are often taken with Arabic coffee).
- Omitting sugar and sugary drinks/foods.

Further suggestions are given in Table 5.1.15.

Physical activity

Physical activity levels are generally low in the UK. Only 35% of men and 24% of women reach the

Table 5.1.15   Dietary modifications for weight reduction diet

Food group	Dietary modifications/suggestions
Bread, rice, potatoes, pasta and other starchy foods	Bread – avoid spread. Check quantity as often taken with rice/couscous as a complement to main dish. Use whole wheat variety
	Potatoes – avoid fried, better consumed in a stew
	Yam/cassava – avoid fried and check quantities consumed
	Rice – boiled or steamed. Avoid boiling with juice from meat/poultry
Vegetables and fruit	Encourage at mealtimes, desserts and snacks.
	Check number of dates consumed and whether they are stuffed (e.g., with nuts)
	Use low-fat dressings on salads; limit/avoid olive oil
	Use unsweetened fruit juices (limit to one glass)
Milk and dairy foods	Choose low-fat varieties and check quantity consumed
Meat, fish, eggs ,beans and other non-dairy sources of protein	Trim visible fat from meat and remove skin from chicken
	Use alternatives to meat (e.g., pulses)
	Limit consumption of nuts – often included in main dishes and desserts
Foods and drinks high in fat and/or sugar	Limit/avoid dessert; often based on sugar, syrups, honey and nuts
	Avoid ghee and butter and limit usage of oils (e.g., in hummus, fool often served with oil
	Check and avoid sugar/honey added to beverages (use sweetener if appropriate)
	Check if sugar/honey added to drinks
Encourage water as fluid	Choose diet/light fizzy drinks if consumed
Cooking methods	Boil, steam, grill or oven-bake. Avoid frying. If oil is used, measure amount rather than pouring liberally

recommended physical activity of five times a week (Miles, 2007). The WHO and Department of Health recommend 30 minutes of moderate-intensity physical activity a day to prevent obesity (WHO, 2003; DH, 2004). The prevention of weight regain in formerly obese individuals requires 60–90 minutes of moderate-intensity activity a day (Saris *et al.*, 2003; Hill & Wyatt, 2005). Activity can be in one session or in several shorter bouts of activity of 10 minutes or more. A combination of increased physical activity and reduced energy intake is the most successful way to weight loss.

Some barriers to physical activity are often cited, including lack of time or motivation. In a Bahraini survey involving 2,013 subjects (both men and women) the majority were found to walk less than 1 km on an average weekday, often the reasons being the weather (too hot) and for cultural reasons, particularly for women, hence an increase in activity requires changes in attitudes in the workplace and at home (Al-Mahroos & Al-Roomi, 2001).

In many Arab League countries women generally undertake the bulk of domestic responsibilities and most wear the *hijab*. In the UK this may also hinder them engaging in physical activity. In the UK, many leisure centres provide women-only activity classes, which can be an acceptable alternative in many cases. Activities in or near the home, such as walking up and down the stairs, can be an acceptable and safe way to undertake additional activity. In the workplace, especially if the job is sedentary, making use of the stairs rather than using a lift, walking part of the way to work by getting off one bus stop early if public transport is used or taking a walk during lunch breaks, are options that can become a routine on most days. Participation in family activities should also be encouraged whenever practical.

Behavioural changes

In Qatar 535 Arab women were interviewed about their attitudes towards eight fad diets related to weight reduction and the effect of education level. In general, 20–54% of women believed in these fads and 45.1–50.6% did not know whether or not these fads were correct (Musaiger, 2002).

In a survey of 526 Kuwaiti adults, the majority of <30 year olds followed diets found in magazines, on the Internet or picked up by word of mouth. The main reasons for attempting weight loss were for health problems and appearance. Stopping a weight loss programme recommended by health professional was due to an inability to resist sweets, the cost and dissatisfaction with the outcome. It appears from the surveys undertaken in the Gulf States that many people are health-conscious and able to obtain nutritional information, although not always from reliable sources, but lacked behavioural management support for effective weight reduction (Al-Qaoud *et al.*, 2007). Slow (0.5–1 kg per week) and sustained weight loss is an important part of weight management although individual may not necessarily see it as rewarding in the short term. It is important to establish the reasons for wanting to lose weight and provide support that takes into account social and cultural requirements. A food diary started before a consultation can be a valuable way to become familiar with a patient's eating habits and lifestyle; however, it is important to bear in mind the patient's level of literacy and ability to write.

The use of interpreters, or having a family member to act as translator, should be considered, if appropriate, otherwise the use of visual aids to demonstrate foods and changes to the diet is a useful way for the patient to understand the health message.

Meals are often family and social affairs with much sharing of a variety of dishes (*mezzeh*). Likewise, eating out, often in fast-food outlets, is enjoyed with friends. It is a sociable time and often food is taken on a help yourself basis rather than the meal being provided on a plate. Self-serving on a small plate before eating rather than 'picking' can heighten awareness of what is being selected and allows the individual to monitor their intake. Serving foods such as salad and vegetable dishes first is good practice and avoidance of extras such as dips and bread should be encouraged. The whole family can join in the education on healthy eating so that meals can be cooked and shared for all to enjoy. It is helpful if the person who prepares the food attends so that more detail can be provided and appropriate advice given.

Evidence of good practice

The Third Arab Conference on Nutrition, which took place in the UAE in December 2007, aimed to promote healthy nutrition in the Arab countries. Various activities were identified, such as supporting awareness programmes to promote healthy nutrition and lifestyle through mass media and preparing or updating the national nutrition plan of action as part of the national health plan in each country (Third Arab Conference on Nutrition, 2007).

In Saudi Arabia, evidence-based guidelines are planned for the management of obesity, along with the best ways to adopt these guidelines. The guidelines have incorporated input from health professionals, such as dietitians, physicians and academic and government representatives (Almajwal *et al.*, 2008).

5.1.6   Diabetes

> **Key points**
>
> - Diabetes is considerably more prevalent in the eastern Mediterranean region than in Europe and North America.
> - Type 2 diabetes has increased due to changes in the environment, such as urbanization, which is often associated with an increase in obesity.

Prevalence

In 2009, more than 220 million individuals were estimated to have diabetes worldwide (WHO, 2009). In the UK the prevalence is approximately 2.6 million (Diabetes UK, 2009). In the eastern Mediterranean region, chronic diseases such as diabetes, cardiovascular disease and cancer account for almost half (47%). Prevalence for both type 1 and type 2 diabetes in the eastern Mediterranean region (excluding Sudan) is reported to be around 10%. There are rural and urban differences. For example, in Egypt a study reported an overall prevalence of 9.3%, but this rose to 20% in population samples taken from higher socioeconomic classes in urban areas. Similarly in Sudan, the highest prevalence was seen in the north (5.5%) and the lowest in the western desert areas (0.9%). Unfortunately, a consistent finding is the low detection rate with the percentage of undiagnosed diabetes ranging from 40% to >60% (Alwan, 1997).

In 2007, six of the ten countries with the highest prevalence of diabetes (in the 20–79 years age group) were from the eastern Mediterranean region, of which four (United Arab Emirates, Saudi Arabia, Bahrain and Kuwait) were in the top five. The largest age group presenting with diabetes were aged 40–59 years (International Diabetes Federation, 2002).

The United Arab Emirates has the highest prevalence, with 19.5% of the population suffering. Diabetes causes 75% of deaths among UAE nationals (Diabetes UK, 2009).

Risk factors

Type 2 diabetes constitutes 85–95% of all diabetes in developed countries and an even higher percentage in developing countries and has evolved in association with rapid cultural and social changes, ageing populations, increasing urbanization, dietary changes and reduced physical activity (WHO, 1994).

Energy-dense diets, along with reduced physical activity, are a major cause of obesity, which itself can contribute to insulin resistance and lead to raised blood sugar levels. Genetic factors also contribute to the increased risk of type 2 diabetes. Approximately 15–25% of first-degree relatives of people with type 2 diabetes develop impaired glucose tolerance or diabetes; however, modifiable risk factors are an important contribution to mitigate genetic risk factors.

The transition of populations from rural to urban areas has been associated with a change in lifestyle and related to an increase in the prevalence of obesity. This has been demonstrated within the same country and ethnic groups but living under different conditions (International Diabetes Federation, 2003).

Average life expectancy has also increased in many of the eastern Mediterranean region countries, and while type 2 diabetes often presents later in life, it has contributed to an increase in prevalence.

Treatments

Diet and lifestyle treatment contribute significantly to maintaining good glycaemic control and reducing microvascular disease in both type 1 and type 2 diabetes.

Treatment may include diet only, diet and tablets, or insulin injections. It is a common misperception that patients treated with tablets or insulin can eat freely as they are taking medications for 'sugar'. Also patients, particularly type 2 diabetics, who initially were treated with tablets and who progress to insulin often feel that moving on to insulin means their diabetes has 'worsened'. An audit of a diabetes clinic in the United Arab Emirates conducted in 2005 showed that although many aspects of treatment were fulfilled, fewer than half of patients were referred to a nutritionist and a relatively small number had advice documented for diet, exercise, smoking status and BMI. It is therefore important to establish whether Arab patients in the UK are aware of these aspects as part of their diabetes treatment and education, especially as 'plumpness' may be well be regarded as a sign of affluence and fertility (Afandi *et al.*, 2006).

Insulin

A major problem today lies in the widespread long-term lack of access to insulin and other diabetes supplies. This poses a serious threat to the lives of people with diabetes in developing countries, especially those in sub-Saharan Africa where there are reports of premature deaths.

The administration of insulin in many of the Arab countries is often via syringes from an insulin vial using long needles. Patients introduced to the pen-like injection usually appreciate this alternative. Insulin treatment should be balanced against the glycaemic effects of consuming carbohydrates. If patients lack knowledge of carbohydrate-rich foods and their effects on insulin, treatment may well not be effective, especially if the diet and timing of meals vary from day to day. The availability of short, intermediate and long-acting insulin administered via pen injections increases the flexibility of regimens. Education on the effects of insulin is important to reduce the risk of hypoglycaemia and enable the patient to change the insulin dose appropriately. Rapid-acting insulin can take effect within 10 minutes and has an onset for 2–4 hours, and hence is useful for patients who have irregular mealtimes. In contrast, long-acting analogues can have an onset of 24 hours and are generally used once a day.

Tablets

Anti-diabetic drugs should be taken as prescribed at the appropriate time intervals in order to prevent hypoglycaemia (in sulphonylureas only, e.g., Glibenclamide, Gliclazide and Glipizide) and maintain good glycaemic control along with an even distribution of food intake. Sulphonylureas can sometimes increase appetite and hunger and can potentially increase body weight. Newer versions of these tablets (Nateglinide and Repaglinide) are taken only if food is eaten and are less likely to cause a 'hypo'. Metformin is often prescribed for people who are overweight as it can help to suppress the appetite. Piolgitazone and Rosiglitazone are usually taken in conjunction with other tablets and may increase body weight, usually around the abdomen.

Dietary modifications

- For people with type 1 diabetes the goal is matching insulin dosage to dietary intake and activity to achieve the best glycaemic control with the fewest hypoglycaemic incidents.
- For people with type 2, maturity-onset diabetes, the major goal is to achieve a healthy BMI (20–$24 \text{kg}/\text{m}^2$) so as to reduce insulin resistance to achieve good glycaemic control and better blood pressure control.
- For all patients with diabetes, the aim is to reduce the risk of early complications (e.g., nephropathy and cardiovascular) by dietary modification and advice on lifestyle (e.g., ceasing smoking and engaging in physical activity).

Dietary knowledge will vary greatly so it is important to establish the patient's knowledge and literacy before written and verbal information is provided.

A study in the United Arab Emirates found 50% of people to be illiterate, only 24% read food labels and 46% reported that they had never seen a dietitian since their diagnosis, resulting in over half in the study having uncontrolled blood sugar levels and presenting with complications, such as hypertension and raised lipids (Al-Kaabi *et al.*, 2006).

In contrast, it is often the case that close relatives will also have diabetes and patients will therefore have good knowledge of treatment. Most urban-living Arabs have adequate literacy including being able to communicate well in English.

Nutritional advice will help the patient make appropriate choices on the type and quantity of food they eat. It is important to integrate physical activity and a healthy lifestyle as part of counselling. The principles of dietary management are no different from UK guidelines but needs to be culturally appropriate (see Table 5.1.16 for healthy eating suggestions).

Other recommendations
- Encourage regular meals.
- Use low-fat cooking methods (e.g., steaming, boiling, baking and grilling).
- Limit or avoid convenience foods which may have 'hidden' fats, sugar and salt.
- Salt intake should be 6 g or less per day. Check whether salt is added in cooking and/or at the table. Encourage the use of herbs and spices as alternatives.
- Discuss and clarify beliefs and misconceptions about diet and diabetes. Common beliefs include that bananas are 'bad', whereas honey

Table 5.1.16 Healthy eating and diabetes for the Arabic diet

Food group	Foods to encourage	Foods to limit/avoid
Bread, rice, potatoes, pasta and other starchy foods (choose high-fibre/ low GI varieties)	Include starchy foods at each meal Bread with grains, bread made with whole wheat flour Basmati rice High-fibre (wholegrain/oat-based) cereals Couscous Potatoes with skins Unrefined grains (e.g., millet, sorghum)	Check portion size; often starchy foods can comprise half or more of plate Bread made with white flour. Croissants Refined/sugar-coated cereals. Refined grains e.g., millet, sorghum Potato chips, crisps
Vegetables and fruit (Aim for 5–9 portions a day)	Vegetables and salads All fresh fruit, spread fruit out during the day	Limit fruit juice to one small glass a day Check intake of dried fruit (e.g., dates – often consumed as a snack or stuffed with a sweet filling)
Meat, fish, eggs, beans and other non-dairy sources of protein (Aim for low-fat varieties, particularly pulses where fibre is also provided)	Lean meat, poultry without skin All pulses (e.g., chickpeas, broad beans, lentils) Oily fish – aim for two portions a week All other fish varieties (excluding shellfish)	Shellfish Fatty meats, processed meat Skin from poultry Coconut (check quantity as often added to sweets and desserts)
Milk and dairy foods (Aim for low-fat varieties)	Skimmed/semi-skimmed milk. Low-fat/sugar plain yoghurt. Low-fat cheese varieties (e.g., 'light' soft cheese, cottage cheese)	Full-cream milk, evaporated or condensed milk Full-fat yoghurt or those with syrup. Hard, high-fat cheeses.
Foods containing fat and or sugar (Aim to reduce total amount of fat added to foods)	Use oils rich in MUFA (e.g. olive or rapeseed oil). Check quantity added to dips, foods (e.g., hummus, *fool*) Oils rich in PUFA (e.g., corn, sunflower oil), use secondary to MUFA-rich oils Spreads based on MUFA Use sweeteners, if necessary to replace sugar in cooking, beverages	Animal-based fats (e.g., ghee, butter) Cakes, biscuits, Arabic sweets (e.g., baklava), dates stuffed with nuts/marzipan Honey Sugar added to beverages or those containing sugar (e.g., fizzy drinks)

has 'natural sugar' and so can be taken liberally, and olive oil contains 'no fat'.

- Where practical and appropriate, members of the family should be included to help achieve the dietary aims; especially other relatives with diabetes or those who are responsible for shopping or cooking at home.
- Avoid diabetic food products.
- Check if alcohol is consumed.
- Encourage physical activity. If little is undertaken, aim to build gradually to 30 minutes of moderate-intensity activity (e.g., brisk walking). Exercise can be split, for example, into two sessions of 15 minutes or three sessions of 10 minutes.
- Provide appropriate diet sheets.

Herbal remedies

Arabs in the Baghdad region were the first known people to separate medicine from pharmacological science – hence the first drug stores were established here. Many medicines originally were derived from plants or animal sources until synthetic drugs were developed, although natural pharmaceuticals are still popular and widely used.

The WHO inventoried over 20,000 medicinal herbs and approximately 250 species have been analysed to identify their bioactive chemical component. In the eastern Mediterranean region more than 700 plant species have been noted for use as medicinal or as botanical pesticides. For those suggested for diabetes (see table 5.1.17)

A medicinal plant is often characterized physically, such that the shape, size, colour and texture may serve as an important selection criteria for therapeutic purpose, for example, seeds with a kidney shape may be used for treating kidney stones. The majority of herbal remedies are taken in the form of tea or other drinks containing the diluted or concentrated chemical ingredients.

Surveys conducted in Arab countries have revealed that most of the herbalists do not have any formal education in the field of medicine and pharmacy. In addition, in some cases inappropriate formulations or lack of understanding of plant and drug interactions or uses has led to adverse reactions. It is noted that surveys conducted in different groups in the Middle East support the need to handle of herbal medicine appropriately. This calls

Table 5.1.17 Plant species and common name used traditionally to treat diabetes

Plant	Common name
Ceratonia siliqua	Carob tree
Cupressus sempervirens	Mediterranean cypress
Juglans regia	Walnut
Mercurialis annua	Annual mercury
Morus nigra	Black mulberry tree
Sarcopoterium spinosum	Thorny burnet
Smilax aspera	Prickly ivy
Teucrium polium	Felty germander
Trigonella foenum-graecum	Fenugreek
Vaccinium myrtillus	Blueberry (leaves)
Momordica charantia	Bitter melon

for suitable regulation and licensing (Azaizeh *et al.*, 2006).

It is not unusual for Arab patients in the UK to ask health professionals about the use of herbal remedies to control blood sugar levels. It is also advisable for health professionals to ask patients if they are taking any herbal remedies. Recently, there have been claims for cinnamon to reduce blood sugar levels.

Although herbal remedies have been used for centuries in Arab countries, many of the products sold are not regulated and one cannot be sure of the ingredients or even if harmful contaminants are present. It would therefore be wise to err on the side of caution and discourage patients' use until guidelines are available to health professionals.

Fasting and its impact on change in dietary intake and medication

Fasting normally occurs during Ramadan and is an obligation for all healthy adult Muslims. A study undertaken in 13 Islamic countries estimated that approximately 43% of patients with type 1 diabetes and 79% of patients with type 2 diabetes fast during Ramadan. No food or drink is taken from sunrise to sunset. As this month advances 11 days each year, the effects of the daytime fast are strongly influenced by the season, being most severe during summer months when the hours of sunlight are longest.

Salti and colleagues' extensive study (2004) showed that severe hypoglycaemic episodes were five times more frequent during Ramadan in type 1 diabetes and three times more frequent in type 2 diabetes, especially if physical activity was modified or if insulin or oral hypoglycaemic agent (OHA) doses were changed.

In contrast, patients who reported an increase in food and/or sugar intake had significant increases in hyperglycaemia (Salti *et al.*, 2004). Dietary changes should not need to differ from a healthy balanced diet, but it is common practice to break the fast with dates, honey, water and fruit juices and to eat large quantities of food rich in refined carbohydrate and fat, especially at sunset (*iftar*).

As well as the risk of hyperglycaemia when breaking the fast, lipid profiles may well be unfavourably altered due to the consumption of a large meal and response to 'starvation'. Foods containing complex carbohydrates should be encouraged at the predawn meal (*sahur*), for example, high-fibre cereals and dal to help stabilize blood sugar levels during the day, while more starchy foods, such as Arabic bread and rice, at the sunset meal to break the fast should be encouraged. Sweets (e.g., baklava or *jallebi*) should be kept to a minimum, along with excessive consumption of dates.

General guidelines when breaking the fast and foods to included

- Choose sugar-free fizzy drinks and squashes or better still, water.
- Limit fried foods.
- Limit or avoid sweets and fruit juices.
- Limit the quantity of dates consumed, especially if they are stuffed with a sweet filling or dipped in honey.
- Base meals on starchy foods, vegetables, dal and plain yoghurt.
- Limit the amount of oil used in cooking.

Medication

If patients are taking a sulphonylurea, they should be made aware that this can cause hypoglycaemia,

in which case the dose may need to be changed – e.g., a bigger dose in the evening (when more is eaten) than in the morning when usually a small meal is taken. Medication may well need to be changed during Ramadan. For example, short-acting secretagogues are useful because of their short action duration.

Patient with poorly controlled diabetes, or those who are unwilling or unable to monitor their blood sugar levels during the day, are at high risk of having hypoglycaemic episodes and should be discouraged from fasting. It is always worth reminding patients that they must break their fast immediately if a 'hypo' occurs and should be educated in treating this with a sweet drink, followed by consumption of starchy foods.

Complications associated with diabetes and information on traditional foods for renal diets

Diabetes has major implications with regard to morbidity and mortality; as well as the cost of suffering there is a considerable financial burden. Macrovascular disease constitutes the major cause of diabetes mortality, with 80% of patients having and/or dying from cardiovascular disease, cerebrovascular or peripheral arterial disease. Although there is an association between improvement in glycaemic control and reduction in microvascular end-organ damage (retinopathy, nephropathy and neuropathy) there is no similar consistent relationship between glycaemic control and macrovascular complications (WHO, 2005).

Microvascular disease can be reduced by good glycaemic control:

- New eye disease risk reduced by 76%.
- Worsening existing eye disease reduced by 54%.
- Early kidney disease probably reduced by 39%.
- Kidney disease risk reduced by up to 33%.
- Nerve damage risk reduced by 60%.
- Heart disease risk reduced by 56%.
- Stroke risk reduced by 44%.

(Diabetes Control and Complications Trial, 2009)

Good glycaemic control should be of the current DCCT HbA1c targets of 6.5% and 7.5%, depending on the patient's medical status. The equivalent new units (from 1 June 2009) are 48 mmol/mol and 59 mmol/mol (NHS Diabetes, Diabetes UK and the Association for Clinical Biochemistry, 2009).

Hypertension

People with diabetes and hypertension have a two-fold increased risk of cardiovascular mortality (see Table 5.1.18). It has been shown that each 10 mmHg decrease in systolic blood pressure leads to a reduction in diabetes-related mortality by 15% and complications by 12%. Hypertension is one element of the metabolic symptoms in patients with type 2 diabetes. Other metabolic abnormalities, such as dyslipidaemia and obesity, are also presented.

Reducing weight (if necessary) and sodium intake, along with exercise and a healthy diet, can lower blood pressure. Smoking should be strongly discouraged. It is often necessary to incorporate drug treatment such as ACE inhibitors and/or beta-blockers. A good target for blood pressure for people with diabetes is <130/80 mmHg (WHO, 2005).

Dyslipidaemia

More than 60% of type 2 diabetic subjects in the eastern Mediterranean region have some degree of dyslipidaemia. More than 40% have hyper-cholesterolaemia and a further 23% have hyper-triglyceridaemia and/or low levels of HDL cholesterol. Hypertriglyceridaemia is also a feature of impaired glucose tolerance and impaired fasting glucose.

Table 5.1.18 Classification of hypertension

Classification	Systolic (mmHg)	Diastolic (mmHg)
Normal	<120	<80
Prehypertension	120–139	80–89
Stage 1 hypertension	140–159	90–99
Stage 2 hypertension	≥160	≥100

(WHO, 2005)

A healthy eating plan, modifying the amount and type of fat consumed, increasing soluble fibre and both plant sterols and stanols will favour the lipid profile. Weight reduction is important in obese patients, along with an increase in physical activity. Most patients with diabetes and dyslipidaemia will also require drug therapy, such as statins, bile acid sequestrants, cholesterol absorption inhibitors, nicotinic or fibric acids (WHO, 2006).

Renal disease

Diabetic nephropathy is characterized by proteinuria and is widely considered as the leading cause of end-stage renal disease, which constitutes a major workload of dialysis centres worldwide. The progression to established nephropathy occurs in several stages, microalbuminuria, defined as urinary albumin excretion rate of 20–200 μg/min on a timed specimen without an alternative clinical explanation or urinary protein excretion rate of 30–300 μg/min, is a known predictor of future developments of overt diabetic nephropathy. A study in a district of the UAE found that the prevalence of microalbuminuria in a sample of 513 diabetic patients was 61%, the rate being higher in males and positively related to BMI, type 2 diabetes and the presence of other complications (Al-Maskari et al., 2008).

In a review of data in Saudi Arabia, one study in a diabetic outpatient clinic found 12.8% of patients had dipstick proteinuria, and of the remaining patients 41.3% had microalbuminuria. An increase in diabetic nephropathy may be explained by the increase in the number of people with diabetes, better survival and increasing age of diabetes (Al-Khader, 2001).

Patients with renal disease are likely to require dietary restriction of potassium, phosphate and sodium. All vegetables should be boiled in a large quantity of water and drained. Potatoes should be peeled and then boiled. The potassium content of common foods are given in Table 5.1.19.

Other foods

• Milk and milk products will require restriction, for example 240 ml milk or 120 ml milk and small natural yoghurt. The restriction should

Table 5.1.19 Average potassium content of foods commonly consumed

Food	Potassium (mg)
Fruit	
10 grapes	93–105
1 medium apricot	105
1 medium orange	237
½ cup diced watermelon	93
½ grapefruit	165
1 medium banana	451
½ cup chopped dates	581
5 dried figs	666
½ cup diced pineapple	88
1 medium plum	118
½ medium avocado	549–742
1 medium mango	323
½ cup strawberries	124
1 medium nectarine	288
1 medium raw tomato	251–273
Vegetables (½ cup)	
Green cooked beans	185
Cauliflower	125
Raw diced onion	124
Sweet raw peppers	89
Steamed aubergine	119
Sliced cucumber	84
Cooked chickpeas	239
Raw chopped spinach	154
Raw mushrooms	130
Cooked sliced okra	257
Cooked lentils	366
Cooked asparagus	279

(Agricultural Handbook No. 8)

be included if these foods are added to dishes, such as *lebneh, mahalabia* and *tzaziki*.
- Sweets and desserts commonly contain dried fruit and nuts and some will need to be avoided or restricted.
- Fruit juices should be avoided.

Check if spices are used and if salt is added to cooking or at the table as sodium intake is likely to require restriction.

Evidence of good practice

In 2006, the Imperial College London Diabetes Centre opened in Abu Dhabi, providing a large multidisciplinary service to the local community. The Centre allows staff to remain up-to-date with evidence-based treatments and research.

5.1.7   Coronary heart disease

Key points

- Coronary heart disease is the major cause of death and of chronic disease in the UK and eastern Mediterranean region.
- Many of the risk factors, such as obesity and diabetes, are prevalent in the eastern Mediterranean region.

Introduction

Cardiovascular disease (CVD) is caused by a combination of atherosclerosis and thrombosis. It results in coronary heart disease (CHD), peripheral vascular disease and stroke, depending on the severity and which arteries are affected.

Prevalence

The WHO Region (WHO, 2006) for the eastern Mediterranean, which includes most countries in the Arab League, estimated that chronic diseases accounted for approximately 51% of all deaths, particularly from CVD at 27%. It is projected that by 2015 deaths from chronic disease will increase by 25%, most markedly from diabetes, which is estimated to increase by 50%.

In the UK, in 2005, it was estimated that chronic diseases accounted for 85% of all deaths, CVD being the highest (38%). In contrast, by 2015, it is estimated that in the UK deaths from chronic diseases will reduce by 0.8% although some will increase, particularly diabetes. Obesity, however, is expected to increase in both the UK and eastern Mediterranean region (WHO, 2005).

Death rates from CHD in the UK have been falling since the late 1970s and in recent years it has been falling fastest in those aged 55 and over (BHF, 2008).

In the eastern Mediterranean region comprehensive data are difficult to obtain, as many countries do not report death by cause. However data from Bahrain, Egypt, Iraq, Jordan, Kuwait and Qatar in recent years have shown that the main CVD encountered included CHD, hypertension and stroke. The data indicate a rising trend in mortality from CVD. The prevalence of hypertension appears to be lower in populations living in rural areas (Alwan, 1997).

Risk factors

Hypertension

Mean systolic blood pressure (mmHg) in 2002 in the UK was 126.6 for women and 132.2 for men (normal systolic pressure in healthy adults should be approximately 120). For most of the eastern Mediterranean countries, systolic pressure appears to be similar to UK values, although countries higher than UK values include Comoros, Djibouti, Mauritania, Somalia and Sudan for both sexes and higher for males in Morocco and Kuwait. It was predicted in 2008 that by 2010 the same countries would continue to have the highest systolic pressure (WHO Global Infobase, 2008). Along with promotion of a healthy diet, reduction in excessive weight, limiting salt to <6g/day and eating a minimum of five portions of fruit and vegetables daily are is recommended, along with lifestyle management.

Hypercholesterolaemia

Total cholesterol >5mmol/l was commonly found in UK in 2002. Within the eastern Mediterranean region prevalence of hypercholesterolaemia (≥5.2mmol/dl cholesterol) between 2003 and 2007 was common, for example adults in Iran (43.6%), Kuwait (38.6%), Iraq (37.5%) and Jordan (36%) have hypercholesterolaemia (WHO, 2010).

In the UK, 21.3% and 18.7% of female and male adults respectively were obese, and these figures are rising. In the eastern Mediterranean region in 2002, there was a prevalence of 20% or more obese females in 11 of the 19 countries and 4 out of the 19 countries for adult males. Jordan and Kuwait had the highest prevalence (WHO, 2008).

Diabetes

Prevalence of both type 1 and type 2 diabetes in the eastern Mediterranean region (except for Sudan) is reported to be around 10%. In 2007, six of the top 10 countries with the highest prevalence of diabetes (20–79 years age group) were from the eastern Mediterranean region of which four were in the top five countries (WHO, 2008).

Smoking

Smoking among adult males is about 40% in the eastern Mediterranean region (Alwan, 1997).

Other contributory causes

- Longevity.
- Male sex.
- Postmenopause.
- Decrease in socioeconomic status.
- Ethnicity.
- Low physical activity.
- Raised serum triglycerides.
- Raised LDL cholesterol and reduced HDL cholesterol.

Dietary modifications

Nutrition recommendations for cardio-protection (primary prevention)

- Eat more starchy foods.
- Eat five or more portions of fruit and vegetables a day.
- Reduce total fat intake.
- Choose oils/spreads higher in monounsaturated fat and low in saturates.
- Eat oily fish at least once a week.
- Reduce salt intake.
- Drink alcohol sensibly.

(Stanner, 2005) See Table 5.1.20 for further information.

Other recommendations

- Encourage cooking methods for which fat is not added (grilling, baking, boiling).
- Replace butter or ghee (if used) with fats providing a good source of monounsaturated fats.
- Trim fat from meat and remove skin from poultry. Substitute with pulses, where possible.
- Reduce or avoid the use of salt in cooking or at the table.

Table 5.1.20 Recommended alternatives to traditional Arabic foods

Food group	Foods to encourage	Foods to eat in moderation	Aim to exclude	Comments
Bread, rice, potatoes, pasta and other starchy foods	Bread made from whole wheat flour	White bread	Sugar-coated cereals	Aim to retain fibre content of starchy foods
	High-fibre cereal Unrefined millet, sorghum	Refined cereals	Pastries and biscuits	
			Crisps	
			Chips	
Vegetables and fruit	Vegetables and salads, all fresh fruit	Fruit juices	Avocados	Provide antioxidants, potassium and fibre
Meat, fish, eggs, beans and other non-dairy sources of protein	Lean meats and poultry	Aim to replace some red meat with alternatives (e.g., pulses)	Fried and fatty meat	Aim to reduce saturated fats and provide a source of omega 3 fats and fibre from pulses
	Fish and oily fish		Shellfish	
	Pulses (e.g., broad beans, chickpeas and lentils)			
	Walnuts	Almonds, hazelnuts and pistachios	Coconut	Encourage higher sources of monounsaturated fats (may need to restrict if obesity presents)
		Eggs		
Milk and dairy foods	Skimmed milk	Semi-skimmed milk	Full-cream milk, cream and evaporated milk	Aim to reduce saturated fat
	Low-fat cheese (e.g., cottage cheese)	Medium-fat cheeses	Full-fat hard cheese	
	Low-fat yoghurt		Full-fat yoghurt	
Fats and oils	MUFA-based oils (e.g., olive oil, rapeseed oil)	Low-fat spreads	Butter, ghee, hydrogenated vegetable oils, fast foods/ convenience foods	Aim to reduce saturated fat
Sugar	Beverages without sugar		Beverages with sugar	Aim to reduce refined sugar
Salt				Aim to reduce salt

In addition to dietary management, lipid-lowering drugs are commonly prescribed, particularly statins.

5.1.8   Nutritional deficiencies

Vitamin D deficiency

Inadequate exposure of the skin to sunlight by wearing clothing (especially black clothing) covering forearms, legs and head and the use of sunscreens have shown minority groups, including Arabs, to be at risk of vitamin D deficiency. In addition, dark-skinned persons are less efficient at producing vitamin D. Studies have reported that Arab women particularly have lower 25-hydroxyvitamin than Caucasians. Major dietary sources of vitamin D include fortified dairy and cereal products and spreads and fish/fish oils. Few studies have shown that Arab women lack dietary vitamin D unless milk is avoided or the do not consume fortified products. Women with vitamin D deficiency or low status are at risk of osteomalacia, bone fractures, osteoporosis and myopathy associated with vitamin D deficiency (Dawodu, 2004). Vitamin D supplementation and encouraging that intake of foods rich in vitamin D for those at risk will help to reduce these complications (Dawodu, 2004).

Iron deficiency

Iron deficiency affects psychological and physical development, behaviour and work performance. Women of childbearing age are particularly vulnerable to low iron status. Flour fortification, as wheat is consumed in many cases daily, is an initiative that has been undertaken in parts of the Middle East and North Africa to control iron deficiency. The compound used for fortification of iron is ferrous sulphate added at the rate of 30 parts of iron per million (ppm) of wheat flour. Where flour is required to be stored for long periods, millers could use elemental iron at the rate of 60 ppm (WHO/UNICEF/MI/ILSI, 1998). Some of the consequences of iron deficiency anaemia include low birth weight and reduced mental performance in children. Maternal severe anaemia

results in intrauterine growth retardation and even maternal deaths, particularly in developing countries (Verster & van der Pols, 1995). In the UK, some 3% of men and 8% of women have haemoglobin levels likely to lead to anaemia (Ruston *et al.*, 2004).

5.2   Somalian Diet

Zelalem Debebe

5.2.1   Introduction

Somalia is situated in the Horn of Africa, and is bordered by Djibouti, Ethiopia and Kenya in the east and south-east, while in the north-west and south-west it is surrounded by the Gulf of Aden and the Indian Ocean respectively (see Figure 5.2.1). It is an arid/semi-arid, sparsely populated (8 million people) country with a fairly homogeneous people who share the same religion, language and ethnic origin. The majority (approximately 60%) of Somalis are pastoralists, 20% are farmers and the rest are urban dwellers. The majority of the population (85%) are Somali; other ethnic groups of Bantu and a non-Somali group make up the rest (UN, 2010).

Migration to the United Kingdom

Migration has been influenced by several factors, including colonialism, a nomadic lifestyle and civil war (Kleist, 2004). Somalis have been migrating in greater numbers to neighbouring countries, Western Europe and North America following the outbreak of civil war in 1991 (Grundel, 2002). More recently the majority of Somalis arriving in the UK have come from other European countries and from North America, to join family members who were separated during their initial migration (RAL, 2006).

Current UK population

The estimated number of the Somali-born population in the UK varies greatly and ranges from 43,691 (Somali refugees ONS statistics 2006 estimate) to 95,000. In 2004 about 80% of the Somali population live in London (Harris, 2004). However,

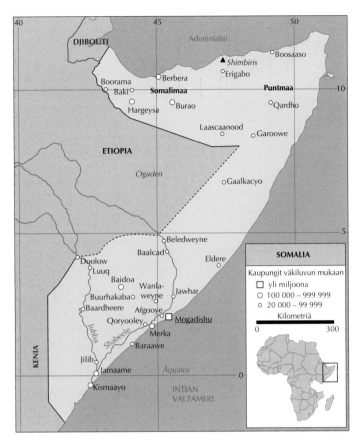

Figure 5.2.1   Map of Somalia

large communities now also live in Cardiff, Liverpool and the Midlands.

Language

Somalia's official language is Somali, although Arabic is also widely spoken. English and Italian are also spoken in the north and south respectively.

5.2.2   Religion and religious dietary restrictions

The majority of Somali people are Sunni Muslims. Religion dictates which foods are allowed or permissible (*halal*) and which are forbidden (*haram*)

(Haq, 2003). All meat or poultry consumed has to be alive and healthy at a time of slaughter and killed according to religious prescription so that it is pure *halal*. All blood should be completely drained. Meat or poultry should be cooked. The main types of meat preferred are camel, goat, lamb, chicken, beef and rarely fish. Pork and all pork products are forbidden, so any slaughtering should not be done where pigs are slaughtered (see Table 5.2.1).

Religious festivals

Eid al-Fitr (festival of the breaking of the fast) commemorates the end of Ramadan, and *Eid al-Adha* (festival of sacrifice) commemorates the story of

Table 5.2.1 List of *haram* foods

Species/animals not acceptable	Pigs
	Lions, wolves, cats, dogs, jackal, hyenas, tigers, foxes, snakes, scavengers
	Animals not slaughtered according to Muslim ritual.
Other ingredients	Animal fat
	Animal shortening
	Pork collagen
	Gelatin
	Lard
	Foods containing alcohol
Drinks	Alcoholic drinks

(HFA, 2010)

Prophet Abraham's willingness to sacrifice his son. These holidays fall on different times of year according to the Islamic calendar. Religious festivals are celebrated by offering special prayers, with family feasts, gatherings and the distribution of alms to the poor (Lancashire Council of Mosques, 2010).

Fasting (Ramadan)

Fasting is a common religious practice and all adult Muslim Somalis are expected to fast. This entails abstinence from eating, drinking and smoking from dawn to sunset every day of Ramadan for 30 consecutive days. People are exempt from fasting if they are ill and during pregnancy and breastfeeding, however most Somalis insist on observing the fast even in such situations (Haq, 2003).

The fast is broken at sunset (*iftar*) with sweet and fatty foods (dates, sambousa, juices), followed by a period of prayer. A big meal (rice and meat with vegetables) is usually taken half and hour to an hour before dawn (*suhur*).

Dietary patterns and commonly eaten foods in Somalia

Apart from religion, location and standard of living also influence dietary eating habits.

Location and livelihood

In Somalia, pastoral communities rely mainly on milk and milk products with some cereal and legumes included, which they obtain by trading livestock, while farmers consume more cereals, legumes, meat, fruits and vegetables. Urban population will have access to a greater variety of cereals, dairy products, fruits, vegetables and meat. Fish consumption is limited to coastal towns. Snacks are not traditionally eaten (Straus *et al.*, 2006). The main beverage is tea, which is drunk very sweet with milk (Wageh, 2005).

Standard of living

According to a focus group of the UK Somali population interviewed in London in 2006 (McEwen *et al.*, 2009), 'In Somalia, those with lower income, couldn't afford to buy fatty food, the well-to-dos ate meat everyday and less fruit and vegetables'. Therefore, the consumption of fruits and vegetables is associated with poverty and a lower standard of living and a meat-based meal at least once a day was considered to be a 'proper meal'.

5.2.3 Traditional eating pattern

> **Key points**
>
> - The traditional diet and lifestyle have undergone a major change in the West.
> - The Somali population in the West tends to have a high-fat/high-sugar diet, with refined carbohydrate used more often.
> - There is an increased use of high-sugar drinks, and sugar is added to tea.
> - The average UK Somali eats only two portions of fruit and vegetable a day.
> - Overweight and obesity are a major concern for the UK Somali population.
> - Physical activity levels in the population are lower than those of the general population.
> - Vitamin D deficiency and osteomalacia have been recorded in a high proportion of Somalis living in the UK. Vitamin D-fortified foods should be recommended.

There is a marked difference between the traditional eating patterns of Somali population in the western world and in Somalia. Migration and westernization have changed some dietary practices. The main staples are milk, sorghum and maize, meat and/or beans. Rice and pasta are also taken regularly. Sugar and vegetable oil or ghee (clarified butter) are used in cooking. Cereals are made into flat bread, and accompanied by milk or meat dishes (Wageh, 2005).

Somalis living in the West try to keep to their traditional foods as much as possible. However, the unavailability of familiar ingredients, uncertainty about food sources and perceived or actual contamination with non-*halal* ingredients have influenced their choice of food. There was an interest in organic foods and 'non-genetically modified' food expressed by a focus group of UK Somalis in London (McEwen *et al.*, 2009). Their diet tends to be high fat and sugar. There is an inrease use of high-sugar drinks, and sugar is added to tea. They also use more refined carbohydrate foods and the average intake of fruit and vegetable is about two portions a day (see Table 5.2.2, page 240 to 241).

5.2.4 Typical meal patterns

Somali families usually eat together at regular times (Maxwell *et al.*, 2006). Somalis usually have three meals a day – two light meals and a main meal, which is substantial. Somalis in the UK also reported long gaps between meals and did not snack (McEwen *et al.*, 2009) (see Table 5.2.3).

Breakfast and evening meal

These tend to be light meals consisting of *anjera*, a soft flatbread traditionally made of sorghum/millet/corn, or porridge made with milk, butter, salt and sugar. In the UK, *anjera* is usually made with wheat flour (self-raising flour) egg, sugar, salt, yeast and water (similar to a pancake but not tossed in the pan). It is usually the size of a chapatti, and an adult may eat 3–4 of these with butter and honey (Woutat, 1998).

The main meal

This is usually eaten at midday or early afternoon. This may be of rice or spaghetti, with meat sauce and mixed vegetables. Having meat with the main meal is considered to be a proper meal. Mutton is the preferred meat, although goat's meat, beef and camel (not in UK) may also be eaten.

Dairy products

Dairy foods are not consumed regularly by adults. Milk is considered to be important for children and given 2–3 times a day as a drink. This could be cow's or goat's milk which substitutes for the preferred camel's milk which is not available in the UK. The most commonly consumed drinks are sweet tea, juice, Vimto or an imported powder mix (juice) mixed with water and sugar.

Sweetened tea may be added to children's milk after they reach the age of three years. Many Somalis avoid most dairy products in the UK because of concerns these may contain pork-derived ingredients (Woutat, 1998; Haq, 2003). Those that do consume milk and margarine preferred products imported from Somalia. The source of margarine and ghee is not fortified with vitamin D.

Vegetables and salad

These may be taken with the main meal. Vegetables are spinach, cabbage, potatoes, carrots, courgettes, green peppers and onions. Salads are made with lettuce, tomatoes and cucumbers. Salads are usually dressed with lemon, lime or vinegar and oil (Woutat, 1998).

Fruits

Bananas, mangos, guavas, oranges and melons are commonly eaten. Bananas accompany most main meals. Apples and grapes are occasionally eaten.

The amount of fruit and vegetable included in the diet was no more than two portions/day

Table 5.2.2   Description of some of the most popular foods in the Somalian diet

Food groups	Examples	Healthier alternatives
Bread, rice, potatoes, pasta and other starchy foods	*Anjera:* like a pancake, made with self-raising flour or corn flour, *teff* (millet) or sorghum mixed with milk or water, eggs (optional) and cooked in a hot, greased pan on one side only (i.e., not tossed)	Use non-stick pan and use less oil
	Malawa: like a pancake (made with wheat flour, sugar, oil and eggs). May be served with honey. It looks like pitta bread without the pocket	Use non-stick pan and less oil Limit amount of honey if used
	Muufo: bread make with corn flour, salt and sugar and baked like a cake	
	Burkaki: dough balls made of *anjera* mix and deep-fried, or rolled out like chapatti, cut into triangles and fried	Use rarely or on special occasions
	Maqhumri: dough made of wheat flour, sugar, eggs and baking powder. Small balls of dough are deep-fried	Use rarely or on special occasions
	Roti (roodhi): pan-cooked bread without oil	Use one without butter
	Roti (Shanai): made with butter	
	Sabaayad: dough made of wheat flour and folded and rolled like puff pastry or *paratha*, then fried in a hot pan with very little oil	Use with a sauce in which more vegetable and less fat has been added.
	Chapatti: pan-fried flat bread using wheat flour and a small amount of vegetable oil or butter	Substitute with *roti* if regularly used
	Iskudahkaris (like pilau rice) is a combination of meat, vegetables and onions fried in oil to which rice and water is added.	Reduce amount of oil used, use rapeseed oil instead of ghee
	May be served with banana on the side.	Increase quantity of vegetables added (fewer potatoes) Smaller portions
	Baasto: spaghetti with meat sauce, served with salad and banana	Smaller portions Reduce oil used to cook sauce Increase portion of salad
Puddings/ sweets	*Halwa:* made with water, sugar, corn starch, butter, oil, cardamom and nutmeg	Reduce portion and frequency eaten
	Aana baraawe (Somali fudge): made with milk, butter, sugar and cardamom	
Meat (goat, lamb, beef and chicken), fish (usually tuna), eggs and beans	*Sugo:* made with onion, garlic, spices, vegetables like carrot and potato, tomato, meat (beef, goat or lamb) and oil (served with rice or spaghetti) Kebab	Increase quantity of vegetables added (fewer potatoes) Trim fat from meat, or boil and skim fat from mince
	Sukhar: beef and tomatoes or vegetable sauce (may be served with bread)	Serve with salad
	Sambosa: dumpling-like pastries with meat (usually lamb) and vegetables, wrapped in filo pastry then deep-fried	Use on special occasions Try baking after spraying or brushing pastry with oil
	Tuna, lentils or cheese and vegetables may be used as alternative fillings	
	Fool is made with pinto beans, tomatoes and fried onions served with any type of bread	Limit amount of butter added before serving
	Ambola: red kidney beans boiled in water with rice and oil added served with sugar and sesame oil	
	Lentils may be used in soups	

Table 5.2.2 (cont'd)

Food groups	Examples	Healthier alternatives
Fruits	Dates, bananas, mangos, guavas, oranges, melons, apples and grapes	Include at least one portion after meals 1–2 times per day
Vegetables	Spinach, cabbages, potato, carrots, courgettes, green peppers, onions, lettuce, tomatoes and cucumbers	Avoid frying. Steam or stir-fry in hot pan with very little oil
		Can use frozen or tinned vegetables
		Increase in meals; add as side-dish or salad
Cooking fats and oil	Ghee: clarified and sometimes spiced butter used for cooking sauces	Use butter less frequently and substitute with vegetable oil whenever possible
	Vegetable oil for frying	Limit oil, measuring and reducing use in cooking

Table 5.2.3   Typical meal pattern for the Somalian diet

Breakfast

Oat porridge is eaten by children and women with cow's milk

Bread (regular or *anjera*) with butter and jam

Eggs – boiled, omelette or scrambled with tomatoes and onions

Baked beans or fried liver with tomato, onions and chilli eaten with pitta bread

Loxoox/Anjera – wheat or millet flour pancake with butter or margarine, served with tea

Mid-morning

Fruit (mainly for children)

Lunch (usually the main meal)

Meat or chicken dishes, including potatoes, with rice or spaghetti, salad and *sabayad*

Fruit may be eaten at the end of the meal

Mid-afternoon

Tea with cakes and/or biscuits

Evening Meal

Similar to breakfast. Tinned baked beans in tomato sauce cooked with fried onions, chilli and tomatoes and served with pitta bread or *sabayad* or omelette

Sweetened fruit squashes or water are drunk with the meal

Bedtime

Milk

(Straus *et al.*, 2006; McEwan *et al.*, 2009) – lower than the general UK population intake of fruit and vegetables (three portions/day) and less than half the recommended five portions/day (DH, 2010).

There is an increasing tendency among children (Haq, 2003) and men, particularly those living alone, to eat takeaway foods (McEwan *et al.*, 2009). Chips, sugary fizzy drinks and increasing amounts of fruit juices are becoming a frequent intake among Somali-born children, reflecting the dietary habits of the children of the host countries (Haq, 2003).

Herbs and spices

Herbs and spices feature frequently in Somali meals and drinks (tea). Cumin, turmeric, coriander, sage and chilli are used to add flavour to most sauces and rice dishes. Cinnamon and cardamom are usually added to tea.

Alcohol

Alcohol intake is reported to be very low as compared to the general UK population. In the Islington study, only 3% of respondent reported to taking alcohol at least once a week and 1% reported the use of cannabis (Straus *et al.*, 2006).

Smoking

The prevalence of smoking among the Somali population in the UK is reported to be higher (31%) than the general population (24%) (Straus *et al.*, 2006). Respondents in the study also felt that smoking among Somalis in the UK was higher than in Somalia. It was also felt that smoking cigarettes was associated with higher probability of chewing qat (also known as Khat).

Qat is a plant that contains a chemical similar to amphetamine, and is chewed slowly to produce a stimulant effect. It is traditionally used in parts of Ethiopia, Yemen and Somalia. The use of qat is legal in the UK. This practice is common among Somali men in the UK (and Somalia). Straus *et al.* (2006) quote studies linking qat chewing with increase use of tobacco, or even with onset of psychotic symptoms with excess use.

Prevalence of chronic diseases

There is lack of data on the prevalence of chronic diseases in the Somali population, both in Somalia and the West.

5.2.5 Overweight and obesity

An interview with a focus group of UK Somalis in Islington indicated that the population were concerned about chronic diseases like diabetes, high blood pressure, high cholesterol, stroke and being overweight. Twelve per cent of the focus group were said to be unhappy with their body size (Straus *et al.*, 2006).

A small sample of Somalis in Australia had a mean BMI of 27.4 kg/m^2, and 60% were classified as overweight or obese (BMI > 25) (Burns, 2004). A study in New Zealand produced a similar result, with 71.4 % of the study having a BMI of >25 kg/m^2 (Guerin *et al.*, 2007). This is markedly different from the projected prevalence of overweight and obesity in men and women in

Somalia for 2005 (18% and 28% respectively) (WHO, 2002).

Physical activity

Planned physical activity and exercise are not common practices in Somalia (Straus *et al.*, 2005). Most Somalis in the UK felt that physical activity was important to maintain good health, but were not familiar with the concept of physical activity that was not part of daily routine. Many Somalis report that they did a great deal of walking when they lived in Somalia and worked harder than they did in UK.

There is a dramatic change in the pattern of daily activity of many Somali people, especially women once they have moved to the West, where most people reported that they were not as active in their daily routines as they had been previously (MIHV, 2005b). Only 38% of the respondents in the UK Somali focus group reported that they did enough physical activity, while 72% of the general UK population reported being fairly active (McEwen *et al.*, 2007).

A focus group of Somalis in New Zealand and Minnesota indicated that the reasons for this reduced activity was lack of a suitable venue (somewhere to walk, a culturally appropriate exercise venue), inclement weather, body pain, weight gain and lack of transportation to gain access to suitable venues, which may be too far from where they reside (Guerin *et al.*, 2003; MIHV, 2005b). A study of Somalis in London revealed that sports facilities were not meeting the needs of the Somali population as it was felt inappropriate for men and women to exercise at the same time (McEwen *et al.*, 2007).

Increasing physical activity is important as part of healthy lifestyle. The Department of Health recommends that all adults should achieve a total of at least 30 minutes of moderate-intensity physical activity on five or more days a week, which could be incorporated in daily activity or be structured exercise or sport or a combination of these (DH, 2004).

Lack of knowledge of the wider benefits of physical activity and inadequate and unsuitable provisions for this ethnic group need to be addressed to enable the community to increase their physical activity and benefit from healthy behaviour change (McEwen *et al.*, 2007).

Infant feeding practices

Infants are breastfed, although exclusive breast-feeding until the age of four months is not common in Somalia (Wageh, 2005) or among immigrants in the West (MIHV, 2005a). Breast milk is not given for the first 24 hours after birth. Instead sugar water or a small amount of cow's or goat's milk diluted with water is given alongside breast milk. Colostrum may be discarded in the belief that it is harmful (Wageh, 2005). Breastfeeding will continue until the child is two years of age as stated in the Qur'an.

Cow's or goat's milk may continue to be given to infants and children alongside breastfeeding for up to 2–3 years. Additional energy in the form of oil and sugar may be added to cow's milk. Sweetened water is also offered regularly to infants, especially in the rural areas (Ibrahim *et al.*, 1992). Solid foods are started after a few months of age (Haq, 2003; Straus *et al.*, 2005; Wageh, 2005).

Most infants are introduced to solid foods before four months of age, the most common complementary food being cereal-based porridges (sorghum, maize) with milk and family food (Wageh, 2005). A study in Minnesota indicated that, although most (94%) infants are breastfed initially, around 40% of mothers reported that they give additional water, formula or other types of milk during the first four months (MIHV, 2005a). In the general population, about 49% of mothers introduce solids after four months of age.

Although the majority of the UK Somali population initiate and continue breastfeeding, exclusive breastfeeding as recommended by WHO (2001) and DH (2007) is not a common practice.

5.2.6 Vitamin D deficiency and osteomalacia

In the Liverpool study, Maxwell *et al.* (2006) reported a high incidence of vitamin D deficiency, with around 34% of those showing signs of osteomalacia. A dietary analysis showed that the intake of foods containing adequate amount of calcium and vitamin D (milk, cheese, yoghurt, cream, fish and eggs) was infrequent, especially in those reporting bone pain (Maxwell *et al.*, 2006).

5.2.7 Suggestions for the way forward

Somalis in UK are aware of the health impact of a sedentary lifestyle and high-fat/high-sugar diet. However, this knowledge is not always translated into behaviour change. Several barriers have been cited as reasons for the limited change in behaviour. Addressing these barriers in a way that is culturally and religiously sensitive is essential to help people change their lifestyle for the better. Some of the following points have been suggested. Recommendations from focus group discussions are also included (MIHV, 2005).

- Provide culturally appropriate educational materials to improve skills (e.g., healthy cooking).
- Incorporate traditional food in healthy diet information messages (e.g., the eatwell plate with pictures of traditional meals).
- Provide/devise a written or picture-based dietary leaflet with information on healthier alternatives/ingredients that are *halal* (e.g., vitamin D-fortified food products, etc.).
- Provide opportunities for men and women to exercise separately (e.g., gyms available for women only on specific days of the week; these may need to provide childcare facilities).
- Use other media to promote activity or healthy cooking (e.g., videos prepared in the Somali language on healthy cooking, exercise, information on infant feeding).
- Encourage Somali mothers to form a breastfeeding support group to promote breastfeeding, appropriate weaning and encourage vitamin D supplementation of breastfeeding women.
- Regular audits of practice of breastfeeding, dietary and lifestyle practices need to be done to ensure messages are being translated to practice.
- A health survey of the UK Somali population needs to be done to assess the health profile and needs of the population and to enable services to be targeted.

Support groups

Arabic Diet

British Heart Foundation
Help line: 0300 330 3311
www.bhf.org.uk
Diabetes UK Central Office Macleod House,
10 Parkway, London NW1 7AA
Tel 020 7424 1000
Email info@diabetes.org.uk

Inspired by Diabetes
http://www.inspiredbydiabetes.com/index.jsp

Further reading

Arabic Diet

Consensus Action on Salt & Health. www.actiononsalt.org.uk.
Department of Health. *Coronary Heart Disease.* www.dh.gov.uk/en/Healthcare/NationalService Frameworks/Coronaryheartdisease.
Food in the Arab World. www.al-bab.com/arab/food.htm.
Food Standards Agency. www.foodstandards.gov.uk.
Imperial College London Diabetes Centre (ICLDC). www.icldc.ae
International Diabetes Federation. www.idf.org.
National Heart Forum. www.heartforum.org.uk/home.aspx.
National Obesity Forum. www.nationalobesityforum.org.uk.
NHS Choices. *Your Health, Your Choice.* www.nhs.uk/Livewell/HealthyRamadan/Pages/Healthyramadanhome.aspx.
Qatar Diabetes Association. www.qda.org.qa/output/page4.asp.
The Multicultural Nutrition Group, British Dietetic Association. www.bda.uk.com
Musaiger, A. & Shahbeek, N.E. (2001) The effect of education and obesity on attitudes towards fad-related diets to weight reduction among Arab women in Qatar. *Nutr and Food Sci*, 31(4), 201–4.
The Muslim Food Board (UK). www.tmfb.net/js/aboutus.html.
Third Arab Conference on Nutrition. Organized by Arab Centre for Nutrition, Abu Dhabi Food Control Authority and Health Authority-Abu Dhabi-UAE; 4–5 December 2007.
WHO Regional Office for the Eastern Mediterranean Region. Eastern Mediterranean Approach to Noncommunicable Diseases Network (EMAN).

www.acnut.com/pdf/2ea.pdf.
www.emro.who.int/ncd/EMAN.htm.
www.halalfoodauthority.co.uk/definitionhalal.html.
www.un.org/Depts/Cartographic/map/profile/somalia.pdf.

Somalian Diet

Abdullahi, M.D, (2001) *Culture and Customs of Somalia.* Greenwood Press, London.
Information Centre for the Office of National Statistics (ONS) (2005) *Infant Feeding Survey: A survey conducted on behalf of The Information Centre for Health and Social Care and the UK Health Departments by BMRB Social Research.* ONS, London.

References

Arabic Diet

Afandi, B., Ahmad, S. *et al.* (2006) Audit of a diabetic clinic at Tawam Hospital, UAE 2004–2005. *Annals of the New York Academy of Sciences*, 1048(1), 319–24.
Agricultural Handbook No. 8 (n.d.) US Department of Agriculture, Washington, DC.
Al-Jalili I. (November 2004) Arab population in the UK. *Study for Consideration of Inclusion of 'Arab' as an Alternative Ethnic Group on Ethnicity Profile Forms.* National Association of British Arabs, British Arab Forum.
Al-Kaabi, J., Al-Maskari, F. *et al.* (Summer 2006) Assessment of dietary practice among diabetic patients in the UAE. *Rev Diabet Stud*, 5(2), 110–15.
Al-Khader A.A. (2001) Impact of diabetes in renal diseases in Saudi Arabia. *Nephrol Dial Transplant*, 16, 2132–5.
Al Lawati, J.A., Barakat, N.M., Al-Lawati, A.M. & Mohammed. A.J. (November 2008) Optimal cut-off points for body mass index, waist circumference and waist to hip ratio using the Framingham cardiovascular disease risk score in an Arab population of the Middle East. *Diab Vasc Dis Res*, 5(4), 304–9.
Al-Mahroos, F. & Al-Roomi, K. (2001) Obesity among adult Bahraini population: impact of physical activity and education levels. *Annals of Saudi Medicine*, 21, 183–97.
Almajwal, A.M., Williams, P.G. *et al.* (2008) *Planning for the Development of Evidence Based Guidelines for the Nutritional Management of Obesity in Saudi Arabia.* Faculty of Health and Behavioural Sciences, University of Wollongong, Australia.
Al-Maskari, F., El-Sadig, M. & Obineche, E. (2008) Prevalence and determinants of microalbuminuria

among diabetic patients in the United Arab Emirates. *BMC Nephropathy*, 9, 1.

Al-Qaoud, N., Prakash, P. & Jacob, S. (2007) Weight loss attempts among Kuwaiti adults attending the Central Medical Nutrition Clinic. *Med Princ Pract*, 16, 291–8.

Alwan A. (1997) Noncommunicable diseases: a major challenge to public health in the region. *Eastern Mediterranean Health Journal*, 3(1), 6–16.

Azaizeh, H., Saad, B., Khalil, K. & Said, O. (2006) The state of the art of traditional Arab herbal medicine in the Eastern Region of the Mediterranean: a review. *Evidence-based Complementary and Alternative Medicine*, 3(2), 229–35.

Bashour, H.N. (2004) Survey of dietary habits in school adolescents in Damascus, Syria Arab Republic. *Eastern Mediterranean Health Journal*, 10(6), 853–62.

British Heart Foundation (BNF) (2008) Statistics database. www.heartstats.org.

Census (various years) HMSO, London.

Dawodu, A. (2004) Vitamin D status of Arab mothers and infants. *J Arab Neonatol Forum*, 1, 15–22.

Dehghan, M., Al Hamad N. *et al.* (May 2005) Development of a semi-quantitative food frequency questionnaire for use in United Arab Emirates and Kuwait based on local foods. *Nutr Journal*, 27(4), 18.

Department of Health (2004) *At Least Five a Week: Report from the Chief Medical Officer*. DH, London.

Department of Health (2011) www.dh.gov.uk/en/Publichealth/Nutrition/DH_126493.

Diabetes Control and Complications Trial 1003; UK Prospective Diabetes Study 1998 (2009)

Diabetes UK, London. www.diabetes.org.uk.

Ethnicity in the 1991 Census (1992) HMSO, London.

FAO (2005) *Sudan Nutrition Profile*. Food and Nutrition Division, Food and Agriculture Association, Geneva.

FAO (2006) *Kuwait Nutrition Profile*. Food and Nutrition Division, Food and Agriculture Association, Geneva.

FAO (2007) *Lebanese Republic Nutrition Profile*. Food and Nutrition Division, Food and Agriculture Association, Geneva.

Goenka, N., Thomas, S. *et al.* (2007) Providing diabetes care to Arab migrants in the UK: cultural and clinical aspect. *Br J of Diabetes and Vasc Dis*, 7, 283–6.

Greater London Authority (June 2005) *London Country of Birth Profiles – The Arab League. An Analysis of Census Data*.

Henley, A. & Schott, J. (2004) *Culture, Religion and Patient Care in a Multi-Ethnic Society: A Handbook for Professionals*. Age Concern, London.

Hill, J.O. & Wyatt, H.R. (2005) Role of physical activity in preventing and treating obesity. *J of Applied Physiology*, 99, 765–70.

HMSO (2003) *The National Diet & Nutrition Survey: adults aged 19 to 64 years*. Her Majesty's Stationery Office, UK.

Institute of Alcohol Studies (IAS) (2008) *Drinking in Great Britain*. IAS Fact Sheet.

International Diabetes Federation (2002) *Diabetes Atlas*. 2nd edition. www.eatlas.idf.org.

International Diabetes Federation (2003) *Diabetes Atlas*. 3rd edition. www.eatlas.idf.org.

Khatib, F.A. & Shafagoj, Y.A. (2004) Metabolic alterations as a result of Ramadan fasting in non-insulin-dependent diabetes mellitus patients in relation to food intake. *Saudi Med J*, 25(12), 1858–63.

Mansour, A.A., Al-Hassan, A.A. & Jazairi, M.I. (2007) Towards establishing normal waist circumference in Eastern Mediterranean and Middle East (Arab) populations. Cut-off values for waist circumference in Iraqi adults. *Int J Diabetes and Metabolism*, 15, 14–16.

McCoy, A. (February 2003) The British Arab. *Focus on NABA*.

Miles, L. (2007) Physical activity and health. *British Nutrition Foundation Nutrition Bulletin*, 32, 314–63.

Mokhtar, N., Elati, J. *et al.* (2001) Diet culture and obesity in northern Africa. *J Nutrition*, 131, 887S–892S.

Moussa, M., Alsaeid, M. *et al.* (2008) Prevalence of type 2 diabetes mellitus among Kuwaiti children and adolescents. *Med Princ Pract*, 17, 270–5.

Musaiger, A.O. (2002) Diet and prevention of coronary heart disease in the Arab Middle East Countries. *Med Principles Pract*, 11(Suppl. 2), 9–16.

NHS Diabetes with Diabetes UK and the Association for Clinical Biochemistry (2009) *A Change in Reporting your HbA1c Results. Information for People with Diabetes*.

Office for National Statistics (2006) *National Diet and Nutrition Survey: Adults aged 19–64 years. Energy, Protein, Carbohydrate, Fat and Alcohol Intake. 2003*. www.statistics.gov.uk.

ONS (2001) *Office for National Statistics, 2001 Census: Special Migration Statistics (United Kingdom)*.

Ruston, D., Hoare, J. *et al.* (2004) *National Diet and Nutrition Survey: Adults Aged 19 to 64 years. Volume 4: Nutritional Status (Anthropometry and Blood Analytes), Blood Pressure and Physical Activity*. The Stationery Office, London.

Salti, I., Benard, E. *et al.* (2004) A population-based study of diabetes and its characteristics during the fasting month of Ramadan in 13 countries. Results of the Epidemiology of Diabetes and Ramadan 1422/2001 (EPIDIAR) study. *Diabetes Care*, 27(10), 2306–11.

Saris, W.H.M., Blair, S.N. *et al.* (2003) How much physical activity is enough to prevent unhealthy weight gain? Outcome of the IASO 1st Stock Conference and consensus statement. *Obesity Reviews*, 4, 101–14.

Stanner, S. (2005) *Cardiovascular Disease Diet, Nutrition and Emerging Risk Factors*. Blackwell, Oxford.

United Nations (2002) *World Population Prospects: The 2002 Revision Population Database (United Nations Population Division)*. esa.un.org/unpp.

Verster, A. & van der Pols, C.J.C. (1995) Anaemia in the eastern Mediterranean region. *Eastern Health Journal*, 1, 64–79.

WHO (1994) *Prevention of Diabetes*. Technical Report Services no. 844. WHO, Geneva.

WHO (1998) *Fortification of Flour with Iron in the Countries of the Eastern Mediterranean Middle East and North Africa*. WHO, Geneva.

WHO (1998) *Obesity: Preventing and Managing the Global Epidemic. Report of a WHO Consultation on Obesity*. WHO, Geneva.

WHO (2003) *Diet, Nutrition and the Prevention of Chronic Disease*. Technical Report 916. WHO, Geneva.

WHO (2005) *Global Comparable Estimates*. www.who.int/infobase.

WHO (2005) *EMRO: The Regional Office and its Partners*. www.emro.who.int/EMROInfo/wrs.htm.

WHO (2005) *Guidelines for the Management of Hypertension in Patients with Diabetes*. WHO, Regional Office for the Eastern Mediterranean Region.

WHO (2005) *Preventing Chronic Diseases: A Vital Investment*.WHO, Geneva.

WHO (2005) *The Impact of Chronic Disease in the Eastern Mediterranean Region*.

WHO (2006) *Guidelines of the Management of Dyslipidaemia in Patients with Diabetes*. WHO, Regional Office for the Eastern Mediterranean Region.

WHO (2006) *Public Health Problems of Alcohol Consumption in the Region*. Regional Office for the Eastern Mediterranean Region, WHO, Geneva.

WHO (2006) *Tobacco Use in Shisha. Studies on Waterpipe Smoking in Egypt*. Regional Office for the Eastern Mediterranean region, WHO, Geneva.

WHO (2006) *WHO in the Eastern Mediterranean Region. Annual Report of the Regional Director 2006*. 1 January–31 December.

WHO (November 2009) *Diabetes Fact Sheet 312*. WHO, Geneva.

WHO (2010) *Eastern Mediterranean Approach to Noncommunicable Diseases Network (EMAN)*. Regional Office for the Eastern Mediterranean Region, WHO, Geneva.

WHO EMRO (2010) *Noncommunicable Diseases. Stepwise Data from Selected Countries in the Eastern Mediterranean Region, 2003–2007*.

WHO FAOSTAT (2003) faostat.fao.org.

WHO Global InfoBase (2008) www.who.int/infobase/comparestart.aspx.

WHO/UNICEF/MI/ILSI Workshop, Beirut, Lebanon 13–16 June 1998.

www.diabetes.nhs.uk/press_and_media/hba1c_leaflets.

www.emro.who.int/ncd/risk_factors.htm#hyper cholesterolemia.

www.emro.who.int/rd/annualreports/2006/chapter1_6.htm

www.london.gov.uk/gla/publications/factsand figures/dmag-2005-19.pdf.

www.who.int/chp/chronic_disease_report/en.

www.who.int/chp/chronic_disease_report/en.

Somalian Diet

Burns, C. (2004) Effect of migration on food habits of Somali women living as refugees in Australia. *Ecology of Food and Nutrition*, 43(3), 213–29.

Department of Health (2004) *At Least Five a Week: Evidence on the Impact of Physical Activity and Its Relationship to Health: A Report from CMO*. www.dh.gov.uk/prod_consum_dh/groups/dh_digitalassets/@dh/@en/documents/digitalasset/dh_4080981.pdf.

Department of Health (2007) *Policy and Guidance, Health and Social Care Topics, Maternal and Infant Nutrition*. www.dh.gov.uk/en/Policyandguidance/Healthand socialcaretopics/Maternalandinfantnutrition/index.htm.

Department of Health (2010) *5 A Day. General Information*. www.dh.gov.uk/en/publichealth/Healthimprovement/FiveADay/FiveADaygeneralinformation/DH_4002343.

Grundel, J. (2002) The migration–development nexus: Somalia case study. *International Migration*, 40(5, special issue 2), 255–81.

Guerin, P.B., Elmi, F.H. & Corrigan, C (2007) Body composition and cardiorespiratory fitness among refugee Somali women living in New Zealand. *Journal of Immigrant Minority Health*, 9, 191–6.

Guerin, P.B., Diiriye, R.O., Corrigan, C. & Guerin, B. (2003) Physical activity programmes for refugee Somali women: working out in a new country. *Women & Health*, 38(1).

Haq, A.S. (2003) *Report on Somali Diet, Common Dietary Beliefs and Practices of Somali Participants in WIC Nutrition Education Groups*. www.ethnomed/clin_topics/Somali_diet_report.html.

Harris, H. (2004) *The Somali Community in the UK: What We Know ad How We Know It*. The Information Centre about Asylum and Refugees in the UK (ICAR), London.

Ibrahim, M.M., Persson, L.A., Omar, M.M. & Wall, S. (1992) Breast feeding and dietary habits of children in rural Somalia. *Acta Paediatrica*, 18(6–7), 480–3. www3.interscience.wiley.com/journal/119986906/abstract.

Kleist, N. (2004) *Nomads, Sailors and Refugees: A Century of Somali Migration*. Sussex Migration Working Paper no. 23.

Lancashire Council of Mosques (2010) *Islamic Festivals*. www.lancashiremosques.com/discovery_islamic_festivals.asp.

McEwen, A., Straus, L. & Ussher, M. (2007) Physical inactivity among a UK Somali population. *Journal of Public Health*, 30(1), 110–15.

McEwen, A., Straus, L. & Croker, H (2009) Dietary beliefs and behaviour of a UK Somali population. *J Hum Nutr Dietetics*, 22(2), 116–21.

Maxwell, S.M., Salah, S.M. & Bunn, J.E.G. (2006) Dietary habits of the Somali population in Liverpool, with respect to foods containing calcium and vitamin D: a cause for concern? *J Hum Nutr Dietet*, 19, 125–7.

Minnesota International Health Volunteers (MIHV) (2005a) *Somali Health Care Initiative. Focus Group Findings. Somali Women's Breastfeeding Practices and Preferences.* Minnesota.

Minnesota International Health Volunteers (MIHV) (2005b) *Somali Health Care Initiative. Focus Group Findings. Diet and Physical Activity in the Somali Community.* Minnesota.

RAL (2006) *Commonwealth Migration and non-European Refugees.* www.researchasylum.org.uk/?lid=1304#13.

Straus, L., McEwen, A. & Croker, H. (2006) *Tobacco Use among the Somali Population in Islington.* A Report for Islington Primary Care Trust by the Cancer Research UK Health Behaviour Unit, University College London.

Tammy's Somali Home. tammyssomalihome.blogspot.com/2008/12/qaxwo-and-somali-sweets.html.

United Nations: Permanent Mission (2010) *Country Facts.* www.un.int/wcm/webdav/site/somalia/shared/documents/statements/1086763821.

Wageh, M.A. (2005) *Somalia Nutrition Profile. Part II. Food and Nutrition Situation.* Food and Nutrition Division, FAO.

World Health Organization (WHO) (May 2001) *54th World Health Assembly: Global Strategy for Infant and Young Child Feeding.* ftp.who.int/gb/pdf_files/WHA54/ea547.pdf.

World Health Organization (WHO) (2002) *Facing the Facts: The Impact of Chronic Diseases in Somalia.* www.who.int/chp/chronic-disease_report/somali.pdf.

Woutat, S, (1998) A bulletin of nutrition, food and health information. *Nutrient*, 12(6). Department of Food Science and Nutrition University of Minnesota Extension Service. www.extension.umn.edu/newsletters/nutrinet/ff1060.txt.

6 West Africa

Arit Ana, Angela Telle (Nigeria), Susanna Johnson (Ghana)

The West African countries included in this section are Nigeria and Ghana. Many of the Nigerians and Ghanaians residing in the UK arrived after 1990, with many coming either to study or as professionals. The downturn in the West African economy, the long-term strength of the UK's, and the primacy of the English language made the UK an easy and attractive place for West Africans to migrate to. Language barriers are few because the majority of West Africans understand and speak English or Pidgin English, but many native languages and dialects are also spoken. The two main religions in West Africa are Christianity and Islam. Muslim and Christian holidays include the end of Ramadan, Easter, Good Friday and Christmas respectively. There is information on migration, traditional diets and changes on migration, religious influences and on dietary considerations for specific disease conditions such as obesity, diabetes and cardiovascular disease.

6.1 Nigerian Diet

Arit Ana, Angela Telle

Key points

- The official language of Nigeria is English, however more than 250 languages are spoken in the country.
- Older generations attach a great deal of importance to their Nigerian backgrounds. They also tend to cling to their traditional diet, which is high in carbohydrates, meat, fish and pulses. It also tends to be high in sodium and low in potassium due to a low consumption of fruits and vegetables.
- Palm oil is the commonest cooking oil in Nigeria. It has no substitute and is often used excessively in soups.
- The most popular cooking method is one-pot cooking, where foods from the five food groups are cooked together.

Multicultural Handbook of Food, Nutrition and Dietetics, First Edition. Edited by Aruna Thaker, Arlene Barton.
© 2012 Blackwell Publishing Ltd. Published 2012 by Blackwell Publishing Ltd.

- Obesity and overweight, the major risk factors for hypertension, diabetes and cardiovascular diseases, have become major health problems and can be attributed to increased consumption of refined and fatty foods and snacks, and decreased physical activity.
- Health promotion education should encourage traditional healthy food habits with the inclusion of healthy local foods and more physical activity.

6.1.1 Introduction

Nigeria is one the most populous countries in Africa and is both physically and culturally diverse. It occupies 923,768 km² on the west coast of the continent, extending 1,450 km from the semi-arid savannah grassland in the north to the humid tropical rainforests of the southern and coastal regions. Nigeria is bounded by Benin, Niger, Chad, Cameroon and the Gulf of Guinea (Figure 6.1.1).

Language

More than 250 languages are spoken in Nigeria and the official languages are English and Pidgin English, which is commonly spoken. Every ethnic group has its own distinct language. Hausa, Yoruba and Ibo are the main languages spoken. These are the main ethnic groups in Nigeria and they are also the main representative groups in UK. There are no language barriers because the majority of Nigerians understand and speak English or Pidgin English. However; some Nigerian visitors to the

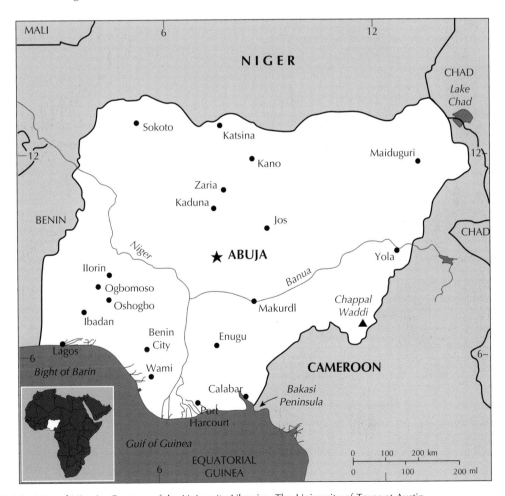

Figure 6.1.1 Map of Nigeria. Courtesy of the University Libraries. The University of Texas at Austin.

UK may have difficulty in being understood or understanding English because of the accent.

Migration to the United Kingdom

Before 1990, most Nigerians were not interested in emigrating permanently but came to the UK for postgraduate studies or on holiday visits. However, the downturn in the Nigerian economy, the long-term strength of the British economy, proximity to the UK and the primacy of the English language made Britain an attractive place for Nigerians to migrate to. The UK is thus home to the world's largest overseas Nigerian community.

Current UK population

Nigerian British is the term given to describe British people of Nigerian descent. The most recent UK census (2001) recorded 88,378 Nigerian-born people resident in the UK. More recent estimates by the Office for National Statistics put the figure at 140,000, with the majority living in London. The Foreign and Commonwealth Office, in its country profile for Nigeria, puts the total Nigerian community in the UK at between 800,000 and 3 million. Nigerian British live throughout the UK, with the largest communities in the principal cities (London, Luton, Birmingham, Cardiff, Liverpool and Manchester). There is also a large student population at the major universities. The vast majority of Nigerians in the UK come from the south of Nigeria and are mainly of Yoruba and Ibo heritage. Nigerians are very tribal – they identify themselves first with their ethnicity, second, with their religion and finally, with their nationality. This mentality is exported to the UK, resulting in the formation of tribal clusters around London. Most are found in Lambeth, Southwark and Peckham (*Country Profile: Nigeria*, 2008).

Older generations attach a great deal of importance to their Nigerian backgrounds, often have very strong ties with their home towns and may regard themselves as temporary residents despite having lived in the UK for many years. They also tend to follow their traditional diet.

The younger generation are generally more integrated into British society. They tend to describe themselves as British-born Nigerian and have adopted UK dietary habits and way of life (Bygott, 1996).

6.1.2   Religion

In Nigeria, Muslims make up about 40% of the population and live mainly in the north. Christians make up about 50% of the population and mostly live in the south. The remaining 10% follow traditional African belief systems. There are also some Born-again Christians.

Religious dietary restrictions

Muslim and Christian holidays include the end of Ramadan (a month of fasting), Easter, Good Friday and Christmas. There are no specific religious practices that impact on nutritional status, except that Muslims and Adventists do not eat pork because it is seen as unclean. Born-again Christians do not drink alcohol. Vegetarianism is not commonly practised by Nigerians. For more information on the Muslim diet, see Chapter 5 section 5.1.2 pages 214–215.

6.1.3   Food production and availability of foods in Nigeria

Nigeria is divided into three by the Niger and Benue rivers:

- The northern section is mainly arid with a monsoon rainfall pattern.
- The middle-belt has a more varied relief and is marked by rugged volcanic highlands, the Jos Plateau.
- The southern and coastal section consists of low-lying plains and comprises the Niger delta in the south-east. This area is made up of mangroves and dense forest and has some of the richest petroleum deposits in Africa.

The north and middle-belt

The geographical pattern of tropical vegetation and animal life corresponds to the zones of rainfall distribution. In the north and middle belt, the smaller rainfall and greater seasonal contrast produce the tropical forests and open grassland known as the Sudan Savannah. Foods grown here reflect the geography (see Table 6.1.1). This area is known as the food basket of Nigeria with the main occupation being farming and animal husbandry (Nason, I999).

Table 6.1.1 Description of foods produced in the north and middle-belt of Nigeria

Food groups	Types of food	Comments
Bread, other cereals and potatoes	Potatoes, wheat, rice, millet, sorghum, yam, cocoyam, corn	Most cereal products consumed in Nigeria are produced in the north and middle-belt
Fruit and vegetables	Mangoes, oranges, grape fruits, water melon, dates Cucumber, lettuce, cabbage, carrots, tomatoes, courgettes, cauliflower, spring onions, peppers, spinach, garden eggs, etc.	
Meat, fish and other sources of protein	Hen and guinea fowl eggs, chicken, beef, mutton, goat, fish, beans, pulses, peanuts	
Milk and dairy foods	Milk, local cheese, *fura*, yoghurt	Milk and milk products are mainly produced in the north but not in commercial quantities to be main source of calcium in the Nigerian diet, especially in the south
Foods containing fats and sugar	Ghee, groundnut oil	Only produced in the north

Table 6.1.2 Description of foods produced in the south and Niger delta of Nigeria

Food groups	Types of food	Comments
Bread, other cereals and potatoes	Yam, cocoyam, water yam, cassava, green plantain, corn, rice	
Fruit and vegetables	Mangoes, oranges, grapefruits, bananas, pineapples, apples, cucumber, okra, squashes, tomatoes, spring onions, spinach, green leafy vegetables, avocado pears, garden eggs, pawpaw, guava, oranges, etc.	Fruits are grown but are not used as part of everyday meal. Fruits are consumed occasionally as snacks A lot of wastage due to lack of appropriate preservation facilities
Meat, fish and other sources of protein	Eggs, chicken, goat, bush meat, beans, fish and other seafood, snails, pulses	Beef and mutton are brought in from the north
Milk and dairy foods		Dairy foods, are not produced in this area
Foods containing fats and sugar	Palm oil and coconut oil, etc.	Only produced in the south

fish, whelks, periwinkles, clams and smoked dry fish (see Table 6.1.2). The geographical diversity in food production also affects the types of food eaten by Nigerians in the UK.

Traditional diet and eating pattern

The traditional diet is high in carbohydrates, meat, fish, pulses and salt. The type of carbohydrate eaten depends on region. Northerners eat more cereals while southerners eat more tubers. Traditional food patterns are interwoven with the culture. They are a response of individuals or groups to social and cultural pressures in selecting

The south and Niger delta

The south is very humid and has all-year rainfall. Foods grown are of the types that require high rainfall.

The main sources of protein, especially in the coastal areas, are various seafoods such as prawns, and consuming foods depending on the food available. Food is very much part of Nigerian culture, and the beliefs, practices and trends in culture affect its eating practices. Nigeria has such a variety of people and cultures that it is difficult to identify one national dish. Each area has its own, which depends on customs, tradition and religion. Nigerians and most Africans often cook the same way and may use similar ingredients but the end product may look or taste different, depending on the tribe, local tradition and cooking methods. Local vegetables and spices used reveal a lot about the cook and the tribe they come from.

Generally, the common staple diet eaten by Nigerians (and other Africans) are starchy foods such as cassava, yam, cocoyam, water yam, plantain, rice, black-eyed beans, millet, corn and sorghum (common among northerners). The cereals are often made into drinks or flour used in puddings (e.g., *ogi*), while the root tubers are usually boiled or made into *fufu* and eaten with soup. The staples are also commonly boiled or fried and eaten with stew or soup, or mixed omelette (egg fried with onion, tomatoes, sometimes sardine or corned beef is included). For some commonly eaten Nigerian foods (see Table 6.1.6).

Nigerian men still believe in 'swallowing' *fufu* at least once a day. This method of eating is often described as 'cut, dip and swallow' because the *fufu* is broken with the fingers, rolled into a small ball, dipped in soup and then swallowed without chewing (those not used to *fufu* may chew it first). This is a common practice among Africans; they cannot enjoy eating *fufu* with a knife and fork as their Caucasian friends do. The average Nigerian eats three large main meals a day bur rarely eats between meals.

Food patterns are based on what the culture considers to be food. Most Nigerians find offal a delicacy and have a variety of recipes for preparing it. No soup is complete without offal (e.g., cow hide, tripe, intestine, brain, liver, kidney, lungs). Meals served with just a few pieces of meat or no meat or fish at all is seen as a sign of poverty and hardship (Ana, 2000).

Northern Nigerians (mainly Muslims) do not eat pork and have diets based on beans, sorghum and brown rice. The Hausas and Fulanis in this region are cattle farmers. They like to eat meat made in the form of *suya* kebabs (chunks of skewered, well-seasoned roasted meat). They also like to drink tea and often frequent coffee houses. Muslims do not drink alcohol.

The Nigerians in the east and south-west eat yams, *gari* (made from cassava), cocoyam and plantain. Yams are eaten instead of potatoes and are important part of the Nigerian diet. Seafoods are the main source of protein.

Alcohol is widely drunk and this is replicated in the life of those who live abroad.

Typical meal patterns

The three main meals (breakfast, lunch and dinner) are often chosen from the staple groups. Dishes such as rice and stew or *moi-moi* may be served at breakfast, lunch or dinner. Most Nigerian foods are cooked as composites (i.e., meat, fish, vegetables, oil, etc., are cooked in the same pot – this is the soup) and then balanced with the missing staple which could be pounded yam *fufu* or boiled rice, so the main meal is usually served without side-dishes. Carbohydrates, proteins, fat and vegetables are also often cooked in one pot as pottage. Nigerians will still want to eat large portions of *fufu* in the evening, irrespective of what was eaten at lunch (Ana, 2000) (see Table 6.1.3). This could result in overconsumption and may lead to obesity.

6.1.4   Traditional foods and healthier alternatives

First-generation Nigerians introduce the traditional diet to their children as early as possible, but the children start rejecting traditional foods as they grow older and start interacting with their Caucasian peers, and become used to eating indigenous foods at school. The children are often embarrassed to share traditional meals with their non-Nigerian friends. Most traditional foods are expensive and this too may be a constraint.

Composite foods

Most foods that are enjoyed are grouped as 'composite' foods. Nigerians, Ghanaians and other West Africans cook more in this way. 'Composite foods are dishes or meals that contain foods from the five food groups.' Examples are green plantain pottage, cocoyam pottage, *ekpangnkukwo*, pizza, soups, casseroles and sandwiches. Sometimes the dish may

Table 6.1.3   Typical Nigerian meal pattern

Meal	Description of foods
Breakfast	*Fufu* with vegetable soup or stew
Traditionally, the type of breakfast eaten depends on the person's profession. Manual workers prefer *fufu* because they believe that this will stay longer in the stomach	Boiled rice or boiled/fried yam, plantain with stew or omelette
In UK, professionals prefer 'lighter' foods like bread, akara or moi-moi served with any cereal of choice. However, due to the time it takes to prepare akara or moi-moi these are often eaten at functions and not at breakfast as is traditionally the case	Moi-moi or akara served with *ogi* (pap) custard made with evaporated milk
	Bread served with fried egg or sardine with tea/coffee or Bournvita
	Any other cereal with full-cream milk
Lunch	
More snacking is done at lunch-time. This could be in the form of sandwiches or leftover meals could be brought in from home	Leftovers
	Sandwiches
	Banana with peanuts
	Roasted corn with ube pear (may not be available in the UK), coconut, peanuts
	Restaurant or fast-food meal
Dinner	
Often a big meal, because most people are away from home at lunchtime. More effort is put into preparing the evening meal. Choice is often from the main staples	Any *fufu* with soup
	Rice, fried plantain with stew
	Rice, fried plantain with stewed beans
Snacks	
Traditional snacks are usually roasted or boiled peanuts, plantain chips	Boiled yam, beans with stew
	Kulikuli (peanut biscuit, popular in north)
In UK, chocolates, crisps and biscuits	*Suya* (hot and spicy barbecued beef, mutton or chicken
Snack foods are an important part of a child's diet. They provide an opportunity for children to eat on their own, without sharing with siblings	Bananas eaten with groundnuts
	'Manpower' (mixture of mature roasted corn/ popcorn and roasted peanuts
	Sliced boiled cassava eaten with peanuts, fish, salted pork or coconut

not be complete without food from one of the main food groups (e.g., vegetable soup completed with *fufu*, boiled rice or yam to make it balanced).

The meal could be made healthier by using less palm or vegetable oil, salt or stock cubes and not overcooking the vegetables.

'The Balance of Good Health'

When planning meals, always choose from the five food groups from 'The Balance of Good Health' plate (see Figure 6.1.2). A popular cooking method is 'one-pot cooking' where foods from the five food groups are cooked together. This gives flexibility in planning meals (see Table 6.1.4).

Food taboos

Food taboos are rife not only in Nigeria but throughout Africa and other parts of the world (see Table 6.1.5). In most cases it is the protein intakes (especially animal protein) of children and of pregnant and lactating women that are affected by native customs. The diet of the population provides approximately half of the protein requirements. The effects of a low-protein diet may be

Table 6.1.4 Traditional Nigerian foods and healthier alternatives

Bread, cereals and other starchy foods	Traditional foods	Healthier alternatives
Rice, millet, sorghum, corn, bread, oat porridge, *ogi* (pap)	Jollof rice: Rice cooked with ground tomatoes, peppers, vegetable oil, sometimes meat, and mixed vegetables Reddish-orange in colour	Balance with mixed vegetables or steamed spinach Use pure vegetable oil in cooking Cook rice with small amount of oil
	Coconut rice: Rice cooked in coconut sauce or cream with ground crayfish, shrimps, meat, dry fish, onions, etc.	Eat coconut rice only occasionally because of saturated fat content which is linked to heart disease
	Tuwo shinkafa: Overcooked rice mashed into dough-like texture and eaten with soup or stew	Reduce portion size
	Sorghum, millet, corn, ground into meal/flour, fermented and made into drinks (*ogi* or pap)	
	Fura de nono: is a northern traditional drink made with millet and full-fat milk	Use low-fat milk instead of full-fat milk in preparing *fura de nono*, porridge and pap
	Corn: Roasted/boiled and eaten with coconut or groundnut, as snack	Eat roasted corn with ube pear or peanuts and not coconut Eat more whole meal bread instead of white bread Sprinkle bran on porridge to increase fibre content
Yam, cocoyam, water yam, plantain, green plantain, cassava **Sweet potato, Irish potato, etc.**	Pounded yam (*fufu*): Peel, softly boil yam, the pound until smooth like dough Eat with soup	Fry yam and plantain less often
	Yam, plantain or cocoyam made into pottage or roast/boiled/fried	Use palm oil sparingly in pottages Boil more often
	Cocoyam/ water yam: made into *ekpang-nkukwo*, peeled, finely grated, wrapped in small portions with cocoyam leaves or spinach, then cooked with crayfish, periwinkles, dried fish, shrimps and palm oil in one pot. Served as a composite food	
	Cocoyam/water yam: made into *ayan-ekpang*, peeled, finely grated, wrapped in plantain leaves or foil, steamed and served with okro soup	
	Cassava: peeled ground, fermented and made into cassava *fufu* or dry-fried into gari	Eat sliced cassava with peanuts or fish, not salted pork or coconut
Meat, fish, eggs and alternatives		
Beef, goat, mutton, pork Chicken, guinea fowl, eggs Bush meat (dried meat from wild animals, e.g., antelope, monkey) Snails	Oven-dry meat, chicken or fish instead of frying for soups, stews and snacks	Oven-dry meat, chicken or fish instead of frying for soups, stews and snacks
	Trim off fat from meat, use lean cuts	Trim fat from meat, use lean cuts
	Soak salted pork overnight, wash thoroughly to remove salt. Too much salt is linked to hypertension and stroke	Soak salted pork overnight, wash thoroughly to remove salt. Too much salt is linked to hypertension and stroke

Table 6.1.4 (cont'd)

Bread, cereals and other starchy foods	Traditional foods	Healthier alternatives
Offals: Cow's foot, cow skin, oxtail, intestines, tripe, lungs, ox tongue, liver, kidney, heart, chicken gizzard	Boil meat, allow to cool, skim off fat or keep overnight in fridge, then remove fat that has set and through away, use stock for soups and stews. Reduce meat portion size	Boil meat, allow to cool, skim off fat or keep overnight in fridge, then remove fat that has set and through away, use stock for soups and stews Reduce meat portion size
Seafoods: Prawns, shrimps, lobster, crab, crayfish, Periwinkles, whelks, clam, catfish, tilapia, eel, croaker, mackerel (icefish), sardines, salmon, smoked dried fish, stock fish, etc.	Aim to have two portions of oily fish like mackerel, sardine, or salmon weekly. Oily fish is high in omega 3 fatty acids which is good for the heart and joints	Aim to have two portions of oily fish like mackerel, sardine or salmon weekly. Oily fish is high in omega 3 fatty acids which is good for the heart and joints
Use palm oil sparingly in vegetable soups and stews	Use palm oil sparingly in vegetable soups and stews Use pure vegetable oil instead of palm oil in moi-moi or frying akara Don't add salt to groundnut before dry frying	Use pure vegetable oil instead of palm oil in moi-moi or frying akara Don't add salt to groundnut before dry-frying
Groundnuts (peanuts) cashew nut, black eye beans and brown beans, egusi (melon seed)	Use groundnut or pure vegetable oil in cooking or frying Limit total daily intake of salt (sodium chloride) to 6 g or less. Limit the use of salt in cooking and avoid adding it to food at the table. Salty, highly processed salty, salt-preserved, and salt-pickled foods should be consumed sparingly Season meat with herbs and spices. If you use stock cubes, do not use salt Eat fried foods occasionally. Eating too much fried foods may result in obesity. Obesity is linked to heart disease, diabetes, hypertension and cancer etc.	Use groundnut or pure vegetable oil in cooking or frying Limit total daily intake of salt (sodium chloride) to 6 g or less. Limit the use of salt in cooking and avoid adding it to food at the table Salty, highly processed salty, salt-preserved, and salt-pickled foods should be consumed sparingly Season meat with herbs and spices. If you use stock cubes, do not use salt Eat fried foods occasionally. Eating too much fried foods may result in obesity. Obesity is linked to heart disease, diabetes, hypertension and cancer, etc.
Milk and dairy foods Evaporated milk, condensed milk, carnation milk, full-cream powdered milk, butter, cheese, yoghurt Milk and milk products are not common in Nigerian cookery, except in baking and on cereals. Evaporated and powdered milk are used in tea and coffee	Use lower fat milk, cheese, yoghurt and butter. Use evaporated, condensed and full fat powdered milk sparingly.	Use lower fat milk, cheese, yoghurt and butter. Use evaporated, condensed and full fat powdered milk sparingly

(Continued)

Table 6.1.4 (cont'd)

Bread, cereals and other starchy foods	Traditional foods	Healthier alternatives
Vegetables and Fruits		
Leafy Vegetables		
Ugu/ikongubong (fluted pumpkin leaves), *afang/okazi, etinyung* (crin-cring), *etinkeni* (hot leaves), *inyangafia* (spinach), *mongmong ikong* (water leaves), *mkpa/oha, atama,* cocoyam leaves, cassava leaves, bitter leaves, okra leaves, editan, etc.	Often used as main vegetables in soups *Edikang ikong* (vegetable) soup *Afang* soup *Abak atama* soup The vegetables give the soup its name. The soup is prepared with the vegetables mentioned above. The soup is a mixture of proteins , vegetables and palm oil	Add to soups about 5 minutes before end of cooking Always add vegetables to soups to increase fibre content Balance boiled yam, rice or plantain and stew with boiled vegetables Do not use potash (*akang*) to tenderize or improve vegetable colour. It destroys vitamin C Do not overcook vegetables. Use very little palm oil in cooking. Use salt or stock cubes sparingly
Other vegetables Carrots, garden eggs, tomatoes, cabbage, salad peppers, runner beans, okra, cucumbers, onions, etc.	Often eaten raw, boiled or used in salads	Boil in small amount of water for about 5 minutes Eat raw for maximum benefit Stir fry vegetables for fried rice for about 3 minutes to retain vitamins.
Fruits Mango, guava, banana, Pawpaw, water melon bush mango, coco fruits, mary fruits (similar to lychees), ube pear, apple, grapefruit, oranges, lime, tangerine, pineapples, avocado pear, canned fruits, fruit juice etc	Fruits are mainly eaten as snack and are not used as main ingredients in cooking Bananas: eaten with peanuts as snacks or made into banana fritters	Aim to eat at least five portions of fruits and vegetables a day.
Fats and oils Palm oil, coconut oil cream, palm kernel oil, palm fruit sauce, ground nut oil, pure vegetable oil, margarine, butter, ghee (used by northern Nigerians)	Palm oil is used liberally in traditional vegetable soups, the more the tastier. Palm oil is bleached and used for frying	Use less oil in cooking soups and stews Use lower fat spread variety on bread Spread margarine sparingly on bread. Do not bleach palm oil, bleaching destroys the vitamin A

Table 6.1.4 (cont'd)

Bread, cereals and other starchy foods	Traditional foods	Healthier alternatives
Foods high in fats and sugar		
Chin-chin, buns, *puff-puff*, cakes, biscuits, sweets, chocolate, crisps, coconut sweets, chocolate, crisps, plantain/banana chips, chocolates, sweets, etc., meat pies, sausage rolls, etc	*Chin-chin:* Flour, egg, milk, sugar mixed together to make a smooth dough, then kneaded, rolled flat, cut into small squares and fried in oil. *Puff-puff:* Flour mixed with yeast, sugar, water, allowed to rise, cut in small balls then fried in oil. Make-me-well (buns): Flour, egg, sugar, margarine, spices (cake mixture) mixed to smooth consistency and fried. Also oven-baked	Limit sweets, snacks to small amounts Use low-fat spread, and reduce sugar in baking recipes Eat coconut sweets occasionally because of saturated fat content. Eat crisps, plantain chips, sweets, pastry, chocolates, biscuits, etc., occasionally. Reduce fat and sugar in pastry or use low-fat spread instead. Use sweetener instead of sugar in home baked snacks. Bake buns instead of frying to reduce fat content
Sugary foods and drinks		
Soft/fizzy/mineral drinks, e.g., Fanta, cola, ginger beer, fruit punch, carrot juice, honey, molasses, brown sugar		Choose diet or no added sugar drinks Use sweetener in drinks and cereal Add less sugar to cereals and avoid in drinks. Brown sugar and molasses are as high in calories as refined white sugar Drink more water instead of soft drinks

Table 6.1.5   Food taboos practised in some parts of Nigeria

Food taboos	Groups who are forbidden to eat them	Reasons	Nutrients affected
Meat	Children	Makes them steal	Protein, B vitamins and minerals
Eggs	Children	Makes them steal	Protein, B vitamins, minerals
Gizzard, chicken drumstick	Children	Only for adult male of the family	Protein, B vitamins, minerals
Liver	Newly delivered mothers	Causes abscess of the liver	Protein, B vitamins, minerals
Fresh meat	Newly delivered mothers	Causes severe abdominal pain	Protein, B vitamins, minerals
Oil	Newly delivered mothers	Causes jaundice in babies	Energy, fat soluble vitamins
Ibaba (a thickening agent for soup)	Men	Makes them impotent	None

(*Am J of Clin Nut*, 1974; Ogbeide, 1974)

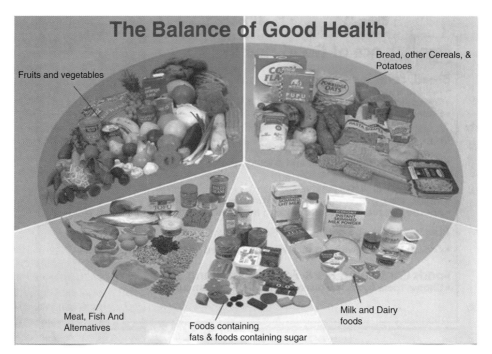

Figure 6.1.2 The Balance of Good Health. Courtesy of Health Information East London and The dept of Nutrition and Dietetics, Barts and The London NHS Trust, Feb. (2001) Adapted from Food Standards Agency (UK)

directly related to public health problems. A lack of adequate protein in the diet, further depleted by food prejudices that forbid eating what is available, can adversely affect the health status of the population (e.g., protein-calorie malnutrition in children, maternal depletion, premature ageing and general malnutrition in women). To prevent these effects from escalating, the lay public should be educated by medical and paramedical personnel who themselves must first be given sound basic nutrition education.

This is not common practice among Nigerians abroad. However, it makes interesting reading and an additional knowledge base for those colleagues who work in Nigeria. These practices are mainly due to ignorance, lack of basic education and poverty.

Starchy staples

White and pink cassava
Cassava is a starchy root with brown skin and firm flesh. There are two varieties of cassava com-monly grown in the southern part of Nigeria. Although tasteless and unappetizing on its own, it is very versatile and can be used to make *gari*, *fufu* or a boiled sliced snack. The pink-skinned variety can be grated and made into traditional dishes like *akara* (fried bean cake), *ekpangnkukwo* (cocoyam pottage) and *ayan ekpang* (a steamed alternative).

Yams
Yams are root tubers and come in many varieties and sizes. The yam is a climbing plant, with white (most common) or yellow flesh. It can be boiled, fried or roasted, but it can also be made into yam pottage which is a complete meal on its own. It can also be cooked and pounded to produce yam *fufu* which is eaten with soup.

Water yam
This has a high water content and is slimy. It can be eaten boiled, but is often used to prepare other traditional dishes.

Cocoyam

These are smaller and tougher in texture. The flesh can be white or pale pink. The leaves grow above the ground on a small shrub. The type used depends on the recipe; the white variety is preferred for traditional dishes, while the pink variety is better for boiling or in making cocoyam pottage. Cocoyam leaves are also used in cooking.

Plantain

This is not a root tuber but a member of the banana family. It can be eaten green (unripe) or ripe. Ripe plantain is often fried and served with rice, stewed beans and stew or omelettes. Plantain can be either shallow- or deep-fried. Fried plantain can be served at any meal. Green plantain is common in Efik cookery, roasted (eaten with palm oil), boiled and eaten with stewed beans, or cooked as pottage.

Green leafy vegetables

Green leafy vegetables form the basis of most Nigerian cookery, in soups or pottages. The ones most commonly used can be found growing wild or cultivated in people's gardens. Most of these vegetables are unique to areas around the former eastern state of Nigeria. Some of these vegetables are listed below with their common (native) and botanical names.

Nutrition information

Vegetables are the main source of the ACE vitamins and minerals in the diet. Vitamin C (ascorbic acid) is widely found in fresh fruits and green leafy vegetables. However, in Nigerian cookery, vegetables cannot be relied on to supply most of the vitamin C requirement, because they are often overcooked. Also the method of processing these vegetables before cooking almost completely destroys the vitamin content due to the oxidative reaction. For example, *afang* leaves are finely shredded and then pounded to tenderize them before adding to soup. Subsequently, what is left of the vitamin C and other nutrients are almost completely destroyed in the processes of sun- or oven-drying the vegetable for export to friends and family. The vitamin C content of the dried vegetable can be improved by using fresh or frozen spinach to cook the soup in the absence of fresh waterleaves. This applies to all the dried vegetables Nigerians use in making soup.

Afang (okazi) (Gnetum africanum)

Afang is a tough, very dark, green leafy vegetable with a strong aroma which is released when cooked. It is a climbing stem which grows wild in the rainforest of the Cross River state but can now be cultivated at home. The vegetable is used in cooking the popular *afang* soup. This vegetable is a rich source of calcium, iron and vitamins especially vitamins A (beta-carotene), E and C, although some of the vitamin C content is destroyed in the process of shredding and pounding/blending or drying.

Afang is often cooked with waterleaves to soften the texture. This vegetable is now available in African and Asian shops in the UK in its fresh, frozen or dry form. Fresh leaves are available on certain market days in shops in areas where there is a large Nigerian community. Fresh spinach or waterleaves increase the nutritional value of the dry leaves.

Atama leaves (Beletientien)

This is an annual herb cultivated in the delta and Cross River areas. It is usually added fresh or dried to *trofai* to make *abak/banga* soup. Dried leaves are used sparingly as the flavour is more intense. It is not readily available but can be found in some Nigerian food shops.

Bitterleaf (Vernonia amygdalina)

This vegetable is commonly found in areas around the eastern part of Nigeria where it is very popular. It is a shrub and is grown in almost every home. It is very bitter and has to be washed in a special way to get rid of some of the bitterness. It is often cooked with *egusi* (melon seed). The leaves have great nutritional value and it is claimed to have herbal and medicinal values too.

Cocoyam leaf (Xanthosoma sagittifolium)

This is the tender leaf of the cocoyam. It is broad and pale green in colour. There are two varieties. The leaves from the pink variety are suitable for cooking and preparing *ekpangnkukwo* because it does not irritate the throat when eaten (an allergic reaction), so always look for this variety. It can be identified by the thin black edge round the whole leaf.

Etinkeni leaf (uzouza)

This is an aromatic vegetable which is rarely used on its own. It is often used in *okro*, *ibaba*, pepper soups, etc., as a flavour enhancer.

Ewedu/Cring-cring (Corchorus olitorius)

Ewedu is a soft-textured green leafy vegetable. It is viscous (sticky) like okro and is often cooked with it. However, it is best cooked with fresh fish and other seafoods. This vegetable is widely available in African and Asian food shops.

Soko (Celosia argentea)

This green leafy vegetable is much preferred in the making of *efo-riro*. It tastes like spinach.

Okro (Okra, ladies' fingers, Hibiscus esculentus)

This is a curved seed pod and is best eaten when young and tender. It is very popular and Nigerians use it in most soups or in pottages to give variety and texture. Okro is widely available and the easiest vegetable to buy in the UK.

Spinach (Spinacia oleracea)

Nigerian spinach is different from European spinach in colour, size and taste. This spinach has pale green leaves and a long thin stalk. It has a very strong flavour. It is commonly used to prepare palm oil rice, or served as a boiled vegetable with yam, rice or plantain. It also features prominently in pottages and *egusi* soup.

Ugu (fluted pumpkin leaves, Telfaria occidentalis)

This dark-green leafy vegetable is grown mainly in the south-eastern part of Nigeria.

Although it has the same name as the European/American pumpkin, it is quite different. The difference lies in the fact that the leaves are eaten whilst the seed are often eaten as snacks. The seeds are found in the large segmented pod, which is completely white when mature. The leaves are eaten when still young and tender. The pumpkin seeds are eaten boiled or dried. This vegetable is the basic ingredient of the famous *edikang ikong* soup.

Waterleaves (Talinum triangulare)

As the name indicates, this has very high water content. It is very soft and slimy when cooked. Waterleaves should always be cooked with other vegetables where it acts as a softening agent for tough vegetables. It is rich in iron, calcium and vitamins A and C.

Ogbono (bush mango seed, Irvingia gabonensis)

This seed is commonly found in the eastern part of Nigeria. The fruit is edible and the seed is found by splitting open the shell. When fresh the seed is white inside with a light-brown outer covering. It becomes sticky and slimy like okro when in contact with water. It has a high fat content. It performs the same function in soups as okro but its main characteristics are its strong flavour and stickiness.

Egusi/Ikon (melon seed)

A high-fat/high-protein seed used as a thickening agent for West African soups (*egusi* soup).

Herbs and spices

Herbs and spices are commonly used in Nigerian cooking as they are considered to have high medicinal values. They are mainly used as flavour enhancers in pepper soups and pottages. The aroma helps to tempt invalids and new mothers to eat, thereby increasing food and nutrient intake.

Iko (basil)

This is a favourite herb and has an aromatic flavour similar to basil. It is used in flavouring soups. The shrub is grown in almost every garden in the Cross River state. It can also be found in Nigerian shops in London.

Ntong (mint)

This herb is grown widely and can be found in the garden of almost every home. It is used to flavour pepper soups and pottages. Fresh mint can be found occasionally in Nigerian shops but the dry leaves are more commonly found. Most sources are brought in from Nigeria as a present.

Hot fresh chilli pepper

Many varieties are grown in West Africa. The most popular one is the fat and segmented variety. This pepper is very hot with a spicy aroma. The yellow variety is hotter with a stronger aroma than the red variety. The pepper is green when young but turns yellow or red when mature. Other varieties are either long and thin or short and thin. They can be used fresh when green or dry (dry chilli pepper). It is very hot when dry, so is used sparingly.

Mfri etinkeni

This is the fruit of the *etinkeni* plant. The fruit grows in clusters and is golden-brown in colour. It is slightly hot with a strong aroma just like the leaves. It is used in flavouring traditional soups and pepper soups. It is ground into very smooth paste if fresh before use, and used sparingly.

Nutmeg (Myristica officinalis)

Nutmeg is the inner kernel of the fruit of *Myristica officinalis*. It is an aromatic spice, stimulating to taste. It is commonly used in flavouring stews, cakes, soups and drinks.

Oyim efik

This spice is native to tropical Asia. It is used in some traditional recipes and native medicine. It is like garlic with a strong flavour and so is used sparingly.

Utazi leaves (Crongromena ratifolia)

This is a bitter, pale green leaf, usually used for flavouring pepper soup. Very sparingly used. It can also be used as a substitute for bitter leaves.

Common cooking oils

Fats and oils are either saturated or unsaturated. Saturated oils, such as butter, coconut and palm oil, are known to increase the amount of cholesterol in the blood, but since regional cuisine is characterized by the type of oil used, lesser quantities in a given recipe could be used. It is not advisable to tell a Nigerian not to use palm oil because they will ignore the advice. It is better to recommend the

quantity to use so that they can make an informed choice.

Groundnut oil

Groundnut oil is made from groundnuts (peanuts). This is the most common cooking oil in Nigeria and is often used in cooking stews and frying. It has a strong and distinctive aroma which distinguishes it from other cooking oils. This oil has a high polyunsaturated fat content and so is healthier than palm oil.

Palm oil

This is a bright orange-red oil extracted from the fruit of the oil palm tree. There is no substitute for it. It is high in saturated fat which can cause heart disease, so use sparingly in cooking. However, this is highly favoured cooking oil and large quantities are used. In fact, it is perceived that some vegetable soups and other foods cooked with it taste better when saturated in palm oil. The oil is rich in beta-carotene, which is converted to vitamin A in the body. Palm oil is easily available in most African-Caribbean and Asian shops. Good quality oil is semi-liquid at room temperature and easily mixed when shaken vigorously. Some may be hard in very cold weather. Avoid oil that is light yellow because it might be rancid.

Palm fruit sauce/stock

This is made by boiling palm fruit until soft which is then drained and pounded in a mortar until the pulp comes away from the nut. It is then mixed with water, drained in a sieve and the sauce used in cooking soup. Trofai is a natural palm fruit sauce produced and canned in Ivory Coast. It has the nutritional properties of palm fruit and should therefore be used sparingly.

6.1.5 Nutritional and health implications in Nigeria and the UK

Obesity

One outstanding Nigerian cultural practice which impacts on a woman's health is the 'Fattening Room'. This is an important practice among the Efiks of Cross River state. Culturally the Efiks see 'fatness' as a sign of beauty, good health and wealth. This is depicted in the cultural practice

Table 6.1.6   Glossary of Nigerian food terms

Food	Description of food
Crayfish	Smoked dried prawns or shrimps used for flavouring soups and savoury dishes. Usually sold whole or grinded.
Dates	Dates are the berry fruits of the date palm of the palm family (Palmae, arecaceae) The sweet, soft varieties (fruit dates) are exported and are eaten raw, while dried dates are highly odour-sensitive and should be stored in an odour-free vicinity.
Ekpang-nkukwo	Traditional Efik dish made with grated cocoyam/water yam, wrapped in cocoyam leaves and cooked with crayfish powder, meat, fish, palm oil, etc.
Foofoo/Fufu	Traditional African food made by boiling starchy foods like cassava, yam, plantain or rice, then pounding them into a dough-like mass and eaten with soup. *Fufu* can also be made with flour from these foodstuffs.
Fura de Nono	Traditional northern Nigerian drink made with fermented millet and full-fat milk and sugar.
Gari	Made from cassava that has been peeled, grated, fermented and dry fried into rough flour which can be made into *fufu* or pudding.
Garden eggs	Also knows as African eggplant a member of the aubergine family. A round shiny green, white or yellow fruit with a slightly bitter taste. Garden eggs are eaten raw as a fruit or diced and added to stews.
Kulikuli	Peanut biscuit, popular northern snack.
Kaun/Akang rock Salt/akang or potash	Usually added to food especially pulses during cooking for faster tenderization and to increase the viscosity in okro and ewedu sauce. Also used for emulsifying oil and water in some soups.
Kuka leaves	Leaves of the baobab tree usually sold dried in powder form and used for kuka soup.
Lucozade	A sparkling drink formulated with glucose syrup, a carbohydrate that provides a concentrated, well-tolerated and readily absorbed source of food. It is a high-energy soft drink.
Millet	Tiny yellow grains obtained from a plant that looks like a bullrush with maize-like stalk. Grows widely in northern Nigeria and used mostly for porridge and gruel.
Ogbono (bush mango seed)	Has a slimy consistency when mixed with water. It is used as a thickening agent in soups.
Ogi (pap)	Porridge made from fermented cornmeal or millet, similar to custard or corn flour in consistency when prepared with hot water and milk.
Porridge	Oatmeal cooked in water.
Pottage	Dish made by cooking tuber, meat, vegetables, etc., together into a thick consistency.
Suya	Hot and spicy barbecued beef, mutton or chicken.
Snail	These are large forest creatures covered with a hard shell. Taste rubbery when overcooked. It is an acquired taste.
Sorghum	Also known as guinea corn, sorghum is cultivated mainly in northern Nigeria. Used for porridge or pap (gruel).
Utazi leaves	This is a bitter pale green leaf usually used for flavouring pepper soup. Very sparingly used. It can also be used as a substitute for bitter leaves.
Ube pear	Native African pear. Grows in south-eastern Nigeria. It is a pink fruit when young, but turns black when ripe. It has to be dipped in hot water or coal to soften it before eating. Tastes like avocado pear.
Yoghurt	Food made with milk that has been thickened with bacteria.

of fattening a young girl before marriage and after the birth of her first baby. To the authors knowledge, this practice is not observed in UK or by enlightened Nigerians because they are aware of the impact that overweight and obesity have on health. Traditionalist in the villages may still practise the 'fattening' tradition on young girls, but the duration of confinement and degree of fatness will depend on the wealth of the family (Ana, 2000).

Obesity and overweight have become major health problems threatening the developing world, and one of the greatest health challenges and risk factor for chronic non-communicable diseases (NCD) such as diabetes mellitus, cardiovascular disease and hypertension worldwide. Recent surveys have demonstrated an alarming increase in the prevalence of obesity in children and adolescents in many countries. This is attributed to increased consumption of refined foods and snacks and decreased physical activity. This has important implications for the physical and emotional health of adolescents, and it also increases the risk of continuing obesity and the development of chronic diseases in adulthood (WHO, 1981; DH, 2006; Ameen & Fawole, 2007).

Coronary heart disease

Coronary heart disease was previously reported to be relatively uncommon among Nigerians in spite of a high prevalence of hypertension. Recent studies have reported increasing occlusive coronary heart disease in Nigerians, especially among elderly, affluent and hypertensive patients exposed to western diets and habits. A similar trend has been reported in other developing countries where diets and lifestyles appear similar to those of the developed countries (National Heart, Lung and Blood Institute, 1994; WHO, 2002; Ameen & Fawole, 2007).

Studies in various parts of the world indicate that people who habitually consume a diet high in plant foods have lower risks of atherosclerotic cardiovascular diseases, probably largely because such diets are usually low in animal fat and cholesterol, both of which are established risk factors for atherosclerotic cardiovascular diseases (INTERSALT, 1988; WHO, 1990; Thomas & Bishop, 2007).

Traditionally, south-eastern Nigerians eat a diet rich in leafy vegetables. However, the preparation and cooking methods, and the use of dried vegetables in soups (by those who live abroad), due to lack of traditional fresh leafy vegetables, reduce the availability of the nutrients especially water-soluble vitamins. Nigerian diets tend to be high in sodium and low in potassium due to the inadequate consumption of fruits and vegetables. The INTERSALT study (INTERSALT Research Group, 1988) suggests that Blacks take less potassium, apparently due to low intakes of fruits and vegetables. Recent studies have shown that a diet containing approximately 75 mEq of potassium (approximately 3.5 g of elemental potassium) daily may contribute to reduced risk of stroke (Claude & Lardoinois, 1995; Akinkugbe, 1996; WHO, 2002) which is especially common among Blacks and older people of all races. Therefore, eating vegetables and fruits, especially bananas which are high in potassium, would help to improve the dietary intake of this mineral. Generally, most Nigerians do not eat fruit as part of their everyday diet. Fruits, though abundant, are quite expensive in the cities but are left to rot in the rural villages. Health education should concentrate on encouraging Nigerians – and especially children – both at home and abroad to eat more fruit and vegetables.

Foods high in fats and foods high in sugar

Fats and oils are used liberally in Nigerian dishes for omelettes, soups and stews. Even the amount of margarine and sugar used in pastry recipes is extremely high when compared with common European recipes. Reducing total fat intake is very important with regard to heart disease and weight management and control, bearing in mind Nigerians' high body mass index and waist circumference index (DH, 2006).

Suggestions for the way forward

This high prevalence is seen as a major contributory factor to the higher prevalence of hypertension, diabetes and stroke (DH, 2006) which is a major health burden for the National Health Service.

Traditionally, Nigerians enjoy their foods. They also like to 'see some flesh on their bones', hence the increased prevalence in overweight and obesity, especially among the older generation.

Meat, fish and alternatives form a very important part of the Nigerian diet. Nigerians, especially the affluent ones, enjoy a diet high in meat and fat; they also prefer full-cream and condensed milk, and consume more eggs, sweets and salty snacks. Excessive intake of these foods increases the risk of certain cancers and coronary heart disease (WHO, 1981; INTERSALT, 1988; National Heart, Lung and Blood Institute, 1994). Reducing the quantity of meat consumed and the liberal use of palm and coconut oil may be a way forward in improving the Nigerian diet.

Nigerians also attach importance to the amount of food on their plate. Giving a guest a small portion is seen as parsimony. Therefore, filling the plate to the brim is often expected, even in restaurants, otherwise customers are driven away. It is therefore important to encourage this target group to attend the basic 'Healthy Eating' awareness workshops, emphasizing the need to reduce carbohydrate and protein portion sizes, reduce salt/sugar/fat intake and introduce healthier cooking methods and some form of physical activity into their lifestyle.

Traditionally, taking exercise is not common, but Nigerians enjoy dancing, which is a good form of exercise. Introducing this as an activity in local community centres may attract them to join some of the healthy living activities available.

6.1.6   Nutritional support

> **Key points**
>
> - Food should be the first step in treating malnutrition.
> - Religious and cultural beliefs should be considered when formulating a care plan for nutrition support.
> - Patient and family involvement aids compliance and can improve the efficacy of nutrition support.

Modification of traditional diet to improve food intake

Nutrition status can be compromised if there is decreased dietary intake, increased nutrition requirements or an impaired ability to absorb or utilize nutrients (Thomas & Bishop, 2007). This can be for a number of reasons, including being physically unable to feed oneself (e.g., in dementia), a symptom of disease (e.g., nausea) or the effect of treatment (e.g., poor appetite/sore mouth).

Following assessment with a suitable screening tool such as the MUST (BAPEN http://www.bapen.org.uk/musttoolkit.html) and the cause of poor intake identified, measures should be taken to address the problem. There is a variety of options available, with modification of diet usually the first approach, as long as an oral intake is not contraindicated. This could be by increasing the amount eaten with small, regular snacks given in addition to meals, or by ensuring the small amounts that are eaten are nutrient- and/or energy-dense. A balanced diet should be encouraged, though less emphasis should be placed on limiting high-calorie foods and drinks (National Advisory Group for Elderly People, 2001).

Food fortification

Increasing the energy and nutrient density of foods and drinks can be achieved using ordinary foods or commercially prepared products which are available on prescription. Simply altering the energy and nutrient density can ensure the volume of the end product remains the same, which is beneficial if there are problems with nausea or poor appetite.

Commercially prepared products can be expensive and should be used as a last resort. Using ordinary household foods to enrich everyday foods is often more acceptable to patients and not seen as medication. Table 6.1.7 lists some practical ways of increasing protein and energy intakes in patients of Nigerian origin.

Sip feeds and religious restrictions

There is a variety of sip feeds on the market and they are divided into two main categories – milk-based and fruit-based. While they can be beneficial in improving nutritional status, they are supposed to supplement food intake and not replace meals. If there are issues with lactose intolerance, then fruit-based sip feeds should be used. If the patient has diabetes, then fruit-based sip feeds and other glucose-based supplements should be used with caution and closely monitored.

Table 6.1.7 Food fortification for Nigerian diets

Food group	Examples	Practical aspects
Starchy carbohydrates	Yam, plantain, rice, yam flour, ground rice, cassava flakes (*gari*)	Use cooking methods requiring oil/fat Add vegetable oil to ground rice/yam flour Add margarine/butter to rice Use slightly more oil than usual in preparation of soups served with these (preferably healthier fats) and other dishes based on these
Meat, fish and other sources of protein	Lamb, beef, chicken, offal, fish, black-eyed beans, *egusi*	Use cooking methods requiring oil/fat Fry fish or meat Black-eyed beans made into fritters are a good snack
Milk and dairy foods	Milk, yoghurts, cheese	Use full-fat versions, e.g., full-fat milk with cereal Evaporated and condensed milk can also be used to make hot drinks
Fruit and vegetables	Ugu, okazi, spinach	Use slightly more oil than usual in preparation of soups containing these (preferably healthier fats)
Fatty and sugary foods and drinks	Lucozade, super malt and nourishment drinks Plantain chips	These should be offered between meals as snacks

In addition to a patient's medical condition, their religious and cultural beliefs play an important role in determining the type of sip feed chosen. For example, a Nigerian Muslim would require products without pork-derived ingredients; similarly, vegetarians (some of whom may be Jehovah's Witnesses or Seventh Day Adventists) would require products without animal-derived ingredients (NHS Education for Scotland, 2007). Awareness of a patient's religious and cultural beliefs is important and should therefore be discussed sensitively as part of the assessment as these can and will influence the type of sip feed used.

Enteral feeding and religious beliefs

Enteral nutrition provides nutrients into the gastrointestinal tract through a tube. Enteral feeding should be considered where oral intake is contraindicated, or insufficient, but the patient's gastrointestinal system is fully functional (NICE, 2006). As the prevalence of hypertension and CVA remains high in patients of Nigerian origin (DH, 2006), enteral feeding post-CVA due to swallowing difficulty may be indicated. Other indications would be increased nutritional requirements for renal disease which could be caused by hypertension or diabetic nephropathy.

The need for enteral feeding, as well as the expected outcomes of the intervention, should be explained to the patient and carers. Length of feeding will determine the route used. Regular input from the dietitian or nutrition support team should prevent any problems and provide solutions to any that may arise. As for sip feeds, choice of feed should take into account the patient's religious/cultural beliefs which are likely to be important, especially if end-of-life issues arise.

Evidence of good practice

There are no specific studies addressing nutrition support in people of Nigerian origin and so good practice guidelines for the general population will apply to this group. Providing sample or starter packs is a good way to prevent waste and reduce costs. Avoidance of repeat prescriptions can also help to prevent waste especially if sip feeds are no longer needed, as well as preventing taste fatigue. Providing a variety of flavours and types of supplement can also prevent taste fatigue and aid patient compliance. Likewise, regular monitoring will ensure that the intervention is effective and enable its aims to be met.

Suggestions for the way forward

Patient preferences need to be taken into account when putting together a nutrition support package. Explaining the rationale behind the chosen nutrition support option(s) to the patient (and, with their permission, to their family) will not only aid compliance but will enable them to feel they are participating in their treatment as well as having a say in how it is carried out. It will also help family and friends express their care to the patient in a helpful and acceptable way as Nigerian culture is traditionally family- and community-oriented and, in many instances, food is specially prepared for loved ones during illness and convalescence.

6.2　Ghanaian Diet

Susanna Johnson

Key points

- The official language is English, but there are many other native languages and dialects.
- The majority (69%) of the population are Christians, 16% are Muslim and some combine the Christian and Muslim faiths in a religion called Zetahil, which is only found in Ghana. Other religions practised in Ghana include Rastafarian, Buddhism and Judaism. There are many religious festivals.
- A traditional meal usually consists of a large portion of starchy foods (e.g., banku and fufu) eaten with a thick stew or soup, often containing meat, fish or groundnuts.
- Many first- and some second-generation Ghanaians eat in the traditional way, by taking a small amount of starchy food in their fingers and dipping it into the stew or soup.
- There have been attempts to review the prevalence of obesity and diabetes among Ghanaians in Africa, Europe and North America, however no studies have been reported. Often data are combined under 'Black African', where increased rates of obesity, cardiovascular disease and diabetes are reported.

6.2.1　Introduction

Ghana is situated in western Africa, on the Gulf of Guinea bordering the North Atlantic between Togo and Côte d'Ivoire (Ivory Coast). It is only a few degrees north of the Equator and as a result has tropical climate Figure 6.2.1.

The current population stands at approximately 23 million of whom 99.8% are Black African. There are many different cultural groups within Ghana depending on the area of the country. The main ethnic/tribal groups are the Akan, Mole-Dagamba, Ewe and Ga-Dangme, although no region is ethnically homogeneous. Like London, all the urban areas are ethnically mixed due to migration from the rural areas to the major cities (www.ghanaweb.com/GhanaHomePage/tribes).

Language

The official language is English, but many native languages and dialects are spoken too.

Migration to the United Kingdom

Well before the commencement of the slave trade, the movement of people around Africa was a way of life. The Trans-Saharan trade routes linked the region to other parts of Africa, permitting the inter-regional movement of traders, scholars and clerics (Anarfi *et al.*, 2003; Bump, 2006). The arrival of Europeans in the 15th century disrupted the traditional patterns, a process exacerbated by the slave trade, which peaked during the 18th century. It is estimated that up to 12 million Africans were transported to the western hemisphere between 1450 and 1850 as forced migrants. Of these, it is estimated that 6.3 million were West African of whom approximately 4.5 million where shipped to North and South America between 1701 and 1810 at a rate of 5,000 a year from the Gold Coast and the coastal region composed of modern-day Ghana, Togo and Benin (Bump, 2006). The slaves took with them their traditions and customs, including dietary habits which are still evident today, for the diet of West Africans has similarities to that consumed by African-Caribbeans and African-Americans. However, there are differences in both

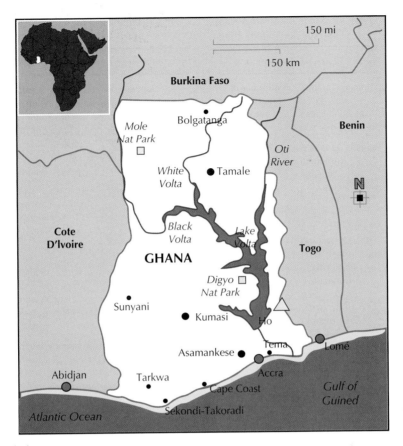

Figure 6.2.1 Map of Ghana

food choices and methods due to other ethnic influences and adaptations over the years. In the UK after the Second World War there was a shortage of manual workers and a recruitment drive was launched to encourage people from Commonwealth countries to migrate to the UK. Small numbers of Ghanaians – predominately students and professionals – had already moved to the UK and other Anglophone countries (Bump, 2006).

By 1874 the British had sole colonial power and had formally established the Gold Coast. The country adopted the name Ghana after becoming the first sub-Saharan African nation to gain independence from colonial rule in 1957.

Shortly after independence, Ghana's economy began to decline as a result of a series of coups which caused political instability. This in turn led to unemployment, shortages of food and medicine, and poor transportation, health and schooling. As a result many people moved to other African countries (e.g., Nigeria) as well as Europe and North America. By the mid-1990s it is estimated that 2–4 million Ghanaians (10–20% of the total population) were living abroad. They included not only professionals and students as before but also semi-skilled and unskilled workers. As a result of colonial ties, Ghanaians represent one of the UK's largest and oldest African migrant communities (Bump, 2006). Today Ghana is often highlighted as a nation struggling with the effects of a brain drain as many Ghanaians continue to emigrate to Europe, North America and other parts of Africa. Particularly in the last three decades, due to political, economic and social problems, there has been another exodus of Ghanaians searching for opportunities elsewhere. Like most African countries, their migration trends are deeply rooted in history (Bump, 2006).

Current UK population

In the 2001 census, the Black ethnic minority population of the UK was 4.6 million (7.9% of the total population). Black African comprised the third largest group, making up 0.8% of these (Thomas & Bishop, 2007). The actual number is unknown as the census categorizes people by continent – Black African – and not country of origin (Hamid & Sarwar, 2004). The number of Ghanaians migrating to the UK has increased steadily over the years. A 1991 census of England and Wales identified 32,277 people who were born in Ghana living in the UK. This had risen by 72% to 55,537 in 2001 (Bump, 2006).

6.2.2   Religion

Religion is an important aspect of the Ghanaian culture and migrants to the UK continue to adhere to their practices. Approximately 69% of the population in Ghana belong to the different Christian denominations (Roman Catholic, Methodist, Anglican, Presbyterian, Evangelical, Mennonite, Church of the Latter Day Saints, Seventh Day Adventist, Born-again Christian, Baptist, African Methodist, Episcopal, Zionist Christian and Lutheran). Some Christians incorporate elements of traditional beliefs into their practices. Sixteen per cent are Muslims, predominantly Sunni, who follow the Maliki version of Islamic law. There are also followers of the other two principal branches: Tijanis and Ahmadis. Other religions practised in Ghana include Rastafarianism, Baha'i, Buddhism, Judaism, Hare Krishna and Zetahil – the last a religion unique to Ghana which combines elements of Islam and Christianity (see Table 6.2.1).

Traditional indigenous beliefs

Traditional indigenous beliefs are practised by 8.5% of the population. Each ethnic group has its

Table 6.2.1   Religious dietary restriction

Religious group	Examples of sects	Dietary restrictions
Christians	Seventh Day Adventists	Alcohol, pork, fish without fins or scales and seafood. Many are vegetarians.
	Born-again Christians	Alcohol (excessive drinking)
Muslims	All	*Haram* foods (pork and seafood without fins or scales)
		Alcohol
		Halal food is permitted
Rastafarians	All	*I-tal* foods are permitted (food that is as pure as possible)
		Avoidance of meat (especially pork)
		Predominantly vegetarian but fish is eaten
		Alcohol, coffee, salt, tobacco ,seafood

own sets of beliefs, however they all believe in a supreme being and lesser gods who act as intermediaries between the supreme being and humankind. The Christian groups incorporate some indigenous traditional beliefs including veneration of ancestors. For example, many Christians will pour a libation of alcohol, water and sweet drinks to the ancestors on occasions such as funerals or the birth of a baby, asking for protection and for them to oversee the occasion. It is also known that Muslims pour libation too, however as alcohol is forbidden water and sweet drinks are used instead.

Religious tolerance is high in Ghana. Apart from the traditional festivals, all major important dates in their calendar are observed depending on one's religious background (e.g., Christmas and Easter for Christians; *Eid-al Fitr* for Muslims). As most of the population are Christians, the Christian dates that are bank holidays worldwide are also observed in Ghana.

Religious festivals

Ghana's culture is depicted in the many festivals that are held at different times of the year. They are held for a number of reasons, such as purification, thanksgiving, ancestral veneration, reunion and dedication. They also cover rites of passage (childbirth, puberty, marriage and death). Highlights of some of these festivals include drumming, dancing, skill contests and the firing of musketry. During these gatherings, in addition to certain foods being used and included in the festival, a vast variety of different dishes and snacks will be prepared for participants and guests.

Aboakyir (deer hunting)

Aboakyir is based on two hunting groups who are sent out to catch a live antelope. The first group to present its catch to the chief at a colourful durbar is declared the winner and is highly regarded for bravery (www.2gsu.edu/~finjws/emma.htm).

Homowo (harvest and thanksgiving)

This festival is celebrated by the Ga people of the greater Accra region in August/September. It commemorates an abundant harvest after a long, severe famine that occurred during the Ga people's migration to present-day Accra. The word *homowo* translates as 'hooted at hunger' (www.ghanaweb.com/GhanaHomePage/tribes/homowo_festival.php). Ceremonies for this festival include processions of chiefs through the principal streets, together with the sprinkling of festive food (*kpokpoi*) to the gods and ancestors of the state. *Kpokpoi* is made from fermented steamed maize and has the texture of couscous. It is consumed with palm nut soup made with fish (Hamid & Sarwar, 2004).

Dipo

This is a puberty festival celebrated by the Krobo people in the eastern region. *Dipo* is also known as the puberty rites and it initiates adolescent girls into womanhood. The *Dipo* girls are covered from the waist to the knees with the upper part of the body decorated with colourful and assorted beads. Exposing their breasts for everyone to see signifies that they are moving into adulthood.

The girls go through a series of rituals, including tasting various foods (e.g., sugar cane and peanuts) and having their feet washed in the blood of a goat

that the girl's family are required to slaughter and present to ward off bad omens that may prevent the girls from having children in the future. Libations are commonly poured (www.travel-to-discover-ghana.com).

Bakatue (fish harvesting)

Bakatue translates as 'the opening of the lagoon' or 'draining of the lagoon' and occurs mainly in the western region. It commemorates the founding of the town of Elmina and to celebrate evoking a deity for the continuous protection of the state and its people. The festival involves a royal procession of chiefs and stool-holders in palanquins through the streets. Rituals are performed on the riverbank and this is followed by the pouring of sacred eggs and mashed yams mixed with palm oil into the lagoon. Prayers are offered to the river god for peace. A fishing net is then cast into the lagoon, after which permission is given to fishermen to open the fishing season following a ban (Hamid & Sarwar, 2004).

Religious festivals and foods

Some of the common foods eaten at special times of the year are also consumed together with a variety of local dishes. Many Ghanaians living in the UK (particularly the first generation) will incorporate both western and traditional dishes (see Table 6.2.2).

Beliefs related to food

Some of the ethnic groups have clan beliefs in which eating certain animals and plants are prohibited as they are regarded as sacred due to their cultural identity. The Ewe Tribal group of Ghana do not eat snails as they believe snails covered their trails during their escape from the wicked King Agadza of Dahomey (the peoples of Benin) (Hamid & Sarwar, 2004). Many of these practices are held by Ghanaians currently living in UK, particularly the first generation of migrants.

6.2.3   Traditional diet and eating pattern

Rice

- Plain boiled rice.
- Jollof: rice cooked in a spicy tomato stew to which vegetables, chicken or red meat can be added.

Table 6.2.2   Religious festivals and food

Religious group	Examples of special dates/ periods	Example of typical foods eaten in UK	Example of foods eaten in Ghana
Christians	Christmas	Roast turkey/ chicken/ duck/goose/ pork/beef Roast potatoes Vegetables (parsnips, brussels sprouts, carrots) Gravy, bread sauce, cranberry sauce	Roast turkey/ chicken/ mutton/ goat, duck, beef, fish Jollof rice, *waakye*, *kenkey*, roast potatoes, yam/cassava, Vegetables (e.g., carrots), gravy, spicy stews, and soups.
Muslims	*Iftar*	Fast is traditionally broken with dates and water	Fast is broken with dates and water
	Eid-Ul-adha	Whole lamb/beef is bought from the butchers ready butchered, prepared and is distributed to family, friends and mosques	Lamb/sheep is commonly sacrificed and many dishes are made from the meat (e.g., stews, soups, roasts) and distributed among family, friends, mosques and the poor,

- *Waakye*: rice cooked with black-eyed beans and a herb (dried rhubarb leaves) that colours the dish and gives it's signature reddish colour.

Rice can also be eaten as a breakfast. Water is added with sugar to make it like porridge. This is known as rice water.

Tubers

Yam
A starchy tuber which can be boiled or fried. Cocoyam is boiled, fried or pulped.

Sweet potato
A starchy tuber which can be boiled, roasted or fried. It is commonly eaten as a fried snack.

Cassava
A starchy tuber which can also be boiled, fried or roasted.

Cassava can be dried and ground into a grainy flour called *gari*. This can be added to soups and used as a thickening agent.

Gari can be eaten as a breakfast food (sugar, water and evaporated milk are added).

Gari is also sprinkled on dishes including *waakye* and a stew cooked with black-eyed peas.

Plantain
Can be eaten ripe (when yellow) or green. Unripe it is usually boiled and served with a stew containing greens, meat and/or fish. It is also cut into thin strips and fried to make plantain chips, which are eaten as a snack.

Ripe plantain is usually boiled, fried or roasted and eaten as a snack or served with *waakye* or a rice dish.

Overripe plantains are mashed and made into dumplings that are deep-fried.

Corn/maize/maize meal

This is one of the most important staples for sub-Saharan Africans. Many starch-based components of a meal are made from cornmeal.

Corn-on-cob is either boiled or roasted and is a common roadside snack, eaten with a piece of coconut.

Most cornmeal-based dishes are made from fermented cornmeal. Fermenting is done by leaving covered dampened cornmeal in a room for 2–3 days. Fermentation takes place using the natural yeast found in the corn. To make a type of porridge it is cooked with water and sugar and eaten at breakfast.

It is commonly made into dumplings (*banku* and *kenkey*). *Banku* is made by cooking fermented cornmeal on a stove where it is continuously stirred to form a glutinous dumpling. *Kenkey* is partly cooked cornmeal mixed with uncooked, fermented cornmeal and then wrapped in dried corn leaves or banana leaves and steamed. Some shops specializing in Ghanaian foods sell ready-made *kenkey*.

Fermenting cornmeal is laborious. Many first-generation migrants use ground rice as an alternative. Ground rice is mixed with water and vinegar and cooked over the stove, stirring continuously to form dumplings. In the UK ready fermented cornmeal is available.

Abolo/ablo
This is a dumpling made from ground rice or maize meal to which yeast or baking powder is added. The mixture is then left to ferment and rise then made into dumplings that are wrapped in banana leaves or foil and then steamed.

Fufu
Fufu is a dumpling made from pounding and beating cooked plantain, cassava, cocoyam and yam.

Making *fufu* is arduous as it involves pounding the ingredients with a large pestle and mortar until a glutinous consistency is achieved and then forming it into dumplings.

Ready-made flours are readily available in the UK. They can be mixed with water and cooked over the stove. Before these became available, many Ghanaians living in the UK made (and still make) *fufu* from farina (potato starch) and instant mashed potato.

Fufu is commonly eaten with soups made from groundnuts (peanuts), palm nut and tomato.

Bread (sugar bread)
Bread is made from flour with sugar added to have a slightly sweeter taste. It is usually eaten with margarine and/or egg at breakfast or served with tea or coffee.

Vegetables and fruits

Vegetables
Commonly eaten vegetables include 'Garden eggs' (white aubergine), pumpkin, okra, greens, tomatoes, corn, onions, chillies. Cucumbers, lettuce and carrots are grown and also used in salads.

Greens are the collective name for various leafy green vegetables commonly used in soups and stew. They include cassava leaves, *aloma* (bitter leaf), jute (West African sorrel), callaloo, cocoyam leaves (*kotomle*) and spinach.

Okra is a very common vegetable and is native to Africa. It is chopped up and added to a tomato-based soup to which fish or meat is added or it is served whole in stew and soups.

Tomatoes are the base of most stew and soup dishes eaten in Ghana. Chillies, spices, herbs, onions, garlic, ginger and other vegetables are added.

Fruits
There is a large variety of tropical fruits in Ghana – pineapple, mangoes, avocado, oranges, pawpaw, guava, passion fruit, watermelons, grapefruit to name just a few. They grow wild, in people's gardens and now are also cultivated. Fruit is not regarded as an important part of the day-to-day food intake and is often eaten as a snack.

Meat, fish, eggs, beans, nuts and seeds
Chicken, mutton/lamb, pork, eggs, beef, goat, fish (dried and fresh), shellfish, snails, offal (tripe and liver), bush meat, duck and corned beef are commonly eaten. Fresh poultry and meats tend to be stewed or fried and then added to stews and soups or roasted/fried/barbecued and served as a side-dish.

Fish and seafood commonly eaten include snapper, tilapia, red and grey mullet, mackerel, sardines, sea bream, barracuda, doctor fish, *tsele* (smoked fish), tuna (fresh, smoked, tinned), *khobi* (dried salted fish), prawns, crab and dried shrimps. They are also added to stews and soups or fried or baked and served with a starchy food and salsa-type condiment (made from ground chillies, onions and tomatoes).

Tinned fish, including sardines and pilchards, are also commonly eaten.

Fish provides a large proportion of protein source to Ghanaians. Fresh fish is predominantly consumed in the coastal regions and dried and smoked fish in the central, land-locked regions.

Smoked, salted and dried fish (used as a traditional means of preserving fish) are common in a lot of dishes and now tend to be added for flavour. They are available in the UK from specialist shops.

Dried fish (e.g., anchovies) are made by drying fresh fish outdoors. Dried salted fish (e.g., *khobi*) is made by placing the fish in salt and then leaving to dry outdoors.

Fish is smoked in a *chorko*. This is a rectangle clay oven divided into two compartments. Trays of fresh fish are either 'wet' hot-smoked or 'dry' hot–smoked. Wet hot-smoking takes 1–2 hours and the fish has a short shelf-life (1–3 days), while dry hot-smoking takes 10–18 hours. As a result most of the moisture evaporates which gives the fish a much longer shelf life of 6–9 months.

Eggs are either boiled or fried and eaten at breakfast, or added to salads or a tomato-based stew to which corned beef has been added.

Black-eyed beans are cooked with rice, added to stew or boiled plain and served with *gari*, stew or palm nut oil, and/or fried plantain.

Kidney beans, red beans and white beans are boiled and ground with spices (chilli, ginger), onion and garlic.

Groundnuts (peanuts) are ground to make soups or roasted or boiled in salted water and eaten as a snack.

Pumpkin seeds (*egusi*) are ground and added to greens and spinach dishes.

Milk and dairy foods

Evaporated and tinned milk is commonly used in Africa and added to tea and some breakfast dishes such as rice water (rice boiled to the consistency of porridge and sweetened).

Ice cream is eaten as a treat.

Ghanaians can have varying degrees of lactose intolerance. Milk and other dairy products were not consumed by first-generation people as it was not commonly eaten in Ghana. Today first-generation Ghanaians commonly incorporate small amounts of dairy products in their diet. This includes fresh milk, cheese and yoghurt. Dairy products are more commonly tolerated in the second generation born and brought up in the UK.

Foods containing fats and/or sugars

Fats and oils

Vegetable oil, palm oil, groundnut oil, coconut oil, sunflower oil and margarine are the main oils consumed.

Stew and soup dishes are cooked with one or more of the oils.

Palm nut oil is commonly used for flavour as well as colour and is commonly used in stews made of greens and okra soup. Margarine is spread on bread.

Sugary foods

The main sources are sugar, honey, fruit juices and fizzy drinks. Although Ghana is a cocoa grower, chocolate is not eaten in large quantities. Cakes, biscuits and African doughnuts are eaten as snacks.

Supermalt (a sweet malted drink) is a favourite with the old and young.

Traditional eating patterns

Eating is a communal affair among Ghanaians. Meal patterns vary with the individual or family. Ghanaians either eat together as a whole family or adults eat together and children eat together.

Most people have three meals a day, although it is not uncommon for some to omit lunch and have a large meal in the evening. A traditional meal usually consists of a large portion of starchy foods eaten with a thick stew or soup. Large quantities of stews and/or soups are cooked so that they last for a few days, but some starchy foods are made daily (e.g., *banku*, *fufu*). As traditional dishes can take time to prepare they are more likely to be eaten in the evening and at weekends and leftovers eaten as lunch during the weekday. Desserts are not usually served after a main meal; instead, sweet foods are eaten as a treat or snack. Many stew and soup dishes have meat, fish, poultry and/or vegetables and often oil is added and they are highly seasoned and spicy.

Many of the first-generation and some second-generation Ghanaians continue to eat in the traditional way, by taking a small amount of starchy food in their fingers and dipping it into the stew or soup.

Herbs and spices

Apart from tomatoes, chilli (fresh and ground), onion, shallots, garlic and ginger form the basis of spices used in many stews and soups. Chillies commonly used are scotch bonnet and bird's eye chillies.

Meats, poultry and fish are frequently marinated in spices before being cooked.

A variety of spices and seasonings are frequently used and include salt, peppercorns, stock cubes, curry powders, thyme, nutmeg, bay leaf, allspice, cayenne pepper, dried and ground shrimps, herring and anchovies.

Cooking methods

Stews and soups are made by slow cooking on the hob and all dishes tend to be cooked in the one-pot style. The starchy accompaniment (e.g., *fufu/banku*) is also prepared on the hob.

In Ghana, non-wealthy Ghanaians generally prepare food on a coal pot as well as most of the starches (rice, boiled starches, *banku*). *Fufu*, if prepared in the traditional method, is pounded using a large pestle and mortar. The coal pot is also used as a barbecue-type grill on which fish, chicken or red meat can be cooked.

6.2.4   Traditional eating patterns and dietary changes on migration

Many first- and second-generation families eat traditional foods but the second generations also choose from the western diet and have more reliance on takeaway and convenience foods. Many specialist food shops (Asian, African and African-Caribbean) sell imported traditional foods, making their availability a lot easier. Prior to this many migrants relied on friends or relatives to bring some of the rarer foods with them to the UK (See Table 6.2.3).

6.2.5   Prevalence of chronic diseases

There have been attempts to review the prevalence of obesity and diabetes among Ghanaians in Africa, Europe and North America, but no studies on Ghanaians or Nigerians in these areas have been reported (Abubakari & Bhopal, 2008). It has been well established, however, that the prevalence of chronic diseases in the ethnic minorities living in the UK is increasing. Over the past 30 years the highest death rates for stroke have been found in migrants from the Caribbean and Africa. They also had the higher prevalence of diabetes and impaired glucose intolerance. Africans were also found to have a higher prevalence of hypertension compared to any other migrant group investigated and hypertension. However, prevalence is lower in Ghana (Harding *et al.*, 2008).

Data specifically regarding Ghanaians are limited as many studies categorize people by continent (i.e., Black African) and not by country; furthermore, reliable national trend data are lacking. However, the prevalence of chronic diseases is becoming more evident and is increasing in many African countries.

Table 6.2.3   Traditional eating pattern in Ghana and dietary changes on migration to the UK

Meal	Traditional	Dietary changes on migration to UK and among second generation	Healthier alternatives
Breakfast	Cornmeal porridge Rice water Bread with margarine (with/without boiled/fried egg) Tea/coffee with evaporated/tinned milk *Kenkey*, fried fish and chilli/stews and soups	Breakfast cereal/porridge with fresh milk Toast with without jam, peanut butter English breakfast Fruit salad Tea with evaporated/tinned/fresh milk	Use semi-skimmed, skimmed or soya milk Low-fat evaporated milk Wholegrain cereals (e.g., Shredded Wheat, Weetabix, porridge) Whole meal bread Reduce sugar Fruit salad Use low-fat margarine Boil eggs rather than fry

(Continued)

Table 6.2.3 (cont'd)

Meal	Traditional	Dietary changes on migration to UK and among second generation	Healthier alternatives
Lunch	Rice dishes (e.g., jollof) with stews *Fufu* and soups *Banku/kenkey* with stews/soups Yam with stew Black-eyed beans with *gari* and stew	Sandwiches, crisps, fruit, pasta dishes, Takeaways (e.g., Indian, Chinese, burger and chips)	Use vegetable/olive oil Use less oil Have plain rice more frequently than jollof Include more vegetables Choose leaner cuts of meat Remove skin from poultry Have more meat-free days Avoid frying meats when making stew/soups Have *fufu* with light soup more frequently than groundnut or palm nut soup Control portion size (particularly of starchy carbohydrates)
Evening meal	As above	As evening meal. Although UK alternatives to *banku* made with ground rice are used. *Fufu* made with farina and mashed potato also used. Boiled potatoes also eaten with stews with greens/spinach stew. Also more commonly with younger people western foods (e.g., roast dinners, burger and chips, pasta dishes). Other ethnic foods (e.g., Indian, Chinese, Thai, Italian)	As above
Puddings/ desserts	Not commonly consumed	Fruit, ice creams, cakes, puddings, yoghurt	Enjoy occasionally Fruit, low-fat yoghurts
Snacks	Plantain (fried/roasted) Peanuts, fruit, ice cream, peanuts, corn, African doughnuts (deep-fried sweet dumpling), cakes, biscuits	Crisps, chocolates, fruit, peanuts and other nuts, crackers, plantain (fried/roasted), plantain chips cake, biscuits	Fruit (fresh and dried) Roast plantain Crackers Roasted corn Handful of plain roasted nuts
Alcoholic drinks	Traditional: Palm wine 7% alcohol by volume, Pito (millet wine) 5% alcohol by volume, akpeteshie (local gin) 40% alcohol by volume Gin, whisky, brandy, wines Beers, draughts	Traditional alcoholic drinks occasionally consumed more by first-generation migrants and for libation/festivals All types of alcoholic drinks available in the UK are consumed.	Keep within recommended units Use diet mixers

(Hamid & Sarwar, 2004)

Nutritional deficiencies

The risk of vitamin D deficiency in the UK population is generally low. It has been established that one of the groups at risk are minority ethnic groups where complete covering up is practised, usually in adult women of Asian (Thomas & Bishop, 2007) and African-Somali origin. (Maxwell *et al.*, 2006). Although no specific data regarding the UK Ghanaian population is available, vitamin D deficiency may be common in Ghanaians Muslim women.

Suggestions for the way forward

- Raise awareness of what healthy eating entails and appropriate portion sizes in relation to chronic disease.
- Target people with chronic diseases and roll out tailored education programmes.
- Raise awareness of the importance and benefits of physical activity, possibly implementing programmes in the community and have them audited.
- Offer education on the implications of obesity to counter the common belief that the bigger one is the better.
- A health survey of the Ghanaian population in the UK needs to be carried out to establish trends in health and so that appropriate action can be undertaken.

Websites

Nigerian Diet

www.ic.nhs.uk/pubs
en.wikipedia.org/NigerianBritish
www.ajcn.org/cgi/reprint/27/2/21
www.uni.edu/gai/Nigeria/Background/why_study_Nigeria.html
www.en.wikipedia.org/wiki/Geography_of_Nigeria
en.wikipaedia.org/wiki/British_Nigerian#population
enwikipedia.org/wiki/united_kingdom_census_2001

Ghanaian Diet

www.ghana.com
www.ghana-com.co.uk
www.ghanaweb.com

www.ghanaweb.com/GhanaHomePage/tribes/
www.nationsencyclopedia.com/Africa/Ghana-RELIGIONS.html
www.travel-to-discover-ghana.com/index.html
www.wikipedia.org/wiki/History_of_ghana
www.WHO.int
www.2gsu.edu/~finjws/emma.htm
www.bapen.org.uk/musttoolkit.html

Further reading

Nigerian Diet

Bowling, T. (ed.) (2004) *Nutritional Support for Adults and Children: A Handbook for Hospital practice.* Radcliffe Medical Press, Oxford.

Department of Health (2001) *Essence of Care: Patient-focused Benchmarking for Health-care Practitioners.* DH, London.

Ghanaian Diet

Matlon, S.M., Isles, C.G. & Higgs, A. (1986) Potassium supplementation in blacks with mild to moderate essential hypertension. *J. Hypertension*, 4, 61–4.

Nason, I. (1991) *Enjoy Nigeria: A Travel Guide.* Spectrum Books, Ibadan.

National Center for Health Statistics. Centers for Disease Control and Prevention (1998) *NHANES III Individual Foods Data File from the Dietary Recall Documentation.* Series 11(2A).

Ojofeitimi, E.O. & Smith I.F. (December 1988) Nutrition support and malnutrition in Nigeria. *Nutr Clin Pract*, 3(6), 242–5.

Okafor, J.C. (1979) Edible indigenous woody plants in the rural economy of the Nigerian forest zone. In D.U.U. Okali (ed.), *The Nigerian Rainforest Ecosystem (Proceedings of M.A.B. Workshop on the Nigerian Rainforest Ecosystem).* University of Ibadan, Nigeria.

Omolou, A. (1972). Malnutrition as a cause of death in children in Nigeria. *The Food & Nutrition Bulletin of the Joint FAO/WHO/OAU Regional Food & Nutrition Commission for Africa*, No. 11.

Shields, A. *Nigeria Background Information: Why Study Nigeria.* www.uni.edu/gai/Nigeria/Background/why_study_nigeria.html.

Shittu, T.A., Ogunmoyela, O.A. & Sanni, L.O, (1999) *Nutrient Retention and Sensory Characteristics of Dried Leafy Vegetables. Proceedings of the 23rd Annual Conference of the Nigerian Institute of Food Science and Technology*, Abuja, 130–2.

Sproston, K. & Mindell, J. (2004) *Health Survey for England. Vol. 1: The Health of Minority Ethnic Groups.* DH, London.

Stroud, M., Duncan, H. & Nightingale, J. (2003) Guidelines for enteral feeding in adult hospital patients. *Gut*, 52(Suppl. VII), vii–vii, 12.

References

Nigerian Diet

Akinkugbe, O.O. (1996) The Nigerian hypertension programme. *Journal of Human Hypertension*, 10(Suppl. 1), S43–6.

Ameen, L.O. & Fawole, O (2007) 1A.3. *Prevalence of Risk Factors for Cardiovascular Disease among Nigerian Youth.* Department of Medicine, UCH, Ibadan, Nigeria; Department of Epidemiology, Medical Statistics and Environmental Health, University of Ibadan, Nigeria. *American Journal of Clinical Nutrition* (1974) 27, 213–16.

Ana, A. (2000) *A Taste of Calabar.* Calabar, Nigeria.

Bygott, D. (1996) *Black and British.* Oxford University Press, London.

Claude, K. & Lardoinois, M.D. (1995) Nutritional factors and hypertension. *Arch Fam Med*, 4(8), 707–13.

Country Profile: Nigeria. Foreign and Commonwealth Office. en.wikipedia.org/wiki/Foreign_and_Commonwealth_Office

Department of Health (2006) *Health Survey for England – The Health of Minority Ethnic Groups 2004.* DH, London.

INTERSALT Cooperative Research Group (1988) INTERSALT; an international study of electrolyte excretion and blood pressure: result for 24 hr urinary sodium and potassium excretion. *British Medical Journal*, 297, 319–28.

National Heart, Lung and Blood Institute (March 1994) *Report of the Working Group on Research in Coronary Heart Disease in Blacks.* BHLBI, Bethesda, MD.

National Institute for Health and Clinical Excellence (2006) *Nutrition Support in Adults: Oral Nutrition Support, Enteral Tube Feeding and Parenteral Nutrition.* NICE, London.

NHS Education for Scotland (2007) *Multi-Faith Resource for Healthcare Staff: Spiritual Care.* Edinburgh.

Nutrition Advisory Group for Elderly People of the British Dietetic Association (2001) *Have You Got a Small Appetite? Your Guide To Eating Well.* BDA, London.

Ogbeide, O. (1974) Nutritional hazards of food taboos and preferences in Mid-West Nigeria. *American Journal of Clinical Nutrition*, 27, 213–16.

Thomas, B. & Bishop, J. (2007) *Manual of Dietetic Practice.* 4th edition. Blackwell, Oxford.

WHO (1981) *Prevention of Coronary Heart Disease. Report of a WHO Expert Committee on Prevention of CHD*, WHO, Geneva.

WHO (1990) *Diet, Nutrition and the Prevention of Chronic Diseases. Report of a WHO Study Group.* WHO, Geneva.

WHO (2002) *The World Health Report 2002 Reducing Risks, Promoting Healthy Life.* WHO, Geneva.

Ghanaian Diet

Abubakari, A. & Bhopal, R. (2008) Systematic review on the prevalence of diabetes, overweight/obesity and physical inactivity in Ghanaians and Nigerians. *Public Health*, 122, 173–82.

Anarfi, J., Kwankye, S., Ababio, O. & Tiemoko, R. (2003) *Migration from to Ghana: A Background Paper.* Development Research Centre on Migration, Globalisation & Poverty, Brighton.

Bump, M. (2006) *Ghana: Searching for Opportunities at Home and Abroad.* Institute for the Study of International Migration, Washington, DC.

Harding, S., Rosato, M. & Teyhan, A. (2008) Trends for coronary heart disease & stroke mortality among migrants in England & Wales 1979–2003: slow declines notable for some groups. *Heart*, doi:10.1136/hrt.2007.122044.

Health Survey for England 2004 (2006) *The Health of Minority Ethnic Groups: Summary of Key Findings.* DH, London.

Maxwell, S.M., Salah, S.M. & Bunn, J.E.G. (2006) Dietary habits of the Somali population in Liverpool, with respect to foods containing calcium and vitamin D: a cause for concern? *J Hum Nutr Dietet*, 19, 125–7.

Hamid, F. & Sarwar, T. (2004) *NHS Global Nutrition: The Republic of Ghana Diet* NHS Telford and Wrekin Primary Care Trust, Understanding Ethnic Communities – Working with African, African-Caribbean, Chinese & South Asian Communities, Telford.

Thomas, B. & Bishop, J. (2007) *Manual of Dietetic Practice.* 4th edition. Blackwell Sciences, Oxford.

7

East and South-East Europe

Elzbieta Szymula (Poland), Stavroulla Petrides (Greece), Thomina Mirza, Tahira Sarwar (Turkey)

The countries included in this section are Poland, Greece and Turkey. They have been chosen due to the high levels of migration to the UK from these countries. Much of the migration took place following the Second World War due to shortages of unskilled workers in the UK. The main religion of the Polish and Greek people is Christianity and for Turkey is Islam. Religion is important in these countries and celebrated with many festivals. The traditional diet of the Greek and Turkish people is the Mediterranean diet, which is high in starchy foods, oily fish, dairy foods, fruit and vegetables, with the major source of oil being olive oil. The traditional diet of Poland is high in saturated fat and very high levels of obesity are common. There is information on migration, traditional diets and changes on migration, religious influences and on dietary considerations for specific disease conditions such as obesity, diabetes and cardiovascular disease.

7.1 Polish Diet

Elzbieta Szymula

Key points

- Migration has often been for political, economic and labour-related reasons. There have been several waves of migration to the UK. The first followed the Second World War and the most recent (2004) after Poland's accession to the European Union.
- Poland is a devout country. Approximately 90% of the population are Roman Catholics. Religious observance is lower in younger generations.
- Obesity levels are high: over 50% of adults and 19% of children are either overweight or obese.
- The major (41%) cause of deaths is from cardiovascular diseases.
- Favourable changes in food composition and eating patterns have been seen since the early

Multicultural Handbook of Food, Nutrition and Dietetics, First Edition. Edited by Aruna Thaker, Arlene Barton.

1990s, including less consumption of saturated fat, increased consumption of unsaturated fat and increased intake of fruit and vegetables.
- Over time consumption of convenience food has increased and physical activity levels have dropped.

7.1.1   Introduction

Poland is located in Central Europe, bordered by Germany to the west, the Czech Republic and Slovakia to the south, Ukraine and Belarus to the east and the Baltic Sea, Russia and Lithuania to the north and north-east (Figure 7.1.1). Poland covers an area of 313,000 sq. km and is the ninth largest country in Europe. Poland has a population of 38.1 million people (GUS, 2007), of whom approximately 61% live in urban areas. After a period of stagnation, the population is currently (2007) increasing at a 0.03% natural increase rate (births less deaths) per year. However, the population is declining due to emigration (GUS, 2007). Poland became a member state of the European Union in May 2004 with Czech Republic, Estonia, Hungary, Latvia, Lithuania, Slovakia and Slovenia the so-called A8 group (HO, 2009).

Until the Second World War Poland was ethnically diverse. The Holocaust, and territorial changes after the war which led to forced migrations, changed the ethnic composition of the country so that today 98% of Poland's inhabitants are ethnic Poles. The remaining 2% are composed mainly of Ukrainians, Belarusians, Germans and to less extent Slovaks, Czechs, Russians, Lithuanians and Jews (MIA, 2009).

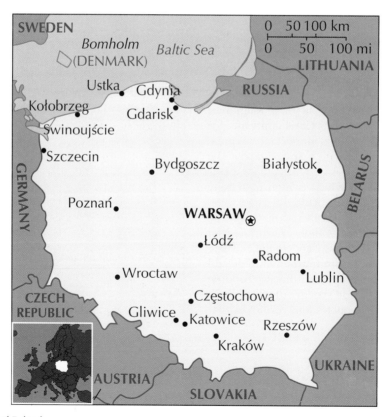

Figure 7.1.1   Map of Poland

Migration to the United Kingdom

The main reasons behind migration are political, economic and labour-related. There have been several waves of Polish migration to the UK during the last 70 years. The first was in the 1940s and 1950s and the second in the 1980s and 1990s. In 1981 martial law was declared, followed shortly afterwards by food rationing. This generated another wave of migration to the West. Postwar Poland was a communist regime until 1989 and many people escaped the regime by emigrating to the West. The third and most recent migration started in 2004, following Poland's accession to the European Union (EU). High unemployment (15–20%) throughout the 1990s until 2006 appears to have been the main reason for migration to the UK at this time (CRONEM, 2007).

Current UK population

It is difficult to establish the number of Poles living in UK due to a lack of statistical data. Some unofficial UK and Polish sources estimate that there are approximately 1 million Poles currently living in the UK. Official UK statistics show that between May 2004 and March 2009 over 600,000 Poles registered for work in the UK (ONS, 2007; HO, 2009). Those who registered constitute approximately 60% of all Polish migrants (CRONEM, 2007). Since 2008 the number of Poles registering for work has steadily declined, reflecting a slowdown in Polish immigration rates. Some Poles have returned home as the economic situation has improved in Poland.

7.1.2   Religion

Poland is a devout country. Approximately 90% of the population are Roman Catholics, followed by 1.3% Orthodox Jews and 0.5% Protestants (GUS, 2007). The remaining population is comprised of other minority faiths. It should be noted that religious observance among the younger generations is not as strong as it was in the past (LSMU, 2009).

Religious festivals and public holidays

Poles have centuries-old customs and traditions, many of which have a religious background. Even those who are not practising Catholics or are non-believers celebrate religious festivals, as these are part of their culture. The most important religious festivals and public holidays are Christmas, Easter, Corpus Christi (June), Assumption Day (15 August) and All Saints' Day (1 November). Other traditional festivals and national holidays include New Year (New Year's Eve also known as Sylwester), Carnival time (New Year to Ash Wednesday), 'Fat' Thursday (the Thursday before Ash Wednesday) and Shrove Tuesday (*Ostatki*), May Day, Constitution Day (3 May), Pentecost Sunday, St Andrew's Day (30 November) and Independence Day (11 November). On 'Fat' Thursday doughnuts filled with jam and *faworki* are eaten, while on Shrove Tuesday the culinary theme is herring and vodka.

Fasting

Poles in general are very family oriented and family gatherings take place during festive times and on national holidays. In Poland Roman Catholics fast during various religious festivals. Fasting means abstinence from meat and sometimes from other luxury items. Fish and vegetarian dishes are permitted. Light meals, often one or two instead of three, are consumed. Good Friday and half of the day on Christmas Eve are the main fast days. Some people do not consume meat on Fridays and eat fish instead.

Religious festivals and foods

Festivals are often associated with overeating; large quantities of alcohol are also consumed. 'Eat, drink and loosen your belt' is a popular Polish saying dating back to the 17th century, when Poland was a very prosperous country. Traditionally, Poles are very hospitable and guests are always made welcome – another Polish saying is 'Guest in the house, God in the house'. It should be noted that it is considered ill-mannered to refuse a meal or snack offered when visiting family or friends, or to leave food on your plate. It may be difficult to make healthy eating suggestions for festive periods, although moderation should always be encouraged.

Easter

Good Friday is the strictest fast day of the year. On Easter Saturday most Poles attend church with a small basket of the traditional Easter foodstuffs: a piece of bread, hard-boiled eggs (dyed yellow-brown with onion skins or painted), Easter cakes, ham, sausages and horseradish or beetroot and horseradish relish. This basket is taken to be blessed by the priest. The basket is often decorated with colourful professionally decorated eggshells, called *pisanki*, and twigs of boxwood. Following this ritual the feast begins, continuing throughout the weekend and ending on the evening of Easter Monday.

Christmas

Christmas Eve (*Wigilia*) is the day most celebrated in Polish homes. Meat is forbidden on that day. Usually, only one small meal is eaten late in the afternoon. Christmas Eve supper, which is eaten at 4–5 o'clock, is a very special meal. Preparations can take several days. Family members share *oplatek* (holy bread in the form of a wafer) and wish each other all the best for the future. The meal consists of fish (carp, herrings) and vegetarian dishes (e.g., beetroot soup, mushroom soup), *pierogi* (Polish ravioli), stewed sauerkraut with beans or mushrooms, poppy-seed cake, gingerbread or baked cheesecake and dried fruit compote. Traditionally, there are 12 courses, reflecting the number of Christ's apostles; however, there are usually 5–8 small dishes. It is the custom to set an extra place at the table for an unexpected guest. After supper, many people attend mass, held at midnight. Christmas Day is celebrated with close family members, Boxing Day with family and friends. Popular traditional dishes served on Christmas Day and Boxing Day include chicken or beef bouillon or tomato soup, followed by breaded pork or veal cutlets. Eaten throughout the day are cold cuts of roast and smoked meats, hams and sausages, a variety of pickles, vegetable and herring salads, and cakes.

7.1.3 Traditional diet and eating patterns

Polish cuisine has been influenced by the culinary traditions of many countries and cultures over the centuries, including German, Russian, Lithuanian, Czech, Austrian, Hungarian, Jewish, Italian,

French, English, Turkish and Tartar. Poland's turbulent history, which encompasses hundreds of years of wars with different nations, foreign invasions, partitions of the country lasting 150 years, several vast territorial changes, as well as trading, cultural and marital exchanges with the royal courts of Europe, has left Poland with a rich cuisine that draws on a multitude of culinary styles and flavours.

Poland has a number of staple dishes which are found all over the country in some form. Local dishes particular to specific regions also abound. In general, Polish cuisine is characterized by a liberal use of meat and sausages, a variety of pickles, herbs and spices, as well as different kinds of pasta and dumplings. It is related to other Slavic cuisines in its use of kasha (*kasza* – buckwheat, pearl barley, millet).

Polish food is rich, substantial and relatively high in fat, including saturated fat, and salt. Typical meals are hearty and often contain a lot of meat or sausages (mostly smoked). The vegetables typically used in Polish cuisine are cabbage (including *sauerkraut*), beetroot, cucumber, carrots, celeriac, parsley, dill, mushrooms and potatoes. Cream and sour cream are common ingredients in soups and sauces, or are added as a topping.

Bread, rice, potatoes, pasta and other starchy foods

Bread is one of the staple foods of Poland. It has a special meaning in the Roman Catholicism and a special place in Polish tradition and homes. Newlyweds are welcomed by their parents on the threshold of their home with bread and salt, bread is blessed at Easter, some people, superstitiously, still do not like throwing it away in case it brings hunger or bad luck. Popular types of bread and rolls include mixed rye and wheat bread, wheat bread, rye bread and wholegrain bread. Poppy seeds, sunflower and pumpkin seeds, and oats are added to some types of bread and rolls. *Chalka* (*challah*) is a special type of slightly sweet, braided bread of Jewish origin commonly eaten at Christmas.

In general, Polish bread is made with a sourdough starter. The most popular bread is mixed rye and wheat bread, although, some people still prefer 'white' bread, which is made from refined flour, with a higher proportion of wheat to rye than that used in wholegrain or rye bread. The older generation of Poles who remember the war associate 'dark' bread with food shortages and poor status.

Kasha or groats (*kasza*) is the general name for buckwheat (*kasza gryczana*), cracked pearl barley (*kasza perlowa*), semolina (*kasza manna*) or millet (*kasza jaglana*). The first two are the most popular. It is sometimes flavoured with mushrooms or chopped fried bacon. Kasha can be used as a stuffing for poultry, ravioli/dumplings or savoury strudel. It is a good source of fibre and therefore should be encouraged as a healthy food alternative.

Semolina boiled with milk is popular with small children as an alternative to oat porridge.

Oats are eaten as rolled oats or oatmeal with milk, often with a sprinkling of sugar. Oats are often added to rolls and bread.

Cereals served with warm or cold milk are becoming increasingly popular as breakfast food.

White or brown rice is used in soups (e.g., tomato or sour cucumber soup), stuffed cabbage parcels and sweet rice dishes. Rice porridge made with milk and little sugar is also popular.

Pasta, noodles and dumplings

Pasta comes in a wide variety of shapes. It is a commonly added to soups, meat, mushroom and vegetable dishes, particularly those that come with a sauce. Pasta can also be served as a sweet dish with fruit, poppy seeds or mixed with farmer's cheese (similar to feta, but less salty), sugar and cream.

Another type of dumpling or pasta are *kluski*. The dough is made from plain wheat flour, eggs and water or mashed boiled potatoes mixed with wheat or/and potato flour and eggs. Other types include yeast dough-based *kluski*, often served steamed. *Kluski* can be stuffed with meat, cabbage, *sauerkraut* or mushrooms. They are served boiled, with similar toppings to *pierogi*. Plain *kluski* (without a stuffing) are usually an accompaniment to goulash or any other meat dish with a sauce, or in a soup.

Dumplings or 'Polish ravioli' (*pierogi*). The origin of dumplings is unknown but it is thought that they came to Poland from the Far East via the Russian Empire around the 13th century. There are hundreds of recipes for Polish dumplings. The standard dough is unleavened and made from plain wheat flour and eggs, similarly to pasta dough. *Pierogi* come in a variety of shapes, mostly crescent or semi-circular, sometimes square like ravioli or folded tortellini shapes. They can have savoury or sweet fillings. Savoury fillings include farmer's cheese with potatoes ('Russian style'), minced meat, *sauerkraut*, cabbage, mushrooms or kasha. Sweet fillings are farmer's cheese or fruit (e.g., apples, cherries, plums, wild blueberries and strawberries). *Pierogi* are either plain boiled or boiled and then fried, and are served with a variety of toppings (e.g., melted butter, sugar, fried breadcrumbs, cream, fried onion, fried bacon pieces).

Meat, fish, eggs, beans, nuts and seeds

Meat

Meat (red meat and poultry) is consumed in large quantities in Poland. It is eaten as sausages, cold meats and hams, hot meat dishes, pâtés, as pasta, dumplings or cabbage stuffing and added to soups. Sausages and hams are generally smoked. Meat is usually fried or stewed, or less often roasted. Grilling is especially popular during the summer months and has become very popular in recent years.

Pork is by far the most popular meat, followed by beef and veal, then poultry. Lamb is rarely eaten apart from in the southern mountainous region of Poland. Offal, including liver, pâtés, tripe and black pudding, is also commonly eaten.

Fish

Preserved fish (i.e., marinated, smoked, preserved in aspic or tinned) is very widely eaten. Fresh fish is quite expensive and therefore frozen or preserved fish is more commonly eaten. Fresh or frozen fish is usually prepared by frying in breadcrumbs, although baking, grilling and steaming are sometimes used. The most popular fish are herring, trout, mackerel, cod, pollock, carp, salmon, sprats and sardines. Pike, perch, eel and roach are available but not commonly eaten. Seafood (prawns, lobster, other shellfish) is very expensive and therefore rarely eaten.

Herrings are usually marinated in oil and/or vinegar with herbs and spices. Sour cream, mayonnaise, plain yoghurt, tomato paste, onion, apple, gherkins, raisins, peppers and mushrooms are the most common ingredients added to marinated herrings.

Carp is traditionally eaten at Christmas. It is fried with or without breadcrumbs. Carp is also served 'Jewish style' in aspic or 'Greek style' in tomato sauce.

Eggs

Eggs are a popular breakfast food, eaten scrambled, fried or boiled. Hard-boiled eggs are added to soups and salads. They are often eaten with mayonnaise or bacon.

Beans

The following are most commonly eaten: butter beans, small white or multi-coloured beans (similar to canellini and pinto beans), yellow split peas, French beans (green and yellow), broad beans and green peas. Beans and peas are common ingredients in soups and as an accompaniment to meat dishes, in traditional dishes made with either *sauerkraut* and beans, or beans and sausage in a tomato sauce casserole ('beans Breton style'). Lentils and chickpeas are less popular, although with the revival of traditional Polish cuisine, they are gaining more interest.

Nuts and seeds

Walnuts, hazelnuts and almonds are used mainly in cakes, biscuits and chocolate products. Peanuts are a popular savoury snack. Sunflower, pumpkin and poppy seeds are frequently used in baking. Poppy-seed cake is widely eaten at Christmas and Easter. Pastries with a poppy-seed-based filling are very popular as a snack food or dessert.

Milk and dairy foods

Full-fat milk and dairy products are very popular, although semi-skimmed, skimmed milk and low-fat dairy products are gaining in popularity.

Cheese is generally divided into 'white' (cottage cheese or farmer's cheese) and 'yellow' (hard cheese) varieties. The majority of 'yellow' cheese is of the Emmental or Cheddar type. Camembert, Brie, Boursin and blue cheeses are eaten by some. Spices and herbs (e.g., paprika, black pepper, mixed herbs) are sometimes added to cheeses. Regional varieties include Oscypki and Bryndza, both smoked.

Plain and fruit yoghurts are popular. Full- and low-fat varieties are available. Cream and sour cream are commonly used in soups, sauces, salads and desserts.

Kefir is similar to natural yoghurt but is more liquid. It is made by the natural process of bacterial and yeast fermentation of milk. It is a popular refreshing drink, especially in the summer months, and can be served on its own or with ravioli, dumplings or potato pancakes.

Maslanka (buttermilk) is less commonly used as a drink.

Vegetables

Summer

During the summer raw vegetable salads are eaten in preference to pickles. Generally, these salads are made of cucumbers, tomatoes and lettuce to which sour cream, yoghurt or mayonnaise is often added. French, flat and broad beans, cauliflower, baby beetroot and cabbages are also popular summer vegetables and are consumed boiled, served with butter, stewed or as a soup ingredient. Root vegetables (beetroot, carrots, parsley, celeriac) and leeks, onions and cabbage are eaten all year round.

Autumn

Mushrooms, especially the wild varieties, are consumed in large quantities in Poland and mushroom picking is a popular pastime. The fresh mushrooms are dried, pickled and stewed. Dried mushrooms are used as an ingredient in soups, meat and vegetable dishes throughout the year.

Winter

In winter pickles and preserves, including the Polish sour or fermented varieties, are more popular due to the unavailability and high cost of many fresh vegetables. Many people pickle their own vegetables, most commonly cucumbers, peppers, beetroot, and mushrooms and mixed vegetable salads (cabbage, carrot, onion and peppers). Additionally, cucumbers and cabbage are preserved by the bacterial fermentation method and are commonly known as 'sour cucumbers' or 'cucumbers in brine' and *sauerkraut* (sour cabbage).

Fruit

Most popular are local and seasonal fruits such as apples, pears, plums, cherries and peaches. However, citrus fruits and bananas are also very popular, as are the increasingly available exotic fruits.

Beverages

Tea is usually drunk with a slice of lemon and sugar, honey or fruit syrup (e.g., raspberry). Herbal teas (camomile, mint, linden tree blossom and many others) are very popular. Some are used for medicinal purposes; indeed, various herbal concoctions are prescribed by doctors while others can be bought in herbal shops and pharmacies without prescription.

Coffee is as popular as tea and often drunk with cream rather than milk.

Popular soft drinks include fruit juices and fruit nectars (sweetened fruit juice concentrate), mineral water, fizzy drinks, fruit compote (*kompot*).

Fats and oil

Butter, margarine and vegetable oils are used in cooking. Olive oil has not been traditionally used due to its comparatively high price. Lard is still used by some for frying. Lard with pork scratchings is served in some restaurants as a spread for bread as part of 'traditional old Polish food'. Red meat, poultry and sausages are most commonly fried, often in a generous amount of oil, as first stage of stew preparation. Sometimes dumplings are fried after being boiled and then fried bacon pieces or melted butter are added as a topping. Some vegetables are boiled and then fried, adding to the overall high fat content of the Polish diet. Mayonnaise and cream are often used in Polish cuisine, in vegetable, egg and herring salads.

Sugar and sugary foods

Sugar is added to tea, coffee, breakfast cereals and porridge. Fruit nectar drinks (thick juice high in sugar), fruit juices and other soft drinks are all very popular. Honey may be added to tea as an alternative to sugar and is regarded as a very healthy natural food. Some dumplings, pancakes and omelettes have sweet fillings (fruit, jam or cheese with sugar) and often have sugar sprinkled on top. Pastries, cakes, ice cream, sweet jelly, biscuits and sweets are all popular snacks or desserts.

Accompaniments

Pickled and sour vegetables, including cucumbers and mushrooms, are eaten with main meals, in sandwiches, salads and with herrings. They are a perfect accompaniment to cold meats and sausages. Relishes, such as horseradish cream, horseradish and beetroot relish, garlic sauce and tartar sauce, all go well with cold meats, ham and sausages. Ketchup and mustard are frequently consumed with these foods.

Herbs and spices

Commonly used herbs and spices include dill, parsley, marjoram, caraway seed, black pepper, mustard seed, garlic, paprika, bay leaf, cinnamon, nutmeg, allspice and herb pepper (a mixture of herbs and spices).

Food production and preservation

A method of bacterial and yeast fermentation is widely used in food production and preservation. This souring (fermentation) technique is a cornerstone of Polish cuisine. The souring technique (*kwaszenie* or *kiszenie*) is a method of natural bacterial or yeast fermentation used in the production of *sauerkraut*, 'sour cucumbers' also known as cucumbers in brine, sour beetroot, sour cream, *kefir*, fermented ryemeal and sourdough starter. Salt and spices, including bay leaf, mustard seed, horseradish and garlic, are used in this method of food production (apart from bread and *kefir* production). Ryemeal is used as a base for *żurek* (a traditional soup). Yeast dough is used in bread and cake baking.

Fat-assisted cooking methods are still very common; however, healthier cooking practices (e.g., baking in foil, grilling and steaming) are becoming increasingly more popular (Ciborowska & Rudnicka, 2007).

Alcohol

Poland has a so-called Northern European drinking pattern, which can be described as 'non-daily drinking, irregular binge drinking episodes (during weekends and at festivities), and the acceptance of drunkenness in public' (Popova *et al.*, 2007). Spirits, liqueurs and beer are the most popular alcoholic drinks, with vodka being the national drink of Poland. Mead is a traditional alcoholic drink made from honey. It dates back many centuries and is mostly drunk in winter months. Over the past 15 years the consumption of beer has increased and it is now consumed on a par with vodka and other spirits in Poland. Wine is not that common but some sweet wine is produced in Poland, including home-made. Imported western wines are becoming more popular, especially among the younger generation. In 2002 consumption of pure alcohol equivalents per capita per annum was estimated at almost 12 litres, which was comparable with the UK (13l), and was twice as high as the global average of 6 litres. 39% of Polish men and 9% of women were heavy drinkers (more than 40g alcohol/day, equivalent to more than 3–4 units) whereas 16% and 34% respectively were abstainers or a very light drinkers (0–0.25 g of alcohol per day) (Rehm *et al.*, 2007). High alcohol consumption and a heavy, irregular drinking pattern have been shown to be very detrimental to health, increasing the risk of cardiovascular disease, liver and hepatobilliary disease, some cancers and alcohol-related deaths and injuries. In 2002, alcohol-attributable mortality was 14% in Polish men and 4% in women. The highest rates of alcohol-attributable deaths were found in younger adults (20–44 years of age). This pattern was similar for men and women in all European countries studied (Rehm *et al.*, 2007).

7.1.4 Smoking

A survey carried out in Poland in 2007 by the Institute of Oncology based in Warsaw showed that 34% of men smoked daily, 2% occasionally, 19% were ex-smokers and 45% never smoked. In women, 23% smoked daily, 3% occasionally, 10% were ex-smokers and 64% never smoked (GUS, 2007). On average Polish men smoked 18 cigarettes and women 13 per day. Smoking prevalence in young women in their 20s has risen by 9% in a 10-year period. Higher prevalence rates were noted among people who were less educated, unemployed and those who came from poor families. Overall, prevalence of smoking in the Polish population is falling.

7.1.5 Physical activity

The majority of Polish adults lead a sedentary lifestyle (Pol Nat Rep, 2006). Only 36% of adults meet the current guidelines of a minimum of 30 minutes of physical activity taken on at least five days of the week. This has increased since the mid-1990s when only 10% of adults and 30% of children and teenagers were physically active (Ruszkowska-Majzel & Drygas, 2007). However, children as young as five still spend on average almost three hours a day watching television and playing computer games. Over 40% of adults are inactive.

In the UK Polish adults and children seem to be more active than some other ethnic minority communities, such as the Turkish or Somali, however, there are no definite numbers for comparison with the data from Poland (LSMU, 2009). Polish adults and children in the UK tend to take part in some structured and unstructured activities, including walking, football, swimming, cycling, dancing and ballet classes, volleyball, karate and Polish scouts.

7.1.6 Traditional and changing dietary patterns in Poland

Traditionally, people ate breakfast, 'second breakfast' (elevenses), dinner and supper. This pattern is still followed by some Poles today, especially those who start work early, school children and the older generation. In this meal pattern, the first breakfast is usually relatively small (e.g., one slice of bread with jam, egg or cheese; a small portion of cereal). This is then followed by a sandwich for second breakfast at 10–11 am, dinner (the main meal) at 2–3 pm and supper at 7–8 pm. With changing working patterns, more similar to those in western countries, young professionals and their families have adapted their meal pattern accordingly. They are more likely to consume three meals – breakfast, lunch and dinner – with small snacks between meals if required. An irregular eating pattern and skipping breakfast are also more prevalent.

Following Poland's transition to a market economy in the 1990s, some favourable changes in food consumption were noted. This included a 10–15% average fall in overall energy intake. Consumption of saturated fat started to fall in favour of an increase in unsaturated fat. Lard and butter were often replaced by rapeseed, soya and olive oil, and spreads made from these vegetable oils. Fruit intake was also noted to have increased (Ciborowska & Rudnicka, 2007; Klosiewicz-Latoszek *et al.*, 2008). Nevertheless, in the mid-2000s Polish people still consumed a diet high in fat, on average 37% of energy in men and 35% in women, with saturated fat intake of about 14% and 13% respectively (Waśkiewicz, 2008). Protein intake was approximately 13% and carbohydrate intake was 52% among adults. Salt intake continues to be very high (approximately 15 g/day) and simple carbohydrates intake is more than 10% energy. Consumption of fruit and vegetables is still considered to be low. It has been found that 'currently over 50% of Polish children and teenagers consume too much fat and their salt intake is on average 12 g per day' (Jarosz, 2007). Less than half of Polish school children eat fruit and vegetables every day and one in three consumes soft drinks and confectionery daily (PorGrow, 2007).

Other dietary characteristics among Poles include a low fish intake, relatively low dairy intake and low intake of beans, pulses and wholegrains. An increase in fast food and ready-made meal consumption has been noted since the early 1990s (PorGrow, 2007) (see Table 7.1.1 and Table 7.1.2).

7.1.7 Dietary changes on migration to the United Kingdom

Polish immigrants in the UK are a diverse group in terms of integration with British society, its tradition, culture and way of life, with diet being an important part. The oldest, postwar immigrants and second- and third-generation Poles are perhaps the most integrated with British society. As one would expect, they have adopted the British diet to the highest degree. There are currently no studies on the diets of Polish people who have moved to the UK. However, one might speculate, based on similarities with other ethnic groups who have migrated, that the majority of recent Polish immigrants follow their traditional diet. In time this may change as they integrate more fully with British society and explore traditional British, Indian, Chinese, Middle Eastern and African-Caribbean food.

It is worth noting that Poles rarely had the chance to travel freely before 1989. At this time Poland was in the Eastern Bloc, behind the Iron Curtain. Under the communist regime, most restaurants were closed and the few that survived were often too expensive for the general population. In their place, self-service cafeterias or eateries (*bar mleczny* or milk bars), appeared in postwar Poland. They were subsidized by the state, cheap and good value for money, serving simple dairy, egg, cereal and flour-based meals.

Since the early 1990s eating out has become much more popular, especially in the larger cities and towns. Unfortunately, besides traditional Polish and other restaurants, many fast-food establishments such as McDonald's, Kentucky Fried Chicken, pizza and kebab houses have become popular, a trend seen in many other countries, including the UK in the 1970s.

Many Polish people are very attached to their traditional home-made food and traditional diet, which is significantly different from the British diet. Poles are very proud of their traditional foods and often express concern about the quality, lack of variety and blandness of British food. They do the majority of their shopping in Polish shops and delicatessens. In the 1980s and 1990s Polish food was quite scarce in the UK and relatively expensive. For these reasons new immigrants to the UK ate more British food than those currently arriving. Many Poles take every opportunity to bring Polish foods such as sausages, hams and sweets to the UK from Poland. This occurs less often nowadays, possibly due to the abundance of Polish shops and supermarkets at cheaper prices, wherever a significant Polish community exists.

One may also speculate that the dietary habits of the most recent Polish immigrants may have changed in terms of the quality of food eaten away from Poland. This could be due to the time constraints of migrant workers who do not have enough time to prepare traditional meals. They

Table 7.1.1 Typical meal pattern for Polish people with guidelines on how to adapt this intake towards healthier eating

Meal	Traditional food	Encourage	Discourage
Breakfast	Bread/bread roll with butter/ margarine and selection of toppings: jam, honey, cheese, ham Eggs: boiled or scrambled (no milk added) plain or with chopped bacon or smoked sausage. Frankfurters or similar. Oat/rice porridge Breakfast cereal Tea, coffee, cocoa	High-fibre bread/bread rolls (e.g., rye, rye and wheat, with seeds, oats, wholegrain) Margarine instead of butter Eggs: boiled. Scrambled: choose plain or with mushrooms, tomatoes or peppers instead of bacon or sausage High-fibre, no added sugar breakfast cereals. Add fruit to cereal instead of sugar Low-fat dairy (e.g., cottage cheese) with radishes, chives	White bread and rolls Use of butter Adding bacon or sausage to eggs. Alternatively use lean sausage or ham Avoid frequent consumption of Frankfurter-type sausages Cereal with added sugar. Adding sugar to cereal/ porridge Full-fat milk and dairy
'Second breakfast' (children, early risers and older generation)	Sandwich Fruit Yoghurt Pastries, doughnuts	Fillings: lean ham or cold meat cuts, tuna salad, cottage cheese mixed with tinned fish Fruit Low-fat yoghurt	Fillings: fatty sausages and pickled cucumbers Creamy yoghurts Frequent consumption of pastries and doughnuts
Dinner (main meal)	Soup: home-made vegetable and meat stock-based. Most vegetable soups contain some meat or sausage. Cream, potatoes, dumplings or pasta may be added Red meat, chicken or fish – stewed, fried or grilled, often served with a cream-based sauce Potatoes/buckwheat/ pearl barley/ dumplings/potato pancakes Vegetables: fresh, stewed, boiled or pickled. Some salads are mixed with cream or mayonnaise (e.g., coleslaw) Other: Dumplings (*pierogi*) with cream/chopped fried bacon/ butter topping Stuffed cabbage Black pudding. Fried liver. Hunter's stew. Pancakes.	Soup: home-made. Choose pure vegetable soups more often. Add beans, pearl barley. Replace cream with yoghurt or *kefir* where possible Choose lean meat and poultry that has been grilled, stewed, steamed, baked, or cooked in foil. Remove skin from poultry. Trim fat off meat. Eat fish more often. Use low-fat yoghurt in salads. Small amounts of olive oil, with herbs and lemon/vinegar as salad dressing/ vinaigrette Choose boiled or fresh vegetables whenever possible Choose low-fat yoghurt or *kefir* as an accompaniment to *pierogi*.	Soup: ready-made. Add less meat and sausages to soups Choose low-fat cream where possible or avoid it all together Frequent consumption of fried meat and excessive amount of oil in cooking Avoid adding butter, sour cream or mayonnaise to salads Avoid frequent consumption of pickled and soured preserves as they are high in salt Avoid excessive amounts of butter, cream, sugar and fried bacon toppings with *pierogi* Avoid frequent consumption of offal. Avoid sugar or cream toppings for pancakes.

Table 7.1.1 (cont'd)

Meal	Traditional food	Encourage	Discourage
Supper	Sandwich with cheese, ham, cold meat, smoked sausage, paté Smoked, tinned or marinated fish (e.g., mackerel, sardines, herrings) Fish, poultry or meat with vegetables in aspic Fish in breadcrumbs Fried or grilled, smoked sausage or Frankfurter-type sausage Pickled cucumbers/ mushrooms Omelette, pancakes, *pierogi*	Choose high-fibre bread and vegetable oil spread Choose low-fat cheese, poultry, cold cuts Drain oil from herrings. Choose tinned fish in tomato sauce or water rather than oil Grilled, baked fish. Choose grilled sausages Choose fresh vegetable salads over pickled more often Choose fruit, vegetable and farmer's cheese fillings more often	Avoid fatty sausages and trim fat off ham and cold cuts Always include vegetables but avoid adding cream, butter or mayonnaise Avoid fried sausages and Frankfurter-type sausages. Fried fish. Frequent use of smoked fish (which is high in salt) Avoid excessive amounts of sugar, cream, bacon and butter as a topping
Desserts	Milk pudding (*budyn*), *kisiel* (non-dairy flavoured pudding) Fruit jelly Yoghurt Fruit Ice cream Pastries, cakes	Choose fruit, low-fat yoghurt *Kisiel* *Budyn* prepared with low-fat milk Fruit sorbet	Avoid full-cream yoghurt, pastries and cakes especially with icing sugar and cream. Avoid whipped cream with desserts. Eat ice cream only occasionally
Snacks	Biscuits, chocolate, cakes, pastry, doughnut, chocolate-coated nuts/fruit Fruit Pretzels, crisps, nuts and seeds	Choose fruit or low-fat yoghurt Moderate intake of plain, unsalted nuts, dried fruit, plain pretzels or popcorn Preferable biscuit choices include plain, without chocolate or cream filling	Avoid frequent consumption of biscuits, cakes, chocolate, pastries Avoid sugar- or chocolate-coated nuts and biscuits Salted crisps, pretzels and nuts.
Drinks	Tea, black, with lemon or fruit syrup Herbal teas with or without honey. Coffee with milk or cream Cocoa Fruit juice, juice drink, fruit nectar, vegetable juice, regular fizzy drinks, mineral water	Try sweetener instead of sugar, honey or fruit syrup Coffee with low-fat milk Choose mineral water, vegetable juice, unsweetened fruit juice and sugar-free fizzy drinks	Adding sugar, honey or fruit syrup to tea Avoid cream in coffee Avoid sugary drinks and juices. Avoid nectars, as they are high in sugar

may rely heavily on ready-made Polish foods and also some UK convenience foods, both of which are higher in energy, saturated and total fat, salt and sugar, compared to the traditionally prepared home-made foods. Polish immigrant families or couples should be in a better position, as family members, often the women, will regularly cook meals for the whole family or their partners, whereas single people, males in particular, may not see the point of preparing complex meals just for themselves. They may also lack the skills to do so (see Table 7.1.3).

Table 7.1.2   Glossary of traditional Polish foods

Name of foods	Description
Soups – *Zupy* (pl.), *zupa* (singl.)	
Barszcz czerwony	Beetroot soup is usually based on vegetable broth with the addition of 'sour beetroot' liquid or brine, or lemon juice, to prevent loss of colour and improve taste. Smoked ribs or smoked sausage may be added for flavour. It is served with sour cream or clear with mushroom ravioli/hard-boiled egg/ *krokiet* (savoury pancake fried in breadcrumbs and stuffed with meat/cabbage/mushrooms). Popular party dish and traditionally eaten on Christmas Eve with mushroom ravioli (a vegetarian version).
Żurek	Sour rye soup made with fermented rye meal. Served with boiled potatoes, hard-boiled egg, 'white sausage' (similar to *Bratwurst*), usually with sour cream and seasoned with marjoram.
Krupnik	Barley soup with vegetables and meat (e.g., ribs).
Kapuśniak	Sour cabbage (*sauerkraut*) soup, made with addition of smoked sausage or meat.
Zupa ogórkowa	Sour cucumber soup based on meat and vegetable stock. Served with rice or potatoes,
Zupa koperkowa	Dill soup, served with cream and potatoes.
Rosół z kurczaka	Chicken consommé with noodles.
Rosół wołowy	Beef consommé with noodles.
Zupa pomidorowa	Tomato soup, served with rice or noodles, often based on meat and vegetable stock, with sour cream.
Zupa grochowa or Fasolowa	Thick pea or butter bean soup often made with smoked sausage and bacon bits.
Zupa jarzynowa	Vegetable soup, served with cream.
Zupa kalafiorowa	Cauliflower soup, served with cream.
Zupa grzybowa or Barszcz grzybowy	Mushroom soup with cream. Served with pasta shapes or boiled potatoes. This dish is traditionally eaten on Christmas Eve.
Zasmażka	Roux made with butter/fat, flour and often bacon. It is added to some soups (e.g., *krupnik, kapuśniak, zupa ogórkowa and grochówka*).
Beef, veal, pork, lamb, rabbit	
Mięso wołowe or wołowina	Beef
Mięso cielęce or cielęcina	Veal
Mięso wieprzowe or wieprzowina	Pork
Galareta	Aspic made with a fish or meat stock.
	Beef and veal are often stewed in a sauce with/without added cream, and mushrooms/horseradish/vegetables/dill and often thickened with flour.
Flaki or flaczki	Beef tripe soup, heavily seasoned with marjoram. A popular dish at parties.
Gulasz	Goulash or beef stew. Can be quite spicy with paprika or cayenne pepper; or mild with mushrooms.
Zrazy	Beef rolls stuffed with bacon, gherkin and onion or red pepper, in a sauce.
Kotlet cielęcy	Veal cutlet, fried in breadcrumbs.
Baranina	Lamb, grilled or roasted.
Sztuka miesa w sosie	Beef chunks in a sauce (horseradish, dill, etc.).

Table 7.1.2 (cont'd)

Name of foods	Description
Kotlet schabowy	Fried pork cutlet/chop in breadcrumbs.
Sznycel	Minced meat cutlet, usually made with pork or pork and beef meat, fried in breadcrumbs.
Kiełbasa	Sausages. Most smoked, apart from 'white sausage', black pudding and Frankfurter-type sausages. Sausages go well with pickled or sour cucumbers, mustard or horseradish. They are eaten in sandwiches, in soups, grilled, fried, with scrambled eggs or as a snack at parties.
Klopsy	Meat balls, made with pork or pork and veal/beef, often served with tomato sauce.
Golonka	Pork knuckle, sometimes cooked in a beer sauce, with horseradish.
Smalec z chlebem	Partially double fried lard with pork scratching, and onion, served with bread.
Gołąbki	Cabbage parcels, originally Lithuanian. They are stuffed with pork mince, mushrooms and rice, served with tomato or mushroom sauce.
Bigos	'Hunter's stew' made from *sauerkraut* and shredded white cabbage, with chunks of various meats (beef, smoked bacon, ribs, sausages and sometimes game), dried mushrooms and prunes. Herbs and seasoning include juniper berries, black pepper, bay leaf, caraway seed nutmeg. A popular dish at parties.
Pierogi	Stuffed dumplings, larger than ravioli, filled with *sauerkraut*/ mushrooms/meat/cheese and potatoes, or with fruit. They are usually boiled, sometimes boiled and then fried. Savoury varieties are often served with melted butter or fried chopped bacon and onion as a topping. Sweet varieties are often topped with melted butter or cream and a sprinkling of sugar.
Kopytka/pyzy/kluski ślaskie	Dumplings made with potato and wheat flour, can be stuffed with meat or plain and served with mushroom sauce, meat stew, goulash.
Placki ziemniaczane	Potato pancakes, eaten plain or with sour cream/mushroom sauce/goulash. Plain *placki* can be served with *kefir*.
Fasolka po bretońsku	French-style bean and sausage casserole in tomato sauce, known as 'beans Breton style'.
Kaszanka	Equivalent of black pudding.
Szaszłyk.	Chunks of meat and onion, grilled on a spit.
Królik	Rabbit. Usually stewed in dill sauce with cream.
Poultry	
Kurczak z rożna	Roast chicken.
Kurczak de volaille	Chicken steaks filled with butter, mushrooms or cheese and fried in breadcrumbs. Similar to chicken kiev.
Potrawka z kurczaka	Chicken stewed in vegetables.
Wątróbki drobiowe:	Chicken liver with onion.
Kurczak w galarecie	Chicken with vegetables in aspic.
Kaczka z jabłkami	Duck baked with apples.
Fish	
Śledzie w śmietanie/w oleju	Herrings in sour cream/in oil. Herrings are usually marinated in vinegar and/or oil, with herbs and spices, and also with onion/apple/pickled cucumbers. They can be very salty.

(Continued)

Table 7.1.2 (cont'd)

Name of foods	Description
Karp po żydowsku	Carp in aspic 'Jewish style', with raisins or vegetables. More popular is carp fried in breadcrumbs. Both traditionally served on Christmas Eve. Carp in aspic is a popular light dish, often served as a starter.
Makrela	Mackerel, eaten mostly smoked.
Pstrąg	Trout. Served grilled, poached or fried.
Łosoś	Salmon, often poached or cooked in a dill sauce.
Dorsz	Cod, usually fried in breadcrumbs.
Ryba w galarecie	Fish in aspic, with carrots, peas, hard-boiled egg. It is a popular light dish, often served as a starter.
Vegetables	
Ogórki kiszone	Cucumbers in brine or sour cucumbers. They can have a very high salt content.
Ogórki konserwowe	Pickled cucumbers. High salt content.
Surówka z kiszonej kapusty.	Sauerkraut salad with freshly grated carrots, apple and onion. Seasoning includes caraway seed and pepper. Sometimes small amount of oil and sugar is added. Relatively high salt content.
Salatka jarzynowa	Vegetable salad with mayonnaise, similar to Russian salad. It is made with boiled vegetables (carrots, celeriac, parsley root, and potatoes), raw apple and onion, pickled and sour cucumbers, pickled mushrooms, hard-boiled egg, and mixed with mayonnaise and sour cream. Herb pepper and other spices are added for flavour. It is traditionally served as an accompaniment to ham, sausages and cold meats at Christmas, Easter and parties.
Ćwikła z chrzanem	Beetroot and horseradish relish.
Desserts, cakes and pastries	
Budyn	Flavoured custard-type dessert.
Drożdżówka	Yeast cake, filled with jam, poppy seeds or farmer's cheese.
Galaretka:	Sweet jelly with fruit, often served with whipped cream.
Faworki or chrust	Sweet crispy deep-fried pastry in the shape of twisted ribbons, sprinkled with icing sugar. Traditionally eaten on Fat Thursday and during Carnival time.
Lody	Ice cream, often served with fruit, nuts and whipped cream.
Makowiec	Poppy-seed cake. Traditionally eaten at Christmas and Easter.
Naleśniki	Pancakes stuffed with jam, fruit, cottage cheese. etc., very similar to crepes.
Pączki	Doughnuts, filled with rose petals or fruit jam/marmalade.
Piernik	Ginger cake with raisins, nuts and honey. Varieties include plum marmalade layer and chocolate coating.
Pierniki or pierniczki	Gingerbreads, often with sugar icing or with chocolate coating, some have a fruit filling.
Sernik	Baked cheese cake.
Szarlotka	Apple charlotte or apple pie, sometimes served with whipped cream.
Kompot	A light sweet drink consumed with dinner. Made from fresh or dried fruit, boiled in water with sugar.

Table 7.1.3   Traditional Polish food choices and healthier alternatives

Foods	Encourage	Discourage
Starchy foods	Traditional foods: Potatoes: boiled plain or with minimal amounts of oil or vegetable based margarine. Boiled as soup ingredient, mashed with vegetable spread and low fat milk. Rye, whole wheat, mixed rye and wheat foods: flour, bread, stuffed dumplings/ravioli, pasta. *Kasha*: cracked pearl barley, buckwheat, millet, semolina, Oats, rice, corn.	Fry foods to a minimum Avoid chips, fried potato pancakes. Avoid adding butter, cream or fried bacon to wheat-based foods (e.g., dumplings, *kasha*) and potatoes. Avoid adding too much salt during cooking or at the table.
Vegetables and fruits	Traditional foods: Cucumbers, tomatoes, beetroot, cabbage, peppers, lettuce, carrots, celeriac, parsley, cauliflower, leek, garden peas, beans and pulses. Mushrooms, including wild varieties. Choose fresh and frozen vegetables. Use small amounts of olive/rapeseed oil or vinaigrette for vegetable salads. Encourage pure vegetable soups. Other vegetables include: courgettes, broccoli, aubergine, sweet corn, Chinese cabbage. Fruit: apples, pears, plums, cherries, peaches, strawberries, raspberries, blueberries, red and blackcurrants, gooseberry, citrus fruit, bananas, watermelon, grapes, pineapple.	Avoid frequent consumption of cucumbers in brine or 'sour' cucumbers (*ogorki kiszone*), pickled vegetables, sauerkraut. They contain high levels of salt. Avoid adding mayonnaise, cream or butter to vegetables/salads. Avoid cream, sausage/meat and roux in vegetable soups and replace with low-fat yoghurt/*kefir* where possible. Avoid tinned fruit in syrup, and adding sugar and cream to fruit salads.
Milk and dairy foods	Traditional foods: Cheese, milk, yoghurt, *kefir*, buttermilk. Choose reduced fat and sugar versions. Milk: 0.5%, 1.5% or 2% (equivalent of semi- and skimmed milk). Cheese: farmer's/cottage cheese – choose *poltlusty* or *chudy* (reduced fat)	Avoid 3.5% milk and 30%, 18% cream. Avoid full-fat cheese, *tlusty* and cream cheese. Avoid condensed and evaporated milk (used mainly in puddings) as they are high in sugar and fat.
Meat, fish, eggs, beans, nuts and seeds	Traditional foods: Choose chicken, turkey, rabbit meat more often than red meat. Lean pork, beef and veal, pork loin, boiled or roast ham, roast meat. Fish: herring, mackerel, trout, carp, cod, sprats, sardines, salmon, halibut, pollock, pike. Beans and pulses. Eggs, nuts and seeds. Healthier methods of meat and fish preparation include boiling, baking, grilling, poaching, stewing (including in vegetables). Use various herbs and spices to flavour foods. Use less salt in cooking and do not use salt at the table.	Offal should be eaten in moderation as it is usually high in fat. Frankfurters, luncheon meat, patés and many sausages are high in fat and salt, and should not be frequently eaten. Salted or marinated herrings should be soaked to remove some salt. Avoid frying fish and meat. Remove visible fat/skin from meat/poultry/ham/bacon before cooking/eating. Avoid adding cream or mayonnaise Many meat and fish seasonings have salt in them, including popular Vegeta and many herb mixes. Eat fewer foods with high salt content such as bacon, ham, luncheon meat, sausages, salted nuts, smoked fish, packet and ready-made soups and sauces. Avoid ready meals as much possible as they are high in fat and salt.

(Continued)

Table 7.1.3 (cont'd)

Foods	Encourage	Discourage
Fat and sugar-rich foods	*Kisiel, budyn* made with low-fat milk, low-sugar fruit jelly, fruit cake (*keks*), ginger cake (*piernik*), *babka* (yeast dough cake with raisins), yeast dough cakes/pastries, *drozdzowka*. No added sugar drinks and fruit juices, diluted *kompot*, low-fat milk/*kefir*-based fruit and vegetable drinks should be chosen instead. Choose low-sugar jams and marmalades. Use tinned fruit in natural juice rather than in syrup.	Avoid cream cakes, gateaux, French pastries, doughnuts, whipped cream with ice cream and desserts. Also avoid sugar icing on cakes. Sugary drinks (e.g., nectars, fruit syrups and canned, sugar fizzy drinks) should be avoided.
Other	Oils such as rapeseed, olive, and sunflower oils are better choices, in small amounts. Use non-stick good quality pans, measure the amount of oil with a tablespoon or use oil spray. Herbs and spices with small amount of oil may be used to marinate fish or meat, and to cut down on salt added to food.	Lard should be completely avoided as it is very high in saturated fat. Salad creams and relishes can be high fat and salt.

7.1.8 Emerging and evolving health problems in Poland and the prevalence of chronic diseases

There are no studies on chronic diseases among Polish migrants in the UK. Available are some emerging health problems and disease prevalence rates including its recent trends in Poland, which should provide some background knowledge about the potential problems among Polish migrant population in the UK.

In 2004 life expectancy in Poland was estimated to be 71 years for men and 79 for women. Although it has increased by four years since the early 1990s, this is still lower than the average life expectancy in the EU (Polish National Health Programme, 2007). The most common causes of death were, and still are, cardiovascular disease (47% of all deaths) and cancer (24%).

Obesity

Obesity has been rising over the past few decades throughout the world, in developed and developing countries. It was estimated that in 2005 there were about 1.6 billion overweight and 400 million obese adults worldwide. Approximately 20 million children under the age of five were estimated to be overweight (WHO, 2007). According to recent estimates, in many EU countries more than half of adults are overweight or obese (PorGrow, 2007). This includes Poland, where over 50% of adults and 19% of children are either overweight or obese (PorGrow, 2007; WHO, 2007). Among adults 41% of Polish men and 29% of Polish women are overweight, whereas a further 16% of men and 20% of women are obese. Abdominal obesity is more prevalent in women than in men. Prevalence of overweight among Polish school children is 17% in boys and 12% in girls, and obesity respectively 4.5% and 4% (Pol Nat Rep, 2006). In common with other EU countries, including the UK, there is an upward trend in obesity among children and adults in Poland. For example, in 2000, 25% of men aged 50–59 years were obese compared to 1991 when 12% of men were obese in this age group. This was confirmed by the WOBASZ study conducted in 2003–5. It found that 21% of men and 22% of women aged 20–74 were obese, and a further 40% and 28% were overweight respectively.

Cardiovascular disease

Before 1991 (1960–90) cardiovascular mortality was very high in Poland and was rising relatively fast. After 1991 it started to fall very quickly. Nevertheless, cardiovascular disease (CVD) remains the main cause of death in Poland. Almost half of deaths are attributed to it, 41% in men and 53% in women. Ischaemic heart disease is the single biggest killer in Poland. It was responsible for 14% of all deaths in 2002 (WHO, 2007). An estimated 17% of Poles suffer from hypertension and almost 10% have established coronary heart disease (GUS, 2007). The reason for the fall in CVD mortality after 1991 is thought to be mainly due to the halving of saturated fat intake in favour of unsaturated fat and also an increase in fruit intake, which almost doubled. Consumption of poultry was also noted to have increased and red meat to have decreased (PorGrow, 2007; Klosiewicz-Latoszek *et al.*, 2008). These changes in food consumption resulted from the introduction of the market economy and changes in the price of foods (Zatonski *et al.*, 2007).

Diabetes

Recent estimates of the prevalence of diabetes in Poland are approximately 2 million people (5% of the population), a further 15% of adults have impaired glucose tolerance. With rising levels of obesity an increase in the rates of type 2 diabetes can be expected in the near future. The Polish National Diabetes Prevention Programme aims to improve diagnosis and treatment and reduce the complications of diabetes; as well as reduce the occurrence of type 2 diabetes.

Cancer

In 2002, 24% of all deaths were attributed to cancer (26% for men and 23% for women) in Poland. Lung cancer is the biggest killer. The risk of dying from stomach or liver cancer is decreasing, whereas colorectal, bladder and prostate mortality rates are increasing (Polish National Health Programme, 2007).

7.1.9   Maternal and infant nutrition

According to a survey carried out by the Polish Office of National Statistics (GUS, 2007) 88% of babies are breastfed and among those, 89% are exclusively breastfed. Polish mothers breastfeed

their babies on average for 3–6 months. There is some recent evidence that this seems to be true for the Polish migrant community in the UK. A qualitative research project carried out by the London Social Marketing Unit (LSMU) among the Polish migrant community living in London showed that many women breastfeed as they consider it best for their babies (LSMU, 2009). The majority of women stop breastfeeding at 3–4 months. Mothers who wean their babies earlier than the recommended six months believe that: their baby is ready, interested in 'grown-up' food and/or that porridge-style food is not 'real food'. Some mothers try to bulk up a baby who may appear small. Many women based their decision to wean early on advice from health professionals, family or friends. It also emerged from the LSMU study that most Polish mothers, although aware of the six-month guideline and the dangers of premature weaning, generally did not consider weaning at 4–5 months as too early and chose to ignore the guidelines.

Mothers gave formula milk to their infants before one year of age and cow's milk, water and tea after one year. Some would bulk up baby milk with semolina (*kasza manna*), a traditional practice commonly seen in Poland. Weaning foods include baby jar food (cereal, rice, meat, fruit and vegetables), soups, yoghurts and puréed or grated fresh fruit and vegetables. For older babies and toddlers mashed family meals are introduced gradually, in addition to branded jar food. Drinks include milk, water, fruit juices and drinks. Older toddlers snack on crisps, chocolate and salty adult foods.

7.1.10   Evidence of good practice and suggestions for the way forward

A healthy, balanced diet is an important factor in maintaining good health throughout life. Many chronic diseases, including obesity, type 2 diabetes and CVD, are related to diet and lifestyle. Unhealthy, energy-dense diets, high in fat and sugar, combined with low levels of physical activity, have led to the current obesity epidemic. It has been recognized that changes in the diet and lifestyle which occur with globalization, economic growth, urbanization and migration are reflected in the health and nutritional status of populations (WHO/FAO, 2003). This can be seen in many countries in 'nutrition transition'. A rise in the wealth of a country is correlated with an increase in food availability, often unfavourable changes in food composition and a decrease in physical activity.

In Poland some favourable changes in food composition and eating patterns have been observed since the early 1990s, including less consumption of saturated fat (e.g., butter, lard, red meat, full-fat dairy products), increased consumption of unsaturated fat (e.g., vegetable oil spreads, rapeseed, soya and olive oils) and increased intake of fruit and vegetables. On the other hand, consumption of convenience food has increased and physical activity levels have dropped. Children as young as five spend on average almost three hours a day watching television. Most adults lead a sedentary lifestyle.

Furthermore, the level of knowledge about the role of a healthy diet and lifestyle in reducing the risk of diet-related conditions such as cardiovascular disease among the general population is poor. Twenty per cent of Poles do not have any knowledge about non-pharmacological methods of CVD prevention and a further 40–50% have poor knowledge of these factors (Bielecki et al., 2005). Among people with a history of CVD less than a quarter of men and women understood the importance of a diet rich in fruit and vegetables and having less salt in their diet, and just over a third were aware that eating less fat would bring health benefits. Approximately half of these people appreciated the role of physical activity, and one third recognized the benefits of weight reduction, if overweight, in disease prevention (Waśkiewicz, 2008).

The Polish National Health Programme 2007–15 aims to reduce saturated fat consumption to <30% of total energy, increase fish consumption, increase the intake of whole grains, fruit, vegetables and pulses, as well as low-fat dairy and decrease intake of salt and sugar. It also aims to improve infant nutrition by encouraging breastfeeding until six months of age and improve physical activity levels among children and adults.

In response to the high prevalence of obesity, the Polish National Food and Nutrition Institute (IZZ) started implementation of POL-HEALTH: Overweight, Obesity and Chronic Disease Prevention Programme in 2007. This programme was created in response to a WHO initiative from the 'Global Strategy for Nutrition, Physical Activity and Health' (2004) and the European Strategy for Obesity Prevention. The main aims of POL-HEALTH are to improve health and reduce the prevalence of chronic disease in the population by improving nutrition and eating habits, raising awareness about the fundamental role of a healthy diet and lifestyle in the prevention of nutrition-related diseases such as obesity and its comorbidities. The goals include revision of dietary and physical activity guidelines for children and adults, healthier school meals, provision of educational material on nutrition, and collaboration with the catering industry, food manufacturers, hospitals and employers to provide healthier food and create an environment conducive to good health. There are also plans to train more health professionals, including dietitians and medical doctors with an interest in nutrition. Mass media campaigns and community-based projects, including health promotion activities, health clubs and workshops in schools, workplaces, leisure centres and academic institutes, are to be implemented.

7.1.11 Barriers to a healthier lifestyle in the United Kingdom

Polish people who recently (i.e., less than 10 years ago) migrated to the UK deal with a range of cultural, social and economic issues that can impact on attitudes and behaviours with regard to diet, health and lifestyle (LSMU, 2009).

Preserving the cultural heritage

Poles, like other recent migrants, have been found to hold on to their cultural foods as a way of preserving their cultural heritage. Western foods seem to have little impact on family meals, however, high-sugar breakfast cereals, high-sugar/high-fat snacks and fast foods are increasingly prevalent among some Polish families.

Food plays an important role in the lives of Polish families. Generally speaking, women spend a great deal of time and effort preparing traditional meals mostly from scratch, using fresh ingredients. Home cooking and baking have always been seen as signs of a good upbringing in Poland. Polish food is considered healthier, especially when meals are fully prepared in the traditional way. Although traditional Polish foods were found to be 'relatively healthy and balanced on the surface' in the LSMU study, there were a number of problem areas identified. The meals seem healthy and balanced due to the range of different foods and fresh vegetables consumed. The unhealthy food practices identified include: high levels of fat consumption (fatty hams, smoked meats and sausages, cream, deep-frying), high levels of 'invisible' snacking on sweet and savoury foods after an evening meal (Polish crisps, sweets, chocolate bars and biscuits); and the regular consumption of high-salt condiments.

Religious observance

Religion can also impact on food choices and the priority given to physical activity. Although religion plays an important role in people's lives in Poland, for many Poles in the UK, free from community pressure, religion fades in importance. They may find that they have more time to spend with their family, in which to relax, go for walks or play sports.

Language skills and education

It seems that some families, in particular those with higher education levels and better English language skills, have a fairly good understanding of the nutritional value of foods and what constitutes a healthy, balanced diet. They, especially women, are more aware of healthy eating guidelines and try to incorporate these in their family's diet.

It has been found that Polish mothers, even those lacking language skills, tend to be outward-looking and are likely to seek health information and advice. Healthy eating messages come from the Polish and English mainstream media, including internet sites, television channels, books and newspapers. Some information comes via children who are taught about healthy eating at school. It has also been found that although Polish people, including parents, are aware of healthy eating messages; they often do not change their eating or lifestyle behaviour. This may suggest that there might be a lack of understanding or confidence in translating these health messages into practice (LSMU, 2009).

Time and financial constraints

For some, lack of time or money can have a negative impact on food choice and physical activity behaviour.

Attitudes to health

According to the LSMU study (2009), although there seems to be some awareness of obesity and related health risks, few Polish people were able to make the link between their diet and lifestyle, and possible future health problems. Some people perceive obesity to be a 'British problem'.

Many believe that their diet is healthy as most of their meals are freshly prepared; they eat vegetables with their dinner or lunch and eat fruit. Children are given fruit drinks and sweetened fruit and vegetable juices on regular basis, which again are considered healthy as they contain vitamins, but they fail to acknowledge the amount of sugar and extra calories their children consume. Adults also underestimate the amount of fat and salt in their diet.

The LSMU study also found that most Polish people have a proactive approach to health and being free from sickness is a key priority. For many, being healthy means eating good quality food, taking part in regular exercise, achieving a work/life balance and emotional well-being. Some seem to be more conscious with regards to their diet and lifestyle behaviour in connection with their health. Many Poles showed knowledge of and interest in the role that vitamins and minerals play in their bodies. Vitamin supplements are often taken by Poles to prevent or help to recover from illness. Many have a relatively high level of medical knowledge and are able to self-diagnose and self-cure minor aliments with medication and herbal remedies.

Suggestions for the way forward

The evidence from the LSMU study suggests that the way forward is to acknowledge and build on existing good diet and lifestyle behaviour. These efforts should concentrate on highlighting the importance of improving the less healthy aspects of the traditional Polish diet. This would include adopting healthier cooking methods when preparing cultural meals, replacing high-fat, high-sugar and high-salt foods and sugary drinks with healthier alternatives, encouraging mothers to breastfeed until their child is six months, and educating on the use of healthier snacks for toddlers and children, as well as adults. Clear, culturally acceptable and direct health messages should target primarily mothers, who, in most cases, dictate the family's diet. Children can act as a source of information, especially for those whose parents' English language skills are poor. Health messages regarding increasing physical activity levels should highlight its benefits in preventing illness and for children in achieving their educational potential.

7.2   Greek Diet

Stavroulla Petrides

> **Key points**
>
> - Migration after the Second World War was to Western Europe, Canada, the USA and Australia. The majority of Greek-speaking people in the UK are from Cyprus.
> - The Greek Orthodox religion stipulates dietary restrictions and three periods of fasting (Easter, Christmas and New Year) amounting to up to 200 days a year.
> - The traditional Greek diet is a 'Mediterranean diet', being high in starchy foods, oily fish, dairy foods, fruit and vegetables, with the major source of oil being olive oil. The Mediterranean diet has been shown to reduce the risk of diabetes, heart disease and stroke.
> - Currently, Greece has the highest smoking prevalence in Europe, with recent epidemiological studies estimating that 40% of the adult population are daily smokers.

7.2.1   Introduction

Greece is part of Western Europe (see Figure 7.2.1). To the north, it is bordered by Albania, Macedonia and Bulgaria and in the north-east shares a border with Turkey (Boatswain & Nicolson, 2001). The term Greek collectively refers to people from mainland Greece the Greek islands, and Greek Cypriots (the ethnic Greek population of Cyprus). Cyprus is sometimes mistakenly believed to be a Greek island and part of Greece. However, while this nation is generally considered to be culturally Greek, it is independent. The island is presently divided into an occupied Turkish area in the north and the Greek-speaking area in the south (Boatswain, 2005).

Language

The official language of Greece and Cyprus is Greek. Greek is spoken by approximately 12 million speakers worldwide, over 10 million of whom live in Greece and over half a million in Cyprus (www.migrationinformation.org). Various organizations have offered support to promote the Greek language and culture. The Church has played a prominent role in teaching the language, often with support from the Greek government and Greek Cypriot authorities (bbb.co.uk/voices). There is a strong emphasis on the need to protect tradition and customs which is highlighted by the numbers of Greeks who send their children to Greek schools in the evenings or weekends to ensure that their cultural identity is not lost (bbb.co.uk/voices). There are more than 100 Greek communities across the UK. A survey of school children published in 2000 reported that Greek was the 12th most commonly spoken language in London.

Migration to the United Kingdom

The most important migration of Greeks took place during the years following the Second World War. Most went from rural areas to northern Europe, Canada, USA and Australia. By far the majority of Greek speakers in the UK, however, come not from Greece but from Cyprus. Such was the scale of migration that one in six Cypriots today reside in the UK. Most came in the 1960s and 1970s, although some arrived after the Turkish invasion of Cyprus in 1974 (www.migration information.org).

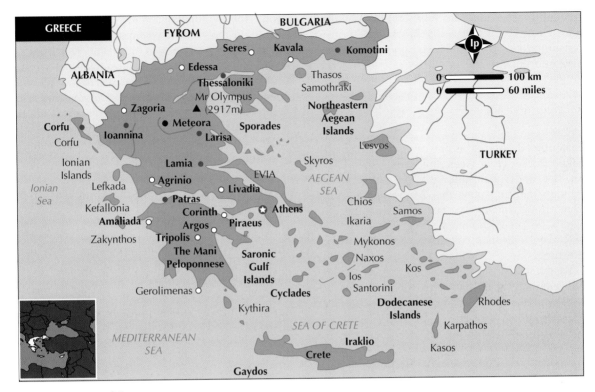

Figure 7.2.1   Map of Greece

Current UK population

Most Greek speakers from the mainland are found in West London; the highest concentrations of Greek speakers from Cyprus are in Enfield, Haringey, Hackney and Southgate (bbb.co.uk/voices). There are nearly as many Greek Cypriots living in London as in the capital of Cyprus (Nicosia), which constitutes the highest number of Cypriots living outside Cyprus. An estimated 40,000 Greeks from Greece (excluding students) also live in the Greater London area, and about 50,000 people of Greek origin live in Birmingham, the rest of the Midlands, Liverpool and Manchester. These numbers probably include a high proportion of people of mixed Greek and Greek Cypriot parentage since. (www.statistics.gov.uk).

7.2.2   Religion

The main religion is Greek Orthodox. Religion was, and remains, a very important influence in

Greek life. The first Greek Orthodox church in London was the cathedral of St Sophia (the Church of the Wisdom of God). Founded in 1877, it still stands in Moscow Road, Bayswater.

Religious dietary restrictions

The Greek Orthodox Church specifies dietary restrictions and fasting on a total of 180–200 days annually. The faithful are advised to avoid olive oil, meat, fish, eggs and cheese every Wednesday and Friday, with the exception of the week after Christmas, Easter and the Pentecost. There are three principle fasting periods annually. The first of these are the 40 days preceding Christmas when meat, dairy products and eggs are not allowed, while fish and olive oil are allowed except on Wednesdays and Fridays. The second is Lent, the 48-day period preceding Easter. During Lent fish is allowed on only two days (25 March and Palm Sunday). Thirdly, there is a total of 15 days in

August (the Assumption) when the same dietary rules apply as for Lent with the exception of fish consumption, which is allowed only on 6 August (Metamorphosis) (Murray, 2010).

Religious festivals

Easter
Easter bread (*tsoureki*) is one of the various breads baked during Holy Week, the week before Easter, for the traditional midnight supper on Easter Sunday morning after the Resurrection service. Three dough plaits together symbolize the Holy Trinity (Kypri & Protopapa, 1997). Eggs are boiled and dyed with food colour, cracked and eaten at this time.

Easter soup (*mayeritsa*) is traditionally eaten at the celebration after the Resurrection service. The main ingredients are lamb, offal, tripe, rice, oil and seasonings.

Easter savoury pastries (*flaounes*) are made with a selection of full-fat cheeses with sultanas, bound with egg and encased in pastry. Traditionally, large trays of *flaounes* are made and eaten after the Resurrection service and on Easter Sunday often in place of bread in the morning and also offered to visitors. *Flaounes* are high in fat and hence energy-dense; the recipe could be modified by using lower-fat cheeses, although this would alter the taste and consistency. *Flaounes* are usually eaten over the 2–3 weeks after the Easter and many households also freeze them and consume them throughout the year. In order to reduce the total fat intake during this period, they could be taken in smaller amounts over a few days of the Easter period.

Christmas
Food at Christmas is plentiful like most occasions when the immediate and extended family get together. Food choices differ between households. A dish often found at this time is *saladina* which can be made from any cuts of meats in aspic. During the Christmas period various cakes are made (e.g., *melomekarouna* and *kourabiethes*). These contain large amounts of butter, sugar and nuts. *Melamekarouna* are drenched with syrup or honey.

New Year
Part of the Greek New Year tradition is to bake and share a cake known as a *vasilopita*. The name is derived from St. Basil, the patron saint of wishes and blessings, whose feast day is celebrated then. A coin is traditionally put in the cake and brings good luck to the person who finds it. All the family gather round the cake, embracing warmly and exchanging good wishes before the cake is consumed.

7.2.3   Traditional diet and eating pattern

Food forms an integral part of the life of Mediterranean people and is not seen as just a 'filler' but a way of sharing. It is rare that a meal will last less than an hour in most households. With more Greek women in the UK working it is not unusual for the grandmother to prepare meals for her adult children and grandchildren and this helps keep many traditional meals on the menu.

Bread, rice, potatoes and other starchy foods

Starchy foods are consumed with most meals and it is common to see bread on the table accompanying meals that may have one or more other sources of carbohydrate.

Bread is mainly white and unsliced and bought from Mediterranean food outlets. Bread can be used to mop up olive oil or sauces and also used to take the wide array of 'dips', including taramasalata, hummus and *tzansiki*.

White pitta bread is usually thicker than the supermarket brands and is taken mostly with grilled meats/barbecues and dips.

Rice is usually long grain. It can be boiled with a stock cube and a popular method is to fry diced onions and vermicelli (fine noodles) in olive oil and add these to the rice. An alternative is to add large handfuls of spinach just before the rice is fully cooked. This is called *spanahoriso*.

Pasta is cooked in a variety of ways. It can be boiled in chicken stock, with chunks of chicken placed on top of the pasta, and halloumi or anari cheese sprinkled on top for taste. A popular dish is *macaronatha tou fournou* (pasta of the oven) which is the Greek alternative to the British pasta bake with mince added to this dish.

Cracked wheat (bulgur) is popular and accompanies dishes like grilled meats and chicken and is often served with full-fat Greek yoghurt. Onions are fried and cracked wheat, water and stock are added. Tomatoes can be used to enhance the flavour.

Potatoes are cooked in many ways. Boiled potatoes are dressed with olive oil, spring onions, lemon, seasoning and large amounts of flat leaf parsley added for flavour.

Meat, fish, eggs, beans, pulses, nuts and seeds

Proteins are plentiful in the Greek diet and the portions are often large. There are no restrictions to the type of meats or fish that can be consumed other than abstinence from some animal products throughout the year for religious observance. Meats are usually seasoned with herbs and grilled, baked, boiled or fried. Chicken skin is rarely removed before or after cooking.

Fish is popular and often fried or otherwise baked or grilled, then dressed with olive oil, lemon juice and parsley. Greek people take all types of fish, and red mullet (floured and fried) is an oily fish which can be regularly found in the weekly diet. Tinned tuna is often taken as a side-dish to pulse based dishes with diced onions, parsley, lemon juice, salt and pepper added to enhance its flavour.

Eggs are eaten mostly at breakfast. These are usually fried or boiled.

Nuts and seeds are generally taken as a savoury snack or used in sweet dishes. They do not usually form a main meal ingredient. Nuts and seeds are usually bought from Mediterranean food outlets. Popular choices include pistachios, almonds, walnuts and pumpkin seeds and can be fried or baked with or without salt.

Pulses are popular in traditional Greek cuisine. There are numerous pulse dishes which can be cooked with or without meat and form main meals. For many, pulses are taken on Wednesdays and Fridays, which are encouraged by the Church as non-meat days. One example is haricot bean casserole (*fasolatha*). The beans are cooked in a rich, tomato-based sauce with or without red meat or chicken. This cooking method is known as *yiahni* and most beans can be cooked in this way.

Another way of cooking haricot beans is with pre-soaked beans cooked in water without tomatoes. Vegetables (e.g., slices of celery and potatoes) are added to the beans and once cooked the beans and vegetables are drained. The dish is then topped with large handfuls of chopped flat leaf parsley, dressed with olive oil, lemon and salt, and eaten with bread which is used to mop up the olive oil from the serving bowls.

Another pulse dish is black-eyed beans with spinach or silver beet, known as *louvvia me lahana.* The beans are boiled and when cooked, large handfuls of green leaves (silver beet or spinach) added to wilt. The beans are then drained and olive oil, lemon juice and seasoning added.

A popular lentil dish, known as *fakes*, is made by cooking lentils with rice then topping with sliced fried onions and seasoning the dish. This is usually eaten as a main dish and can be served with fried or grilled continental sausages, olives, tomatoes and plain yoghurt.

Milk and dairy foods

Consuming three portions of dairy products daily is an achievable target as dairy foods are taken liberally. Milk is usually taken in tea and is used in many Greek desserts.

Cheese may be taken daily. Popular varieties include halloumi, feta, *kefalodiri* (a hard cheese, like Cheddar) and can now be found in most major supermarkets in the UK.

Yoghurt is mostly consumed as plain, natural, full-fat yoghurt with rice or cracked wheat dishes, or with honey as a dessert.

Vegetables and fruit

Greek people tend not to have difficulty in achieving the recommended five portions of fruit and vegetables daily. Vegetables can be boiled or form part of a dish often cooked in a tomato-based sauce. Salads are made with different leaves and include coriander for taste. Olives and feta can be added and the salad is dressed with olive oil, lemon juice and seasonings.

Fruit is usually fresh and taken as a dessert or as a snack. During the summer watermelon is served with halloumi as a light meal.

Fats and oil

Olive oil is the main oil used in cooking, however vegetable oils are also used, especially for deep-fat frying. Margarine or butter is not usually spread on bread unless toasted. Generally speaking, fat-rich foods are pastry-based and/or foods which have large amounts of oils added to them or deep-fried. The pastry used for savoury dishes can be filo, puff or shortcrust.

Sugar and sugary foods

The majority of sugar in Greek cuisine comes in the form of honey and syrups used in sweet pastries and desserts. *Gliko* are a variety of fruits and vegetables preserved in syrup which are offered to guests as a sign of welcome and hospitality. Declining these would insult the host.

Beverages

Fizzy drinks and juices are consumed and the amounts vary between households. Sweet cordials include *triantafillo* (rose cordial), a sugary cordial which is mainly taken in the summer with rose essence or the almond equivalent, *sumatha*. Freshly squeezed fruit juice is also popular and may be taken daily.

7.2.4   Traditional meal pattern

Breakfast

This is an important meal and usually consists of fresh, unsliced white bread (with or without sesame seeds) consumed with cheese – often halloumi, a medium-fat goat cheese, *kefalodiri* or hard cheeses and sometimes feta. The cheese and bread are accompanied by olives, tomatoes and cucumber. Eggs and continental sausages are also taken, but not usually as a daily choice. Savoury pastries can also be consumed. It is not common to see Greek people taking breakfast cereals as their first choice, however this is more acceptable to the

second and third generations in the UK. Tea is taken with milk and some like to take Greek coffee with or without sugar.

Lunch and evening meal

There is usually one main hot meal and one lighter meal. The first generation often take their main meal in the early afternoon whereas this may be the evening meal for the younger working generation. As in many other cultures, women will be the main housekeepers and much of the cooking will be in their hands and recipes are passed down through the generations and adapted as time goes by (see Table 7.2.1).

Herbs and spices

Herbs and spices are widely used in Greek cuisine. Popular herbs and spices include cinnamon, cloves, coriander seeds, oregano, dill, flat leaf parsley, fresh coriander, rosemary and mint.

Salt

Salt is added in cooking and at the table. Foods which are high in salt include olives, feta and smoked products.

Encourage salt and salty foods in moderation only. For those with established hypertension or strong family history of stroke, discourage salty foods. Less salt in cooking and at the table is also advisable.

Cooking methods

Greeks use a wide array of cooking methods from roasting, boiling, grilling and frying. Barbecues are very popular, as is the use of clay ovens in mainland Greece and Cyprus for dishes like *kleftiko*. Olive oil is the oil of choice and is used in cooking and added to liberally dishes and salads. Much of the 'sweetness and body' of the dish is thought to be due to the large amounts of oil.

Alcohol

The main form of alcohol is red or white wine, usually taken with the meal in moderate amounts

Table 7.2.1   Foods to encourage and discourage in the Greek Diet

	Encourage	Discourage
Bread, rice, potatoes and other starchy foods	A variety of carbohydrates within the diet and higher-fibre choices wherever possible.	Large amounts of oil in cooking and in the use of dressings. Discourage large portions of carbohydrates if a reduction in energy intake would be beneficial.
Meat, fish, eggs, beans, pulses, nuts and seeds	A wide range of proteins, particularly the inclusion of oily fish twice a week and pulses for their cardio-protective factors. If pulses are cooked with meat, encourage lean cuts and skin taken off the chicken.	Large amounts of oil either in cooking or at the table. Excessive intake of energy-dense nuts as snacks.
Milk and dairy foods	Three portions of dairy foods daily (preferably lower-fat products) and recommend calcium-enriched soya milk and soya products for those who are fasting (and generally following a vegan diet) if not contraindicated. If dairy foods are limited or abstained from for long periods, there could be an increase risk of developing osteoporosis. Lower-fat dairy products should be encouraged (e.g., lower-fat plain yoghurts), in order to reduce the risk of hyperlipidaemia and obesity.	Large amounts of salty cheese (e.g., feta) if hypertensive.
Vegetables and fruit	Five portions or more daily.	Adding large amounts of salt. Many vegetables are fried with olive oil; the total fat content can be reduced if the vegetables are brushed with olive oil and grilled or baked rather than deep-fried.
Fats and oils	Use of fats and oils in moderation in line with healthy eating guidelines. Pastries and savoury snacks should be taken in moderation.	Large amounts of fried or fatty foods. Recipes can be adapted using lower-fat products and also less oil and healthier cooking methods.
Sugar, sugary foods and beverages	Use in moderation as part of a balanced diet. Encourage more fresh fruit and desserts made with less sugar and pastry.	Large amounts especially for those with chronic health conditions, including diabetes and obesity. Those with diabetes should be encouraged to abstain from very sweet desserts and pastries. Large amounts of sweet beverages, especially for those with chronic health conditions including diabetes and obesity. Those with diabetes should be encouraged to avoid sweet cordials.

(up to two glasses per day) and mostly with the main meal. Wine and other spirits may be taken with small snacks (*meze*). Popular spirits include ouzo and raki (white spirit). Local beers include Keo or locally brewed Carlsberg. Brandy is also locally sourced (e.g., V.S.O.P. and Anglias).

Encourage drinking alcohol within safe recommended levels. Discourage consuming alcohol above the safe recommended levels for all the population.

Smoking

Currently Greece has the highest smoking prevalence among members of the European Union. Recent epidemiological studies estimate that 40%

of the adult population are daily smokers, with 50% of adolescents in certain areas also current smokers. Although anti-smoking policies do exist and have been enforced over the years, many factors have contributed to their failure with a pro-tobacco culture and an increasing number of adolescent smokers exacerbating the problem (Vardavas & Kafatos, 2007).

7.2.5 Traditional meal pattern and dietary changes due to migration

With migration of any culture, there is always a risk that some of the traditional eating habits and meal patterns will change, however Greek and Greek Cypriots in the UK are fortunate to be able to purchase all the foods used in their homeland. For those who enjoy home-cooked foods without the trouble of cooking and preparation, there is an ever-increasing number of restaurants/cafés (*psistayies*, roughly translated as oven-cooking establishments) where home-cooked foods can be purchased providing a healthier alternative to fast-food outlets in the UK (see Table 7.2.2).

Main courses

Kebabs are very popular among Cypriots. They are made from lamb, chicken or pork skewered with tomatoes, onions and peppers, grilled over charcoal and served with pitta bread.

Kebabs are always served with salad and can also be served with rice or fried potatoes (see Table 7.2.3 and Table 7.2.4).

7.2.6 The Mediterranean diet and chronic diseases

The term 'Mediterranean diet' refers to the dietary patterns found in olive-growing areas of the Mediterranean region. Although there are several variants of this diet, the main principles are that it has a high monounsaturated: saturated fat ratio, alcohol is drunk in moderation, mainly in the form of wine: vegetable, fruit, legume and grain consumption is high; milk and dairy products consumption is moderate, and meat and meat products consumption is low (Trichopoulou et al., 2007).

The Mediterranean diet has been shown to have major positive implications in reducing the risk of chronic health conditions so much of the western world is encouraged to follow this pattern of eating (Martinez-Gonzalez et al., 2002). It has been noted that with Greek children and adolescents consuming a more westernized diet and moving away from the traditional Mediterranean diet, there could be major health implications among this community (Kontogianni et al., 2009).

Obesity

A systematic review of obesity and the Mediterranean diet indicated that exploring the relationship between the Mediterranean diet and obesity is complex. However, the evidence points towards the Mediterranean diet's positive role in preventing overweight and obesity (Buckland et al., 2008).

A study of childhood obesity concluded the Mediterranean diet is inversely associated with obesity in a sample of 9–13 year olds; however, physical activity and maternal obesity, dietary beliefs and behaviours seem to be more significant (Lazarou et al., 2010).

Diabetes

Much is known about the value of a low glycaemic index being correlated with improved glycaemic control. It is suggested that the preventive effect, especially with respect to diabetes, might be the low glycemic index of the Mediterranean diet. However, nutrients with a high GI are more frequently consumed in the Mediterranean diet than in other European countries. The major difference seems to be the higher amount of fibre and a higher intake of unsaturated fat, together with a higher intake of fruits and vegetables. Based on recent studies from the Nurses Health and Physicians Health Study, a diet which is similar to the Mediterranean diet, physical exercise and a BMI < 25kg/m^2 protects against the development of type 2 diabetes (Biesalski, 2004).

Coronary heart disease and stroke

Cardiovascular disease is the leading cause of morbidity and mortality in the western world. Adherence to a Mediterranean diet has been associated with a reduced risk of cardiovascular disease

Table 7.2.2 Traditional meal pattern and dietary changes in the Greek diet due to migration to the UK

Meal	Traditional meal	Dietary changes on migration to the UK	Healthier alternatives
Breakfast	Bread: traditionally white, unsliced, served with cheese (e.g., *kefalodiri*), *halloumi* with olives, cucumber, fresh tomatoes. Boiled eggs, grilled or fried, continental sausages (e.g., *loukanika*, not usually consumed daily). Savoury pastries	Same as traditional meal. Breakfast cereals are also consumed but not usually the first choice. Butter and margarine are not always spread on bread. Tea or coffee with cow's milk	Encourage whole meal and granary bread with small amounts of medium fat cheese or boiled egg and tomatoes, cucumber. Reduce intake of olives if hypertensive and rinse these well in water. Select high-fibre cereal or oats and use soya or semi-skimmed milk
Lunch	Main meal taken in late afternoon, consisting of the three main food groups. Proteins: meat, poultry, fish and pulses served with potatoes, rice, bulgur, wheat or pasta, salad and/or vegetables. Bread usually is taken with the meals	Same and/or light meal (e.g., sandwiches with cheese and ham/cold meats, salad)	If main meal, reduce the use of oil and if overweight/obese, advise on portion control. Encourage oily fish, pulses and lean meats with carbohydrates and lots of salad and/or vegetables. Whole meal or granary bread sandwiches with lean meats, fish, pulses and salad. Fruit, fruit and low-fat Greek yoghurt
Evening meal	Smaller main meal, usually another type of meal freshly made or light snack meal	Same and/or light meal (e.g., sandwiches with cheese and ham/cold meats, salad)	If main meal, reduce the use of oil and if overweight/obese, advise on portion control. Whole meal or granary bread sandwiches with lean meats, fish, pulses and salad. Fruit, fruit and low-fat Greek yoghurt
Puddings/ Desserts	Fruit: usually fresh Greek pastries and/or cakes. Milk-based puddings	Fruit: usually fresh Greek pastries and/or cakes. Milk-based puddings, etc.	Encourage fruit in all forms. Consume fewer cakes and pastries. Milk-based puddings made with semi-skimmed milk and less sugar, low-fat Greek yoghurt
Snacks	Nuts, fruit, *meze* (selection of cheeses, cold meats, breads, fresh vegetables)	Nuts, crisps, biscuits fruit, bread and cheese, cakes, savoury and/ or sweet pastries. *Meze* (selection of cheeses, cold meats, breads, fresh vegetables)	Select fruit as the main snack. Take pastries, nuts, crisps and biscuits sparingly
Drinks	Fruit juice, fizzy drinks. Tea, coffee, Greek coffee	Fruit juice, fizzy drinks. Tea, coffee, Greek coffee	Unsweetened juices, water, tea, coffee. Sugar-free fizzy drinks or squashes

Table 7.2.3 Glossary of *meze* or starter courses from the Greek diet

Name of foods	Description
Mezethes/Meze	Little hors d'oeuvres which are very important in the Cypriot cuisine. Each restaurant can create its own *mezethes/meze* and recipes are passed from mother to daughter.
Tzatziki	Cucumber with yoghurt.
Kolokouthakia	Fried courgettes.
Vazania	Fried aubergines.
Fasiolia plaki	Boiled bean salad.
Piperies ghemistes	Stuffed peppers.
Koupepia	Vine leaves stuffed with mince, rice, tomatoes and herbs.
Houmi	Chickpea spread (hummus).
Yaourti	Yoghurt.
Elies mavres	Black olives.
Elies tsakistes	Crushed green olives with garlic and oil.
Fetta	White cheese made from sheep's milk.
Halloumi	Halloumi (soft white cheese).
Avyo ortikiou	Hard-boiled quail's egg.
Tashi	Tahini dip.
Melintzanosalata	Aubergine salad.
Khoriatiki salata	Mixed salad.
Anari	Goat's milk curd.
Patatosalata	Potato salad.
Hot delicacies	
Halloumi tighanito	Fried halloumi (cheese).
Halloumi sti skhara	Grilled halloumi (cheese).
Sheftalies	Minced meat, onions, herbs made into a sausage and grilled.
Keftedhes	Meat balls (fried).
Kalamarakia	Squid, usually fried in batter or grilled.
Pourekia me halloumi	Small pasties stuffed with halloumi.
Pourekia me kaima	Small pasties stuffed with minced meat.
Pourekia me spanakhi	Small pasties stuffed with spinach.
Koupes	Minced meat wrapped in crushed wheat and fried.
Pastoumas	Traditional spicy sausage.
Ravioles	Ravioli with cheese.
Soups	
Trakhanas	Soup with crushed wheat dried in yoghurt.
Louvana	Lentil soup.
Avgholemono	Soup with chicken, lemon, egg and rice.
Khortosoupa	Vegetable soup.
Psarosoupa	Fish soup.

Table 7.2.4   Glossary of main courses and desserts

Name of foods	Description
Meat and beans	
Souvlakia	Lamb kebab.
Kotopoulo souvlaki	Chicken kebab.
Afelia	Fried pork with coriander seeds, garlic and red wine.
Mousakkas	A dish with layers of aubergine, potatoes, courgettes, mince meat covered with a béchamel sauce.
Pastitiou (makaronatha to fourno)	Minced meat with pasta topped with a béchamel sauce.
Psito or kleftiko	Chunks of lamb, which is usually wrapped in foil, with potatoes, onions, tomatoes and baked in a brick oven for about three hours. Used to be baked kebab underground or in a clay oven.
Sheftalies	Minced meat, onions, herbs made into a sausage and grilled.
Keftedhes	Meat balls (fried).
Koupepia	Vine leaves stuffed with mince, rice, tomatoes and herbs.
Kounelli stifado	Rabbit stew with onions.
Fasiolia yiahni	Haricot bean stew, either with or without meat in a tomato-based sauce.
Fakes	Brown lentils with rice and onions.
Fish	Fish is very popular and either fried or grilled/baked and topped with large amounts of olive oil, lemon juice and flat leaf parsley with a side-dish or fried potatoes and salad.
Mbarpouni	Red mullet.
Sorkos	White bream.
Fangri	Sea bream.
Lavraki	Sea bass.
Tonos	Tuna.
Kefalos	Grey mullet.
Tsipoura	Porgy.
Pakayiaros	Cod.
Kalamaraki	Squid.
Oktabothi	Octopus.
Fruits and sweets	
Lokmadhes	Lokma, similar to doughnut soaked in syrup.
Halouvas	Sweet dish made with semolina, roasted almonds and rose water.
Rizoghalo	Rice pudding.
Katiefi	Layers of shredded filo pastry with honey, nuts and syrup.
Paklavas	Layers of filo pastry with honey, nuts and syrup.
Paghoto	Ice cream.
Loukoumi	Turkish delights.
Katimeri	Sweet made with flour, oil, butter, almonds and cinnamon.
Gliko siko	Preserved figs (in syrup).

(Pangiotakos *et al.*, 2008), diabetes (Martinez-Gonzalez *et al.*, 2008) and overall mortality in European (Trichopoulou *et al.*, 2003) and non-European (Mitrou *et al.*, 2007) populations.

Two large randomized trials have provided evidence that the Mediterranean diet can significantly reduce mortality in patients who have suffered a myocardial infarction or patients diagnosed with angina pectoris, myocardial infarction or surrogate risk factors for coronary heart disease (Trichopoulou *et al.*, 2007; Martinez-Gonzalez *et al.*, 2009). The latter paper showed that there was a reduction in the mortality rates for both coronary heart disease and cancer. A Mediterranean diet was associated with a 40% reduction in the risk of CHD. Olive oil consumption was not associated with weight gain and the intake of vegetables and olive oil was inversely associated with hypertension.

The inverse link between stroke and the Mediterranean diet was well illustrated in a study of over 74,000 female nurses followed for a period of >20 years. Those with a greater adherence to a Mediterranean diet had a significantly lower risk of CHD and stroke (Fung *et al.*, 2009).

Cancer

The Mediterranean diet is rich in omega 3 fatty acids and there is strong evidence that the consumption of these fatty acids has anti-inflammatory, anti-apoptotic, anti-proliferative and anti-angiogenic effects (Spencer *et al.*, 2009). The rich intake of vegetables reduces the incidence of endothelial cancers, and a diet rich in olive oil and low in saturated fat is inversely associated with cancers of the upper respiratory-digestive tract (Pelucchi *et al.*, 2009). Fruit intake is inversely associated with digestive tract and laryngeal cancers. Flavanoids and polyphenols present in fruit and vegetables have anti-oxidant properties and are inversely related to upper respiratory tract and upper digestive tract neoplasms, as well as gastric cancers (La Vecchia *et al.*, 1999). Evidence indicates that foods containing lycopene as well as selenium found in fruits and vegetables protect against prostrate cancer (Itsiopoulos *et al.*, 2008). Compared with many western countries Greece has a lower prostrate cancer mortality and Greek migrant men in Australia have retained this lower risk of prostrate cancer (Itsiopoulos *et al.*, 2008).

Other diseases

Recent evidence has shown the positive benefits of a prenatal and childhood Mediterranean diet in the development of asthma and allergies in children (Chatzi & Kogevinas, 2009). Adherence to the Mediterranean diet may positively affect not only the risk of Alzheimer's disease but also the subsequent disease course (Scarmeas *et al.*, 2007). Adopting the Mediterranean diet is positively related to bone mass, suggesting the potential bone-preserving properties of this diet throughout adult life (Kondoyianni *et al.*, 2008).

7.3 Turkish Diet
Thomina Mirza, and Tahira Sarwar

Key points

- Almost all (98%) of the Turkish population are Muslim, of whom two-thirds are Sunni and one-third Shiites.
- Halal foods are consumed, but the following are forbidden (haram): pork and pork products, fish without fins and scales, all commercially made products if the source of the fat in it is not known, alcohol (observance varies according to the level of devoutness), jelly or sweets or puddings made with porcine or gelatin.
- During Ramadan most adult Muslims (with the exception of the very sick, those on some drug treatments and pregnant or menstruating women) fast from dawn to dusk.
- There are many religious festivals throughout the year. Food plays a major part in these celebrations.
- Most Turks follow Mediterranean-style diet principles, which may reduce rates of heart disease and diabetes, however few data are available relating specifically to the Turkish population.

7.3.1 Introduction

Turkey is located at the eastern end of the Mediterranean. It covers around 779,452 sq km and has borders with Armenia, Bulgaria, Georgia,

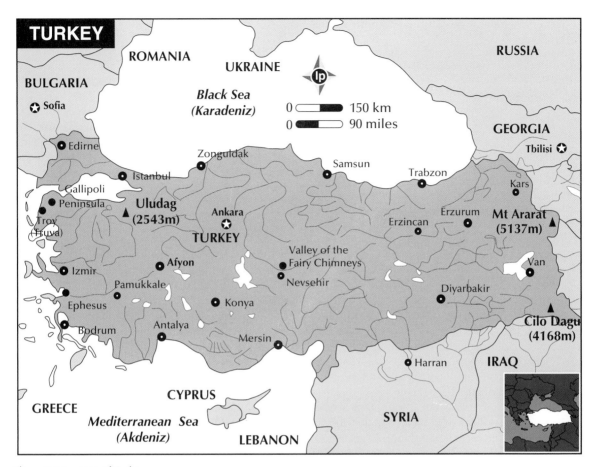

Figure 7.3.1   Map of Turkey

Greece, Iran, Iraq, North Africa, Russia and Syria (see Figure 7.3.1). Modern Turks are the descendants of nomadic people who migrated from the Altay Mountains in Central Asia towards Anatolia. Turkey has a very long history of almost 10,000 years and has been influential since the Roman era and early Christianity, before the birth of Islam. About 80% of the people in Turkey are Turks who originally came from Central Asia, while 17% are Kurds who comprise the majority in the southeastern territories. The remaining 3% are made up of other ethnic groups, including Greeks, Armenians and Jews.

While most Turkish citizens are Muslims, the government is both democratic and secular. Turkey has always been the meeting point for its European and Middle Eastern neighbours, hence it has been called the crossroads of Europe. Consequently, its customs and cuisine are both modern and traditional. Over the centuries the Hittites, Persians, Greeks and Romans have ruled the area. Although Ankara is the capital, Istanbul is the largest city and is the industrial, commercial and intellectual heart of the country. Mustafa Kemal Ataturk was the founder of the modern Turkish republic.

Climate

The summers are very hot. In the west, near Iran and Iraq, winters are very cold (−10° C), and in the south, near Africa and Middle East, it is very hot in summer and cold in winter. Turkey has a very varied landscape and for every 2–4 hours of travelling by car you can expect to experience changes in scenery, temperature, altitude, humidity and vegetation.

Language

Turkish is the official language, although Kurdish and Kurmenji are also spoken.

Migration to the United Kingdom

As a legacy of the Ottoman Empire, there are significant Turkish minorities in Europe such as the Turks in Bulgaria, Cyprus, Greece, Kosovo and the Republic of Macedonia. The postwar migration of Turks to Europe began with 'guest workers' who arrived under the terms of a Labour Export Agreement with Germany in October 1961, followed by a similar agreement with the Netherlands, Belgium and Austria in 1964; France in 1965 and Sweden in 1967. As one Turkish observer noted: 'It has now been over 40 years and a Turk who went to Europe at the age of 25 has nearly reached the age of 70. His children have reached the age of 45 and their children have reached the age of 20.'

Despite the UK not being a signatory to the Labour Export Agreement, it is still a major hub for Turkish emigrants, with a population of quarter of a million Turks (an estimated 100,000 Turkish nationals and 130,000 nationals of the Turkish Republic of Northern Cyprus currently live in the UK). This figure, however, does not include the much larger numbers of Turkish speakers born in Britain or who have obtained British nationality), and the UK is in fact home to Europe's third largest Turkish community. High immigration has resulted in Turkish being the seventh most commonly spoken language in the UK (en.wikipedia.org/wiki/Turkish_people).

Current UK population

The estimated number of Turkish nationals living in the UK (students, au pairs, illegal immigrants included) is around 500,000. They mostly live in London (Islington, Hackney, Harringey, Stoke Newington, Turnpike Lane and Newington Green in the north and Peckham and Lewisham in the south), Birmingham, Manchester, Liverpool and Leeds.

7.3.2   Religion

Ninety-eight per cent of the Turkish population are Muslim, of whom about two-thirds are Sunni and one-third Shiites. The Turks converted to Islam on their way to Anatolia from Central Asia. Although Turkish laws and other social structures are not based on Islamic principles as Turkey is officially a secular state, Islam exerts a continuing influence on society, especially in rural areas. Most Turks observe the Islamic calendar and fast during Ramadan.

Religious dietary influences

In Islam, personal appearance and physical cleanliness are considered to be as important as spiritual purity. There are Islamic instructions on cleanliness and health, which include every aspect of everyday life. These come from Qu'ranic teachings and Prophet Muhammad's practices known as the Sunnah. All the prohibitions (e.g., eating animals found dead, blood and pork, drinking alcohol, gambling, abortion, etc.) were designed to protect the health and well-being of the individual.

Halal meats are preferred as animals are slaughtered in the Islamic way, by reciting the name of God (Allah). Once the animal is slaughtered the blood is allowed to drain out.

The following foods are prohibited:

- Pork and pork products (e.g., pork fat or lard).
- Fish/seafood without fins and scales.
- All commercially made products if the source of the fat in it is not known.
- Alcohol (observance varies according to the level of devoutness).
- Jelly or sweets or puddings made with gelatin.

Some foods are specially recommended in the Qu'ran, such as honey, dates and milk (also olives and figs, but these do not feature in the Turkish diet). In general, Islam recommends eating and drinking in moderation. Islamic teaching also encourages Muslims to wash their hands before and after meals, and to wash fruit before eating it. They are also encouraged to take small mouthfuls and chew them well, to keep food and water covered in storage, to avoid eating food while it is too hot, to avoid eating unless one is hungry and to stop eating before feeling full. Many of these instructions correspond with current health education recommendations. See Chapter 5 section 5.1.2 for more detail on Islamic dietary practices.

Religious dietary restrictions

During Ramadan, Muslims fast from dawn to dusk for one month. Ramadan is the ninth month of the Islamic lunar calendar, and falls on different dates every year. All Muslim adults (those who have reached puberty) are expected to fast. Before the fast begins, a meal (*suhoor*) is eaten before dawn. The Muslim will fast during daylight hours and break the fast immediately after sunset. The fast is usually broken (*futoor* or *iftaar*) with dates and water. If dates are not available, then other fruits can be used. A meal then follows.

The very sick (acutely ill), the sick (those dependent on drug therapy, e.g., Type 1 diabetics), women who are menstruating, pregnant or breastfeeding, or have postpartum bleeding, are exempt from fasting. The latter group will make up their days of missed fasting at a later date, when they are able to do so. Muslims who are acutely ill will be reluctant to break their fast whatever their condition and may not wish to take foods or medicines, even in hospital. While in hospital the chaplain services can be contacted to ensure that the Muslim patient will not be committing a sin by not observing the fast. Hospital patients who are able to fast may require meals to be served outwith standard meal times.

Religious festivals and foods

Eid-al-Adha (Kurban Bayrami, Sacrifice Holiday)

This is a three-day celebration marking the climax of the *hajj* pilgrimage. It commemorates the Prophet Abraham's readiness to sacrifice his son, but God sent him a ram so sparing the boy's life. The act of sacrificing an animal, usually a sheep, represents repentance. The meat is given to neighbours and the needy. It also marks the season of pilgrimage to Mecca (*hajj*).

Eid-al-Fitr

A celebration marking the end of Ramadan.

Seker Bayrami (Sugar Holiday)

Celebrated at the end of Ramadan. A favourite treat at this time is *rahat lokoum* known in the West as Turkish delight.

Muharrem

This commemorates the time when the biblical floodwaters receded and Noah and his family were able to land. It is believed they cooked a meal using whatever remained of their supplies. This event is celebrated by cooking *ashure* (Noah's pudding), which is made of wheat, berries, dried legumes, rice, raisins, dried figs, dates and nuts.

7.3.3 Traditional diet and eating pattern

The foundations of the Turkish diet were laid by its nomadic ancestry. Turkey's diverse geography provides a seasonal climate that allows tea cultivation in the cool north and hot pepper and melon growing in the south. Today's Turkish cuisine reflects the extent of Ottoman Empire, which extended from North Africa, through parts of Middle East, the Balkans and in Europe as far as Vienna.

The cuisine includes a varied selection of appetizers, soups, meat dishes, vegetable dishes, elaborate desserts and Turkish coffee. The seas provide a wealth of fish and shellfish. In the 1900s there was extensive migration from villages to the cities and also from other countries, the migrants bringing their eating habits and cooking styles with them. It is one of the few countries in the world that is self-sufficient, producing all its own food. Partly as a result of this, a huge emphasis is placed on using fresh ingredients. Dishes tend to be simply presented, with food not masked by sauces or elaborate garnishes (see Table 7.3.1).

In Turkey, as in many Mediterranean countries, the main meal is eaten in the evening. Leftovers are uncommon in any household. Traditionally, many foods are eaten with the fingers, but cutlery is now widely used. To begin or end a meal, one might say 'Afiyet olsun' (May what you eat bring you well-being).

Cooking methods

Food is cooked in large quantities. Often it is prepared over few days as it is very labour-intensive and requires a long time to prepare.

- Pulses are stewed.
- Meats, fish, chicken are grilled, fried or baked.
- Meat in the form of kebab are grilled, and *kofta* is fried or baked.
- Vegetables are fried.

Table 7.3.1 Traditional foods in the Turkish Diet

Food groups	Description and names of foods
Bread, rice, potatoes, pasta and other starchy foods	Leavened and unleavened breads: *manti, borek, pide*, whole meal bread, pitta, sliced bread *Fragella*: Like a French baguette, but bulkier Bulgur (buckwheat), often boiled with tomatoes, onions; chicken stock may also be added. Rice pilaf and bulgur pilaf Breakfast cereals (mainly Cornflakes, Weetabix) Potatoes, pasta and pizza
Vegetables	Winter: spinach, leeks, cauliflower, black cabbage, beet. Vegetables are often added to stews. Summer: green beans, marrow, peppers, aubergine, carrots Dolmas: stuffed vegetable in a vine leaf rolled into cigar shape, fried or grilled Salad with olive oil
Fruits	Spring: strawberries, cherries and apricots, Summer: peaches, watermelons, melons, grapes, figs, plums, apples, pears guava, pomegranate, quince (late summer) Winter: oranges, mandarins and bananas; also preserved as dried fruit, compotes and jams, e.g., quince and rose petal preserve
Salted or preserved foods	Pickled vegetables are preserved in vinegar or lemon with salt and eaten in the winter with pulses Jam *Hushaf* – prune juice made with water and sugar. Drunk in summer, chilled.
Meat, fish, eggs, beans and other non-dairy sources	Meat: lamb, beef, chicken (pork not eaten by Muslims); fish; eggs and pulses. Steak tartar was introduced by nomadic Turks who carried spiced and raw meat in their saddle bags. In the UK it is made by kneading double ground raw meat with thin bulgur and hot spices. Bite-sized portions are served with *chilantro*, known for its stomach-protecting properties. Fish: many species of fish migrate from the Black Sea to warmer waters in winter when most fish reach their maturity. Fish, including cod, *tarma* (cod's roe dip), jack, are mainly grilled. Small fish are fried, and eaten as part of meal or as snack Hamsi is considered the prince of all fish. Oily fish like mackerel, trout, and sardines are used. Fried mussels are also hugely popular. Every month has its own preferred fish along with specific vegetables which complement the taste. Offal: liver and heart are fried; tripe is used in soup. Beans: white, black-eyed, butter beans, lima, *bette locher* (white and red striped beans), green and red lentils, chickpeas. All are stewed or cooked with olive oil. Lentils are eaten as soup in the summer with bread. Pulses are used for making hummus or lentil dip.
Milk and dairy foods	Milk, traditionally skimmed but as wealth increases so does the richness of foods, therefore more people now prefer full-fat milk. Cheese: feta, kashar, Cheddar/full-fat cheese. Cheese is often eaten at breakfast. *Tulum*: goat's cheese, crumbly, more mature than cottage cheese, eaten as a snack. *Iyran*: salty drinking yoghurt, consumed with meals especially with kebabs and potatoes or as a snack. *Olik*: diluted yoghurt with cucumber and garlic, eaten as a dip with salad.
Fats and oils	Butter is associated with wealth and status. Most Turkish prefer to cook with *mergnnes* (salted butter). Rice or bulgur with butter eaten at breakfast. Olive oil and vegetable oil also used in cooking.

Table 7.3.1 (cont'd)

Food groups	Description and names of foods
Sugar and sugary foods	Sugar, is sugar added to tea/coffee. Turkish delight, baklava. *Locma* (hard dough fried then added to sweet syrup). *Akide sekeri* (boiled sweets). Milky puddings, rice pudding, semolina (*helva*). *Tahini.* *Pigmies* (boiled grape paste with sugar) Milkshakes (especially banana).
Beverages	Coffee: Turkish with no added milk. Milk is added to instant coffee. Tea: *Elam chai* (powdered apple tea), linden, flower (lime tree) tea, mint, marigold. Cocoa and alcohol also consumed. Men drink more than women.
Herb and spices	Salt, red pepper, black pepper, cinnamon, allspice, paprika, ginger, garlic powder, basil, thyme, oregano, sumac, saffron, cumin, chilli, dill.

- Fat is often left on the meat, especially if it is grilled.
- Whole or quartered, chicken will be cleaned and cooked with its fat on.
- Large fish are cleaned and cooked with scales, fins and head.
- Small fish may be just washed and then cooked whole.

Typical meal pattern

An example of a typical Turkish meal is rice with *kofte*, salad and bread. Traditional foods are generally accessible in Britain, but foodstuffs such as fish are more expensive. Turkish cuisine puts huge emphasis on fresh fruit and vegetables, thus requiring frequent shopping trips. Cost may also influence how much fruit and vegetables is consumed. Eating traditional dishes such as cold *mezes* on a cold day in the UK may appeal less than in the warm climate of Turkey. Therefore more convenience foods may be adopted. Also takeaways and fast-food outlets are now opening in Turkey and are also popular cuisine in the UK (see Table 7.3.2).

Breakfast

- Tea, feta, bread, butter, olives, jam, egg sausage, fish, peppers, pasta, cake, *burik*.
- *Sujuk* (cooked breakfast).
- Breakfast cereals are preferred by younger generation.

Mid-morning

- Coffee.

Lunch

- Pulses, bread, bulgur, soup, pasta, meat, fish, egg, vegetables.
- Two-course meal.
- Desserts are eaten occasionally.

Mid-afternoon

- Tea, biscuit, *berek* (pasty made with cheese/potato wrapped in filo pastry and baked).

Evening meal

- Like lunch.

Snacks

- Nuts (e.g., almonds and pistachios), fruit, bread and cheese, *meze*.

Foods eaten regularly

- Bread, bulgur, potatoes, rice and pasta.
- Stews, meat, chicken, mince (beef, lamb or chicken).
- Kebabs.
- All vegetables.
- Halva.

Foods eaten occasionally (on special occasions, etc.)

- Baklava.
- Fish.
- Veal, expensive meats.
- Dates.

Traditional diet

Meze

In spite of the Islamic prohibition against wine and anything alcoholic, there is a rich tradition in Turkey associated with liquor. Similar to Spanish tapas, *meze* is the general category of dishes that are taken in small quantities to start the meal. These are eaten along with wine or Raki, the anise-flavoured national drink, sometimes referred to as 'lion's milk'.

The bare minimum *meze* is slices of honeydew melon and feta cheese with freshly baked bread. Other *meze* include: dried and marinated mackerel, fresh salad greens in a thick yoghurt sauce with garlic, plates of cold vegetable dishes cooked in olive oil, fried crispy savoury pastry, deep-fried mussels and calamari (squid) served in sauce,

tomato and cucumber salad, and roe in sauce. The main course that follows this would be fish or grilled meat.

When the main course is kebab, then the *meze* spread is different. In this case several plates of different types of salad greens and tomatoes in spicy olive oil, mixed with yoghurt or cheese, hummus, bulgur and red lentil balls, marinated stuffed aubergine, peppers with spices and nuts, and pickle.

Vegetables

The simplest and most basic vegetable dish is prepared by slicing a main vegetable such as courgette or aubergine, combining it with tomatoes, green peppers and onions and cooking it slowly in butter and its own juices, and eaten with a chunk of bread. Vegetables such as fresh string beans, artichokes, root celery, aubergines, pinto beans and courgettes are also cooked in olive oil. These are generally served at room temperature and may be eaten with a tomato or yoghurt sauce. Any vegetable that can be stuffed with, or which can be wrapped round, rice or meat can be used to make dolmas. Aubergines are probably the most popular Turkish vegetable.

Table 7.3.2 Traditional eating pattern and dietary changes on migration

Meal	Traditional	Dietary changes on migration to the UK	Healthier alternatives
Breakfast	Fresh tomatoes, bread, white cheese, olives, egg, marmalade or honey	As traditional: Cereal with milk	Bread (1/2 whole meal, 1/2 white flour). Low- fat cheese, jam, marmalade Cereal with low-fat milk
Lunch	Fresh tomatoes, bread, white cheese, olives, egg, marmalade or honey	As traditional: Sandwiches, takeaways (e.g., pizza)	Rice with chicken and vegetables Sandwich with low-fat filling
Evening meal	Fresh tomatoes, bread, white cheese, olives, egg, marmalade or honey	As traditional (depending on availability): Takeaways (e.g., chips, doner kebab)	Salad with low-fat dressing Soup Rice with meat/chicken and vegetables
Puddings/ Desserts	Baklava, Fresh fruit *muhallebi* (milk pudding)	Fruit Ice cream Cake	Fruit Milk pudding made with low-fat milk, reduced sugar
Drinks	Tea Turkish coffee (*kahve*) Alcohol (drunk by some)	Tea/coffee Alcohol Soft drinks Fruit juice	Water Sugar-free/diet soft drinks Tea/coffee with less/no sugar/ sweetener
Snacks	Fruit roll-ups (sheets of dried, mashed apricots and grapes) Trail mix (nuts and raisins)	Baklava Chocolates, crisps, nuts	Fruit Bread with salad Dried fruit

Desserts

The two most well-known sweets associated with the Turkish cuisine are Turkish delight and baklava. However, the dessert most commonly eaten after a meal is fresh seasonal fruit. Milk desserts (*muhallebi*) are also popular. These are made with rice flour.

Grain-based desserts include baked pastries, fried yeast-dough pastries and the pan-sautéed desserts. The baked pastries can also referred to as the baklava family. These are paper-thin pastry sheets (filo pastry) brushed with butter and folded, layered or rolled after being filled with ground pistachios, walnuts or heavy cream, and baked. Syrup is then poured over the baked pastries. Different types (e.g., the sultan, the nightingale's nest, the twisted turban) vary according to the amount and placement of nuts, size, shape and dryness (see Table 7.3.3).

Table 7.3.3   Glossary of common Turkish foods

Name of food	Description of food
Ashure	A pudding made of cereals, dried and fresh fruits, nuts, sugar and spices, referred to as 'Noah's pudding'.
Ayran	A drink of beaten yoghurt, cold water and salt.
Borek	Thin sheets of pastry filled with cheese or meat mixes and baked or fried. Eaten on special occasions.
Cacik	Grated cucumber with diluted yoghurt, garlic, salt, sprinkled with dill and olive oil.
Doner kebab	A roll of lamb on a vertical skewer turning parallel to a hot grill.
Dolma	Any filled or stuffed vegetable.
Emek	White bread.
Gorp	Mixed nuts and raisins.
Helva	A dessert of flour, semolina, butter, sugar, milk and nuts.
Hummus	Chickpeas mashed in *tahini*.
Kadayif	Finely shredded pastry used to make a dessert. Looks like Shredded Wheat.
Kavurma	Lamb cut into small cubes, braised and browned for use in stews.
Kofte	Any dish made with ground meats, or bulgur and rice mixture; skewered, baked or fried.
Leblebi	Roasted and dried chickpeas eaten as an appetizer. Salted or unsalted.
Lokum	A gelled sweet often mixed with hazelnuts or pistachios, cut into cubes and rolled in powdered sugar. Called Turkish delight in English-speaking countries.
Manti	Small pastries filled with minced meat, similar to ravioli, but very small.
Oturma	Similar to stuffed vegetables, but fried and filled with browned spices then simmered.
Pasturma	Spicy, sun-dried beef.
Pekmez	Grape molasses.
Pide	Flattened oval bread served plain or meat filled.
Pilaki	A bean dish cooked in olive oil, served cold with lemon.
Pilaf	Made from cracked wheat or rice.
Piyaz	Dried bean salad with egg and vegetable.
Sarma	Vine or cabbage leaves filled with minced meat or rice.
Simit	Sesame seed rings.
Sish kofte	Commonly known as shish kebab in the West, pieces of meat or *kofte* spit-roasted.

7.3.5   Prevalence of chronic diseases

There are few data available looking specifically at the prevalence of chronic diseases among the Turkish population.

Overweight

Relatively few data concerning the health status of migrants are available. However, the risk of overweight in children and women is high among the Turkish in comparison to, e.g., the Dutch (eurodiet.med.uoc).

Protective effects of the Mediterranean diet

The Mediterranean diet is promoted as being healthy. In comparison to other ethnic groups such as Caucasians and Asians, diseases such as heart disease and diabetes are not common. However, they can be found and so appropriate advice should be given to follow a healthy lifestyle. (See section 7.2.6 for more detail on the benefits of a Mediterranean diet).

Websites

Greek Diet

www.bbc.co.uk/london/content/articles/2005/05/27/greek_london_feature.shtml
www.bbc.co.uk/voices/multilingual/greek.shtml
www.greeka.com/greece-religion.htm
www.migrationinformation.org

Turkish Diet

www.turkconsulate-london.com
www.geocities.com/resats/culture.html
www.pilot.co.uk/destinations/food/turkey.html
www.banihan.freeserve.co.uk/turkish_cuisine.html
www.turizm.gov.tr/engbakanlik/cuisine/contem.htm
www.focusmm.com/tr_ye_mn.htm
www.turkey.org/artculture/cuisine.htm
www.anatolia.com
www.sallys_place.com/food/ethnic_cuisine/turkey.htm
eurodiet.med.uoc
en.wikipedia.org/wiki/Turkish_people

Further reading

Turkish Diet

Algar, A.E. (1999) *Classical Turkish Cooking.* HarperCollins, New York.

Halici, N. (1989) *Turkish Cookbook.* Dorling Kindersley, London.
Hamid, F. & Sarwar, T. (2004) *Global Nutrition, A Multicultural Resource Pack for Developing Multicultural Dietary Competencies.* Brent and Westminster Primary Care Trust, London.

References

Polish Diet

Bielecki, W. *et al.* (2005) Świadomość zasad zapobiegania chorobom układu krążenia w populacji dorosłych mieszkańców Polski. Wyniki programu WOBASZ. *Kardiologia Polska*, 63: 6 (|Suppl. 4).
Ciborowska, H. & Rudnicka, A. (2007) *Dietetyka.* Warszawa.
CRONEM (Centre for Research on Nationalism, Ethnicity and Multiculturalism) (2007) *Polish Migrants Survey Results.* University of Surrey for BBC Newsnight. www.surrey.ac.uk/Arts/CRONEM/CRONEM_BBC_Polish_survey%20_results.pdf.
GUS (Polish Central Statistics Office) (2007) www.stat.gov.pl/english.
GUS (Polish Central Statistics Office) (2007) *Report on Health of the Population.* www.stat.gov.pl/cps/rde/xchg/gus.
HO (Home Office) (2009) *Accession Monitoring Report, 2004–2009.* www.bia.homeoffice.gov.uk/sitecontent/documents/aboutus/reports/accession_monitoring_report.
Jarosz, M. (2007) *Epidemiologia otylosci wsrod dzieci i doroslych. Zwalczanie otylosci I innych przewleklych chorob niezakaznych.* Report of the Polish Institute of Food and Nutrition. www.izz.waw.pl.
Klosiewicz-Latoszek L. *et al.* (2008) Konsensus Rady Redakcyjnej PFP dotyczący zasad prawidłowego żywienia. *Forum*, 1(10). www.pfp.edu.pl.
LSMU (London Social Marketing Unit) (2009) Childhood Obesity & Infant Weaning Practices. Findings of Qualitative Research Project with Somali, Polish and Turkish Communities in London. Commissioning Support for London.
Ministry of the Interior and Administration (MIA). www.mswia.gov.pl/portal/en/10/54/Ethnic_and_national_minorities_in_Poland.html.
ONS (2007) *Migrants from Central and Eastern Europe: Local Geographies*, No. 129. www.statistics.gov.uk.
Polish National Health Programme (2007) *Narodowy Program Zdrowia 2007–2015.* www.mz.gov.pl/wwwfiles/ma.../zal_urm_npz_90_15052007p.pdf.
Popova, S., Rehm, J. *et al.* (2007) Comparing alcohol consumption in central and eastern European countries. *Alcohol and Alcoholism*, 42(5), 465–73.

PorGrow (2007) *Project Summary Report: Policy Options for Responding to Obesity: Evaluating the Options.* University of Sussex, Brighton. www.sussex.ac.uk/spru/1-4-7-1-8.html.

Rehm, J. *et al.* (2007) Alcohol accounts for a high proportion of premature mortality in central and eastern Europe. *International Journal of Epidemiology*, 36, 458–67.

Ruszkowska-Majzel, J. & Drygas, W. (2007) Effective methods of active lifestyle promotion as a challenge for public health worldwide (Abstract). *Zdr Publ*, 117(2), 225–31.

Szponar, L., Ciok, J., Dolna, A. & Otarzewski, M. (2006) *Polish National Report. Policy Options for Responding to the Growing Challenge from Obesity.* National Food and Nutrition Institute. Poland. www.sussex.ac.uk/spru/documents/poland_english.pdf.

Waśkiewicz, A. (2008) Quality of nutrition and health knowledge in subjects with diagnosed cardio-vascular diseases in the Polish population – National Multicentre Health Survey (WOBASZ). *Kardiol Pol*, 66, 507–13.

WHO (2007) *The Challenge of Obesity in the WHO European Region and the Strategies for Response.* www.euro.who.int/docu.

WHO/FAO (2003) *Expert Consultation on Diet, Nutrition and the Prevention of Chronic Diseases.* ftp.fao.org/docrep/fao/005/ac911e/ac911e00.pdf.

Zatonski, W., Campos, H. & Willett, W. (2007) Rapid declines in coronary heart disease mortality in Eastern Europe are associated with increased consumption of oils rich in alpha-linoleic acid. *Journal of Epidemiology* 23(1), 3–10.

Greek Diet

Biesalski, H.K. (2004) Diabetes preventive components in the Mediterranean diet. *European Journal of Nutrition*, 43(Suppl. 1), 26–30.

Boatswain, T. (2005) *A Traveler's History of Greece.* 1st edition. Interlink Publishing, Northampton, MA.

Boatswain, T. & Nicolson, C. (2001) *A Traveler's History of Cyprus.* 4th edition. Interlink Publishing, Northampton, MA.

Buckland, G., Bach, A. & Sera-Majem, L. (2008) Obesity and the Mediterranean diet: a systemic review of observational and intervention studies. *Obesity Reviews*, 9(6), 582–93.

Chatzi, L. & Kogevinas, M. (2009) Prenatal and childhood Mediterranean diet and the development of asthma and allergies in children. *Public Health Nutrition*, 12(9A), 1629–34.

Fung, T.T., Rexrode, K.M. & Mantzoros, C.S. (2009) Mediterranean diet and incidence of mortality from coronary heart disease and stroke in women. *Circulation*, 119(8), 1093–100.

Itsiopoulos, C., Hodge, A. & Kaimakamis, M. (2008) Can the Mediterranean diet prevent prostrate cancer? *Molecular Nutrition and Research*, 53(2), 227–39.

Kondoyianni, M.D., Vidra, N. *et al.* (2008) Adherence rates to the Mediterranean diet are low in a representative sample of Greek children and adolescents. *Journal of Nutrition*, 138, 1951–6.

Kontogianni, M.D., Melistas, L. *et al.* (2009) Association between dietary patterns and indices of bone mass in a sample of Mediterranean women. *Nutrition*, 25(2), 165–71.

Kypri, T. & Protopapa, K. (1997) *Traditional Pastries in Cyprus. Their Use and Importance in Customary Life.* Ellas Press, Cypress.

La Vecchia, C.,Chatenoud, L. & Franceschi, S. (1999) Vegetables and fruit in human cancer: update of an Italian study. *Int J Cancer*, 82, 151–2.

Lazarou, C., Panagiotakos, D.B. & Mataslas, A.L. (2010) Physical activity mediates the protective effect of the Mediterranean diet on children's obesity stutus: The CYKIDS study. *Nutrition*, 26(1), 61–7.

Martinez-Gonzalez, M., Bes-Rastrollo, M. & Serra-Majem, L. (2009) Mediterranean food pattern and the primary prevention of chronic disease: recent devoplements. *Nutr Rev*, 67(Suppl. 1), 111–16.

Martinez-Gonzalez, M.A., de la Fuente-Arrillaga, C. *et al.* (2008) Adherence to a Mediterranean diet and risk of developing diabetes: prospective cohort study. *British Medical Journal*, 33, 1348–51.

Martinez-Gonzalez, M.A., Sanchez-Villagas, A., De Irala, J. & Martinez, J.A. (2002) Mediterranean diet and stroke: objectives and design of the SUN project. *Nutritional Neuroscience*, 5, 65–73.

Mitrou, P.N., Kipnis, V. *et al.* (2007) Mediterranean dietary pattern and prediction of all-cause mortality in a US population. *Arch Intern Med*, 167, 2461–8.

Murray, G. (2010) *Five Stages of Greek Religion.* Kindle Publishing Group, New York.

Pangiotakos, D.B., Pitsavos, C. *et al.* (2008) ATTIXA Study. *Vasc Med*, 13, 113–21.

Pelucchi, C., Bosetti, C. & Rossi, M. (2009). Aspects of the Mediterranean diet and cancer risk. *Nutr Cancer*, 61(6), 756–66.

Scarmeas, N., Luchsinger, J.A., Mayeux, R. & Stern, Y. (2007). Mediterranean diet and Alzeimer disease mortality. *Neurology*, 69(11), 1084–93.

Spencer, L., Mann, C. *et al.* (2009) The effect of omega-3 FAs on tumour angiogenesis and their therapeutic potential. *Eur J Cancer*, 45(12), 2077–86.

Trichopoulou, A., Bamia, C. & Norat, E. (2007) Modified Mediterranean diet and survival after myocardial infarction: the EPIC-Elderly study. *Eur J Epidemiol*, 22(12), 871–81.

Trichopoulou, A., Costacou, T., Bamia, C. & Trichopoulos, D. (2003). Adherence to a Mediterranean diet and survival in a Greek population. *New Engl J Med*, 348, 2599–608.

Vardavas, C. & Kafatos, A.G. (2007) Smoking policy and prevalence in Greece: an overview. *Eur J Public Health*, 17(2), 211–13.

8 Maternal and Child Nutrition

Eulalee Green, Maureen Lee, Lindy Parfrey, Rita Žemaitis

This chapter will describe current recommendations for maternal health (preconception and during pregnancy) before moving onto nutrition in childhood (breast feeding, bottle feeding and weaning). Cultural and religious influences on maternal and child health will then follow. A final section on oral health will complete this chapter.

8.1 Introduction

Preconception, pregnancy and the first few years of a child's life are critical periods which can have life-long health implications. Therefore, appropriate, consistent support and advice on nutrition and nutrition-related health issues for mothers and advice for infants and children under five years old is important. This will help service providers to see how their actions with women, families and children at particular points can be effective.

The health of a foetus and newborn depends mainly on the well-being and nutritional health of the mother before pregnancy, during pregnancy and while breastfeeding.

8.2 Preconception

Women who are planning to become pregnant, or are at risk of becoming pregnant, may wish to consider their own health to help to improve the chance of delivering a healthy baby. The following factors should be considered.

Healthy eating and healthy lifestyle

- When planning to become pregnant, women should follow a healthy diet as described by the eatwell plate model with particular emphasis on good sources of folic acid and iron.
- Women should be advised to begin taking a folic acid supplement and continue until at least the 12th week of gestation.
- Women with no previous history of a neural tube defect-affected pregnancy should take 400 µg/day folic acid supplements. However, some women require the higher 5 mg/day folic acid supplement (NICE, 2010) if they have:
  - A family history of neural tube defects or their partner has.
  - A baby with a neural tube defect.
  - A history of diabetes (and perhaps gestational diabetes).
  - A BMI > 30 kg/m².
- Oily fish is a good source of essential fatty acids (EFA); however, women trying to become pregnant should restrict themselves to two portions

Multicultural Handbook of Food, Nutrition and Dietetics, First Edition. Edited by Aruna Thaker, Arlene Barton.

a week. Women wanting to become pregnant should avoid eating shark, swordfish or marlin due to the levels of mercury found in these fish (Scientific Advisory Committee on Nutrition, 2004). EFAs can be metabolized from plant fatty acids such as alpha-linoleic acid (ALA). Eicosapentaenoic acid (EPA) and docosahexaenoic acid (DHA) are not essential fatty acids for adults because they can be produced if enough alpha-linoleic acid is consumed; 21% of dietary ALA is converted into EPA and 9% is converted to DHA (Burdge & Wootton, 2002). Therefore, to produce the recommended levels of DHA women need to consume at least 2.3 g of ALA a day. This is much greater than the Institute of Medicine (2002) and Department of Health (1991) recommendations for ALA in pregnancy and lactation.

- Daily moderate physical activity should be a part a healthy lifestyle and therefore this should be encouraged. However, women with a medical condition, hypertension or severe obesity should be advised to consult their doctor before significantly increasing their physical activity level.
- Women who are planning to conceive are advised to avoid alcohol. However, should they choose to drink alcohol they should limit their intake to 1 or 2 units a day and avoid intoxication.
- Women who smoke or chew tobacco should be supported to stop (DH, 2000; NICE, 2006).

Body weight

Overweight (BMI > 25 kg/m^2) or obese (BMI > 30 kg/m^2) women are at greater risk of problems during pregnancy, including diabetes, hypertension and complications during pregnancy and delivery. The risks to their babies include preterm deliveries and birth defects (Centre for Maternal & Child Enquiries, 2010). These women may have difficulty getting pregnant. Therefore, these women should achieve and maintain a healthy weight before planning to become pregnant.

Having a BMI < 18 kg/m^2 increases the risk of low birth weight babies (<2.5 kg) due to pre-term delivery or intrauterine growth retardation (small-for-date) babies, or babies with congenital malformations. Women planning to have a baby should be supported to achieve and maintain a health

body weight before conceiving (Institute of Medicine, 1990; Kumari, 2001).

Pre-existing conditions

Women with pre-existing medical conditions that affect their nutritional status or diet, or which require them to take regular medication, should plan their pregnancy with the help of their GP or obstretician (NICE, 2010). These conditions include:

- Cardiac disease, including hypertension.
- Renal disease.
- Endocrine disorders.
- Diabetes.
- Psychiatric disorders requiring medication.
- Haematological disorders.
- Haemaglobinopathies.
- Autoimmune disorders.
- Epilepsy requiring anticonvulsant drugs.
- Malignant disease.
- Severe asthma.
- Use of recreational drugs such as heroin, cocaine (including crack cocaine) and ecstasy.
- HIV or HBV infection.

Maternal oral health during pregnancy

Due to hormonal changes, a mother may notice her gums appear inflamed and may bleed more easily. Pregnant women need to keep a high standard of oral hygiene and should visit a dentist.

Good dental health is important to prevent preterm babies. The risk of delivering a baby before 35 weeks' gestation is three times higher (23.4%) in women continuing to have periodontal disease after scaling and root planning than women who were successfully treated (7.2%) and had no periodontal disease after treatment (Jeffcott, 2010). However, there are a number of reviews and interventions studies that show that scaling and root planing for periodontal disease had no effect on birth outcomes. Niederman (2010) suggests that studies that show no effect between treated and untreated women may be due to the authors not including course antibiotics and checking that the periodontal disease was no longer present after treatment. Therefore, Niederman (2010) recommends that women who are planning to become pregnant should visit their dentist to ensure that they do not have dental caries or periodontal disease. If treatment is required, the women should receive a course of antibiotics and the absence of periodontal disease should be confirmed after treatment.

NHS dental treatment is free for pregnant women and those who have had a baby in the 12 months before dental treatment starting.

Risk of developing complications during pregnancy

Women should be made aware of their risk of developing complications during pregnancy and encouraged to seek medical advice when they become pregnant. These risk factors include risk for:

- Pre-eclampsia: age >40 years, history of pre-eclampsia, hypertension, renal disease or BMI $\geq 30\,\text{kg}/\text{m}^2$.
- Diabetes: BMI $\geq 30\,\text{kg}/\text{m}^2$, previous baby $\geq 4.5\,\text{kg}$, previous gestational diabetes, family history of diabetes, or an ethnic group at high risk of diabetes (Asian, Afro-Caribbean or Middle Eastern) (NICE, 2010).

Healthy timing and spacing of pregnancy

Birth spacing is the time from the birth of one child to the conception of the next. Birth spacing of less than two years has been shown to have a high risk of miscarriages, stillbirths, pre-term births, birth defects and learning difficulties (WHO, 2006).

Over the last 30 years there have been a significant number of studies that confirm that short birth spacing increases the risk of foetal, child and maternal morbidity and mortality. The reason for this is unclear. Several studies have indicated acute maternal nutritional deficiency (e.g., folic acid, vitamin B_{12} and iron). However, most serum levels of nutrients, except iron, return to their pre-pregnancy levels within three months.

The advice for birth spacing after miscarriage or abortion is less clear. There was only one large-scale study on over 2,500 women from South America that suggested that women should wait at least six months before attempting to conceive (WHO, 2006).

USAID (2008) recommend that women should delay their first pregnancy until they are at least 18 years old to reduce the risk of maternal eclampsia, puerperal endometritis and maternal death.

Table 8.1 Obstetric complication by maternal age 35–39 and ≥40 years compared with maternal age ≤ 35 years

Women 35–39 years old (percentage birth complications)	Women ≥ 40 years old (percentage birth complications)
Caesarean delivery (31.4)	Caesarean delivery (40.5)
Chromosomal abnormalities (0.8)	Chromosomal abnormalities (1.9)
Gestational diabetes (5.3)	Gestational diabetes (7.3)
Miscarriage (1.5)	Low birth weight (7.5)
Placenta previa (0.9)	Miscarriage (2.2)
	Placenta previa (1.9)
	Preterm delivery (11.8)

(Cleary-Goldman et al., 2005)

A number of studies have found that there is an incremental increase in the risks for mother and baby with increasing maternal age beyond 35 years. One of the latest studies looked at 36,000 women (Cleary-Goldman et al., 2005) found the following maternal age-related risks (see Table 8.1).

8.3   Pregnancy and lactation

During the first two trimesters, lower activity levels compensate for the increase in requirement for maternal energy. During the third trimester and lactation, there is a small increase in nutritional requirements (DH, 1991). This section provides a summary the nutritional and dietary needs of pregnancy and lactation.

Healthy eating and lifestyle

Most of the advice to women planning to conceive applies during pregnancy and lactation. There are increased requirements during pregnancy and lactation for energy and protein, as well as some vitamins and minerals (DH, 1991).

- Bread, breakfast cereals, pasta and starchy root vegetables – a small portion at each meal. Women should choose wholemeal breads and pasta, and whole grain breakfast cereals which are very good sources of B vitamins and iron.

- Meat, chicken, fish, lentils and beans – three portions a day. These foods are good for protein and minerals, such as iron (14.8 mg/day) and zinc (pregnancy 7–9 mg/day, lactation 13–15 mg/day).
- Milk, yoghurt, cheese and alternatives – three portions a day (700–800 mg/day calcium) of the low-fat variety every day before and during pregnancy. These foods are good for protein, calcium and B vitamins. Breastfeeding women will need at least six portions a day (1,250–1,350 mg/day calcium).
- Fruit and vegetables – at least five portions a day. These foods are good for vitamins, such as vitamin C (pregnancy 50 mg/day, lactation 70 mg/day) and folic acid (400 µg/day). Pregnant and lactating women should have at least three portions of fruit and two portions of vegetables a day. The fruit or vegetables may be fresh or frozen.
- Fatty foods and sugary foods – avoid these foods. Many of these only provide empty calories and have very little nutritional value.

Drinks

Women should drink often during the day, to have at least 2,000 ml/day (8–10 cups) of alcohol-free fluid. In addition, they should avoid drinking tea with meals or supplements because this affects the body's ability to use the iron.

Body weight

The expected weight gain for women with a BMI between 19.6 kg/m^2 and 24.9 kg/m^2 is 11.5–16 kg. Most of this weight gain will occur during the third trimester. This is associated with the lowest risk of complications during pregnancy and labour and with a reduced likelihood of having a low birth weight infant (IOM, 2009). To meet the energy costs of pregnancy, a modest increment of 200 kcal/day above the estimated average requirement (EAR) is suggested in the third trimester only (DH, 1991).

There are no additional recommendations for obesity levels II (BMI 35–39.9) and III (BMI > 40); or for women with additional problems such as breathing difficulties, diabetes, high blood pressure and high cholesterol. These women may need to hold their weight at the pre-pregnancy level or lose some weight (see Table 8.2).

Table 8.2 Weight gain during pregnancy

Pre-pregnancy BMI (kg/m^2)	Total weight gain kg (lb)	Weight gain during 2nd and 3rd trimesters g (lb)
Underweight (<18.5)	12.7–18.2 (28–40)	450–590 (1 – 1.3)
Normal weight (18.5–24.9)	11.4–15.9 (25–35)	360–450 (0.8–1.0)
Overweight (25.0–29.9)	6.8–11.4 (15–25)	230–320 (0.5–0.7)
Obese (≥30.0)	5.0–9.1 (11–20)	180–270 (0.4–0.6)

(Institute of Medicine, May 2009)
(ABM 2010)

Obese women with a BMI greater than 30 kg/m^2 with diabetes or hypertension should contact their medical team and registered dietitian for advice and monitoring during the antenatal and postnatal periods.

Safe exercising in pregnancy

The Royal College of Obstetricians and Gynaecologists advise that:

- All women should be encouraged to participate in aerobic and strength-conditioning exercise as part of a healthy lifestyle during their pregnancy.
- Reasonable goals of aerobic conditioning in pregnancy should be to maintain a good fitness level throughout pregnancy without trying to reach peak fitness level or train for athletic competitions.
- Women should choose activities that minimize the risk of loss of balance and foetal trauma.
- Women should be advised that adverse pregnancy or neonatal outcomes are not increased for exercising women.
- Initiation of pelvic floor exercises in the immediate postpartum period may reduce the risk of urinary incontinence.

Healthy, lactating women should not be encouraged to follow weight-reducing diets. However, as breastfeeding may help to use up body fat that has been accumulated in pregnancy, this will help women return to their pre-pregnancy weight.

Table 8.3   Warning signs of excessive exercising

Signs of breathing difficulty	Signs of over-exercising	Signs of foetal distress
Excessive shortness of breath	Headache	Leakage of amniotic fluid
Difficulty in breathing before exertion	Muscle weakness	Vaginal bleeding
Light-headedness	Calf pain or swelling	Painful uterine contractions or preterm labour
Feeling of fainting	Excessive tiredness	Reduced foetal movement
Dizziness	Pelvic girdle (hips) pain	Abdominal pain, particularly in back or pubic area
Chest pain or palpitations		

(RCOG, 2006)

Women need to be made aware that limiting their intake of food may result in a decrease of the nutrient content and volume of their breast milk and nutrient deficiencies may occur in women who are eating very low-calorie or unconventional diets (IOM, 1990).

Overweight or obese (BMI > 25 kg/m^2) lactating women who wish to lose weight may be reassured that a modest weight loss (0.5–1 kg a week) should not affect lactation (Lovelady et al., 2000). These women should eat a healthy, balanced diet, limit the amount of fat and sugar intake, and take moderate activity. This will help to lose any weight gained during pregnancy. Exclusive breastfeeding, combined with a low-fat diet and exercise, will result in more effective weight loss than diet and exercise alone. Poor appetite may indicate poor milk production, as milk production would appear to drive diet rather than the reverse (Dewey et al., 1994; Dusdieker et al., 1994).

Women who have recently had a baby should receive support to achieve a healthy weight. CMACE/RCOG report that weight loss of at least 4.5 kg before the next pregnancy will reduce the risk of a woman developing gestational diabetes by 40%. Warning signs of excessive exercise can be seen in Table 8.3.

Folic acid

All women should take 400 μg/day or 5 mg of folic acid a day before pregnancy and throughout the first 12 weeks.

Supplementation above 5 mg/day masks vitamin B$_{12}$ deficiency-associated anaemia. The effect of doses between 1 mg/day and 5 mg/day on masking vitamin B$_{12}$ deficiency is unknown. Therefore, it may be prudent to assess the vitamin B$_{12}$ status of women before they take 5 mg/day folic acid to exclude vitamin B$_{12}$ deficiency in these women.

There have been reports that folic acid supplements increase the risk of breast cancer and multiple births. However, at the recommended levels studies found no association between folic acid supplementation and an increased risk of breast cancer.

Research has found that a slightly increased number of multiple births is correlated with folic acid supplementation. However, it is unclear if this association is due to folic acid improving the survival rate of twin foetuses beyond the first few weeks of gestation or if it causes the development of more twins.

Vitamin B$_{12}$

Vitamin B$_{12}$ (cobalamin) helps maintain healthy nerve cells and red blood cells, and is needed to make DNA (the genetic material in every cell). It helps the cells to use folic acid. It only occurs naturally in meat, fish, milk, yoghurt, cheese and eggs. It may also be found in fortified cereals and yeast products. Therefore, deficiency is common in people that exclude these foods from their diet (i.e., eat a vegan diet) (see Table 8.4). The requirements for pregnancy are 1.5 μg/day and for lactation is 2.0 μg/day.

Table 8.4   Vegetarian sources of Vitamin B_{12}

Foods	µg/d
Bread, whole meal, 2 slices	0.3
Bread, white, 2 slices	0
Bran flakes, 3 tablespoons (25 g)	0.5
Fortified cereals, 3 tablespoons (25 g), e.g. special K, Cheerios, Weetabix (2 biscuits)	0.5
Yeast extract (1 g)	0.01

Deficiency can give rise to:

- Tiredness, weakness, nausea, constipation, wind, loss of appetite and weight loss.
- Nerve damage, such as poor memory, numbness and tingling in the hands and feet.
- Loss of balance, depression, confusion and soreness of the mouth or tongue.
- In pregnant and lactating women can cause nerve damage in the foetus.

Vitamin B_{12} deficiency is shown by large, pale red blood cells that look identical to folic acid deficiency. Also, people taking more than 4 mg/day of folic acid will have normal-looking red blood cells even if they are B_{12}-deficient. Therefore, people with this type of blood cell should be tested for B_{12}. Women requiring 5 mg/day folic acid supplement for pregnancy should also be tested for B_{12} deficiency.

Vitamin A

Vitamin A is an essential vitamin for everyone, including pregnant women. Women require 600 µg/day (Scientific Advisory Committee on Nutrition, 2005). The early sign of deficiency in adults is night blindness (an inability to adapt to night-time light). Persistent deficiency causes xerophthalmia of the eyes. Symptoms include dryness and thickening of the conjunctivae and corneas, and foamy white patches (Bitot's spots). In severe deficiency the cornea breaks down (keratomalacia). In addition to changes in the eye, all mucus skin areas (lungs, gut and urinary tract) may become dry, hard and scaly. Immunity becomes impaired.

Most people in the UK have sufficient vitamin A from meat products, or make enough from beta-carotene in fruit and vegetables. High levels of vitamin A can cause miscarriage and birth defects. In adults, an intake >1,500 µg/day was found to cause bone demineralization. Therefore, pregnant women should avoid foods high in vitamin A, such as liver and liver products, including cod liver oil supplements.

Vitamin D

Women of Caucasian origin who are not pregnant will make sufficient vitamin D in the summer months to meet their requirements for the year. The incidence of vitamin D deficiency among these women ranges from 2% to 4% (Pal & Shaw, 2001; Nesby-O'Dell et al., 2002). Pregnant Caucasian women should be advised take a supplement containing 10 µg/day during pregnancy and lactation (DH, 1994). Black and Asian women living in the UK do not make sufficient vitamin D during the summer months. The incidence of vitamin D deficiency among these women ranges from 28% to 88% (Pal & Shaw, 2001; Nesby-O'Dell et al., 2002; Sachan et al., 2005).

The Department of Health (2008) advises that during pregnancy all women should take a 10 µg/day supplement of vitamin D, especially women at high risk of deficiency such as:

- Women of South Asian, African, Afro-Caribbean or Middle Eastern descent.
- Women with limited skin exposure to sunlight.
- Women with a pre-pregnancy BMI > 30 kg/m².

A review by Hollis and Wagner (2004) found that dark-skinned pregnant and lactating women who were vitamin D-deficient required supplement of 25–50 µg/day to produce normal circulating maternal levels of vitamin D and a sufficient supply to the breastfed infant. This may be achieved by a combination of Calfovit (a prescription calcium with vitamin D supplement) in combination with the Healthy Start Women's supplement to provide 30 µg/d. This is 2–5 times higher than the current DH recommendation of 10 µg/day. However, there are currently no DH recommendations for higher level of vitamin supplementations for these women.

Table 8.5 Recommended maximum portions* of oily fish per week during pregnancy and lactation

Fish	Children up to 16 years	Pregnant, planning pregnancy and girls	Breastfeeding
Mackerel, sardines, trout, fresh tuna	2 portions	2 portions	2 portions
Tinned tuna	6 portions	2 portion tuna steaks or 4 portions tinned	2 portion tuna steaks; no limit on tinned
Fresh or tinned shark, swordfish and marlin	Avoid	Avoid	1 portion

*1 portion = 140 g

Table 8.6 Recommended daily intake of essential fatty acid in pregnancy and lactation

	Alpha-linoleic acid		Linoleic acid	
	IOM* g/day	DH** % energy	IOM g/day	DH % energy
Pregnancy	1.4	0.2 ($\approx$ 0.48 g)	13	1.0 ($\approx$ 2.4 g)
Lactation	1.3	0.2 ($\approx$ 0.56 g)	13	1.0 ($\approx$ 2.8 g)

*Institute of Medicine (2002);
**DH = Department of Health (1991)

Fish

Eating oily fish provides eicosapentaenoic acid (EPA) and docosahexaenoic acid (DHA) which are omega 3 fatty acids and essential for visual and neurological development in the foetus. The recommended daily intake for DHA is 0.2 g/day (DH, 1991) (i.e., two portions a week of oily fish). However, oily fish is contaminated with mercury and dioxins. The Scientific Advisory Committee on Nutrition (2004) advises pregnant and lactating women to limit their intake (see Table 8.5).

EPA and DHA are not essential fatty acids for adults because they can be produced if enough alpha-linoleic acid (ALA) is consumed (21% of dietary ALA is converted into EPA and 9% is converted to DHA; Burdge & Wootton, 2002). Therefore, to produce the recommended levels of DHA women need to consume at least 2.3 g of ALA a day. This is much greater than the IOM and DH recommendations for ALA in pregnancy and lactation (see Table 8.6). A list of dietary sources of essential fatty acids can be seen in Table 8.7.

Peanuts and food allergy

The Committee on Toxicity (2008) states that in the light of new evidence from human studies it is less clear if eating peanuts during pregnancy and lactation increases or reduces the risk of babies developing a peanut allergy. Animal studies indicate that low maternal intake of peanut products increases the risk of peanut allergy in infants and high maternal intake reduces the risk. They concluded that the previous advice that pregnant and lactating women should avoid peanuts was over-cautious and that it is not necessary to advise women with a family history of allergies to avoid peanuts.

Food-acquired infections

The following bacteria and parasites found in some foods can be unsafe in the pregnant woman and her foetus. Safe food hygiene and handling is required to reduce the risk of exposure to bacteria/parasites that may harm the foetus or cause pre-term delivery or stillbirth.

Table 8.7 Dietary sources of essential fatty acids

Foods	Energy (kcal)	Alpha-linoleic acid g	Linoleic acid (g)
Nuts and seeds			
Walnuts – 6 nuts	138	1	8
Sunflower seeds – 1 tablespoon	96	0	4
Brazil nuts – 3 nuts	68	0	3
Sesame seeds – 1 tablespoon	72	0	3
Pumpkin seeds – 1 tablespoon	91	0	3
Peanut butter (smooth) – thinly spread on 1 slice of bread	73	0	2
Peanuts (groundnuts) – 10 nuts	73	0	2
Almonds – 6 nuts	80	0	1
Hazelnuts – 10 nuts	65	0	1
Oils (1 tablespoon)			
Safflower	99	0	8
Evening primrose	99	0	8
Grapeseed	99	0	7
Sunflower	99	0	7
Soya	99	1	6
Walnut	99	1	6
Wheat germ	99	0	6
Corn	99	0	6
Cotton seed (linseed or flaxseed)	98	0	6
Sesame	99	0	5
Peanut (groundnut)	99	0	3
Rapeseed	99	1	2
Hazelnut	99	0	1
Palm	99	0	1
Olive	99	0	1

Listeriosis

Listeria bacteria are found in soil, water and on vegetation. Listeria infection can cause severe problems during pregnancy as the bacteria can cross the placenta to infect the baby. In early pregnancy listeriosis may cause miscarriage; later in the pregnancy it may cause premature labour and result in a stillbirth.

To reduce the risk of listeriosis, pregnant women should avoid the following foods:

- Soft, mould-ripened cheeses.

- Unpasteurized cheeses and milks.
- Chilled foods or ready-made meals unless thoroughly reheated.

Toxoplasmosis

Toxoplasmosis is caused by the parasite toxoplasmodium. It is not usually dangerous for a healthy individual, but in pregnancy a woman's immunity is lowered. The parasite can be passed on to the foetus and cause foetal abnormalities.

To reduce the risk of exposure to toxoplasmosis pregnant women should avoid the following foods:

- Raw or undercooked meats and poultry.
- Unwashed fruits and vegetables.

Salmonellosis

The salmonella bacterium is one of the commonest causes of food poisoning and its incidence is rising every year in the UK. Salmonella differs from listeriosis and toxoplasmosis because it affects the mother and does not pass across to the baby. In pregnant women it may cause severe vomiting and diarrhoea which can lead to maternal dehydration.

To reduce the risk of exposure to salmonellosis pregnant women should avoid the following foods:

- Raw or partially cooked eggs (soft scrambled eggs, home-made mayonnaises, hollandaise sauce).
- Undercooked meats and poultry.
- Soft ice creams (i.e., sold from ice cream vans and machines).

Raw shellfish should also be avoided during pregnancy as they can contain harmful bacteria and viruses that could cause food poisoning.

For details of food hygiene and safety in pregnancy guidelines and in general see National Collaborating Centre for Women's and Children's Health (2008).

Caffeine

Pregnant and lactating women should limit their caffeine intake to not more than 200 mg (about 1 or 2 drinks) per day (see Table 8.8). Higher intakes have been associated with an increased risk of having a miscarriage or low birth weight infant (2010).

Table 8.8 Caffeine content of common drinks and foods

Drinks	
Mug of instant coffee	140 mg
Mug of filter coffee	100 mg
Mug of brewed coffee	100 mg
Cup of tea	75 mg
Can of energy drink	up to 80 mg
Can of cola drink	up to 40 mg
Foods	
50 g bar of milk chocolate	up to 50 mg
50 g bar of plain chocolate	up to 25 mg

Alcohol

There is no known safe limit for alcohol in pregnancy. With increasing alcohol intake there is an increase risk of miscarriage during pregnancy and having a baby affected by foetal alcohol syndrome (learning difficulties and congenital malformations). Therefore, NICE (2010) recommends that all women who are planning to become pregnant or who are pregnant should avoid drinking alcohol, especially in the first trimester.

Moderate to heavy alcohol consumption may interfere with the let-down reflex, inhibit milk intake, affect infant motor development, slow weight gain and cause other side-effects in the baby (Mohrbacher & Stock, 2003). It is also important for women to be aware that the baby might reject the breast if they do not like the smell or taste of the breast milk which can be affected by maternal alcohol intake. In this instance, the mother should not drink alcohol. However, the current DH recommendations are that breastfeeding mothers who wish to drink alcohol should express breast milk prior to drinking alcohol and then avoid breastfeeding for at least two hours after drinking.

At all other times, alcohol should be limited to 1–2 units, once or twice a week. (A unit is a pint of ordinary strength beer, lager or cider, a small glass of wine, or a single 25 ml measure of spirit) (see Table 8.9).

Smoking

Pregnant and lactating women should be encouraged to stop smoking (2006). Nicotine, like other

Table 8.9 Alcoholic beverages providing 1 unit of alcohol

Drink	Volume
Beer, lager, cider (3–5%)	240 ml (½ pint)
Spirits (e.g. gin, vodka, whisky)	Pub measure (25 ml)
Wine	125 ml glass
Fortified wine (sherry, port)	50 ml

toxins, passes to the baby through breast milk. As nicotine suppresses prolactin levels it can have a negative effect on breast milk supply. Studies show that lactating women who smoke have reduced duration of breastfeeding (Amir & Donath, 2002).

Passive smoking is detrimental to the baby's health as there is an increased risk of chest infections and Sudden Infant Death Syndrome (SIDS). Therefore, smoking in the same room as the baby should be avoided (Golding, 1997).

Medications and drugs

Use of prescription medicines should be limited to circumstances where the benefit outweighs the risk during pregnancy and lactation. Advice should be always be sought from a doctor about the use of any medications during pregnancy and lactation.

Illegal drugs (amphetamines, ecstasy, cocaine, heroin, marijuana, etc.) can harm babies if the mother is using them during pregnancy or lactation. Drug-dependent women should be supported to stop using by their local drug addition support services.

8.4 Childhood nutrition

In 2004 the UK accepted the WHO/UNICEF (2003) 'Global Strategy for Infant and Young Child Feeding' recommendation that infants should be exclusively breastfeed up to six months (26 weeks) old. The earliest introduction of mixed feeding should be at four months (17 weeks). (Refer to WHO/UNICEF (2003, Section 3.5) for more information.)

The World Health Organization's (1991) definitions related to breastfeeding are:

- Breastfeeding: The child receives breast milk directly from the breast or expressed breast milk.
- Exclusively breastfeeding: The infant has received only breast milk from his/her mother, milk donor or expressed breast milk and no other liquid (including water or other milks) or solids, with the exception of vitamin supplements or medicines.
- Mixed or complementary feeding: The infant has received both breast milk and solids or semi-solid foods (such as purée).
- Bottle-feeding: The infant has received no breast milk in the 24 hours before the data collection.
- Combined breastfeeding. Breastfed plus mixed (complementary) feeding.

These recommendations are designed to prevent infant sickness and death from lack of hygiene, and secure the positive health benefits of breastfeeding. However, the WHO/ UNICEF (2003) recommendations acknowledged that the number of infants being exclusively breastfed for six months could be maximized by recognizing and overcoming the following problems:

- Poor nutritional status of the breastfeeding mother.
- Communities where there is a high prevalence of nutritional deficiencies, such as iron, zinc and vitamin A.
- The routine primary health care of infants should include the assessment of growth and signs of nutrient deficiencies.

In addition, the delay in introducing solids until six months would require a shortened period for the introduction of a good mixed diet. That is a diet that contains a good range of flavours, food combinations and textures to ensure a nutritionally adequate diet, prevent food neo-phobic behaviours (Birch, 1998; Johnson, 2002) and to encourage age-appropriate biting and chewing skills necessary for good oral development by 12 months.

The following section provides guidance to help practitioners support successful breastfeeding, safe bottle-feeding, appropriate weaning and a healthy diet for children under five years old.

8.5   Breastfeeding

Antenatal support

The antenatal period is an ideal time to promote the benefits of breastfeeding and advise on aftercare and local postnatal support services. This opportunity should aim to assist expectant women to address any fear and embarrassment they may feel at touching or handling their breasts and develop confidence, which will assist with both breastfeeding and expressing milk. This is the time to explain that breastfeeding is the healthiest way for a woman to feed her baby and there are important health benefits for both mother and baby.

Breast milk from a healthy, well-nourished mother provides the ideal balance of nutrients for an infant. Therefore, the antenatal period is the best time to improve the nutritional status of the mother to reduce the risk of foetal and infant nutritional deficiency during pregnancy and lactation.

Women who are anaemic should be encouraged to take iron supplements as advised by their doctor.

All women should be encouraged to take folic acid and vitamin D in accordance with the NICE (2008) recommendations (see section 8.3).

During the antenatal period, the practitioner should take the opportunity to discuss the following advantages to the mother of breastfeeding for at least 12 months (Ip *et al.*, 2007):

- 4–12% less type 2 diabetes in women with no history of gestational diabetes.
- 28% less breast cancer.
- 21% less ovarian cancer.

The advantages to the baby of exclusive breastfeeding for at least six months are:

- 23% fewer ear infections (acute otitis media) when compared with mixed breast- and bottle-feeding, and 50% when compared with babies who were exclusively bottle-fed for six months.
- 42% less atopic dermatitis, despite having a family history of allergies.
- 64% less gastroenteritis.
- 72% fewer hospitalizations due to lower respiratory tract disease in infants.
- 27% less asthma in children without a family history of asthma, and 40% in children with a history of asthma.

- 7–24% less adult obesity and 4% less adult obesity for each month of breastfeeding in infancy.
- 19–27% less type 1 diabetes in children; 39% less type 2 diabetes in adulthood.
- 19% less acute lymphocytic leukaemia.
- 15% less acute myelogenous leukaemia.
- 36% less Sudden Infant Death Syndrome.

(Ip *et al.*, 2007)

Advantages of colostrum to the baby

Colostrum is in the breasts when a baby is born. It is very important for babies to receive colostrum for their first few feeds. It is all that most babies need before the mature milk comes in, because:

- Colostrum contains more antibodies, white blood cells and other anti-infective proteins than mature milk. These anti-infective proteins and white cells provide the first immunization against the diseases that a baby meets after delivery, therefore colostrum helps to prevent the bacterial infections that pose a risk to the newborn. The antibodies probably also help to prevent a baby from developing allergies.
- Colostrum has a mild purgative effect, which helps to clear the baby's gut of meconium (the first rather dark stools). This clears bilirubin from the gut and helps to prevent jaundice.
- Colostrum contains growth factors, which help a baby's immature intestine to develop after birth. This helps to prevent the baby from developing allergies and intolerance to other foods.
- Colostrum is richer than mature milk in some vitamins, especially vitamin A. Vitamin A helps to reduce the severity of any infections the baby might have (WHO, 2006).

Disadvantages of formula feeding

The benefits gained for both mother and child when breastfeeding are further enhanced by avoiding the following disadvantages of formula feeding:

- An increased risk of gastroenteritis from contaminated formula powder or from poor hygiene during preparation of feeds.

- Cow's milk formula may trigger insulin-dependent diabetes mellitus in later life (Dosch *et al.*, 1994)
- An increased risk of developing an allergy to cow's milk (Kull *et al.*, 2002).
- The cost involved in purchase of formula and equipment.
- The increased time and effort required to prepare feeds and clean and sterilize all equipment required (The commonly used term 'sterilize' is used here. 'Home sterilization' using sterilizing solutions and techniques in fact disinfect equipment, they do not clinically sterilize it.)
- The use of preservatives and other ingredients to prolong shelf-life of the formula.

If a woman chooses not to breastfeed her baby, then support, advice and guidance on appropriate alternatives should be available.

Post-delivery and breastfeeding the newborn

Women should be encouraged to have skin-to-skin contact with their baby as soon as possible after the birth. It is not recommended that women be asked about their proposed method of feeding until after the first skin-to-skin contact.

- Babies should be put to the breast within the first hour after the birth. After the first two hours babies become sleepy, therefore, early breast-feeding should be encouraged. Unrestricted, skin-to-skin contact during breastfeeding increases successful breastfeeding, reduces baby's anxiety and stabilizes its heart rate.
- From the first feed, women should be offered skilled breastfeeding support from a healthcare professional and mother-to-mother or peer support to enable comfortable positioning of the mother and baby and to ensure that the baby attaches correctly to the breast to establish effective feeding and prevent concerns, such as sore nipples.
- Separation of a woman and her baby within the first hour of the birth for routine postnatal procedures (e.g., weighing, measuring and bathing) should be avoided unless these measurements are requested by the woman or are necessary for the immediate care of the baby.

- Breastfeeding on demand should be unrestricted and should be facilitated whenever the baby shows signs of hunger, such as increased alertness, activity, mouthing, rooting or crying.
- Women should be supported, in a hands-off manner, to achieve the correct positioning and attachment for successful breastfeeding. A copy of the description of positioning and attachment, for practitioners and mothers is available from the UNICEF UK Baby Friendly Initiative 'Breastfeeding your baby'.
- Babies should be kept with the mother by 24-hour rooming-in and continuing skin-to-skin contact when possible. Privacy, adequate rest for women without interruption caused by hospital routine, and access to food and drink on demand should be provided.
- A woman's experience with breastfeeding should be discussed at each contact to assess if she is on course to breastfeed effectively and identify any need for additional support. Breastfeeding progress should then be assessed and documented in the postnatal care plan at each contact.
- Women who believe they have insufficient milk should have the attachment and positioning reviewed. The baby's health should also be evaluated. Reassurance should be offered to support the woman to gain confidence in her ability to produce enough milk for her baby.
- If the baby is not taking sufficient milk from the breast and supplementary feeds are necessary, expressed breast milk should be given by a cup or bottle.

Supplementation with fluids other than breast milk is not recommended. Formula milk should not be given to breastfed babies unless medically indicated. The type, amount and method should be a joint decision between the mother, dietitian, nursing staff and the medical team (NICE, 2006).

Expressing breast milk

Women may wish to express and store breast milk for a number of reasons. These may include: if the baby is having difficulty attaching to a full breast; if the breasts feel full and uncomfortable; if the baby is too small or sick to breastfeed; if the mother needs to be away from her baby for more than an hour or two.

Women should be shown how to express breast milk using the three main methods – by hand, hand pump or electric pump. It is vital parents are shown how to safely sterilize the equipment and how to store expressed breast milk (NICE, 2008).

Preparing breast milk for storage

- Wash hands with soap and warm water.
- Sterilize storage containers.
- If using a pump, sterilize the pump according to the manufacturer's instructions.
- Express milk by hand or pump and put in storage container.
- Do not add milk to already cooled or frozen milk.
- Leave space at the top to allow expansion during freezing.
- Seal storage container to prevent contamination.
- Label the container with the date.

(Academy of Breastfeeding Medicine Protocol Committee, 2010).

Storing expressed breast milk

- Store breast milk at the back of the fridge or freezer to prevent intermittent rewarming when the fridge or freezer door is opened. (Storage times are given in Table 8.10.)

Using stored breast milk

- Use the oldest milk in the fridge or freezer first.
- If frozen, defrost in the fridge overnight, or by running under warm water or by standing the container in warm water.
- Do not heat the milk above 40°C.
- Do not use a microwave to heat milk because it does not heat the milk evenly and it reduces the anti-infective qualities of the milk.
- Milk that has been defrosted overnight in the fridge should be used within a few hours after being warmed or brought to room temperature.
- Once the baby has started drinking the milk, it should be discarded after 2 hours.
- Do not feed the milk to the baby if the milk appears stringy, foul or purulent.

(Academy of Breastfeeding Medicine Protocol Committee, 2010)

Hypotonic babies – Down's syndrome or Prader Willi

Infants with low muscle tone (hypotonia), such as Down's syndrome or Prader Willi, are often sleepy and may have a poor suck. It is possible to successfully breastfeed an infant with these conditions and as these children are more susceptible to upper respiratory tract infections, the mother should be encouraged to breastfeed where possible. Patience is required as the baby may be a slow feeder. Mothers should be encouraged to feed in different positions to find their baby's preference.

Babies with Down's syndrome may have a small oral cavity which may cause the tongue to protrude and push against the nipple. This can cause pain. Mothers with a hypotonic baby should be referred to a lactation specialist in order to help establish her milk supply. The mother may also need to express breast milk after each feed to prevent her supply from drying up. This can be given to the baby from a cup or syringe.

Babies with poor muscle tone are best held in the football hold where weight is supported on a pillow underneath the mother's arm. This allows the mother to support her baby's head and neck and she can observe him latching on and any problems with sucking. Applying gentle, steady pressure to the back of the baby's head will help him suck without tiring. When supporting the establishment of breastfeeding, the lactation specialist can confirm good attachment by checking that the baby's tongue is supped under the breast, and is visible between the breast and the baby's gum.

Babies with hypotonia are often sleepy, so should be put to the breast every two hours (i.e., 8–12 times a day). Even so, often weight gain can be slow. It may be easier to feed the baby when in light sleep cycle when there is rapid eye movement (REM), arm or leg movements or sucking motions (La Leche League International, 1997).

Breast surgery and breast implants

After breast surgery it is still possible to breastfeed. However, successful breastfeeding can depend on the procedure and where the surgical incisions were made.

- Women who have had incisions around the areola are five times more likely to have insufficient

Table 8.10 Safe storage of expressed breast milk

Location	Temperature	Duration	Comments
Table	Room temperature (up to 25° C)	6–8 hours	Containers should be covered and kept as cool as possible; covering the container with a cool towel may keep milk cooler.
Insulated cooler bag	−15 to −4° C	24 hours	Keep ice packs in contact with milk containers at all times, limit opening cooler bag.
Refrigerator	4° C	5 days	Store milk at the back of the main body of the refrigerator.
Freezer			Store milk towards the back of the freezer, where temperature is most constant. Milk stored for longer durations in the ranges listed is safe, but some of the lipids in the milk undergo degradation resulting in lower quality.
Freezer compartment of a refrigerator	−15° C	2 weeks	
Freezer compartment of refrigerator with separate doors	−18° C	3–6 months	
Chest or upright deep freezer	−20° C	6–12 months	
Defrosted			
Defrosted in refrigerator		Use within 24 hours	
Defrosted outside refrigerator		Use immediately	

(ABM, 2010)

milk than women who have not had breast surgery (Hurst, 1996). When milk ducts and nerves are cut, milk production can be affected.

- If during breast reduction surgery the nipple areola is moved with the milk ducts and nerves still attached, there is a lower rate of post-surgery milk insufficiency.
- The amount of breast tissue removed can affect breastfeeding as can breast augmentation (implant) if the implant is placed under the breast tissue rather than under the muscle as it may put pressure on the milk-producing glands (Hurst, 1996).
- Scar tissue may be painful.

If the mother had surgery because the breasts developed, she may not have enough milk-producing glands to produce a full supply of milk.

Nipple injury or burns can also affect the mother's ability to breastfeed as the route for the breast milk may be obstructed.

HIV-positive women

In WHO/UNICEF/UNAIDS' recommendations on the prevention of mother-to-child transmission of HIV infection previous infant feeding guidelines were endorsed (WHO, 2000), that is 'when feeding with infant formula milk is acceptable, feasible, affordable, sustainable and safe avoidance of all breastfeeding by HIV-infected women is recommended from birth'. In the UK there are safe and uninterrupted supplies of infant formula; therefore, in 2004 the Department of Health endorsed the WHO/UNICEF/UNAIDS position and recommended that HIV-infected women should be advised not to breastfeed their babies.

Breastfeeding beyond 12 months

Mothers should be encouraged to breastfeed for as long as they wish. The World Health Organization (2003) and the Department of Health (2004) recommend that breastfeeding for a minimum of six months (26 weeks) is the ideal for most healthy babies. The introduction of complementary foods (i.e., weaning) should not be delayed beyond six months and breastfeeding should continue at least until 12 months. Many mothers carry on breastfeeding beyond 12 months but may only do so at certain times of the day. How ever long mothers decide to feed, their efforts should always be applauded.

Returning to work

Some mothers may need or wish to return to work within months of having their baby and may want to provide breast milk in their absence. In order to do this, mothers need to build up a supply of expressed milk, especially if the woman is returning to work within the first six months.

Expressing milk at about the same time every morning may produce more milk as supply is encouraged by expression. Mothers may be able to express milk at work and store it in the staff kitchen fridge or in a cooler bag with an ice block until it can be frozen at home.

8.6   Bottle feeding

While breastfeeding is recommended as the best form of nutrition for infants (WHO, 2001), some mothers will choose not to breastfeed exclusively or not to breastfeed at all. Some women may have been advised not to breastfeed by their medical team (e.g., HIV-positive women), or are unable to breastfeed (e.g., women who have had radical breast surgery, or are taking prescription medications unsafe for the baby).

NICE (2006) recommends that most healthy women should not be asked about their decision to breastfeed until after the first skin-to-skin contact after birth.

Health professionals must support a woman's right to choose not to breastfeed. However, some women may benefit from help and support to overcome some of the perceived barriers.

For mothers choosing to formula feed, there are many infant formulas available and it is important that parents make educated decisions on which is most appropriate for their child. This section provides information on the type of infant formula, and how to prepare, use and store them safely.

Standard infant formula

Standard infant formulas are produced from modified cow's milk. The Infant Formula and Follow-on Formula Regulations (DH, 1995) regulate the nutritional composition and ingredients of infant formula.

There are three main types of standard infant formulas:

- Whey-dominant infant formula.
- Casein-dominant infant formula.
- Follow-on formula.

Whey-dominant infant formula
Whey-dominant infant formula has a protein ratio of 60/40 whey to casein and is the closest in composition to human breast milk. For this reason they are easier for babies' gastrointestinal systems to digest and are gentler on the infant's kidneys (lower renal solute load) than the casein-dominant formula. Whey-dominant infant formulas are suitable to be continued throughout the first year of life and should be recommended over other standard formula.

Casein-dominant infant formula
Casein-dominant infant formulas have a protein ratio of 20/80 whey to casein resulting in a higher renal solute load than whey-based formulas. They are promoted as being more 'satisfying' for the hungry baby. This is based on the theory that casein forms a curd in the baby's stomach. Manufacturers claim that is more slowly digested and therefore stays in the stomach for longer and satisfying the hungrier baby. There is no research to support this.

Whey- and casein-dominant formulas have equivalent energy density so poor weight gain should not a reason to change from one type of formula to the other and parents should be discouraged from changing formulas without professional advice and support.

Follow-on formula

Follow-on formulas are not suitable for infants under six months of age. Follow-on formulas are higher in protein and electrolytes, and usually slightly higher iron and vitamins A and D, and therefore have a higher renal solute load.

For most babies, a follow-on formula offers no advantage over whey- or casein-based standard infant formula. It is not known if the extra electrolytes (e.g., iron) are absorbed (DH, 1995) or if these formulas offer any advantage over an adequate mixed diet plus 350–500 ml of a standard infant formula in the infant aged over 6 month.

In a few cases, follow-on formula may be advantageous such as for assisting older infants to reach dietary requirements for iron if their food intake is poor. There may also be an advantage to changing an infant to a follow-on formula if this formula is used in preference to changing to fresh cow's milk between 6 and 12 months of age.

There are now several 'growing up formulas' on the market. These are targeted at the older toddler as part of a mixed diet and are not necessary.

Specialist infant formula

There are several specialist, prescription or over-the-counter infant formulas available to manage nutritional disorders. These include:

- Elemental formula.
- Extensively hydrolysed formula.
- Partially hydrolysed formula.
- High-energy formula.
- Pre-thickened formula or thickeners.

Extensively hydrolysed and elemental infant formula

Babies and children with proven cow's milk protein intolerance should receive a prescribed extensively hydrolysed or elemental formula, under the guidance of a doctor and dietitian.

The extensively hydrolysed formulas are based on cow's milk protein, treated so that the protein is broken down (hydrolysed) into smaller protein portions (extensively hydrolysed) that are no longer recognized by the body as a toxin and therefore do not cause a reaction in the intolerant child. The elemental formulas are made from amino acids (the building blocks of protein) and are used for babies and children that react to the small protein portions in the hydrolysed formula. Very few children require an elemental formula.

There are also hydrolysed feeds that also have MCT (medium chain fats) which are easily absorbed and therefore suitable in the management of infants that have diarrhoea and abdominal pain due to problems absorbing fats.

Partially hydrolysed infant formula

There are several infant formulas available without prescriptions which are designed to help prevent allergy in at-risk infants (those with atopic family history; see the Food Allergy and Intolerances section p346). These formulas are partially hydrolysed which aims to reduce the allergenic substances atopic babies may react to.

Partially hydrolysed formulas are intended for use in at-risk infants when breastfeeding is not possible.

High-energy infant formula

Specialized high-energy formulas are available on prescription for children with faltering growth due to poor intake or increased requirements.

Specialized high-energy formulas are higher in energy than standard formulas. The extra energy may come from additional fats and/or carbohydrates. Good dental hygiene is essential due to the additional sugars in these formulas. Parents should be advised to encourage the use of a feeder cup rather than a bottle from six months to limit the risk of dental caries.

High-energy formulas should not be used without medical and dietetic supervision.

Pre-thickened infant formula and formula thickeners

Some medical conditions, such as gastro-oesophageal reflux or dysphagia, may indicate the use of a thickened feed or a feed that thickens in the gut.

Standard formulas may be thickened by the addition of a feed thickener. The amount of thickener required is individual for the child and thickeners should only be used under the supervision of a medical doctor and paediatric dietitian, speech and language therapist or health professional.

More recently, formulas have been made to thicken once they reach the acidic environment of the stomach. These formulas are as thin as normal formulas when flowing through the bottle or cup, and thicken in the stomach to prevent reflux.

Thickeners and thickened feeds should not be used without supervision from speech and language therapist or dietitian.

Special ingredients
In recent years, manufacturers have fortified infant formula with ingredients found in human breast milk. Some of these include:

- Long chain polyunsaturated fatty acids – omega 3 and omega 6 long chain fats, which contribute to the development of the brain and the retina in the eye.
- Nucleotides – proteins associated with growth and antibody (immune) response.
- Beta-carotene (vitamin A) – an anti-oxidant that plays a role in the development of the immune system, skin and tissue growth.
- Prebiotics – non-digestible carbohydrates that can selectively stimulate the growth of healthy bacteria present in the gut.

(NHS Greater Glasgow and Clyde Guidelines).

There is insufficient evidence to confirm the benefit of the addition of these substances and their use in the body (bio-availability) is uncertain. Therefore, these formulas should not be promoted as beneficial over those without the additional substrates until more research is available.

Alternative formula and fresh milks

The use of alternative milks is increasing, and many healthcare practitioners receive enquiries about their safety and suitability for infants. These include:

- Soya infant formula.
- Organic cow's milk formula.
- Goat's milk infant formula.
- Fresh goat or sheep's milk.
- Fresh cow's milk.
- Unpasteurized or unhomogenized cow's milk.

Soya infant formula
Soya infant formulas are not recommended for infants (particularly those under six months old) unless required for medical or religious reasons (Scientific Advisory Committee on Nutrition, 2003).

There are three main reasons why soya infant formulas are not recommended as first-choice infant formula. These include:

- Phytoestrogens – soya milks include high levels of phytoestrogens. There is concern about the possible long-term health implications due to the high doses of the phytoestrogens consumed by an infant fed solely on soya formula at a developmental age when permanent changes due to the phytoestrogens are most likely to occur (see below).
- Sensitivity and allergy to soya protein. The risk of protein sensitization is likely to be greatest in the first six months of life and therefore the use of soya infant formula during this period is not recommended for allergic infants. In addition, infants who are intolerant to cow's milk protein are at risk of cross-reactivity to soya protein (British Dietetic Association, 2004).
- Increased risk of peanut allergy. Infants fed soya-based formula may have increased risk of peanut allergy (Lack et al., 2003).

There is ongoing debate about the effects of high-dose phytoestrogens (such as the doses an infant would receive if fed solely on soya infant formula for the first six months of life) on sexual development and immune function. A retrospective cohort study conducted in 1999 (Strom et al., 2001) found no statistically significant evidence from the available data between groups (men or women) who had been fed soya formula or cow's milk formula. However, they did report that women who had been fed soya formula reported slightly longer duration of menstrual bleeding (with no difference in severity of menstrual flow) and greater discomfort with menstruation.

There are animal studies that show changes in the number of Leydig (testosterone-producing) cells in the testes. Suppression of the testosterone rises in neonatal marmosets fed soya formula (Sharpe *et al.*, 2002).

As a consequence of the lack of convincing evidence regarding the safety of soya formula phytoestrogen levels the recommendations from the British Dietetic Association are that infants should not receive soya formula as first-line treatment for food allergies, especially for infants under six months old (British Dietetic Association, 2004).

Cases where the use of soya infant formula may be indicated include:

- Infants with cow's milk protein allergy or intolerance who refuse extensively hydrolysed/ elemental formulas.
- Vegan mothers, who cannot or choose not to breastfeed.
- Galactosaemia where the lactose of low-lactose formulas is considered too high and the use of extensively hydrolysed formulae are not appropriate.

(British Dietetic Association, 2004)

Organic infant formula

Organic infant formulas meet the criteria set out by the Infant Formula and Follow-on Formula Regulations (1995) and are therefore safe to feed to infants; however, they provide no nutritional advantages over standard infant formula (DH, 1995).

Goat's milk infant formula

On 1 March 2007 goat's milk infant formula was removed from the UK market and is no longer sold. This is due to a lack of available scientific data to establish the suitability of goat's milk as a protein source in infant and follow-on formula. In addition, there is not enough research evidence to support the belief that the incidence of allergic reaction is lower when feeding goat's milk-based formula compared to cow's milk-based formula (European Food Safety Authority, 2005).

Fresh goat's and sheep's milk

Fresh goat's and sheep's milk are unsuitable for infants and children for the following reasons:

- Goat's milk and sheep's milk contain lactose so are also unsuitable for babies who are lactose-intolerant.
- Goat's milk is low in folic acid and vitamin B_{12} so is not nutritionally sound.
- Sheep's milk is significantly higher in protein, fat, energy and minerals than cow's milk, and is the least similar to breast milk.
- Goat's milk and sheep's milk may not be pasteurized and so are unsafe for children. If parents cannot be persuaded not to feed their child with these milks, advice on food safety and boiling the milk is important, as is advice on appropriate vitamin and mineral supplements.

For the above reasons, fresh goat's milk and sheep's milk should not be given to children under two years old (DH, 1994; COT, 1996).

Fresh cow's milk

It is well accepted that fresh cow's milk is not a suitable main drink for infants (DH, 1994). It is high in protein and sodium, resulting in a high renal solute load. Cow's milk is inadequate in some nutrients, such as iron, for the needs of young infants.

Cow's milk is safe to use in small amounts to mix into solid foods (see section 8.7) in babies from six months of age who are not sensitive to cow's milk protein.

Children who are over 12 months may have cow's milk as their main milk, as part of a mixed diet. Semi-skimmed and skimmed milks should not be given to children under two years, because the lower fat content reduces the energy density and the fat-soluble vitamins of the milk (DH, 1994). Semi-skimmed milks may be given to children over two years and skimmed milks to children over five years if they are consuming an adequate diet and growing well (DH, 1994; COT, 1996).

Evaporated, condensed or powdered cow's milk is not suitable for infants as they are nutritionally inadequate and high in sugar.

Unpasteurized or unhomogenized milk

Animal milks that have not been pasteurized are not safe for children. Milks that have not been homogenized may have uneven distribution of fat and therefore are not suitable for infants under two years (DH, 1995).

Is the baby getting enough feed and fluid?

Infant formula

Healthy newborn infants require approximately 150 ml of feed per kg body weight by the end of the first week of life (Shaw & Lawson, 2002). For low birth weight babies this may increase up to 200 ml per kg body weight. This is approximately 600–700 ml every 24 hours for a newborn baby but will vary for each individual baby. Bottle-fed babies, like breastfed babies, should be fed when they are hungry (i.e., on demand). In the first few days after birth, this may be as frequent as every 2–3 hours. After the first couple of weeks, they usually settle down to feed every 3–4 hours.

Overfeeding, force-feeding or the use of a bottle as a pacifier should be discouraged as this may lead to vomiting and, in the longer term, an inappropriately high energy intake (Shaw & Lawson, 2002).

Fluids

Bottle-fed infants may require additional fluids in the form of cooled, boiled water during hot weather (Thomas & Clayton, 2001). This should not replace formula volume.

Once solids are introduced from six months of age (see section 8.7), formula intake will reduce as the appetite is partly satisfied by solid foods. At this age the fluid requirement is approximately 120 ml/kg body weight.

By 12 months a child's thirst will dictate the fluid requirements and children should be encouraged to drink water and milk as their main drinks at this age. It is recommended that children over 12 months should have two or three milk drinks a day and additional water drinks throughout the day (Thomas & Clayton, 2001). If a child refuses cow's milk, three servings of a calcium-rich alternative, such as yoghurt or cheese, should be included in the diet.

Too much cow's milk and dairy products in the diet may lead to iron deficiency due to a reduced intake of iron-rich foods, so a variety of foods is important.

Signs the baby is getting enough feed and fluid

In young infants it is generally accepted that regular wet nappies (6–8 very wet cloth nappies or 5–6 wet disposable nappies as well as 2–5 bowel movements/day) indicate that the baby is getting enough fluid (La Leche League, 2006).

Growth plotted on a growth chart by a doctor, health visitor or other health professional is a good way of monitoring whether a child is receiving adequate feed (energy) intake.

It is noteworthy that a formula-fed baby will grow at a different rate from a breastfed baby and different growth charts are now available.

Preparation of infant formula feeds

Powdered infant formula is not a sterile product and may be contaminated with bacteria which can cause serious illness. Correct preparation and handling, and following the manufacturer's guidelines, reduces the risk (FSA, 2005).

Personal hygiene

Good personal hygiene is vital when preparing and handling infant feeds. Hands should be thoroughly washed before preparing or handing formula feeds. The area used for preparing bottle feeds should be cleaned with hot soapy water and be uncluttered.

Cleaning and sterilizing equipment

All equipment used in the preparation of infant formula should be thoroughly cleaned with hot soapy water, rinsed and then sterilized. This includes bottles, teats, teat caps and dummies (if used). Bottles, teats and teat caps should be scrubbed using a bottlebrush to ensure all feed has been removed and then all items should be rinsed with fresh water before sterilization.

There are various sterilization techniques:

- Sterilizing solutions – require dilution and sterilizing by soaking the equipment for a specified length of time. Sterilizing solutions should be changed every 24 hours and all equipment must be completely immersed in the solution (with no air pockets present).

- Electric sterilizing systems – produce steam to sterilize the equipment.
- Microwave oven steam sterilization systems – specifically designed for microwave ovens and produce steam to sterilize the equipment (i.e., it is steam and not microwaves that sterilize).
- Boiling in water – requires a vessel large enough to submerge the equipment fully. The vessel must then be covered with a lid and the water boiled for 10 minutes.

It is essential that manufacturers' instructions are carefully followed as the time taken for the method to kill bacteria will vary.

Following sterilization, all equipment should remain in the sterilizing chamber until ready to be used.

All equipment used to feed a child should continue to be sterilized until the child is six months of age. This includes any equipment used to clean and prepare bottles and any utensils used for feeding the baby solids if a parent chooses to feed their child solids before six months of age (see section 8.7 for information on the recommended age for the introduction of solids).

After six months of age, bottles, teats and caps, as well as any equipment used to prepare formula milk or bottles (of expressed milk), should continue to be sterilized. However, utensils used to feed the child solid foods or other drinking vessels (cups/beakers) do not need to be sterilized but should be washed thoroughly with hot soapy water, rinsed and dried (Line, 1992).

It is recommended that each bottle of formula be made up fresh at the time of the feed. Storing prepared formula may increase the risk of a baby becoming ill and should be avoided (FSA, 2005).

The following steps (including those outlining 'preparing feeds for use later', 'rewarming stored feeds' and 'transportation of feeds') are new recommendations by the Department of Health and the Food Standards Agency (FSA, 2005, 2006).

- Clean the surface on which to prepare the feed thoroughly.
- Wash hands with soap and water and then dry.
- Boil fresh tap (not mineral) water in a kettle. Alternatively, bottled water that is suitable for infants (sodium content < 20 mg/l) can be used for making up feeds and should be boiled in the same way as tap water. Mineral water and bottle waters should not be used for formula preparation unless the sodium content is <20 mg/l.
- Allow the boiled water to cool to no less than 70°C. This means in practice using water that has been left covered for less than 30 minutes after boiling.
- Pour the boiled water required into the sterilized bottle.
- Add the amount of formula as instructed, always using the scoop provided with the powdered formula by the manufacturer. Adding more or less powder than instructed could make the baby ill.
- Reassemble the bottle following the manufacturer's instructions.
- Shake the bottle well to mix the contents.
- Cool quickly to feeding temperature by holding under a running tap or placing in a container of cold water.
- Check the temperature by shaking a few drops onto the inside of the wrist – it should feel lukewarm, not hot.
- Discard any feed that has not been used within two hours.

It must be stressed that the concentration (i.e., how much powder and water to use) of powdered infant formula must be prepared according to the manufacturer's instructions, unless otherwise advised by a dietitian or doctor. Adding too much powder to the volume of water (over-concentrating) can put pressure on the kidneys (high solute load), lead to dehydration and, in the longer term, lead to obesity. Preparing diluted formula (using less powder than recommended) can lead to an inadequate intake of energy and nutrients which may result in malnutrition and/or faltering growth.

Preparing bottles of infant formula for later use

If feeds are prepared in advance for any reason (such as for babies in care), the following guidance should be followed:

- Prepare a minimum number of bottles only.
- Prepare formula in individual bottles and not one large batch.

- Keep the storage time of the prepared formula to a minimum (i.e., prepare the feeds in the morning rather than the night before).
- Store in a fridge at a temperature of less than 5°C in the back of the fridge, not the door, and check the temperature of the fridge regularly.
- Never store feed for longer than 24 hours.
- Follow the advice on rewarming stored feeds below.

Rewarming stored feeds
- Remove stored feed from the fridge just before it is needed.
- Rewarm using a bottle warmer or by placing in warm water.
- Microwaves should never be used for rewarming a feed.
- Never leave a feed warming for more than 15 minutes.
- Shake the bottle to ensure the feed has heated evenly.
- Check the feeding temperature by shaking a few drops onto the inside of the wrist – it should be lukewarm, not hot.

It is preferable that ready to feed liquid infant formula is used if feeds cannot be prepared at the time needed.

Transporting feeds

Because of the potential for growth of harmful bacteria during transport, feeds should first be cooled in a fridge (<5°C) and then transported as follows:

- Prepare feeds and place in the fridge (as outlined above).
- Ensure feed has been in the fridge for at least one hour before transporting.
- Remove feed from the fridge immediately before transporting.
- Transport feeds in a cool bag containing an ice brick.
- Feeds transported in a cool bag should be used within four hours.
- Rewarm at the destination (see above).

Alternatively, if the destination is reached within four hours, feeds transported in a cool bag can be placed in a fridge and kept for up to a maximum

of 24 hours from the time of preparation. This though this is not ideal as the risk of illness increases the longer it is stored.

Demonstration is important when educating parents on the preparation of formula feeds. It is important to emphasize that the formula powder should be added to the water and not the other way around.

Vitamins
Infants and young children having less than 500 ml of infant formula a day require vitamin drops to provide vitamins A, D and C (DH, 1994; NICE, 2008), such as the Healthy Start Vitamin drops.

8.7   Weaning

Definition

Weaning is the gradual introduction of semi-solid foods to the baby's diet. Weaning is a staged process occurring over a period of months, whereby the amount, range and textures of foods are introduced and increased.

Weaning is necessary because, when a baby reaches approximately six months of age, breast milk or infant formula is no longer sufficient to meet nutritional requirements, particularly for nutrients such as iron. The weaning process introduces the baby to the tastes and textures of family foods. Also, chewing, biting and moving food around the mouth using the tongue is important for early motor skills for speech development (Thomas & Clayton, 2001).

When to wean

The timing and method of weaning is important and will vary according to infants' individual development.

The current recommendations are that babies should be exclusively breastfed for the first six months (26 weeks) of life (DH, 1994, 2004). Most infants who are exclusively milk fed (breast or formula) for the first six months receive adequate nutrition. Infants should never receive solid foods prior to four months (17 weeks) of age (DH, 1994).

For preterm babies, the recommendations are to introduce solids according to actual age, not gestational age (see section 8.8).

Infants aged 4–6 months will display a readiness to start solid foods. The developmental signs that a baby is ready to try solids include the ability to:

- Hold up the head unsupported.
- Bring the hands to the midline.
- Put objects in the mouth.

Other signs include:

- Hunger that is not satisfied with an increased breast or formula feed.
- Reduced time between feeds or waking through the night if previously sleeping through.
- Loss of the (forward) tongue thrust.
- Slowed growth rate.
- Interest in others eating and their foods.

Early weaning

Parents should be encouraged not to introduce complementary foods before four months (17 weeks). The possible problems with the early introduction of solids should be discussed. These include (Thomas & Clayton, 2001):

- The immature gastrointestinal system of a young infant may be susceptible to food allergy and infection.
- The secretion of digestive enzymes by the immature gastrointestinal may not yet be adequate.
- The immature kidneys of a young infant cannot cope with the increased solute load of a solid diet until at least four months.
- The oral motor skills may not be adequately developed for safe oral control of food. This is a choking risk.
- The early introduction of solids has been associated with the following:

    - Increased risk of food allergy and intolerance and eczema (see Allergy and Intolerances section).
    - Persistent cough or wheeze (Wilson et al., 1998).
    - Obesity (DH, 1984, 1988).

Early weaning may also lead to a reduced intake or absorption of nutrients from breast or formula milk before the quantity of solid food is adequate to replace this. This can lead to nutritional deficiencies.

It is important to educate parents choosing to introduce solids before six months on the correct foods to choose as first foods (see below), and that the progression through the stages will need to be slower than for infant starting solids at six months.

In babies with gastro-oesophageal reflux, the early introduction of solids may be recommended by health professionals as the baby may tolerate solid foods better than easily regurgitated liquids. This should be undertaken with the support and guidance of a health professional.

Late weaning

Delaying the introduction of solids beyond 26 weeks may also cause problems. The issues that may arise from late weaning include:

- Inadequate intake of energy and/or nutrients such as iron and zinc, as breast or formula milk is not longer providing adequate amounts to meet requirements.
- Faltering growth.
- Delayed development of feeding skills.
- Behavioural feeding problems.
(DH, 1994).

How to wean

When planning to introduce solid foods into a baby's diet, parents should be guided as follows:

- Babies should be in an upright position. Supporting the back and feet to allow controlled eating is important. This may be achieved in a carer's arms or a suitable baby chair.
- Chose a quiet, relaxed time when the baby is not sleepy.
- Ensure the baby is hungry, but settled. To ensure the baby is not too hungry it may be best to try solid foods following a small milk feed.
- At first, a small rubber teaspoon of food should be offered (see 'Foods to give' below for texture advice) once in the day.
- Each new food introduced should be offered individually to allow identification of any food sensitivity and to allow the baby to become

accustomed to the new taste. This can take 10–12 trials of a new food.

- It is important never to force-feed a child. Instead, be guided by the baby's appetite.
- Relax and allow the baby to enjoy the introduction of solids with food play. Parents should be encouraged to allow mess and fun.
- Never leave a baby unsupervised during feeding.
- Solids should never be added to an infant's bottle. This is a choking risk, may lead to dehydration and hinders the establishment of good weaning practices. Food in the bottle also adds calories to the milk and may lead to obesity and tooth decay.
- It may be useful to warn parents that a baby's stools will change with the introduction of solid foods.

Baby-led weaning

Baby-led weaning is based on the idea that normal babies appear quite capable, with the right support from their parents, of managing their own introduction to solid food. Baby-led weaning suggests that the child's development will set the pace of the introduction to solids and that a child who is not able to get food to his or her mouth is unlikely to be ready to manage the food in the mouth or digest it. Baby-led weaning suggests that putting food to a baby's mouth overrides the child's ability to lead weaning at his or her own pace and increases the risk of choking (Rapley, 2008). Guidelines have been produced regarding baby-led weaning. These include a list of 'do' and 'do not' suggestions. However, these guidelines are not evidence-based.

This method is not supported by sufficient evidence. Speech and language therapists do not support baby-led weaning as there are concerns about its safety.

Foods to give

There are many names given to the different 'stages' of weaning (as used by commercial baby foods). These names usually refer to the progression through increasing food textures, variety and the volumes of food offered at each developmental step. The rate at which each child progresses through the stages of weaning is individual.

Foods to avoid

Before six months

If parents decide to introduce solids before six months (26 weeks) they should be advised to avoid the following foods in their child's diet (Food Allergy and Intolerance Specialist Group statement, 2005):

- Gluten-containing breads/cereals (including rusks and barley).
- Wheat-containing breads/cereals (including rusks).
- Eggs and egg products (custards, biscuits, cakes).
- Cow's milk.
- Soya and soya products.
- Nuts, nut pastes and seeds.
- Fish and shellfish.
- Citrus fruits, including juices.

While whole meal and high-fibre foods are healthy for children, extracted fibre (e.g., bran cereals) can overfill a child and lead to a lower energy intake. This may lead to a reduced absorption of some important nutrients such as iron and zinc.

Before 12 months

Children should continue on breast or infant formula milk until they are at least 12 months old. From 12 months of age, children may be given cow's milk as a drink. Until a child is 12 months old it is important to avoid the following foods:

- Honey – due to the risk of infection (clostridium botulinum).
- Nuts – due to the risk of choking, children should not be given whole nuts of any kind until they are five years of age. Smooth peanut butter may be given from six months of age if there is no family history of atopy or food allergy.
- Sugar – due to the risk of dental caries and of developing a preference for sweet foods.
- Salt and processed foods high in salt – due to the infant's immature kidneys and the high solute load of added salt.
- Tea – due to the tannins in tea reducing the absorption of iron.
- Unprocessed bran – as it reduces iron absorption.

Fluids from six months

Breastfed infants under six months do not need any fluids in addition to breast milk. Bottle-fed babies of this age need only formula milk and cooled boiled water.

The following points should be noted when giving babies water or using water to prepare foods/formula (Thomas & Clayton, 2001):

- Cooled, boiled tap water is suitable for babies.
- Bottled water should be boiled before use and has no advantage over tap water.
- Mineral waters must have sodium (salt) < 20 mg/l.
- Carbonated waters are not recommended.
- Flavoured or sweetened water or those with vitamins and minerals added are not recommended.
- Fruit juices are not required for children, but if used should be diluted with water 1 part juice to 10 parts water. Juice contains fruit sugar increases the risk of dental caries, provides 'empty' calories (energy without other nutrients, which may decrease a child's appetite for more nutritious foods) and may encourage a preference for sweet flavours.

Home-cooked and commercially prepared infant foods

Parents should be encouraged to home-prepare baby foods if possible. There are many advantages to home-prepared food, including:

- Lower cost.
- More control over texture progression.
- Flavours can be separated to allow taste development.
- Babies can be introduced to and develop a taste for the flavour of family foods.
- No added salt or sugar.

Barriers to home preparation of weaning foods may be parents' cooking skills and lack of equipment (e.g., fridge space, hob and oven). Lack of time is also a reported barrier, however if a baby's meal is prepared from selections of the family meal there should be minimal extra work required.

Preparing baby foods at home in bulk and freezing in small (ice cube) labelled portions is a time-efficient way to have baby foods at hand.

Commercially prepared baby foods may be convenient to use on occasions, such as when away from home, travelling or when the child is in occasional care. While jarred baby foods may play a role in the young child's diet, the disadvantages include:

- Price.
- Salt and sugar content.
- The flavours of different food ingredients are mixed, limiting the experience for the child.
- The texture is predetermined and does not allow grading up from purée through mashed to finger foods.

Parents need to be aware that the texture of jarred or tinned baby foods referred to as 'stage 2' or 'from 7 months' can create problems for the baby. The texture of these foods can be a smooth purée, or semi-liquid, with lumps. This requires a high level of skill to hold the food in the mouth, while swallowing the liquid, then chewing the lumps, and finally swallowing. Infants do better with gradual progress from smooth purée to a more lumpy consistency rather than lumps within purée.

If parents choose to use commercially prepared baby foods, they should be encouraged to buy the savoury choices over the sweet and those with 'no added sugar' and 'no added salt'.

Parents should also be educated regarding the food safety requirements for commercially prepared baby foods. Jars and tins should be checked for the 'use by' date and once opened should be stored in the fridge for no longer than 24 hours.

Cultural and religious influences on weaning

The following guidance on vegan, vegetarian, ethnic minority and cultural diets have been adapted from Shaw and Lawson (2002).

The multicultural society of the UK brings many and varied cultural and ethnic diets. The extent of adoption of traditional dietary customs varies between families, as does the availability of traditional foods in a western environment.

Each ethnic group will have its own traditions with regard to breastfeeding and weaning practices; therefore, practitioners should try to understand the family's context when supporting them.

The discussion with the family should focus on practices surrounding the following areas of infant nutrition:

- Breastfeeding practices and duration.
- Family and other support.
- Age of introduction to solids.
- Method of solid introduction.
- Suitable weaning foods.
- Practice around adding anything to the bottle other than breast or formula milk (i.e., solids, sugars, flavours).

Vegetarian and vegan diets

Vegetarian and vegan diets are common among many religious, cultural and ethnic groups. Individuals may also restrict their dietary intake of meat and animal products for humanitarian, ethical or health reasons.

There are many variations of diets within vegetarianism and veganism, from complete abstinence from all animal foods (including eggs and dairy foods) to partial avoidance of selected animal-based foods (see Table 8.11).

Careful attention should be given to ensuring a well-balanced diet within these dietary restrictions to achieve a nutritionally balanced diet that meets the needs of a child's normal growth and development. With greater dietary restriction there is an increased risk nutritional deficiency.

Nutrients at risk of deficiency
Children weaned onto a vegetarian diet need the same considerations as those weaned onto a non-vegetarian diet. The main nutrient at risk is iron and vegetarian alternatives should be included in the diet. Non-animal sources of iron include mashed lentils/beans/chickpeas, tofu, smooth nut pastes (if no allergy) and fortified cereals.

Suitable dietary alternatives need to be sourced to replace those foods excluded to provide the nutrients that are at risk of deficiency (see Table 8.12).

Special dietary considerations
The following dietary considerations should also be considered for infants and children weaned onto a vegan (or highly restricted vegetarian diet):

Table 8.11 Vegetarian or vegan diet

	Foods excluded	Animal protein source	Non-animal protein source	Nutrients at risk of deficiency
Part-vegetarian	Red meat Offal	Poultry Fish Milk Cheese Yoghurt Eggs	Beans Pulses Nuts Seeds	Iron
Lacto-ovo-vegetarian	Red meat Offal Poultry Fish Eggs	Milk Cheese Yoghurt	Beans Lentils Nuts Seeds	Iron
Lacto-vegetarian	Red meat Offal Poultry Fish Eggs	Milk Cheese Yoghurt	Beans Lentils Nuts Seeds	Iron Vitamin D
Vegan	Red meat Offal Fish Poultry Eggs Milk Cheese Yoghurt		Beans Lentils Nuts Seeds	Protein Energy Iron Fat-soluble vitamins Vitamin B_2 Vitamin B_{12} Calcium Zinc

- Infants should continue to receive frequent breastfeeds or at least 500 ml of soya-based infant formula (Farley's Soya Infant Formula being the only acceptable formula for vegans as it contains vitamin D which is not derived from sheep's wool).
- A minimum of 350 ml breast or formula milk per day should be offered until the age of two years.

Table 8.12   Nutrients at risk of deficiency during vegetarian and vegan weaning

Nutrient	Suitable dietary alternative sources
Protein	Pulses (soya, tofu, tempeh, beans and lentils), grains (wheat, rice, rye, millet, etc.), seeds, groundnuts*, nuts and nut spreads*. Meals should have a combination of grains with seeds or grains with pulses to get the right balance of essential amino acids to ensure the best use of the availability protein.
Energy	Vegetable oils/margarine, groundnuts*, nut spreads*.
Iron	Iron-fortified cereals, wholegrain cereals, whole meal bread, pulses, dried fruit, nuts*. Dark leafy green vegetables and legumes are not a suitable source of iron for infants and young because they would have to eat 120 g to get 2 mg. Foods rich in vitamin C, such as fruits and vegetables, aid the absorption of non-animal sources of iron.
Fat-soluble vitamins	In England white Caucasians make enough vitamin D for the year from 30 minutes a day of moderate sunlight from April to October. Blacks and Asians living in England do not make enough, and must rely on dietary sources or supplements. Vegetable oils/margarines, fortified soya milk and fortified cereals.
Vitamin B$_2$	Wheatgerm, almonds, green leafy vegetables, yeast extract** (e.g., Marmite, Tastex), avocado, soya beans, fortified soya milk.
Vitamin B$_{12}$	Fortified yeast extract (e.g. Marmite, Tastex), fortified cereals, fortified soya milk, tofu.
Calcium	Fortified soya products (soya milk and yoghurt), seaweed products (*kombu, wakame, nori*), nuts* and seeds. Other sources (bread, leafy green vegetables, pulses) are not suitable sources of calcium for infants and young children because they would need to eat over 120 g to get 100 mg.
Zinc	Some soya products (flour, miso, cheese and tempeh), nuts*, seeds, wheat germ, wholemeal bread, fortified breakfast cereals, seaweed, hard cheeses.

*Nuts should be introduced with care if there is history or evidence of nut allergy, and nuts should not be given to children under two years of age unless finely ground due to choking risk.
**Yeast extracts should be used with care in children under 2 years of age due to the high salt content.

- Unsweetened soya milk (supermarket bought) fortified with calcium and B vitamins may be introduced in cooking from six months but should not be used as a main drink until after two years of age.
- Vitamin drops containing vitamins A and D should be encouraged.

The growth and development of infants and children following a vegan diet should be carefully monitored.

Due to the complexity of the vegan diet and the more restricted vegetarian diets and risk of nutrient deficiencies, a specialist dietitian should be consulted to assess dietary adequacy and assist in constructing a suitable diet plan.

South Asian diet

The South Asian community represents the largest ethnic minority group in the UK and consists of people who have migrated from India, Pakistan and Bangladesh and those via East Africa. Dietary customs are largely based on the religious and cultural beliefs of the three main religious groups: Hindus, Muslims and Sikhs. Diets vary widely between these groups (see Table 8.13).

Typical breastfeeding or bottle feeding practices
Breastfeeding rates are higher among Asian mothers than Caucasian mothers in the UK. However, Bangladeshi and Pakistani mothers are less likely to continue beyond eight weeks of life. Increased education to promote the importance of breastfeeding up to six months is required within Asian communities.

Typical weaning practices
Late weaning and prolonged breastfeeding are commonly practised in infants who have parents

Table 8.13 Religion and dietary customs

Religious group	Religion	Staple	Dietary customs and restrictions
Hindus	Hinduism	Millet	No beef
		Wheat	Often no pork
		Rice	No alcohol
			Often vegetarian or vegan
Moslems	Islam	Rice	No pork
		Millet	*Halal* meat
		Wheat	No alcohol
			No fish without scales
Sikhs	Sikhism	Wheat	No beef
			Often no pork
			No *halal* meat

Table 8.14 Suitable South Asian weaning foods

6 months, puréed	Cauliflower and potato
	Cauliflower and pea
	Pea and potato
	Aubergine and potato
	Green vegetable and potato
	Lentil and rice
	Chickpeas and marrow
	Porridge
	Fruit purée
7–12 months, mashed	Meat, fish or poultry may be added (if eaten by family)
	Introduce small lumps to the above foods
	Mild spices (e.g., cumin and coriander) may be added
	Mashed pulses such as chickpeas, kidney beans

born outside the UK and parents who have recently migrated to the UK. Traditional practices considered it safer to leave the infant on breast milk and wean straight to family foods. In the UK late weaning may be partly due to the poor availability of suitable foods and the lack of adequate or appropriate advice.

Some Asian infants born in the UK are weaned earlier and are commonly given sweet, commercially produced baby foods, which are low in iron and protein. Mothers should be encouraged to cook suitable savoury foods at home (see Table 8.14).

The practice of adding foods such as rusks, honey and cereals to bottles of milk is also common and should be discouraged. There is often a delay in feeding development due to the late switch from bottle to cup and the late progression to family foods.

Cow's milk is introduced from the age of five months in some Asian families. This can lead to nutritional problems, such as high saturated fat and salt intake, and low vitamin D and iron status.

Nutrition problems commonly found in Asian children
- Iron-deficiency anaemia.
- Rickets.

African-Caribbean diet

The African-Caribbean community is the second largest ethnic minority group in the UK.

A minority of the African-Caribbean community in the UK are Rastafarians. Many Rastafarians avoid animal-derived foods (i.e., have a vegan diet) and some avoid foods 'from the vine', such as grapes, sultanas, raisins and wine.

Typical breastfeeding or bottle-feeding practices
Over 90% of African-Caribbean women breastfeed their babies, however this is often for a short duration and rarely exclusive.

Many women avoid giving their babies colostrum and give water instead, because they believe that colostrum is 'stale' breast milk and water will cleanse the baby's body prior to giving the breast milk. This practice may reduce breast milk production and may also contribute to the low exclusive breastfeeding rates.

Typical weaning practices
African-Caribbean infants may be weaned as early as one month of age. In contrast, late weaning is

Table 8.15 Suitable African-Caribbean weaning foods

6 months, puréed	Rice or oat porridge, cornmeal
	Root vegetables (e.g., yam, potato)
	Rice with vegetables (e.g., peas, okra, pumpkin)
7–12 months, mashed	Introduce small lumps to the above foods
	Meat, fish or poultry
	Lentils, kidney beans, gungo peas

commonly observed within the orthodox Rastafarian community.

Common weaning foods include high-starch foods with low nutrient density, such as corn meal, oats and rice porridge, which may lead to deficiencies in energy, protein, vitamins and minerals. It is also common practice to add thin porridge to bottles. This can lead to a delay in the weaning process and obesity. It is also a choking risk and should be discouraged (see Table 8.15).

Nutrition problems commonly found in Afro-Caribbean children
- Iron-deficiency anaemia.
- Rickets.
- Obesity.

Chinese diet

Chinese people are the third largest ethnic minority group in the UK. Dietary habits vary according to the country and region from which the family originates. Chinese in the UK may be British, Caribbean, Hong Kong, Taiwan, China, Malaysia or Singapore born.

The Chinese diet is based on Yin and Yang foods which are cold or hot (in terms of female or male energy, not temperature), which limits and guides this community as to what foods can be eaten, by whom and at what stage of life.

Typical breastfeeding or bottle-feeding practices
In the UK, Chinese women often return for work soon after childbirth, which has led to a decrease in the rate and duration of breastfeeding.

Soya bean oil is a poor source of docosahexaenoic acid (DHA) and arachidonic acid (AA), essential fatty acids that are found in fish. Soya oil is a major source of fat in the Chinese diet. Because of this, their breast milk has been found to have a low concentration of DHA and AA and it has been suggested that mothers who are breastfeeding their infants should supplement their diet with a good source of DHA and AA, such as fish oil.

Nutrition problems commonly found in Chinese children
The main dietary-related health concern for Chinese people is the high salt intake due to the use of many preserved foods and the high fat and sugar intake associated with the increasing intake of western foods.

A high incidence of lactose intolerance due to hypolactasia (low levels of lactase) is also becoming apparent with the consumption of milk and other dairy products.

West African diet

Many of the traditional foods of the West African communities are similar. Common foods are rice, yam, cassava, coco, *gari*, plantain, *kenke* and couscous. Preparation methods may differ from country to country. The majority of West Africans are Muslim or Christian.

Typical breastfeeding or bottle-feeding practices
Although most West African women will breastfeed from birth, it is rare to find exclusive breastfeeding. Mixed feeding, combining breastfeeding with a bottle, is common. Women may breastfeed at home, but bottle-feed in public. Health professionals should continue to encourage mothers to continue breastfeeding.

Typical weaning practices
There tends to be an over-reliance on manufactured weaning foods within the West African families, particularly in the early stages of weaning. This reliance may come from the belief that commercial baby foods meet the baby's nutritional

requirements. Mothers may lack knowledge of how to prepare family foods in a way suitable for young babies.

Many West African babies are often introduced to solids earlier than recommendations, with foods being added to bottles due to the baby not being ready to take solids from a spoon. Adding sugar to food is also a common practice that should be discouraged. Another practice that should be discouraged is a prolonged period of giving purée-consistency foods.

There are many traditional family foods that make suitable weaning foods if the texture is appropriate. These include yams, green bananas, plantains, ground rice, sweet potato, cassava and maize flour (cornmeal) and should be encouraged to use these as weaning foods and instructed on how to prepare them to a suitable form for their baby's developmental stage.

Somali diet

The following information on Somali diets has been taken from the Kings College Hospital *Breastfeeding and Nutrition for Under 5s Guidelines* and is a guide from the Somali Women's Group in Camberwell, south London (2003).

Although the following is a guide on the typical diet of those from northern Somalia, those from southern Somalia will have the same foods and drinks, but use a lot more beans and pulses in their dishes.

Many Somalis will only eat beef in Somalia, believing that the *halal* process is not carried out correctly in the UK. Fish may be consumed, but infrequently as meat is more popular. It is rare to find a vegetarian Somalians.

Typical breastfeeding or bottle-feeding practices

Breastfeeding is traditionally thought to be the best milk for all babies, so they are all breastfed. Babies are breastfed up to six months and many continue until two years of age. The majority of women choose to breastfeed until the child is two years old as a form of birth control. Breastfeeding usually stops when the milk dries up.

Some children will be combination-fed (i.e., breast and bottle feeds). However, this is uncommon. From six months some babies will be given goat's milk in addition to breast milk. Goat's milk is not recommended (see section 8.6).

Typical weaning practices

Weaning usually starts between four and five months of age. The first foods are usually home-cooked potato, vegetables and *halal* meat (lamb, goat, camel).

The practice of adding high-sugar baby cereals to bottles should be discouraged, as should the inclusion of high-sugar and high-fat foods (e.g., crisps, chocolates, biscuits, cakes and fizzy drinks), which are common in the Somalian diet.

8.8   Preterm infant nutrition

Preterm infants have limited stores of nutrients as building nutritional stores occur predominantly during the last trimester of pregnancy. Therefore, a preterm infant's energy and nutrient requirements are higher than that of the term infant to allow for catch-up growth and to compensate for the stressful period post-delivery.

Suitable milks

Mothers are encouraged to demand breastfeed their preterm infants whenever possible.

During the inpatient stay breast milk fortifier (BMF) (e.g., Nutriprem BMF, SMA BMF or Milupa Eoprotin) may be used to increase the protein, calorie and micronutrient content of breast milk. In rare cases this may be continued after discharge. BMF is high in vitamins and minerals (particularly calcium and phosphate) but low in calories. It does not provide iron. Breast milk fortifier is not available on prescription and therefore will need to be supplied by the hospital dietitian or neonatal unit.

For mothers who choose not to breastfeed, an appropriate formula will be recommended by the medical or nutrition team, taking account of the infant's gestational age, birth weight and growth. This may either be a term formula or a nutrient-enriched preterm formula.

Preterm formulas are higher in protein, energy, vitamins and minerals than standard term infant formula. The calcium and phosphorus content is higher to aid bone mineralization. Infants should be kept on this formula until six months corrected age unless weight gain is excessive or if growth is poor and a higher calorie formula is required (McGuire *et al.*, 2004).

Vitamin and mineral supplementation

Each neonatal unit will have a policy on vitamin and mineral supplementation for preterm babies. Guidance should be taken from the discharging hospital, however common practice follows these basic principles:

- Babies who are discharged home fully breastfed should receive a multivitamin and mineral (containing vitamin D and an iron supplement).
- Babies who are discharged home on preterm formula should not require any supplements until they transfer to a term formula when usual vitamin and mineral guidelines apply.

Weaning for the preterm baby

The government currently recommends that term babies be fed solely on breast milk or infant formula for the first six months of life. Each baby should, however, be considered as an individual as to when solids are introduced.

In the past, preterm babies may have been introduced to solids at a corrected age; it is now advisable to wean preterm babies onto solids 5–7 months after birth. The same signs that the baby is ready for solids should be observed in the preterm baby and the same guidance should be followed as to what foods and textures, their quantities and how to introduce them.

A weaning leaflet has been written for preterm infants by dietitians, a speech therapist, neonatologists, a research nutritionist and a psychologist. It is available free of charge from the UK neonatal charity BLISS (www.bliss.org.uk).

8.9 Food allergy and intolerance

There are two types of adverse reactions to food: food allergy and food intolerance.

Food allergy

Food allergy is an immune system response in response to a certain food or foods. This causes an antibody response and is immediate onset, or directly following the ingestion of the reactive food. The most common foods to cause allergic reactions in children are:

- Cow's milk.
- Soya.
- Eggs.
- Wheat.
- Peanuts.
- Nuts.
- Fish.
- Citrus fruits.

(COT, 1998; 2008)

Food allergy can be detected by a skin prick test, patch tests, blood tests (*in vitro* blood tests or radio allegro sorbent tests, RAST) clinical history and exclusion diet with food challenges (Thomas & Clayton, 2001).

Food intolerance

Food intolerance (sensitivity) is a reaction to food which does not involve the immune system but is reproducible when the causal food is eaten repeatedly.

As intolerance reactions do not involve the immune system they are not detected on skin prick tests or blood tests. They rely on taking good clinical history and food exclusion and challenges for the detection and identification of the causal foods. The causal food may be difficult to detect due to the possibility of delayed response of up to 48 hours or more (Thomas & Clayton, 2001).

Allergy prevention

During pregnancy mothers should be encouraged to eat a normal, healthy, balanced diet. There is insufficient evidence to support restricted maternal diet to reduce the risk of food allergies in children from the non-atopic families. Also, avoiding foods major foods groups may place the mother and foetus at nutritional risk.

Infants with a family history of atopy (an inherited tendency to develop allergies such as asthma, eczema, rhinitis, urticaria, allergic dermatitis) are at greater risk of developing food allergies. The following are the current recommendations on maternal and infant diet to prevent the development of food allergy in these at-risk children (British Dietetic Association, 2005):

- Government advice is that in families with an atopic history, the mother may wish to avoid eating peanuts during pregnancy and breast-feeding (COT, 1998). There is no clear evidence to support this, however excluding peanuts will not alter the maternal diet significantly and so mothers may be happy to avoid peanuts given the possible severity of childhood nut allergy. These mothers are also recommended to avoid introducing peanuts into the diet of their child before three years of age (COT, 1998).
- Exclusive breastfeeding should be encouraged for six months. The mother should continue to eat a normal, healthy range of foods while she is breastfeeding.
- Where breastfeeding is not possible, the child should not be given a formula based on cow's milk or soya before six months of age (British Dietetic Association, 2005). An extensively hydrolysed protein formula with proven effect or elemental formula is recommended.
- Weaning onto solid foods should not begin before six months of age. If the child is introduced to solids prior to six months (26 weeks) of age it should never be done before four months (17 weeks) and care should be taken to choose low allergen foods (see section 8.6).
- Typical allergen foods should be delayed until after six months. These foods include cow's milk, wheat, soya, egg, nuts, sesame seeds and citrus fruits. There is not adequate evidence to support that delaying the introduction of these foods until after six months of age has any effect on preventing the development of allergy (Zutavern *et al.*, 2004) and may in fact lead to nutritional deficiencies if not supervised by a dietitian.

8.10   Oral health

Improving oral health is part of the government's wider public health strategy and many of the key factors that lead to poor oral health are risk factors for other diseases (DH, 2005).

There are two main types of dental diseases:

- Tooth decay or dental caries.
- Gum disease.

Tooth decay

The main cause of tooth decay is the frequent consumption of sugars. The plaque bacteria on the surface of the teeth turn sugars into acid. The acid causes demineralization (an acid attack) which can lead to cavities, tooth destruction, pain and infection (Levine & Stillman-Lowe, 2004).

Gum disease

Gum disease is swelling, soreness or infection of the tissues supporting the teeth caused by the plaque bacteria on the gums (Levine & Stillman-Lowe, 2004).

Dental disease can cause pain and the need for dental treatment sometimes requiring general anaesthetic which can be a risk to the general health, especially if medically compromised. Dental disease is preventable.

Children

The points to consider for the protection of children's teeth include the following.

Dental erosion

Dental erosion is caused by tooth wear and loss of enamel and sometimes dentine. This is caused by the direct action of food chemicals on the tooth surface. These food chemicals are found in acidic drinks such as juices, squashes and carbonated fizzy drinks which contain phosphoric acid (including sugar-free varieties).

It is commonly accepted among dental health workers that acidic drinks lead to a softening of the tooth enamel which can then thereby damaged. Therefore, tooth brushing should be avoided for an hour following the consumption of these drinks. Taking milk or cheese may be beneficial to protect the enamel. Parents should be advised about the effect these drinks can have on their infants' teeth.

Sugar types

Sugars which have the potential to cause tooth decay are called non-milk extrinsic sugars (NMES). These sugars are added to foods and drinks when they are manufactured (e.g., glucose syrup, dextrose). Natural sugars (e.g., honey, syrups and sugars in fruit juices) can also cause tooth decay. Sugars which are found naturally in fruit and vegetables contained within the plant cells are not considered to be responsible for tooth decay (Levine & Stillman-Lowe, 2004).

Milk

Breast milk is the best form of nutrition for infants, or cow's milk formulas if this is not the option.

Soya

Soya-based infant formula contains sugars that cause decay. Parents need to be especially vigilant with their baby's tooth brushing as the teeth appear (Levine & Stillman-Lowe, 2004).

Adding substances to milk

Adding any type of sugar or honey to milk should be avoided. Sweetened milk drinks, milkshakes and manufactured bedtime drinks should not be given to children. These expose the teeth to sugars which can lead to dental diseases.

For the same reasons parents should be advised to avoid adding any solids to baby's drinks including cereals, risks, baby rice. This is also a choking risk and may lead to obesity through an excess caloric intake.

Drinks

Water

Cooled boiled water needs to be encouraged if a (non-breastfed) baby or child is thirsty. Plain water is the safest drink as far as the teeth are concerned (Levine & Stillman-Lowe, 2004).

Drinks to avoid

The following drinks should not be offered to babies or young children:

- Pure fruit juices contain high levels of sugars and are very acidic which can lead to decay and erosion. If using fruit juices they need to be diluted 1 part juice to 10 parts water and given in a cup preferably at meal times when drinking times are kept short (Levine & Stillman-Lowe, 2004).
- Baby juices contain high levels of sugars (fructose, glucose). They are made from manufactured fruit syrups (British Nutrition Foundation, 2009).
- Squashes contain sugars and acids and have no nutritional benefit. They may also contain colourings, preservatives and sweeteners.
- Fruit and herbal teas are acidic, and can be sweet and so cause erosion and tooth decay. Added sugar or honey can increase risk of tooth decay (British Nutrition Foundation, 2009).
- Flavoured waters can contain up to 10% NME sugars (sucrose) (Levine & Stillman-Lowe, 2004).
- Adult-type drinks (e.g., tea and coffee) can reduce iron absorption and if they contain sugar can lead to tooth decay (British Nutrition Foundation, 2009).

Drinking habits

'Early childhood caries', formerly known as 'nursing bottle caries', is a rapidly progressing decay, usually of the upper front teeth. This is caused by prolonged contact between sugar in sweet drinks and the teeth. There is increased risk of early childhood caries if the bottle is used as a comforter.

Parents need to be aware that early childhood caries are usually caused by teeth being bathed for prolonged periods of time in the sugars from drinks taken through bottles and valve-type feeder cups (Levine & Stillman-Lowe, 2004).

Sugary drinks and snacks should be avoided one hour before bed as there is low salivary flow during sleep and it is unlikely that brushing before bedtime will remove all traces of any sugary snacks and drinks (Levine & Stillman-Lowe, 2004).

Cups

A free-flow lidded feeding cup, without a valve, or an open-topped cup should be introduced at the weaning stage (six months of age). Cup feeds will initially complement breast- or bottle-feeding until the child reaches an age where larger volumes can efficiently be taken from a cup.

Breastfed babies may not need to be introduced to a bottle as the baby can be weaned from the breast onto the cup (depending on the age of complete weaning).

By the baby's first birthday the cup needs to be used exclusively (with the breast if still breastfeeding) and bottles should be stopped completely.

Free-flow non-valved or open-topped cups encourage a sipping action as liquid flows freely from them. This offers health benefits, including helping to protect baby's teeth from tooth decay.

For older children, parents need to be aware of the issues surrounding cups with valves which prevent spillage. These 'no-spill' cups allow children frequent access to drinks and discourage sitting down to drink, which keeps drinking times shorter. In some cases children sip at drinks all day, which can be problematic if the drink is a sweet and sugary as this places the child at risk of dental decay. The National Oral Health Promotion Group advise that constant sipping on high-calorie, sweet drinks may also reduce the child's appetite for nourishing meals.

Foods

Manufactured foods with added sugar should not be included in children's diets. The frequency and quantity of the sugars consumed are strongly linked to health risks, including dental decay. Sugary foods need not be introduced at the weaning stage. No sugar needs to be added to any food. There are natural sugars present in whole fruits, vegetables and milk. Fruit juice and dried fruit have a high concentration of sugars so are not recommended for consumption between meals (Levine & Stillman-Lowe, 2004).

Dummy use

Parents need to be advised if their baby is using a dummy that it should never be dipped in any type of sugary substance as this increases the risk of tooth decay (British Nutrition Foundation, 2009).

Teething products

When the baby is at the teething stage from around six months, parents need to be aware of avoiding rusks and any other teething product containing sugar to prevent the risk of tooth decay as the teeth appear (British Nutrition Foundation, 2009).

Medicines

Advise parents to use sugar-free medicines where possible, especially for children on long-term medication, to prevent tooth decay (British Nutrition Foundation, 2009).

Tooth brushing and fluoride

There is currently no fluoride added to the local water. Parents need to be strongly advised to introduce tooth brushing with a fluoride toothpaste as soon as the first tooth appears in order to help prevent tooth decay.

A small, soft, age-appropriate toothbrush and a smear of fluoride toothpaste should be used for babies and a pea-sized amount of toothpaste from the age of three years. It is important to discourage children from eating toothpaste or swallowing excessive amounts so parents should help with tooth brushing until children are about seven years old. A gentle scrub technique should be used to ensure a systematic brushing of all tooth surfaces.

Low-fluoride toothpastes give only limited protection against tooth decay. Unless the baby and any siblings are caries free and in good health, a regular family fluoride toothpaste should be used. Advise parents to ask their dentist for further advice (Levine & Stillman-Lowe, 2004).

Websites

www.dentalhealth.org.uk/faqs/leafletdetail.
    php?LeafletID=23.
www.healthystart.nhs.uk/en/fe/vitamin_supplement_
    recommendations.html.
www.nice.org.uk/nicemedia/live/10936/29269/
    29269.pdf.
www.nice.org.uk/nicemedia/live/10988/30144/
    30144.pdf.
www.nice.org.uk/nicemedia/live/11000/30365/
    30365.pdf.
www.nice.org.uk/nicemedia/live/11180/31411/
    31411.pdf.
www.nice.org.uk/nicemedia/live/11943/40097/
    40097.pdf.
www.nice.org.uk/nicemedia/live/11946/41342/
    41342.pdf.

Further reading

Aucherbach, K. (1990) The effects of nipple shields on maternal milk volume. *Journal of Obstetric and Gynaecological Nursing and Neonatal Nursing*, 19(5), 410–27.

Burdge, G. *et al.* (2002) Eicosapentaenoic and docosapentaenoic acids are the principal products of alpha-linoeic acid metabolism in young men. *British Journal of Nutrition*, 88(4), 355–64.

Centre for Maternal & Child Enquiries (CMACE)/Royal College of Obstetrics & Gynaecology (2010) *Joint Guidelines: Management of Women with Obesity in Pregnancy*. London.

Clayden, G.S. *et al.* (2005) The management of chronic constipation and related faecal incontinence in childhood. *Archives of Disease in Childhood – Education and Practice*, 90: 58–67.

Conde-Agudelo, A. *et al.* (2006) Birth spacing and risk of adverse perinatal outcomes: a meta-analysis. *Journal of the American Medical Association*, 295(15), 1809–23.

Coutsoudis, A. & The Breastfeeding and HIV International Transmission Study Group (BHITS) (2004) Late postnatal transmission of HIV-1 in breast-fed children: individual patient data meta-analysis. *Journal of Infectious Diseases*, 189(12), 2149–53.

Craig, W.R. (2005) Metoclopramide, thickened feedings, and positioning for gastro-oesophageal reflux in children under two years. *Cochrane Review*, 2, Wiley, Chichester.

Cumming, R.G. & Klineberg, R.J. (1993) Breastfeeding and other reproductive factors and the risk of hip fracture in elderly women. *International Journal of Epidemiology*, 2(4), 684–91.

de Rooy, L. & Hawdon, J. (2002) Nutritional factors that affect the postnatal adaptation of full-term, small and large-term gestational age infants. *Paediatrics*, 109(3), e42.

Edwards, A.G. *et al.* (1990) Recognising failure to thrive in early childhood. *Archives of Diseases in Childhood*, 65(11), 1263–5.

European Commission Directorate General for Health and Consumer Protection (2001) *Eurodiet: Nutrition and Diet for Healthy Lifestyles in Europe*. EC, Strasbourg.

Expert Group on Vitamins and Minerals (2003) *Safe Upper Levels for Vitamins and Minerals*. FSA, London.

Friedman, L (1993) Commentary on breast feeding and risk of breast cancer in young women [original article by United Kingdom National Case-Control Study Group appears in BR MED J 1993;307(6895):17–20]. *ONS Nursing in Oncology*, 2(6), 18–19.

Holmes, V.A. *et al.* (2005) Homocysteine is lower in the third trimester of pregnancy in women with enhanced folate status from continued folic acid supplementation. *Clinical Chemistry*, 51(3), 629–34.

Huang, R.C. *et al.* (2002) Feed thickener for newborn infants with gastro-oesophageal reflux. *Cochrane Database Systematic Reviews*, 3, CD003211 (abstract).

Klougart, N. *et al.* (1989) Infantile colic treated by chiropractors: a prospective study of 316 cases. *Journal of Manipulative Physiological Therapy*, 12(4), 281–8.

La Leche League (1997) *Breastfeeding a Baby with Down's Syndrome*. La Leche League, Nottingham.

La Leche League International (2004) *The Womanly Art of Breastfeeding* (7th edition). Plume Publisher, New York.

National Institute of Health and Clinical Excellence (2004) *Fertility: Assessment and Treatment for People with Fertility Problems*. NICE, London.

National Institute for Health and Clinical Excellence (2005) *Division of Ankyloglossia (Tongue-tie) for Breastfeeding*. Interventional procedure guidance 149. NICE, London.

Office of Population, Census & Statistics (1992) *Mortality Statistics Perinatal and Infant*. HMSO, London.

Quan, R. *et al.* (1992) Effects of microwave radiation on anti-infective factors in breast milk. *Pediatrics*, 89(4), 667–9.

Scientific Advisory Committee on Nutrition (2006) *Folate and Disease Prevention*. The Stationery Office, London.

Shelton, K. (1994) Empowering women to breastfeed successfully. *Breastfeeding Review*, 2(10), 455–8.

Sigman, M. *et al.* (1989) Effects of microwaving human milk: changes in IgA content and bacterial count. *Journal of American Dietetic Association*, 89(5), 690–2.

Srinivasan, R. & Minocha, A. (1998) When to suspect lactose intolerance: symptomatic, ethnic, and laboratory clues. *Postgraduate Medicine*, 104(3), 109–11, 115–16, 122–3.

World Health Organization (2000) *Preventing Mother-to-Child HIV Transmission*. Press Release WHO/70 from the WHO Technical Consultation. WHO, Geneva.

World Health Organization (2001) *The Optimal Duration of Exclusive Breastfeeding: Report on an Expert Consultation*. WHO, Geneva.

World Health Organization Report (2005) *Make Every Mother and Child Count*. WHO, Geneva.

World Health Organization, Department of Reproductive Health and Research and Department of Making Pregnancy Safe (2006) *Policy Brief on Birth Spacing: Report from a World Health Organization Technical Consultation*. WHO, Geneva.

World Health Organization, Department of Reproductive Health and Research (WHO/RHR) and Johns Hopkins Bloomberg School of Public Health/Center for Communications Programs (CCP), INFO Project (2007) *Family Planning: A Global Handbook for Providers*. CCP, Baltimore, MD and WHO, Geneva.

World Health Organization, Maternal Health, Safe Motherhood Programme, Division of Family Health (1992) *The Prevalence of Anaemia in Women* (2nd edition). WHO, Geneva.

Wright, C.M. (2000) Identification and management of failure to thrive: a community perspective. *Archives of Diseases in Children*, 82(1), 5–9.

Xiong, X. et al. (2006) Periodontal disease and adverse pregnancy outcomes: a systematic review. *British Journal of Obstetricians and Gynaecologists*, 113(2), 135–43.

Zhu, B.P. (2005) Effect of interpregnancy interval on birth outcomes: findings from three recent US studies. *International Journal of Gynaecology and Obstetrics*, 89(Suppl. 1), S25–S33.

References

Academy of Breastfeeding Medicine Protocol Committee (2010) Human milk storage information for home use for full-term infants. *Breastfeeding Medicine*, 5(3), 127–30.

Amir, L. & Donath, S. (2002) Does maternal smoking have a negative physiological effect on breastfeeding? The epidemiological evidence. *Birth*, 29(2), 112–23.

Birch, L (1998) Development of food acceptance patterns in the first year of life. *Proceedings of the Nutrition Society*, 57, 617–24.

British Dietetic Association (2004) *Paediatric Group Position Statement on the Use of Soya Protein for Infants*. BDA, Birmingham.

British Dietetic Association (2005) Food Allergy and Intolerance Specialist Group Consensus Statement, *Practical Dietary Prevention Strategies for Infant at Risk of Developing Allergic Diseases*. BDA, Birmingham.

British Nutrition Foundation (2009) *Nutrition through Life*. BNF, London.

Burdge, G. & Wootton, S. (2002) Conversion of alpha-linoleic acid to eicosapentaenoic, docosapentaenoic and docosahexaenoic acids in young women. *British Journal Nutrition*, 88(4), 411–20.

Cleary-Goldman, J. et al. (2005) Impact of maternal age on obstetric outcome. *Obstetrics & Gynaecology* (The American College of Obstetricians and Gynecologists) 105(5, part 1), 983–90.

Committee on Toxicity of Chemicals in Food (COT) (1996) *Consumer Products and the Environment*. FSA, London.

Committee on Toxicity of Chemicals in Food (COT) (1998) *Peanut Allergy*. HMSO, London.

Committee on Toxicity of Chemicals in Food (COT) (2008) *Consumer Products and the Environment: Statement on the Reproductive Effects of Caffeine*. FSA, London.

Committee on Toxicity of Chemicals in Food, Consumer Products and the Environment (2008) *Statement on the Review of the 1998 COT Recommendations on Peanut Avoidance*. FSA, London.

Department of Health (1984) *Diet and Cardiovascular Disease: Report on Health and Social Subjects*, 28, HMSO, London.

Department of Health (1994) *Weaning and the Weaning Diet: Report of the Working Group on the Weaning Diet of the Committee on Medical Aspects of Food Policy (COMA)*. Report on Health and Social Subjects No 45. HMSO, London.

Department of Health (1995) *The Infant Formula and Follow-on Formula Regulations*. HMSO, London.

Department of Health (2004) *HIV and Breastfeeding: Guidance for Chief Medical Officers*. DH, London.

Department of Health (2004) *Infant Feeding Recommendation*. HMSO, London.

Department of Health (2005) *Choosing Oral Health: An Oral Health Plan for England*. DH, London.

Department of Health (2008) *Healthy Start: Vitamin Supplement Recommendations*. HMSO, London.

Department of Health, Committee on Medial Aspects of Food Policy 41 (1991) *Dietary Reference Values for Food, Energy and Nutrients for the United Kingdom*. HMSO, London.

Department of Health, Committee on Medial Aspects of Food Policy 45 (1994) *Weaning and the Weaning Diet*. HMSO, London.

Department of Health Committee on Medial Aspects of Food Policy 50 (2000) *Folic Acid and the Prevention of Disease*. HMSO, London.

Department of Health and Social Security (1988) *Present Practice in Infant Feeding: Third Report*. Report on Health and Social Subjects 32. HMSO, London.

Dewey, K.G. et al. (1994) A randomized study of the effects of aerobic exercise by lactating women on breast-milk volume and composition. *New England Journal of Medicine*, 330(7), 449–53.

Dosch, H.M. et al. (1994) Lack of immunity to bovine serum albumin in insulin-dependent diabetes mellitus. *The New England Journal of Medicine*, 330(22), 1616–17.

Dusdieker, L.B. et al. (1994) Is milk production impaired by dieting during lactation? *American Journal of Clinical Nutrition*, 59(4), 833–40.

European Food Safety Authority (EFSA) (2005) *Statement of the Scientific Panel on Dietetics Products, Nutrition and Allergies Replying to Applicant's Comment on the Panel's Opinion Relating to the Evaluation of Goat's Milk Protein as a Protein Source for Infant Formulae and Follow-on Formulae*. www.efsa.europa.eu.

Food Allergy and Intolerance Specialist Group (FAIG) (2005) The British Dietetic Association. *Practical Dietary Prevention Strategies for Infants at risk of Developing Allergic Diseases*. www.bda.uk.com.

Food Standards Agency (2005) *Guidance for Health Professionals on Safe Preparation, Storage and Handling of Powdered Infant Formula*. DH, London.

Food Standards Agency (2006) *Revised Guidance on Powdered Infant Formula*. DH, London.

Golding, J. (1997) Sudden infant death syndrome and parental smoking – a literature review. *Paediatric and Perinatal Epidemiology*, 11(1), 67–77.

Greater Glasgow and Clyde Infant Feeding Policy and Guidelines for Health Professionals (2006) *Breastfeeding Formula Feeding and the Introduction to Complementary Foods (Weaning)*. NHS, Glasgow.

Hollis, B.W. & Wagner, C.L. (2004) Assessment of dietary vitamin D requirements during pregnancy and lactation. *American Journal of Clinical Nutrition*, 79(5), 717–26.

Hurst, N.M. (1996) Lactation after augmentation mammoplasty. *Obstetrics and Gynecology*, 87(1), 30–4.

Institute of Medicine (1990) *Nutrition during Pregnancy*. National Academies Press, Washington, DC.

Institute of Medicine (2002) *Dietary Reference Intake for Energy, Carbohydrate, Fibre, Fat, Fatty Acids, Cholesterol, Protein, and Amino Acids*. National Academies Press, Washington, DC.

Institute of Medicine (2009) *Weight Gain in Pregnancy – Re-examining the Guidelines*. National Academies Press, Washington, DC.

Ip, S. *et al.* (2007) Breastfeeding and Maternal and Infant Health Outcomes in Developed Countries. Evidence Report/Technology Assessment No. 153 (Prepared by Tufts-New England Medical Center Evidence-based Practice Center, under Contract No. 290-02-0022) AHRQ Publication No. 07-E007. Rockville, MD: Agency for Healthcare Research and Quality.

Jeffcott, M. (2010) *Risk of Preterm Birth is Reduced with Successful Periodontal Treatment*. 39th Annual Meeting of the American Association for Dental Research, Washington, DC.

Johnson, S.L. (2002) Children food acceptance patterns: The interface of ontogeny and nutrition needs. *Nutrition Reviews*, 60(5, part 2), s91–s94.

Kull, I., Wickman, M., *et al.* (2002) Breastfeeding and allergic diseases in infants – a prospective birth cohort study. *Archives of Disease*, 87, 478–81.

Kumari, A.S. (2001) Pregnancy outcome in women with morbid obesity. *International Journal of Gynecology and Obstetrics*, 73(2), 101–7.

La Leche League (29 August 2006) *La Leche International Offers Support for Mothers Concerning Dehydration and Inadequate Milk Supply*. Media Release. La Leche League, Nottingham.

Lack, G., Fox, D., *et al.* (2003) Factors associated with the development of peanut allergy in childhood. *New England Journal of Medicine*, 348, 977–85.

Levine, B. & Stillman-Lowe, C. (2004) *The Scientific Basis of Oral Health Education*. British Dental Association, London.

Line, S. (1992) Sterilising feeding bottles in the home. *Professional Care of Mother and Child*, 2(8), 249–50.

Lovelady, C.A. *et al.* (2000) The effect of weight loss in overweight, lactating women on the growth of their infants. *The New England Journal of Medicine*, 342(7), 449–53.

McGuire, W., Henderson, G. & Fowlie, P. (2004) Feeding the preterm infant. *British Medical Journal*, 329, 1227–30.

Mohrbacher, N. & Stock, J. (2003) *The Breastfeeding Answer Book*. La Leche League, Nottingham.

National Collaborating Centre for Women's and Children's Health (2008) *Antenatal Care Routine Care for the Healthy Pregnant Woman*. London, sections 5.6, 10.1

National Institute for Health and Clinical Excellence (2006) Obesity. NICE, London.

National Institute for Health and Clinical Excellence (2006) *Postnatal Care of Women and Their Babies*. NICE, London.

National Institute for Health and Clinical Excellence (2008) *Diabetes in Pregnancy*. NICE, London.

National Institute for Health and Clinical Excellence (2008) *Improving the Nutrition of Pregnant and Breastfeeding Mothers and Children in Low-income Households*.

National Institute for Health and Clinical Excellence (2010) *Antenatal Care: Routine Care for the Healthy Pregnant Woman*. www.nice.org.uk/nicemedia/live/11947/40115/40115.pdf.

National Institute for Health & Clinical Excellence (2010) *Donor Breast Milk Banks: The Operation of Donor Breast Milk Bank Services*. www.nice.org.uk/nicemedia/live/11000/30365/30365.pdf.

Nesby-O'Dell, S. *et al.* (2002) Hypervitaminosis D prevalence and determinants among African American and white women of reproductive age: third National Health and Nutrition Examination Survey, 1988–1994. *American Journal of Clinical Nutrition*, 76(1), 187–92.

Niederman, R. (2010) Periodontal treatment did not prevent complications of pregnancy. *Evidence-Based Dentistry*, 11(1), 18–19.

Pal, B.R. & Shaw, N.J. (2001) Rickets resurgence in the United Kingdom: improving antenatal management in Asians. *The Journal of Pediatrics*, 139(2), 337–8.

Rapley, G. (2008) *Guidelines for Implementing a Baby-Led Approach to the Introduction of Solid Food*. www.rapley-weaning.com/assets/blw_guidelines.pdf.

RCOG (2006) *Recreational exercise and pregnancy: information for you*. Available from www.rcog.org.uk/files/rcog-corp/uploaded-files/PIRecreationalExercise2006.pdf.

Sachan, A. *et al.* (2005) High prevalence of vitamin D deficiency among pregnant women and their newborns in northern India. *American Journal of Clinical Nutrition*, 81(5), 1060–4.

Scientific Advisory Committee on Nutrition (2003) *Paper for Information: The Committee on Toxicology of Chemicals in Food, Consumer Products and the Environment (COT) Statement on Phytoestrogens and Soy-Based Infant Formula*. Food Standards Agency, London.

Scientific Advisory Committee on Nutrition (2004) *Advice on Fish Consumption: Benefits and Risks*. Food Standards Agency, London.

Scientific Advisory Committee on Nutrition (2005) *Review of Dietary Advice on Vitamin A*. The Stationery Office, London.

Sharpe, R., Martin, B. *et al.* (2002) Infant feeding with soy formula milk: effects on the testis and blood testosterone levels in mammoset monkeys during the period of neonatal testicular activity. *Human Reproduction*, 17(7), 1692–1703.

Shaw, V. & Lawson, L. (2002) *Clinical Paediatric Dietetics* (2nd edition). Blackwell, Oxford.

Strom, B., Schinnar, R. *et al.* (2001) Exposure to soy-based formula in infancy and endocrinological and reproductive outcomes in young adulthood. *Journal of the American Medical Association*, 286(19), 2403–13.

Thomas, B. & Clayton, B. (2001) *Manual of Dietetic Practice* (3rd edition). Blackwell Science, Oxford.

United States Agency for International Development (2008) *Healthy Timing and Spacing of Pregnancy: A Trainers' Reference Manual*. Catalyst Consortium, USA

Wilson, A.C. *et al.* (1998) Relation of the infant diet to childhood health: seven-year follow-up cohort of children in Dundee Infant Feeding Study. *British Medical Journal*, 316(712), 21–5.

World Health Organization (2006) *Infant and Young Child Feeding Counselling: An Integrated Course*. whqlibdoc. who.int/publications/2006/9789241594752_eng.pdf.

World Health Organization (2006) *Report of a WHO Technical Consultation on Birth Spacing*. whqlibdoc. who.int/hq/2007/WHO_RHR_07.1_eng.pdf.

World Health Organization & United Nations Children's Fund (2003) *Global Strategy for Infant and Young Child Feeding*. WHO, Geneva.

Zutavern, A. *et al.* (2004) The introduction of solids in relation to asthma and eczema. *Archives of Diseases in Childhood*, 89(4), 303–8.

9 Nutritional Management of Disease

Damyanti Patel, Sarah Toule (Cancer), Yvonne Jeanes, Suzanne Barr (Metabolic Syndrome and Polycystic Ovary Syndrome), Kashena Mohadawoo, Shahzadi Uzma Devje (Vitamin D Deficiency)

There are some conditions that are prevalent in many of the cultural groups, so rather than include a section within each of the chapters some of these conditions are brought together in this general chapter on disease states. This chapter includes sections on cancer, metabolic syndrome, polycystic ovarian syndrome and vitamin D deficiency.

Cancer can affect anyone, but in this section we draw together the evidence for specific cancers in Black and minority ethnic groups and also discuss the dietary treatment for these and the support that is available.

Metabolic syndrome and polycystic ovarian syndrome are conditions that are being reported more commonly in all westernized countries. The prevalence is particularly high in the South Asian population.

The section on Vitamin D highlights the occurrence of rickets and osteomalacia in the black and minority ethnic groups in the UK and some recommendations to overcome this condition.

9.1 Cancer in the different BME groups
Damyanti Patel, Sarah Toule

9.1.1 Introduction

Cancer is characterized by uncontrolled cellular growth, when the normal division, differentiation and death of cells become unregulated. There are over 100 different types of cancers, named according to the site at which cancerous cells are identified. Researchers have long attempted to discover the factors that affect why and how cancer develops, as well as how risk can be reduced. Alongside developments in understanding biological and environmental factors, trends have emerged that indicate varying risks according to ethnicity. Such patterns have been invaluable in helping understand preventable and non-preventable risk factors and in indicating high-risk groups in need of targeted efforts to reduce cancer incidence.

Multicultural Handbook of Food, Nutrition and Dietetics, First Edition. Edited by Aruna Thaker, Arlene Barton.
© 2012 Blackwell Publishing Ltd. Published 2012 by Blackwell Publishing Ltd.

9.1.2   Incidence and ethnic variations

Cancer trends are changing across the world and the varying risks for cancers among different ethnic groups highlight significantly raised risks in broad regions of the world.

The information is categorized by cancer type rather than by ethnicity and draws on risks to both black and minority ethnic (BME) and non-BME group for comparison. Risk factors that are specific to particular ethnic groups, regions or cultures are also discussed.

Cancer: no longer a disease of the affluent

Previously considered mainly a disease of the developed, White or affluent world, there is evidence of increasing incidence of cancer across the world, as well as raised risks in certain developing countries or BME groups for certain cancers. This rise may be influenced by improved data collection through cancer registries and improved detection and diagnosis in less developed countries, but there is no doubt that the prevalence of cancer in these groups is increasing. Furthermore, overall mortality from cancer is higher in poorer countries (Ward *et al.*, 2004). These populations face several issues; not only are migrant groups from developing to developed regions demonstrating assimilation of the cancer trends of their new environment, but most regions in the developing world are also adopting the lifestyles of the developed world in terms of dietary habits and reduced activity. They are showing are increasing incidence in those cancers previously associated mainly with the western world (Popkin, 2007).

Industrialization and its effect on cancer trends

Industrialization in most parts of the world has allowed for better food security due to improved technology in food production, preservation, storage and transport. Although this positively reduced food poverty, malnutrition and infectious disease, it soon caused concern due to a rise in overweight and obesity and other associated chronic diseases. Overweight now exceeds underweight in most middle- and low-income countries, including North Africa, the Middle East, Central Asia, China and Latin America. In Africa, sub-Saharan Africa is the only area which is not demonstrating this trend. By nature, urban/industrialized food systems tend to be relatively energy-dense, while low in dietary fibre and starchy staple foods, and have also led to increased consumption of animal products in many areas where historically most dietary energy came from plant sources, such as roots, tubers, cereals and fruits (World Cancer Research Fund/American Institute for Cancer Research (WCRF/AICR), 2007).

Changes in these food systems affect people's dietary habits, levels of activity, body composition and patterns of various diseases. Such changes, whether due to local industrialization or migration to more developed regions, appear to be greatly affecting cancer demographics across the world, where incidence of cancer rises after contact with industrialized and urbanized ways of life (Popkin, 2004; WCRF/AICR, 2007).

These dietary changes have been rapid in recent years and as a result, cancer incidence, predicted to double by 2030, is likely to see the greatest increases in the middle- and low- income countries of Asia, Africa, the Middle East and Latin America (Popkin, 2004; WCRF/AICR, 2007).

International variations

Incidence rates vary widely between countries and some broad regional trends can be identified. Middle- and low-income regions, countries within Africa, Asia, Latin America, generally show higher rates of cancers of the upper aero-digestive tract (mouth, pharynx, larynx, nasopharynx and oesophagus). Exceptions to the rule are parts of China, where cancer of the oesophagus is 100 times more common than in Europe and North America (Key *et al.*, 2002; Parkin *et al.*, 2005). The economy of most regions are still peasant agriculture-based and although prevalence and incidence of various cancers in traditional rural societies are often uncertain due to less efficient recording, there is reasonable evidence that relatively common cancers in such regions include those causally associated with chronic infection, such as cancers of the stomach, liver and cervix (WCRF/AICR, 2007).

High-income countries, urbanized and industrial areas of middle- and low-income regions and countries have higher rates of colorectal cancer and of hormone-related cancers such as of the breast, ovary, endometrium and prostate.

Research is increasingly demonstrating the importance of environmental factors on cancer risk. The first indications that risk is associated with environmental and dietary factors came from studies that demonstrated changes in cancer risk and incidence following migration of populations from their native regions to other geographical areas (WCRF/AICR, 2007). These studies show that adoption of local lifestyle behaviours often leads to assimilation of local cancer risk and incidence, with remarkable changes in some of the most common cancers, including stomach, colorectal, breast and prostate, as quickly as in one generation. It is now accepted that a large proportion of cancers are associated with environmental and dietary factors and that a large percentage can be prevented by lifestyle change (WCRF/AICR, 2007).

Overall cancer rates

The number of new cancer cases ranges from 2.2 million cases in China (20.3% world total) and 1.6 million in North America (14.4%) to about 1,400 in Micronesia/Polynesia. Although the cumulative risk of developing any cancer before the age of 65 years is highest in North America for both sexes, the risk of dying from cancer before this age is highest in Eastern Europe for men and in East Africa for women (Parkin *et al.*, 2005). Indeed, if compared in terms of mortality, there is little difference between rates in developed and developing countries despite disparities in cancer incidence. One reason for this, aside from differences in screening, diagnostic and treatment services, is that the cancers most common in developing countries, such as cancer of the liver, stomach and oesophagus, are those with poor prognoses. On the other hand, for cancers most common in the western world (colorectal and breast), prognosis can be influenced by earlier diagnosis and treatment, thus improving survival (Parkin *et al.*, 2005).

BME groups and cancer rates in the United Kingdom

Caucasians generally tend to show increased incidence of all combined malignancies compared to other ethnic groups, although there are no differences when comparing overall risk for men only from White and Black groups. However, differences in risk between ethnic groups emerge when comparing risk for specific cancers (National Cancer Intelligence Network (NCIN), 2009).

Asian subgroups in the UK show increased risks of cancer of the liver, mouth and cervix, but lower incidence of cancer of the breast, prostate, lung and bowel (NCIN, 2009). The latter is also found in Blacks, although this group does show higher rates of stomach, liver, prostate and cervical cancers.

Differences in survival have also been identified, with both Black and Asian women showing poorer survival from breast cancer despite lower incidence rates. However, Asians and Black males show improved outcomes for lung cancer compared to Caucasians (NCIN, 2009).

9.1.3 Specific cancers and risk by ethnicity

Lung cancer

Lung cancer is the most common cancer in the world. Previously reported as more common in the developed world, the past 25 years have seen a steady catch-up in developing countries, and despite higher rates being observed in North America and Europe, especially Eastern Europe, almost half the cases are now occurring in the developing world. Moderately high rates are seen in Australia and New Zealand, as well as China and Japan. Despite evidence suggesting the beginning of a decline in lung cancer incidence in men in some of the high-risk regions, incidence and mortality are increasing rapidly in Southern and Eastern Europe (Parkin *et al.*, 2005).

Geographic patterns are strongly linked with exposure to tobacco smoking (WCRF/AICR, 2007). There also appears to be a higher risk in certain ethnic groups, such as African-Americans and Latinos, where engagement in multiple-risk behaviours such as at-risk drinking and being overweight is higher than in Caucasian populations (Kendzor *et al.*, 2008). Only in low-risk areas of East and West Africa is smoking tobacco not thought to be the cause.

There is strong evidence that arsenic in drinking water is a cause of lung cancer and possibly high-dose supplements of beta-carotene (20 mg/day) or retinol (25,000 international units/day). On the other hand, consumption of fruits and other foods containing crytenoids may offer a protective effect (WCRF/AICR, 2007).

Differences between ethnic groups are also reflected in survival from lung cancer in the UK, with Black men and Asian showing improved outcomes compared to Whites (NCIN, 2009).

Breast cancer

Breast cancer is the second most common cancer worldwide, and the most common cancer in women. More than half of breast cancer cases are in Europe and North America. The rates are high in most developed areas except for Japan, where it ranks as the third most common cancer. Even in many moderate-risk areas it remains the most common cancer in women. In most of Africa and Asia rates are low, with the exception of South Africa. The lowest incidence is found in central Africa (Parkin et al., 2005).

Incidence rates are increasing in most countries, with the sharpest increases being recorded in countries with previously low rates. China in particular is showing a 3–4% annual increase in breast cancer cases, which is six times the annual increase of about 0.5%. Similar rates are seen in other parts of eastern Asia (Parkin et al., 2005).

In older women, although rates of breast cancer are generally higher in White women, some studies have shown that in women aged 35 and under, incidence rates are slightly higher in African-American women. Furthermore, despite improvements in survival rates among women of all races and ages due to earlier detection and treatment, death rates in African-American women remain higher than in Caucasians, despite the lower overall incidence (Ghafoor et al., 2003; Chlebowski et al., 2005; Smigal et al., 2006) and this trend is mirrored in the UK (National Cancer Intelligence Network, 2009).

Differences in survival may partly be explained by the varying rates of screening uptake observed in different ethnic groups, leading to certain groups presenting with poorer prognosis breast tumours. For example, African-American women are more likely to be diagnosed with large tumours and distant-stage disease (Ghafoor et al., 2003) and the

same has been observed in Asian-American women (Hedeen et al., 1999).

A further study found that Black and Hispanic women were less likely to be diagnosed with early-stage breast cancer than their White counterparts (Lantz et al., 2006). This effect remained even after controlling for study site, age and socioeconomic factors. However, method of disease detection appeared to be an important factor affecting stage of diagnosis in certain groups. Other studies have identified significantly lower uptake of screening mammography in women with lower levels of education and access to healthcare and insurance, higher levels of deprivation, and in recent immigrants (Qureshi et al., 2000; McKenzie et al., 2008).

Improved screening can reduce late diagnosis and poorer prognosis. It is important that high-risk groups are identified and offered appropriate referrals and treatment (Smigal et al., 2006).

Reproductive history may also affect risk. The higher rates seen in women in developed countries may be explained by the fact that, on average, these women have fewer children and breastfeed for shorter durations, thus benefiting less from the protective effect thought to be conferred by breast-feeding (Collaborative Group on Hormonal Factors in Breast Cancer, 2002).

Colon and rectum cancers

Worldwide, colorectal cancer is the fourth and third most common cancer in men and women respectively. Rates vary greatly across regions and are highest in more developed regions with a significantly high incidence in men in Japan (Flood et al., 2000; Parkin et al., 2005). Incidence tends to be intermediate in southern parts of South America and low in Africa and Asia. There is strong evidence to suggest a correlative effect between risk of large bowel cancers and per capita consumption of meat, fat (specifically animal fat) and fibre (Armstrong & Doll, 1975; Prentice & Sheppard, 1990; McKeown-Eyssen, 1994). Higher levels of physical inactivity, excess body weight and waist adiposity also increase the risks of colon cancer (Giovannucci, 2002).

Migrant studies provide further evidence for the importance of diet and environmental factors, showing that the incidence of colorectal cancer increases rapidly within the first generation of populations moving from low- to high-risk regions (McMichael *et al.*, 1980; Parkin *et al.*, 2005). Stark examples are the increased risk observed in Japanese individuals born in the USA who now show higher risks than White Americans, while rates for Japanese individuals living in Hawaii and Los Angeles are among the highest in the world (Parkin *et al.*, 2002). Unfortunately, while rates of colorectal cancer are showing slowed rises or stabilization, in higher-risk areas the incidence is increasing rapidly in those countries where risk was previously low (i.e., Japan and other parts of Asia) (Parkin *et al.*, 2005). Currently, in the UK, Whites show the highest risk of developing colorectal cancers compared to other ethnic groups (National Cancer Intelligence Network, 2009).

Embarrassment and lack of interest in colorectal cancer screening seem to be partly responsible for low uptake of screening services among Bangladeshi and African communities in the UK (Robb *et al.*, 2008). South Asian men and women in particular are far less likely to return an initial test kit for bowel cancer or complete the screening process (Szczepura *et al.*, 2008), all important in addressing mortality rates in high-risk groups.

Stomach cancer

Stomach cancer is the second most common cause of death from cancer and international rates show large variations in incidence. Almost two-thirds of cases occur in developing countries. Very high incidence rates are seen in Eastern Europe, parts of Central and South America and particularly in East Asia, where cases in China account for 42% of all cases. Rates tend to be generally low in Africa, although the incidence in women in Central Africa approaches that of Eastern Europe (Parkin *et al.*, 2005).

Again, migrant studies show strong evidence for an environmental factor, where risk reduces rapidly following movement from high- to low-risk regions. However, childhood environment is also an important factor and the migration factor is therefore affected by age at migration (McMichael *et al.*, 1980; Parkin *et al.*, 2005). In the UK Black men show the highest rate of stomach cancer compared to other ethnic groups (National Cancer Intelligence Network, 2009).

Infection with *Helicobacter pylori* infection, which is very common in the developing world, is a risk factor for stomach cancer. It is also considered an indirect carcinogenic factor by causing gastritis, a precursor of other gastric disorders (Peek & Blaser, 2002; Vyse *et al.*, 2002, Huang *et al.*, 2003, Wong *et al.*, 2004). It is estimated that 76% of adults in developing countries are infected with the bacterium (Sitas *et al.*, 1992).

Diet plays an important role, with risk of stomach cancer increasing with high consumption of some traditionally preserved salted foods, especially meats and pickles, and with salt (Goh *et al.*, 2007). It appears, however, that the effect a high salt intake has on risk is stronger when stomach disorders are also present (Shikata *et al.*, 2006).

Improved food preservation may have contributed to reduced risks in some countries by improving hygiene and reducing infections. Risk is also inversely correlated with intake of fruit and vegetables, and a Mediterranean-style diet has been found to reduce stomach cancer risk (Popkin, 2004; Parkin *et al.*, 2005; Goh *et al.*, 2007; Buckland *et al.*, 2010).

Other carcinogens include smoking tobacco (Mao *et al.*, 2002, González *et al.*, 2003), and possibly the capsaicin in chilli-type peppers, which are a common ingredient in the cuisines of many regions showing higher rates of stomach cancer (Archer & Jones, 2002).

Prostate cancer

Prostate cancer is the fifth most common cancer worldwide and risk is generally higher in more developed countries. Increased screening and diagnosis of asymptomatic prostate cancers, however, may account for some of the increased incidence rates seen in areas such as the USA and UK where prostate cancer is now the most common cancer in men (Brewster *et al.*, 2000; Office for National Statistics, 2008).

Data from the UK, USA and Caribbean show significant ethnic variations for prostate cancer risk (Glover *et al.*, 1998; Parkin *et al.*, 2003; Aus *et al.*, 2005). Migrants from low- to high-risk countries show quite marked increases in incidence rates, some of which can be attributed to increases in screening and diagnosis (Parkin *et al.*, 2005). In the UK, Asian men have the lowest rate (Jack *et al.*, 2007; Ben-Shlomo *et al.*, 2008).

African-Caribbean men have a greater risk of prostate cancer than White men in both the USA and UK – African-Caribbean men in the UK are three times more likely to develop prostate cancer than their White counterparts (Ben-Shlomo et al., 2008; National Cancer Intelligence Network, 2009) and some evidence suggest they are also typically diagnosed 5.1 years younger (Metcalfe et al., 2008). Such higher relative risks may in fact be underestimated, due to possibly lower uptake of prostate screening services among Black men (Etzioni et al., 2002). Inter-ethnic differences may be related to environmental factors such as diet, as well as the possibility of genetic or metabolic differences (Shibata & Whittemore, 1997; Platz et al., 2000; Skinner & Schwartz, 2009; Van Cleave et al., 2010).

Improved survival rates in higher-risk areas are being observed, possibly due to increases in overall uptake of screening services, with more cases being diagnosed at earlier, more treatable stages. In the USA, for example, relative survival rates in 2000 were reported to be 99% (Parkin et al., 2005). However, mortality rates remain highest in African-Caribbean men and in other areas including the Caribbean and Central Africa, although it is low in North Africa and Asia (Parkin et al., 2005; Evans et al., 2008). Again, risks may be the consequence of racial differences in cancer biology, with Black men having a more aggressive phenotype, but will also undoubtedly be associated with differences in health behaviour, screening uptake and clinical management (Evans et al., 2008).

Studies in the USA which have examined several factors, such as education, income, access to insurance and healthcare, also demonstrate that socio-demographic factors and ethnicity are highly correlated variables suggesting that multiple factors may be contributing to the poorer outcomes observed in Black men with prostate cancer (Grossfeld et al., 2002).

Liver cancer

Liver cancer is the sixth most common cancer, but is the third most common cause of death due to poor prognosis. Survival rates vary from 3% to 5% across the world (Parkin et al., 2005).

Most cases occur in developing countries (82%), with 55% of cases recorded in China alone. Other areas of high risk are sub-Saharan Africa, eastern and south-eastern Asia and Melanesia. Lower incidence is seen in Latin America and south-central Asia as well as most developed regions, although Southern Europe presents a substantial risk (WCRF/AICR, 2007).

In the UK, higher rates of liver cancer have been found in Asians compared to Whites, for both sexes and for all ages (National Cancer Intelligence Network, 2009).

Infection with hepatitis B and C viruses are major risk factors for liver cancer worldwide, where 85% cases are caused by these viruses. International variation in hepatitis B infection (which is more prevalent) largely mirrors patterns of liver cancer incidence. In Japan infection with hepatitis B is relatively low, but risks of liver cancer are not reduced due to a relatively high rate of hepatitis C virus (Parkin et al., 2005).

Exposure to aflatoxins is also a probable contributing factor in high-risk tropical areas where contamination of food grains with Aspergillus fumigatus is common. Furthermore, there is a multiplicative interaction between aflatoxin exposure and chronic hepatitis B virus infection, suggesting different carcinogenic mechanisms (Parkin et al., 2005; WCRF/AICR, 2007).

Cervical cancer

Cervical cancer is the second most common cancer in women worldwide, with 83% of cases occurring in developing countries. This stark regional difference is mostly due to the introduction of screening programmes in the 1960s and 1970s in developed counties, before which incidence rates were similar to those seen in developing countries (Parkin et al., 2005). The highest incidence rates are seen in sub-Saharan Africa, Melanesia, Latin America, the Caribbean and south-east and south-central Asia. In most of these areas, it is the most common cancer to affect women.

Very low rates are observed in China and western Asia. However, in the north-west of China, the minority Uigur women have a high incidence of cervical carcinoma compared to majority Han women in the same region, suggesting a possible genetic factor for susceptibility (Zheng et al., 2008).

A recent survey in the UK found that cervical cancer was significantly higher in Asian women than all other ethnic groups, when comparing incidence in women aged 65 years and over (National Cancer Intelligence Network, 2009).

The major risk factors for cervical cancer are oncogenic subtypes of the human papilloma virus (Parkin *et al.*, 2005) and molecular pathways for some mucosal cancers induced by the human papilloma virus may vary according to ethnicity (Li *et al.*, 2004).

Oesophageal cancer

Oesophageal cancer is the eighth most common cancer worldwide and the sixth most common cause of death from cancer. Large international variations are observed, with a 20-fold variation between high-risk China and low-risk western Africa. High risks are also observed in southern and eastern Africa, south-eastern Asia and, in men only, Japan (Parkin *et al.*, 2005).

A genetic predisposition may account for some of the increased risk in Japan and Japanese individuals in the USA, although environmental factors play an important role (Parkin *et al.*, 2005). Alcohol is the main carcinogen (Zambon *et al.*, 2000; Zeka *et al.*, 2003; Freedman *et al.*, 2007; Weikert *et al.*, 2009) and risk is multiplied when alcohol drinkers also smoke tobacco (Key *et al.*, 2002; Wild & Hardie, 2003; WCRF/AICR, 2007). Over 90% of cases may be attributed to these causes (Engel *et al.*, 2003). In the Indian subcontinent, chewing tobacco and betel quid is an important causal factor (Lee *et al.*, 2005; Parkin *et al.*, 2005; WCRF/AICR, 2007).

There is also convincing evidence of increased risk of adenocarcinoma with increasing BMI (Lagergren *et al.*, 1999). Adenocarcinoma of the lower third of the oesophagus is steadily increasing in the USA and Europe, and is likely to be linked to increasing incidence of acid reflux as a result of obesity (Lagergren *et al.*, 2000; Parkin *et al.*, 2005; WCRF/AICR, 2007).

It is also probable that the traditional herbal infusion maté, which is drunk scalding hot through a metal straw in parts of South America, adds to the high rates in this region (Castellsagué *et al.*, 2000; Sewram *et al.*, 2003; Parkin *et al.*, 2005; WCRF/AICR, 2007).

Micronutrient deficiencies may also play a role in the high risks seen in Central Asia, China and southern Africa. Other dietary factors in these areas include high consumption of pickled vegetables, nitrosamine-rich foods and mycotoxins (Parkin *et al.*, 2005). A protective effect may be achieved through increased consumption of non-starchy vegetables and fruits, particularly foods containing beta-carotene or vitamin C (WCRF/AICR, 2007). It is estimated that most cases of oesophageal cancer can be prevented through healthy eating, weight control and by reduction in tobacco and alcohol use (Engel *et al.*, 2003).

Oral cancer

The incidence rates for oral cancers are highest in Melanesia, with almost two-thirds of cases occurring in men. In men alone, rates are high in many developed countries, although rates are also high in southern Asia where the highest incidence for women is recorded. Laryngeal cancer rates are higher in South America, south-central and west Asia, while rates tend to be low in many African countries (Parkin *et al.*, 2005).

Causal factors for oral cancers are tobacco and alcohol use, infection with the human papilloma virus and gastric reflux. Consumption of alcohol is a strong factor in risk of cancers of the mouth, pharynx and larynx and the risk is multiplied when drinkers also smoke tobacco (WCRF/AICR, 2007).

High rates of oral cancer in South Asian populations are strongly linked to chewing tobacco or betel quid (*paan*). The risk is increased when betel quid is chewed with or without tobacco but the effect is stronger with betel quid containing tobacco (Bedi, 1996). In the UK, chewing tobacco is particularly common in the Bangladeshi community, and even more so among women (NHS Information Centre (2006) Health Survey for England, 2004).

Smoking *beedi* (tobacco rolled in a tendu leaf) is also common in the South Asian community and is another risk factor for oral cancer (Rahman *et al.*, 2003). Reverse *chutta* smoking, where the lighted end of a cigar is in the mouth, is popular among Indian women and rates of cancer of the palatal mucosa are high in this group (Gupta *et al.*, 1984). Indeed, Asian women have been found to have the highest rate of mouth cancer in parts of the UK, while Asian men may have lower rates compared to Whites (National Cancer Intelligence Network, 2009).

Consumption of maté may also be linked with oral cancers (Parkin *et al.*, 2005; WCRF/AICR, 2007).

It is estimated that 50% of oral cancers could be prevented by improved dietary and smoking habits, with evidence suggesting a protective effect with consumption of non-starchy vegetables and fruits, particularly foods containing carotenoids (Pavia *et al.*, 2006; WCRF/AICR, 2007).

Nasopharyngeal cancer

Nasopharyngeal cancer is relatively rare on a world scale, but has a very specific geographical distribution. Very high incidence is seen in southern China, as well as in communities that have migrated from southern China to other countries. It is also relatively high in populations in other parts of China, south-east Asia, north-east India, North Africa and native peoples of Canada and Alaska. Trends are showing gradual decreases in incidence in high-risk regions such as Hong Kong and Singapore (WCRF/AICR, 2007).

There is strong evidence that consumption of Cantonese-style salted fish increases the risk of nasopharyngeal cancer (WCRF/AICR 2007). This applies only to the specific Cantonese method of preservation, whereby fish is salted as well as fermented. Migrant studies also suggest a genetic factor, with migrant populations from China and North Africa showing elevated risks in host countries, even in the second generations (Parkin *et al.*, 2005).

Other strong factors increasing the risk of nasopharyngeal cancer are smoking tobacco, occupational exposure to formaldehyde and infection with Epstein-Barr virus (WCRF/AICR, 2007).

9.1.4   Conclusion

It is clear that despite biological factors affecting cancer risk, there are numerous environmental and lifestyle factors that affect the risks of particular cancers. More importantly, such factors are modifiable and are therefore crucial in the challenge of reducing cancer rates.

The recent WCRF/AICR recommendations to reduce cancer risk included maintaining a healthy body weight, engaging in physical activity, eating a balanced diet (including reduced consumption of red/processed meat, energy-dense foods, highly processed foods and alcohol) and encouragement of breastfeeding.

In addition to diet, behaviours specific to particular ethnic groups must be addressed. The subject of cancer is still a taboo, or even an oblivious, health concern within many ethnic groups and these groups are seldom reached by the standard methods used by health promotion services to raise awareness of the risks, signs and symptoms and services for detection and treatment of cancer. Particularly as these groups age and their cancer risks increase, it is important that health services along the cancer pathway take action to provide culturally specific and appropriate information and services.

Where cancer diagnosis and survival can be improved by screening, it is important that services are tailored to the needs of specific BME communities to encourage uptake. The concept of screening, or the mere use of health services when 'well', is less understood and accepted among some BME communities compared to the general public, as is the understanding of entitlement to information and services (Hill, 2006).

Socioeconomic status is also an important issue and should be considered alongside cultural factors. Effective communication is vital and undertaking training by health professionals, in order to improve communication about the importance of cancer screening, has been found to have a positive effect on uptake by BME groups (Atri *et al.*, 1997).

While the fact that behaviours are ingrained in traditional cultures adds to the challenge of bringing about behaviour change, this can also serve as an advantage in providing useful information about the likely behaviours of specific groups and the cancers for which they are most likely to be at risk, enabling health promotion activities to be tailored for and directly aimed at high-risk groups.

It is also worth noting that the practice of ethnic coding and recording is neither complete nor standardized. Inaccuracies and misinterpretations are therefore unavoidable when utilizing such registries to identify trends and risk factors (Gomez & Glaser, 2006). Improvements in the accuracy and comprehensiveness of ethnic recording are vital to our understanding of the current cancer demographics and our ability to respond to the needs of specific groups and populations.

9.1.5   Support for individuals with cancer in the UK

Cancer affects many people. One in three of us will be diagnosed with the illness during our lifetime and two million people are living with cancer in the UK today. As the population ages and as treatments improve, this number will grow. People living with cancer not only need medical help, they and their families also need practical, emotional and financial support.

Macmillan Cancer Support is a charity which helps to improve the lives of everyone affected by cancer, no matter who they are, where they live within the UK or what kind of cancer they may have.

Macmillan is a source of support

Macmillan is a source of support, helping with all the things that people affected by cancer want and need. We guide people through the system, supporting them every step of the way. We fund nurses and other specialist health care professionals and build cancer care centres. But we give so much more than medical help.

People need practical support at home, so we provide anything from time off for a carer, to a lift to hospital. People need emotional support, so we listen, advise and share information though our phone service, website and trained professionals. People need financial help to cope with the extra costs cancer can bring, so we give benefits advice and grants for anything from heating bills to travel costs. Together we listen, we learn, we act to help people live with cancer.

Macmillan is a force for change

We listen to people affected by cancer and work together to improve cancer care. People who live with cancer are experts by experience. Together we use this knowledge to make a positive difference to the lives of people affected by cancer. This could be anything from getting a coffee machine installed in a waiting room to bringing about changes in the law.

We fight discrimination – from challenging unfair travel costs and insurance policies to improving the national benefits system. Together we challenge the status quo, we push for change, we lead the way.

Cancer self-help support groups

Macmillan supports 900+ independent cancer self-help support groups and organizations across the UK. By joining a group, people affected by cancer can spend time with others who share and understand their experience. It's an opportunity for people to talk about their deepest concerns and know they will be met with acceptance and understanding. This simple act of sharing can make an enormous difference to the way they feel.

We can provide grants to help with the initial set-up costs of a new group and to support established groups. We offer a range of free publications, support and advice, and have worked with cancer self-help support groups across the UK to develop our good practice guidelines. We also run workshops to provide training on setting up and running a group and can tailor these courses to meet a group's specific needs.

Self-help support groups have been set up within BME communities. But it has been a struggle to get people from these communities to come to these groups due to stigma attached to the word 'cancer'. Those groups that exist are very positive in building relationships and empowering their members to work as a team to raise awareness about cancer in the communities. Language, culture and religious barriers prevent people affected by cancer from joining these groups.

The National Diversity Coordinator has been involved in setting up these groups and working with the community champions to build relationships with the voluntary organizations from BME communities to further Macmillan's Outreach Programme. (Visit macmillan.org.uk/selfhelpand support for more information.)

Macmillan's phone service (0808 808 00 00) is staffed by cancer support specialists. They are there for everyone affected by cancer, whatever they need. They can answer questions about cancer types and treatments, provide practical and financial support to help people live with cancer, and are there if someone just wants to talk.

We also have an interpretation service in over 200 languages. People just need to state, in English, the language they wish to use when they call.

Damyanti Patel (National Diversity Coordinator)
Macmillan Cancer Support
89 Albert Embankment
London SE1 7UQ

For cancer information resources in various languages and details of local support groups contact:

Macmillan Cancer Support
89 Albert Embankment
London, SE1 7UQ
Tel: 020 7840 7840
Fax: 020 7840 7841
Website: www.macmillan.org.uk

If someone is deaf or hard of hearing, they can use the textphone service on 0808 808 0121, or the Text Relay system.

Visit macmillan.org.uk/howwecanhelp for more information.

9.2   Metabolic Syndrome and Polycystic Ovary Syndrome (PCOS) in BME groups

Yvonne Jeanes, Suzanne Barr

Key points

- There is a high prevalence of metabolic syndrome and polycystic ovary syndrome (PCOS) in South Asians and African-Caribbean groups.
- Weight management, incorporating a healthy balanced diet and physical activity, is an important and integral part of the treatment for metabolic syndrome and PCOS. These positive changes to lifestyle will reduce the likelihood of people developing type 2 diabetes and vascular disease at an earlier age compared with Europeans.

9.2.1   Introduction

Polycystic ovarian syndrome (PCOS) is the most common endocrine disorder in women of reproductive age, affecting up to 10% of the population (Lindholm *et al.*, 2008). The clinical and biochemical features of the syndrome are diverse, including central adiposity, insulin resistance, menstrual irregularity and fertility problems, excess hair (hir-

sutism) and acne (ESHRE, 2004; Diamanti-Kandarakis, 2008). Although the precise aetiology of PCOS is unknown, it involves a combination of genetic and environmental factors (Franks *et al.*, 2006). There is no single diagnostic criterion; however, the most recent definition is the Rotterdam criteria (ESHRE, 2004), which are defined by the presence of any two of the three following features:

1. Oligoovulation, leading to oligomenorrhoea (infrequent menses), or anovulation leading to amenorrhoea (absence of menses) (ESHRE, 2004).
2. Clinical and/or biochemical signs of hyperandrogenism.
3. Polycystic ovaries and exclusion of other aetiologies.

As women with PCOS are more likely to be overweight and have an increased likelihood of central adiposity and insulin resistance, these women have a subsequent increased risk of developing metabolic syndrome, type 2 diabetes and cardiovascular disease (Ehrmann *et al.*, 1999; Escorbar-Morreale & San Millan, 2007; Essah, 2007; Dokras, 2008; Westerveld *et al.*, 2008). In PCOS, insulin resistance is exacerbated by weight gain, particularly in the abdominal region, which is common in women with PCOS, with up to 50% of patients overweight or obese (Moran & Norman, 2004; Barr *et al.*, 2007). Even though obese women with PCOS are generally thought to be more symptomatic and at greater health risk, normal weight women with PCOS are also at increased disease risk (Chang *et al.*, 1983; Dunaif *et al.*, 1989; American Association of Clinical Endocrinologists, 2005) and suffer debilitating symptoms (Sheehan, 2004).

Women with PCOS often present to healthcare professionals due to reproductive complications such as infrequent menses and infertility. It is at this stage that these women need to be educated of the increased long-term risk of metabolic complications of the syndrome in order to make appropriate lifestyle modifications.

Metabolic syndrome is a clustering of metabolic abnormalities centred on insulin resistance. The two criteria used most frequently are shown in Tables 9.2.1 and 9.2.2.

Table 9.2.1 Adult Treatment Panel III metabolic syndrome is defined by the presence of three or more of the following components

Central obesity as measured by waist circumference (women > 88 cm)

Fasting blood triglycerides ≥150 mg/dl

Blood HDL cholesterol (Women < 50 mg/dl)

Blood pressure ≥130/85 mmHg

Fasting glucose ≥110 mg/d

(ATP III, 2001)

Table 9.2.2 Diagnostic criteria for metabolic syndrome

Insulin resistance identified by the presence of:

- Type 2 diabetes, impaired fasting glucose or impaired glucose tolerance

With any two of the following:

- Blood pressure ≥140/ ≥95 mmHg and/or antihypertensive
- Triglycerides ≥150 mg/dl (≥1.7 mmol/l)
- HDL cholesterol (women <39 mg/dl (1 mmol/l))
- BMI > 30 and/or waist/hip ratio >0.85 (women)
- Urinary albumin excretion rate ≥20 ug/min or albumin/ creatinine ratio ≥30 mg/g

(WHO, 1999)

9.2.2 Prevalence of metabolic syndrome and PCOS

The incidence of metabolic syndrome is higher in certain ethnic subgroups, including South Asian and African-Caribbean groups. South Asians have a higher prevalence of metabolic syndrome (29–46%), compared with Europeans (9–19%) (McKeigue et al., 1988, 1991; Tillen et al., 2005). Central adiposity and metabolic disturbances related to insulin resistance are more prevalent in South Asians (Forouhi, 2000; Raji et al., 2001). The reasons for this remain unclear, however it has been linked with an insulin receptor polymorphism, indicating there is a strong genetic component to the development of insulin resistance in this population (Abate et al., 2003), in addition to lifestyle factors. Non-centrally obese individuals of any ethnicity maintain lower insulin levels, but as levels of central obesity increase, the proportionate increase in insulin resistance is greater in South Asians compared with Europeans (Forouhi, 2000; Raji et al., 2001).

PCOS is more prevalent in South Asian women residing in the UK than in Caucasians (52% compared with 20–33% having polycystic ovaries) and of these 70–80% have symptoms of PCOS (Rodin et al., 1998). Women with PCOS originating from Asia are more insulin resistant and are at a greater risk for developing type 2 diabetes compared with White women (Wijeyaratne et al., 2002). Lo et al. (2006) reported that South Asian women with PCOS were younger and had greater severity of symptoms than Caucasians. A large representative study carried out in the USA found the prevalence of PCOS to be 8% in Black women compared with 4.8% in White women (6.6% in the total population) (Azziz, 2006). There is a paucity of studies involving African-Caribbean groups or South Asian women with PCOS.

In the UK, an estimated 25% of the general population show features of metabolic syndrome (Tonkin, 2004), with an increased prevalence in women with PCOS of 35–47% (Glueck et al., 2003; Dokras et al., 2005; Azziz, 2006; Ehrmann et al., 2006). It is likely that the shared features of the metabolic syndrome and PCOS (e.g., central obesity, hypertriglyceridemia, low high-density lipoprotein (HDL) cholesterol, hypertension and elevated fasting plasma glucose concentrations) are responsible for the increased risk of type 2 diabetes in women with PCOS rather than the syndrome *per se* (Ehrmann et al., 2005).

9.2.3 Treatments

Weight management and lifestyle modification are fundamental in the treatment of metabolic syndrome and reducing the risk for diabetes and vascular disease. In addition to lifestyle advice, treatment for metabolic syndrome encompasses medication for an individual's presenting traits (e.g., antihypertensives, statins, insulin sensitizers).

Strategies targeting obesity and abdominal adiposity, insulin resistance and hyperandrogenism, alone or in combination, in women with PCOS are effective in ameliorating the signs and symptoms of hyperandrogenism while improving the metabolic comorbidities in most cases (Escobar-Morreale & San Millan, 2008). Research has shown that as little as 5% weight loss in women with PCOS can reduce insulin levels, improve menstrual function and reduce serum testosterone (Moran *et al.*, 2003; Stamets *et al.*, 2004; Qublan *et al.*, 2007).

Use of drugs

The use of metformin may prove beneficial in a subset of the population of women with PCOS. Hyperinsulinemia is an important parameter in deciding whether or not to initiate metformin therapy to women with PCOS with the hope of preventing or delaying the onset of type 2 diabetes. Cardiovascular risk factors including markers of subclinical inflammation, and dyslipidemia may also be improved by metformin therapy. For ovulation induction, metformin is not as effective as clomiphene citrate as first-line therapy for women with PCOS (Mathur *et al.*, 2008).

Combined oral contraceptives containing synthetic progestogen such as cyproterone acetate (Yasmin®) and ethinyl oestradiol (Dianette®) are commonly prescribed for the treatment of androgenic symptoms (e.g., acne and hirsutism) and also act to induce regular shedding of the endometrium. Other anti-androgenic medications include androgen-binding receptor inhibitors such as spirononolactone, flutamide or finasteride. Prescribable treatments for acne include systemic therapies such as isotretinoin (Roaccutane®) and topical treatments including retinoids and antimicrobials such as benzoyl peroxide or antibiotics. A topical treatment for hirsuitism, eflornithine (Vaniqa®), has recently been made available on prescription. Norethisterone (synthetic progesterone) can be prescribed to induce menses in amenorrhoeic women.

Dietary modification

The dietary modification for metabolic syndrome and PCOS are similar – weight management is key in their treatment. However, there remains debate on what the macronutrient contribution of the diet should be (Marsh & Brand-Miller, 2005). It should be noted that there are many women with PCOS who are lean, but despite having a normal BMI may still be insulin resistant and display abdominal fat distribution (Herriot *et al.*, 2008). In addition to the potential short-term benefits of diet and lifestyle modifications for symptom control, women with PCOS are an important population group for health promotion, with appropriate dietary interventions having the potential to impact on future diabetes and vascular disease in this group.

Dietary intervention studies have made some progress in recommending a suitable diet for women with PCOS; however there remains no clear consensus as to the optimum dietary management strategy primarily due to a lack of evidence in this population group. A number of review articles have been published proposing dietary management strategies that go beyond weight loss (Marsh & Brand-Miller, 2005, Farshchi *et al.*, 2007, Liepa *et al.*, 2008). In the majority of the dietary studies conducted in women with PCOS, improvements in metabolic and reproductive outcomes have been closely related to improvements in insulin sensitivity, suggesting that dietary changes designed to improve insulin resistance may produce greater benefits than those achieved through energy restriction alone (Kiddy *et al.*, 1992; Holte *et al.*, 1995; Moran *et al.*, 2003; Gamberini *et al.*, 2004).

Dietary modification needs to focus on the macronutrient contribution of the diet to minimize the risk of developing diabetes and cardiovascular disease. Two large prospective studies have shown positive changes to diet and lifestyle in men and women to be successful in preventing diabetes (Lindström *et al.*, 2003). Dietary interventions to improve insulin resistance and reduce hyperinsulinaemia may be of greater benefit for short-term symptoms and long-term disease risk compared with weight loss alone. There is some evidence to show that by reducing the consumption of saturated fat (Galgani *et al.*, 2008) and reducing the glycaemic index (GI) and glycaemic load (GL) of the diet (McMillan-Price *et al.*, 2006; Barclay *et al.*, 2008), insulin sensitivity can be improved in insulin-resistant populations, however there remains a paucity of studies in women with PCOS. GI has been shown to be positively associated with the prevalence of metabolic syndrome and insulin resistance in a cross-sectional study of 2,834 subjects from the Framingham offspring cohort (McKeown *et al.*, 2004). In addition to dietary modifications, increasing physical activity has been shown to improve insulin sensitivity in insulin-resistant populations (Hayes & Kriska, 2008; Jeanes *et al.*, 2009).

Studies in the general population have focused on manipulating the type of fatty acids rather than quantity to improve metabolic parameters (Sanders, 2009), with intake of n-3 polyunsaturated fatty acids (PUFA) shown to be associated with improved cardio-protection (Russo, 2009); however the role of n-6 PUFAs in CVD prevention remains controversial. A high MUFA diet significantly improves insulin sensitivity compared to high saturated fat diets. However, these benefits are not demonstrated when total fat intake exceeds 38% of total energy (Riccardi & Rivellese, 2000) Barr *et al.* (2007) reported the dietary intake of 200 women in whom the mean total fat intake was found to be 38% of energy, with half of the women in this study having a total fat intake above this value. It would be sensible to incorporate dietary advice to improve the fatty acid composition of the diet, although the relationship between dietary fatty acid modification and cardiovascular disease risk has not been widely studied in women with PCOS (Kasim-Karakas *et al.*, 2004; Douglas *et al.*, 2006).

9.2.4   Evidence of good practice

The increased risk for the development of metabolic syndrome in BME groups highlights the importance of identifying those at risk early, using appropriate diagnostic and screening criteria, which will in turn improve the management of this common yet multifaceted syndrome.

It will be important to detect glucose tolerance in women with PCOS, because type 2 diabetes in PCOS occurs in young, asymptomatic women (Weerakiet *et al.*, 2001). South Asian women with reproductive abnormalities of PCOS have greater insulin resistance and therefore should be advised about reducing the risk of future diabetes and vascular disease.

A survey of current practice by UK dietitians reported that women with PCOS are consulted in a variety of clinical settings with very few specialist clinics, or specialist dietitians (Jeanes *et al.*, 2009).

9.2.5   Suggestions for the way forward

Women with PCOS often present to healthcare professionals with cosmetic or reproductive/menstrual symptoms. However, their attention should be drawn to their future risk for type 2 diabetes and related metabolic complications.

PCOS is a common disorder and healthcare professionals should be aware of the condition and possible dietary management approaches. Dietary intervention studies investigating the effect of reduced GI diets on symptom control and disease risk profile in women with PCOS are required.

9.3   Vitamin D deficiency in BME groups

Kashena Mohadawoo, Shahzadi Uzma Devje

Key points

- Severe vitamin D deficiency presents as rickets and osteomalacia in children and as osteomalacia in adults.
- Vitamin D is important for calcium and phosphate metabolism and deficiency can lead to poor mineralization of the skeleton.
- There are very few dietary sources of vitamin D. The main source is exposure to short wavelength ultraviolet light.
- Several factors can potentially affect vitamin D status, including seasonal variations, altitude, genetics, adiposity, skin pigmentation, melanin concentration, use of sunscreen, clothing and age.
- 25(OH)D concentration can be related to ethnic group and factors such as a vegetarian diet and low exposure to sunlight.
- There is a need for further national surveys of vitamin D status, particularly in BME groups in order to fully quantify the problem in the UK.

9.3.1   Introduction

This section highlights the recurrence of rickets and osteomalacia in Black and minority ethnic (BME) groups in the UK and some recommendations to overcome this problem.

Background

Severe vitamin D deficiency generally presents as rickets and osteomalacia in children and as osteomalacia in adults. Although it is now rarely reported among the White UK population, there is a significant incidence of its re-emergence in the UK South Asian and Afro-Caribbean groups.

The main source of vitamin D is usually considered to be skin photosynthesis following irradiation with short wavelength ultraviolet (UV) light. Dietary vitamin D exists as either ergocalciferol (vitamin D_2) or cholecalciferol (vitamin D_3). The fat-soluble vitamin is absorbed through the lymphatic system from where it is transported to and stored in the liver. The liver enzyme 25-hydroxylase converts dietary and endogenously synthesized vitamin D_2 and D_3 to 25(OH)D 25hydroxyvitamin D (Update on Vitamin D, 2007).

Plasma or serum 25(OH)D concentration are used to assess vitamin D status (Update on Vitamin D, 2007). Generally, there is no accepted criterion for vitamin D deficiency and moreover the measurement for plasma 25(OH)D is not well standardized (Hirani & Primatesta, 2005). Serum vitamin D concentrations <20nmol/l have been regarded as indicative of severe vitamin D deficiency, clinically associated with rickets and osteomalacia (Heaney, 2003; Wharton & Bishop, 2003).

Cases of South Asian and Afro-Caribbean origins are widely reported, but there are no National Diet and Nutrition Survey (NDNS) data for the ethnic minorities (Update on Vitamin D, 2007).

9.3.2 Function of vitamin D

The parathyroid hormone (PTH) promotes the process of vitamin D to be metabolized to the steroid hormone 1,25-dihydroxyvitamin D. 1,25-dihydroxyvitamin D regulates calcium and phosphate metabolism via three target tissues: kidney, small intestine and bone. In the kidney, 1,25-dihydroxyvitamin D regulates calcium transport in the proximal tubule; in the small intestine, it regulates calcium and phosphate uptake from the gut. 1,25-dihydroxyvitamin D is also involved in the maintenance of plasma calcium levels via bone restoration and formation (www.food.gov.uk/multimedia/pdfs/evmd.pdf).

9.3.3 Dietary recommendations

The Dietary Reference Values (DRVs) as defined in the 1991 COMA report do not set a Reference Nutrient Intake (RNI) for vitamin D for adults or children over four years of age who receive adequate sunlight exposure. The RNI for children under the age of four years is 7–8.5µg/day. For 4–65 year olds, it is assumed that the action of summer sunlight will provide adequate vitamin D status, except for specific at-risk groups who are not exposed to sufficient sunlight (e.g., women whose clothing conceals them fully (the Muslim community) and those who are confined indoors (the elderly)). The RNI for these at-risk groups is 10µg/day. For the majority of people in this group, as well as the majority of pregnant and lactating women, people aged 65 years or more, infants and children aged up to three years, vitamin D supplementation will be needed to achieve the Department of Health (1998) RNI (Update on Vitamin D, 2007).

9.3.4 Sources of vitamin D

Exposure to sunlight

The main source of vitamin D is exposure of the skin to sunlight. It has been suggested that 15 minutes three times weekly from April to September, with hands, arms and face uncovered, is adequate for fair-skinned people. Darker-skinned people will need more sunshine. However, there is no clear recommendation on the length and intensity of exposure. The UK population relies on their body stores during the winter months (www.privatehealth.co.uk/diseases/arthritic-bone-muscle/rickets).

Dietary sources

There are few dietary sources of vitamin D. In the UK rich sources are fortified foods such as margarines (~7µg/100g) and some breakfast cereals (3–8µg/100g), oily fish (e.g., salmon, mackerel, sardines) (5–10µg/100g), egg yolk (~5µg/100g) and red meat (~1µg/100g) (Update on Vitamin D, 2007). Supplemental vitamin D contains either ergocalciferol or cholecalciferol.

Vitamin D food fortification

In most industrialized countries, including the UK, processed milk, some powdered milks, infant formulas, margarine, breakfast cereals and bread are fortified with vitamin D (COMA, 1980).

9.3.5   Assessment

The main controversy has been the lack of standardization. Different laboratories and different methods have yielded varying results from the same sample to measure serum or plasma 25(OH) D. Plasma 25(OH)D concentrations in rickets and osteomalacia range from the undetectable to around 20 nmol/l (DH, 1998, Update on Vitamin D, 2007). A plasma 25(OH)D concentration of 25 nmol/l has been used as a conventional cut-off for defining the lower limit of adequacy of vitamin D status (DH, 1998); however, this approach has been questioned and higher thresholds have been proposed (Update on Vitamin D, 2007).

It has been suggested, for example, that vitamin D insufficiency or hypovitaminosis D without clinical signs or symptoms occurs at a plasma 25(OH) D concentration of less than 40 nmol/l (Hanley & Davison, 2005) but there is no agreed definition. Based on associations between plasma 25(OH)D concentration and plasma PTH concentration, calcium absorption, bone turnover markers and bone mineral density, it has been suggested that a plasma 25(OH)D concentration of >75 nmol/l is more appropriate to define vitamin D sufficiency or physiologically optimal concentrations (Update on Vitamin D, 2007).

The concept of establishing a reference range for plasma 25(OH)D concentration based on a threshold at which plasma PTH concentration starts to rise is complicated by the large variation between individuals, the observation that this threshold varied between 30 and 78 nmol/l in several studies and the fact that that no threshold could be identified in some studies (Update on Vitamin D, 2007).

9.3.6   Factors affecting the cutaneous synthesis of vitamin D

Several factors potentially affect vitamin D status. These include seasonal variations, latitude, genetics, adiposity, skin pigmentation, melanin concentration, clothing and age (Update on Vitamin D, 2007).

Seasonal variations in vitamin D status are observed in the UK where the 2000/1 National Diet and Nutrition Survey reported average plasma 25(OH)D concentrations to be highest in July–September and lowest in January–March. During the winter, the UK population relies on body stores and dietary vitamin D to maintain vitamin D status (Update on Vitamin D, 2007).

The cause of low serum 25(OH)D levels among South Asians is likely to be multifactorial. Within the UK, ultraviolet light of the appropriate wavelength to synthesize serum 25(OH)D is available only between April and October. South Asians have the same capacity as lighter-skinned people to make serum 25(OH)D, however, the length of time exposed to UV light needs to be longer to produce a similar response (Roy et al., 2007). It is also important to appreciate that as vitamin D synthesis is mostly via sunshine exposure this comes with other risks, such as eye and skin disease; it may also play a role in reactivating some viral diseases (McKinlay, 2006). The WHO/Euroskin Workshops met in 2005 to discuss the growing controversy on how best to optimize vitamin D status while minimizing these risks.

Research has shown that 25(OH)D concentration can be related to the ethnicity of the individual (Harris & Dawson-Hughes, 1998). A negative relationship has been demonstrated between 25(OH)D concentration and skin pigmentation. It is well recognized that certain ethnic groups are at greater risk of developing 25(OH)D deficiency and subsequently osteomalacia and rickets (Harris & Dawson-Hughes, 1998; Lawson et al., 1999). In ethnic groups with increased melanin, a lower 25(OH)D status has been found, such as in populations of Asian origin (O'Hare et al., 1984; Awumey et al., 1998; Lawson et al., 1999). As melanin functions as a UV light filter, it determines the amount of UVB photons that are able to penetrate the skin (Norman, 1998). The underlying mechanism has yet to be fully elucidated, although it has been shown that melanin absorbs UVB photons in competition with 7-dehydrocholesterol (the presence of this compound in human skin enables the manufacture of vitamin D_3 from UV rays in sunlight), thus reducing the capacity for vitamin D production (Holick, 1995).

Cultural differences such as diet and clothing may also influence 25(OH)D status. Asian populations are known to consume chapattis, for example, which have a high phytate content (thought to interfere with the entero-hepatic circulation of vitamin D metabolites) and often have vegetarian diets, thus obviating their vitamin D intake from animal sources (Clemens, 1989).

In some ethnic groups, such as the Muslim community, the clothing worn almost completely covers the body, so reducing exposure to UVB light. It is often found, therefore, that non-Caucasian populations, such as Asian Indians (Henderson et al., 1990; El-Sonbaty & Abdul-Ghaffar, 1996; Awumey et al., 1998) have lower 25(OH)D levels than their Caucasian counterparts (Awumey et al., 1998; Lawson et al., 1999; Hampson et al., 2003). Also, the 25(OH)D levels for the subjects from the NDNS are significantly higher for both the Caucasian boys ($P < 0.0001$) and girls ($P < 0.0001$) compared with the other ethnic groups (categorized as Indian, Pakistani or Bangladeshi) in all seasonal study waves (Willett, 2004).

Another important factor is that as a person ages the amount of 7-dehydrocholesterol in the epidermis begins to decline. A person 70 years of age exposed to the same amount of sunlight as a 20-year old person would only make 25% of the vitamin D_3 of the younger person (Update on Vitamin D, 2007). Therefore, if they are elderly Asian or Afro-Caribbean they are at even more risk.

9.3.7   Vitamin D deficiency and its prevalence in the UK

Vitamin D deficiency impairs the absorption of dietary calcium and phosphorus, which results in poor bone mineralization. Severe vitamin D deficiency generally presents as rickets and osteomalacia in children and osteomalacia in adults. Rickets and osteomalacia are conditions characterized by pathological defects in growth plate and bone matrix mineralization (Update on Vitamin D, 2007).

In children, failure of bone mineralization gives rise to bone deformities; bones are painful and linear growth is reduced. In adults, bone pain and tenderness are the most prominent features of osteomalacia, and proximal myopathy (progres-

sive muscle weakness and wasting) may also develop. Rickets can be precipitated by dietary calcium or phosphorus deficiency (Update on Vitamin D, 2007).

In children with vitamin D deficient rickets, plasma 25(OH)D concentrations <20 nmol/l have been observed, and in adults with osteomalacia concentrations <10 nmol/l have been recorded (DH, 1998; Update on Vitamin D, 2007).

A lack of national data for certain population subgroups, particularly South Asian and Afro-Caribbean, pregnant and breastfeeding women and infants, makes it difficult to ascertain the prevalence of low vitamin D status in the UK population. Further national surveys of vitamin D status are required, particularly in BME groups, in order to fully quantify the problem and to monitor prevalence into the future (Update on Vitamin D, 2007).

Over the past few years there have been several reports of clinically apparent vitamin D deficiency in UK children. Most, though not all, of the cases that occur in the UK are seen in patients of Afro-Caribbean or South Asian origin. Although skin pigmentation is a factor, other factors, such as a vegetarian diet and low exposure to sunlight (either by staying indoors or by covering the skin), are also accountable.

Breastfeeding exclusively without vitamin D supplementation for periods longer than six months also appears to be important, particularly when associated with inadequate maternal status during pregnancy. It should be noted, however, that there is the possibility of a detection bias in reporting the link between ethnic group and South Asian children, as most of the reports come from areas with high South Asian populations; furthermore, national data are available for South Asian but not Black children (Update on Vitamin D, 2007).

A prospective survey conducted from May 2000 to April 2001 in the West Midlands reported 24 cases of clinically apparent vitamin D deficiency among children aged 0–4 years; only one child was of White ethnic origin; the rest were either of South Asian or Afro-Caribbean origin. It was estimated from census data that the overall incidence was 7.5 per 100,000 children, with children of South Asian origin having an incidence of 38 per 100,000 and of Afro-Caribbean origin children having an incidence of 95 per 100,000. Another survey of children under the age of 16 years presenting to three Birmingham hospitals between June 2001 and June 2003 identified 65 cases (Update on Vitamin D, 2007).

A study in three London hospitals examined 65 children who presented with either rickets or hypocalcaemia and a plasma 25(OH)D concentration <25 nmol/l; 39 children were of Asian origin, 24 Afro-Caribbean and two were Eastern European. Forty-five per cent ($n = 29$) had hypocalcaemic symptoms, of whom 55% ($n = 17$) had no radiological evidence of rickets; 48 children had radiological evidence of rickets, with or without other clinical signs (Ladhani et al., 2004). Children who presented with hypocalcaemia were either under the age of two years or adolescents. The authors speculated that during rapid bone growth hypocalcaemia develops before rickets can ensue (Update on Vitamin D, 2007).

A study in a Leicester hospital observed significant numbers of South Asian mothers having vitamin D deficiency at the end of pregnancy and substantial numbers of children having infantile and adolescent rickets, some of whom have extremely severe bony deformities. Increasing numbers of hypocalcaemic newborns, presenting predominantly with seizures, were also reported. A survey conducted at the Burnley Health Care NHS Trust between 1994 and 2004 identified 14 cases of children presenting with clinically apparent (hypocalcaemia, rickets) vitamin D deficiency. Thirteen of the 14 patients were of South Asian origin. From 1994 to 2001 there were three cases, but from 2002 to 2004 11 cases were reported, highlighting the rising incidence of clinically apparent vitamin D deficiency in the British Asian child community (Update on Vitamin D, 2007).

Hamson et al. (2003) showed an increased prevalence of low serum vitamin D in a Gujarati population (50–60% of subjects) in Leicester. It is possible, however, that the normal range for vitamin D is lower in Gujaratis because the subjects did not have any clinical or biochemical features of osteomalacia. This hypothesis is supported by a community-based study, where elderly Asians were compared with control groups of elderly and young Whites and young Asians. Levels of 25(OH)D were significantly lower in elderly Asians (21/37) and young Asians (7/17) compared with White controls. The difference in parathyroid hormone (PTH) between Asians and Whites was also significant, as was that between young and the elderly (Solanki et al., 1995). Abnormal PTH and 25(OH)D (high PTH and low 25(OH)D), indicative of a high risk of osteomalacia, occurred in 22% of elderly Asians compared with 6% of elderly Whites. Assessing the vitamin D status of South Asians in the UK (Roy et al., 2007) highlighted increased prevalence of hypovitaminosis in 18–36-year-old Pakistani women in Greater Manchester (McKinlay, 2006). In these women, a decrease in serum 25(OH)D level ≤15 ng/ml was associated with a progressive reduction in bone mass at the hip and wrist (Roy et al., 2007).

9.3.7 Prevention of vitamin D deficiency

Over the last few years there has been a growing interest in the specific healthcare needs of ethnic minority groups as Britain has a growing population of ethnic origin.

In the UK, there are specific recommendations to avoid Vitamin D deficiency in vulnerable groups such as pregnant and lactating women, infants, the elderly and BME groups.

The UK RNI (DH, 1998) for vitamin D for all pregnant and breastfeeding women is 10 µg of vitamin D daily and for breastfed babies 7–8.5 µg daily from the age of six months, or earlier if there is increased risk of deficiency by virtue of low maternal status. It is essential that pregnant women receive sufficient vitamin D to build up their own stores and foetal stores to ensure adequate supply to infants during the first six months of life. Vitamin drops for children under five years of age (included in Healthy Start) contain 7.5 µg of vitamin D and supplements for pregnant and nursing mothers contain a daily dose of 10 µg (Update on Vitamin D, 2007).

There is concern that these recommendations are overlooked by health professionals (DH, 1998; Callaghan et al., 2006), as well as by the general public. The Review of the Welfare Food Scheme identified that uptake of vitamin drops in the UK is very low even among those entitled to receive free supplies. The Review concluded that the provision of free vitamin supplements offers a simple and potentially effective means of preventing adverse nutritional outcomes, particularly rickets. Rickets remains evident in the UK and it is likely that the prevalence would increase among high-risk groups if the Scheme were withdrawn.

It has been questioned whether relying on vitamin D supplements given to infants or vitamin D supplementation of formula feeds is adequate to overcome the impact of maternal vitamin D deficiency (Shaw & Pal, 2002). This was reinforced in a survey by Callaghan *et al.* (2006), which highlighted that recommendations for vitamin D supplementation were being ignored and that 50% of those presenting with hypocalcaemic convulsions were formula-fed, implying that these infants had low stores of vitamin D at birth. There appears to be lack of awareness in high-risk groups of the recommendations to take vitamin D supplements (Allgrove, 2004; Shenoy *et al.*, 2005; Callaghan *et al.*, 2006). Furthermore, an audit in the Leicester area reported that while health professionals were aware of the issue, there was no clear policy to resolve it. The antenatal guidance from NICE states clearly that vitamin D supplementation should not be offered routinely to pregnant women due to the risk of abnormalities in the unborn baby (Update on Vitamin D, 2007).

There is a need to state clearly the length and intensity of exposure necessary to balance maintenance of vitamin D status with the risk of developing skin cancer. The Committee also explicitly reiterates that all pregnant and breastfeeding women should consider taking a daily supplement of vitamin D in order to ensure their own requirement for vitamin D is met and to build adequate foetal stores for early infancy. A clear public health strategy and guidance on vitamin D supplementation is necessary to overcome poor understanding and advice among health professionals and at-risk groups of the population (Update on Vitamin D, 2007).

There is an urgent need to standardize laboratory methodologies for the measurement of plasma 25(OH)D concentration. There is also a need to identify markers of functional outcome in different age and vulnerable groups to refine the interpretation of plasma 25(OH)D measurements (Update on Vitamin D, 2007).

Under the Healthy Start scheme, free vitamins containing 70 mg vitamin C, 10 μg vitamin D and 400 μg folic acid are available for women who receive Healthy Start vouchers while they are pregnant and for one year after the birth of their child.

However, this is only prescribed to women who are entitled for it and some may not be aware of its necessity (Update on Vitamin D, 2007).

The response rate for participation among the South Asian target population tends to be low, particularly in the Pakistani and Bengali populations. Thus, it is difficult to undertake epidemiological studies involving invasive and time-consuming procedures in population groups in whom concerns about bone health are not manifested (Falch & Steihaug, 2000; Goswani *et al.*, 2000). Furthermore, the difference in prevalence reported between studies may relate to differences in assays used for 25(OH)D, the definition of 25(OH)D deficiency, latitude or other characteristics of the group being studied. Monitoring of 25(OH)D levels in subjects can only be advocated after clarification of a nationally or internationally agreed 'deficient range' for 25(OH)D and the optimum time to screen within the seasonal fluctuations seen over the year (Pal *et al.*, 2003).

It is also important to note that the current criteria used for establishing vitamin D deficiency and for the diagnosis of osteoporosis based on a normal adult White population cannot necessarily be extrapolated to ethnic populations (Update on Vitamin D, 2007).

Thus researches are required to ascertain the 'normal' levels of vitamin D among South Asians and the Black community nationally. This may then initiate discussions and further research potentially to establish a different set of cut-off values for diagnosing vitamin D insufficiency and deficiency that are more relevant to these population groups. Another argument that lends strong support for this research is that data on a large number of South Asians are already available for analysis and will not only add new knowledge but advance our understanding of vitamin D status among South Asians.

9.3.8   Public health measures to tackle vitamin D deficiency

In the 1980s, when vitamin D deficiency was first recognized as a problem in the South Asian community, various preventative strategies were suggested. These included daily or annual supplementation (Stephens *et al.*, 1981) and fortification of chapatti flour with vitamin D (Pietrek *et al.*,

1976) The Department of Health Working Party rejected the idea of fortification of other foods, though margarine was fortified (COMA, 1980). Currently, there is no policy about the special needs of the South Asian and Black communities with respect to their high incidence of vitamin D deficiency (Iqbal *et al.*, 2001).

There is no doubt, however, that the widespread and sometimes severe consequences of vitamin D deficiency in this subgroup continue and is now regarded to be endemic (Henderson *et al.*, 1990). In spite of the continual political, socioeconomic and medical consequences, there still seems to be a gap in implementing some sort of preventative 'nutritional' policy and many consider that the time for action is long overdue (Compston, 1998). A lack of national data for this group makes it difficult to estimate precisely the prevalence of low vitamin D status in the UK population (Update on Vitamin D, 2007).

There is a need for more research in South Asians and black communities regarding their vitamin D status as this could subsequently have an impact on the delivery of healthcare in areas with high ethnic populations. There is currently little evidence based on research to give any real understanding of the problem of vitamin D deficiency and its consequences among the ethnic minorities living in the UK.

The research should establish the level and extent of vitamin D deficiency among the already identified vulnerable groups such as Indian, Pakistani and Bengali and the Afro-Caribbean populations, as there is lack of good quality and consistent data. The study could form the basis for further research into levels regarded to be 'normal', 'sufficient' and 'deficient' and thresholds of plasma 25(OH)D could be suggested, based on associations with chronic endpoints (e.g., osteoporosis in South Asians). This research could be useful in the decision-making process at a practice level, for instance in arriving at a clinician-oriented decision as to whether or not to treat subjects at risk, thus implementing useful preventative measures before fractures occur (Hampson *et al.*, 2003). Furthermore, progress towards selected health targets can be monitored, as well as the identification of the most vulnerable target groups. Such important information may therefore be used to support the development of policy and also to design and implement appropriate interventions tailored to meet the needs of this population group. Potential interventions could include greater awareness among targeted communities and among health professionals, dietary and lifestyle guidance to prevent vitamin D deficiency, and supplementation trials with calcium and vitamin D where appropriate. Such preventative strategies could potentially save the NHS and related service providers significant money that could be better spent elsewhere.

Support groups

Metabolic Syndrome and Polycystic Ovary Syndrome (PCOS) in Black and Minority Ethnic Groups

Verity (www.verity-pcos.org.uk) A self-help group for women with PCOS

PCOS UK (www.pcos-uk.org.uk) Information for healthcare professionals

Further reading

Cancer in the Different BME Groups

Buckland, G., Agudo, A. Luján, L Jakszyn, P *et al.* (2010) Adherence to a Mediterranean diet and risk of gastric adenocarcinoma within the European Prospective Investigation into Cancer and Nutrition (EPIC) cohort study. *Am J Clin Nutr*, 91(2), 381–390.

Wild, S.H., Fischbacher, C.M. *et al.* (2006) Mortality from all cancers and lung, colorectal, breast and prostate cancer by country of birth in England and Wales, 2001–2003. *Br J Cancer*, 10, 94(7), 1079–85.

Metabolic Syndrome and Polycystic Ovary Syndrome (PCOS) in Black and Minority Ethnic Groups

Byrne, C.D. & Wild, S.H. (2006) *The Metabolic Syndrome*. Wiley, Chichester.

Elsheikh, M. & Murphy, C. (2008) *The Facts: Polycystic Ovary Syndrome*. Oxford University Press, Oxford.

Kovacs, G. T. & Norman, R. (2007) *Polycystic Ovary Syndrome*. Cambridge University Press, Cambridge.

Clayton, R.N., Hogkinson, J. *et al.* (1992) How common are polycystic ovaries in normal women and what is their significance for the fertility of the population? *Clinical Endocrinology*, 37, 127–34.

NCEP/ATPIII (2001) Executive Summary of the Third Report of the National Cholesterol Education Program (NCEP) Expert panel on Detection, Evaluation, and Treatment of High Blood Cholesterol in Adults (Adult Treatment Panel III). *Journal of the American Medical Association*, 285(19), 2468–97.

References

Cancer in the Different BME Groups

Archer, V.E. & Jones, D.W. (2002) Capsaicin pepper, cancer and ethnicity. *Medical Hypotheses*, 59(4), 450–7.

Armstrong, B. & Doll, R. (1975) Environmental factors and cancer incidence and mortality in different countries with special reference to dietary practices. *Int J Cancer*, 15, 617–31.

Atri, J., Falshaw M. *et al.* (1997) Improving uptake of breast cancer screening in multiethnic populations: a randomized controlled trial using practice reception staff to contact non-attenders. *British Medical Journal*, 315, 1356–9.

Aus, G., Abbou, C.C. *et al.* (2005) EAU guidelines on prostate cacner. *Eur Urol*, 48, 546–51.

Bedi, R. (1996) Betel quid and tobacco chewing among the United Kingdom's Bangladeshi community. In *The Proceedings of the CRC/DoH Symposium on Cancer and Minority Ethnic Groups*. BJC, 74(Suppl.).

Ben-Shlomo, Y., Evans. S. *et al.* (2008) The risk of prostate cancer amongst black men in the United Kingdom: The PROCESS Cohort Study. *European Urology*, 53(1), 99–105.

Brewster, D.H., Fraser, L.A., Harris, V. & Black, R.J. (2000) Rising incidence of prostate cancer in Scotland: increased risk or increased detection? *BJU Int. Mar*, 85(4), 463–72; discussion 472–3.

Castellsagué, X., Muñoz, N. *et al.* (2000) Influence of maté drinking, hot beverages and diet on esophageal cancer risk in South America. *Int J Cancer*, 88(4), 658–64.

Chlebowski, R.T., Chen, Z. *et al.* (2005) Ethnicity and breast cancer: factors influencing differences in incidence and outcome. *Journal of the National Cancer Institute*, 97(6), 439–48.

Collaborative Group on Hormonal Factors in Breast Cancer (2002) Breast cancer and breastfeeding: collaborative reanalysis of individual data from 47 epidemiological studies in 30 countries, including 50,302 women with breast cancer and 96,973 women without the disease. *Lancet*, 360(9328), 20 July: 187–95.

Engel, L.S., Chow, W.H. *et al.* (2003) Population attributable risks of esophageal and gastric cancers. *JNCI Cancer Spectrum*, 95(18), 1404–13.

Etzioni, R., Berry, K.M., Legler, J.M. & Shaw, P. (2002) Prostate-specific antigen testing in black and white men: an analysis of Medicare claims from 1991–1998. *Urology*, 59, 251–5.

Evans, S., Metcalfe, C. *et al.* (2008) Investigating Black/White differences in prostate cancer diagnosis: a systematic review and meta-analysis. *International Journal of Cancer*, 123, 430–5.

Flood, D.M., Weiss, N.S. *et al.* (2000) Colorectal cancer incidence in Asian migrants to the United States and their descendants. *Cancer Causes & Control*, 11(5), 403–11.

Freedman, N.D., Abnet, C.C. *et al.* (2007) A prospective study of tobacco, alcohol, and the risk of esophageal and gastric cancer subtypes. *Am J Epidemiol*, 165(12), 1424–33.

Ghafoor, A., Jemal, A. *et al.* (2003) Trends in breast cancer by race and ethnicity. *CA: A Cancer Journal for Clinicians*, 53(6), 342–55.

Giovannucci, E. (2002) Modifiable risk factors for colon cancer. *Gastroenterol Clin North Am*, 31, 925–43.

Glover, F.E. Jr., Coffey, D.S. *et al.* (1998) The epidemiology of prostate cancer in Jamaica. *J Urol.*, 59(6), June, 1984–6; discussion 1986–7.

Goh, K.L., Cheah, P.L. *et al.* (2007) Ethnicity and *H. pylori* as risk factors for gastric cancer in Malaysia: a prospective case control study. *American Journal of Gastroenterology*, 102(1), 40–5.

Gomez, S.L. & Glaser, S.L. (2006) Misclassification of race/ethnicity in a population-based cancer registry (United States). *Cancer Causes & Control*, 17(6), 771–81

González, C.A., Pera, G. *et al.* (2003) Smoking and the risk of gastric cancer in the European Prospective Investigation into Cancer and Nutrition (EPIC). *Int J Cancer*, 107(4), 20 November, 629–34.

Grossfeld, G.D., Latini, D.M. *et al.* (2002) Is ethnicity an independent predictor of prostate cancer recurrence after radical prostatectomy? *Journal of Urology*, 168(6), 2510–15.

Gupta, P.C., Mehta, F.S. & Pindborg, J.J. (1984) Mortality among reverse chutta smokers in south India. *Br Med J (Clin Res Ed)*, 289(6449), 865–6.

Hedeen, A.N. White, E. & Taylor, V. (1999) Ethnicity and birthplace in relation to tumor size and stage in Asian American women with breast cancer. *American Journal of Public Health*, 89(8), 1248–52.

Hill, S. (2006) *Ethnicity and Cancer Prevention Information* (An internal report for Cancer Research UK). Cancer Research UK, London.

Huang, J.Q., Zheng, G.F. *et al.* (2003) Meta-analysis of the relationship between cagA seropositivity and gastric cancer. *Gastroenterology*, 125(6), December, 1636–44.

Jack, R.H., Davies, E.A. & Moller, H. (2007) Testis and prostate cancer incidence in ethnic groups in South East England. *Int J Androl*, 30(4), 215–20; discussion 220–1.

Kendzor, D.E., Costello, T.J. *et al.* (2008) Race/ethnicity and multiple cancer risk factors among individuals seeking smoking cessation treatment. *Cancer Epidemiology, Biomarkers & Prevention*, 17(11), November, 2937–45.

Key, T.J., Allen, N.E., Spencer, E.A. & Travis, R.C. (2002) The effect of diet on risk of cancer. *Lancet*, 360, 861–8.

Lagergren, J., Bergstorm, R. & Adami, H. (2000) Association between medications that relax the lower esophageal sphincter and risk for esophageal adenocarcinoma. *Annals of Internal Medicine*, 133(1), 165–75.

Lagergren, J., Bergstrom, R. & Nyren O. (1999) Association between body mass and adenocarcinoma of the esophagus and gastric cardia. *Ann Intern Med*, 130(11), 883–90.

Lantz, P.M., Mujahid, M. *et al.* (2006) The influence of race, ethnicity, and individual socioeconomic factors on breast cancer stage at diagnosis. *American Journal of Public Health*, 96(12), 2173–8.

Lee, C.H., Lee, J.M. *et al.* (2005) Independent and combined effects of alcohol intake, tobacco smoking and betel quid chewing on the risk of esophageal cancer in Taiwan. *Int J Cancer*, 113(3), 475–82.

Li, W., Thompson, C.H. *et al.* (2004) The site of infection and ethnicity of the patient influence the biological pathways to HPV-induced mucosal cancer. *Modern Pathology*, 17(9), 1031–7.

Mao, Y., Hu, J., Semenciw, R. & White, K. (Canadian Cancer Registries Epidemiology Research Group) (2002) Active and passive smoking and the risk of stomach cancer, by subsite, in Canada. *Eur J Cancer Prev*, 11(1), February, 27–38.

McKenzie, F., Jeffreys, M., 't Mannetje, A. & Pearce N. (2008) Prognostic factors in women with breast cancer: inequalities by ethnicity and socioeconomic position in New Zealand. *Cancer Causes & Control.* 19(4), 403–11.

McKeown-Eyssen, G. (1994) Epidemiology of colorectal cancer revisited: are serum triglycerides and/or plasma glucose associated with risk? *Cancer Epidemiol Biomarkers Prev*, 3, 687–95.

McMichael, A.J., McCall, M.G., Hartchorne, J.M. & Woodings, T.L. (1980) Patterns of gastrointestinal cancer in European migrants to Australia: the role of dietary change. *Int J Cancer*, 5, 431–7.

Metcalfe, C., Evans, S, *et al.* (2008) Pathways to diagnosis for Black men and White men found to have prostate cancer: the PROCESS cohort study. *British Journal of Cancer*, 99, 1040–5.

National Cancer Intelligence Network (2009) *Cancer Incidence and Survival by Major Ethnic Group, England, 2002–2006*. NCIN, London.

NHS Information Centre (2006) Health Survey for England 2004: Health of Ethnic Minorities-Full Report. Available from www.ic.nhs.uk/statistics-and-data-collections/health-and-lifestyles-related-surveys/health-survey-for-england/health-survey-for-england-2004:-health-of-ethnic-minorities-full-report.

Office for National Statistics (2008) *Cancer Statistics Registrations: Registrations of Cancer Diagnosed in 2005*. England Series MB1, no. 36. ONS, London.

Parkin, D.M. Ferlay J. *et al.* (2003) *Cancer in Africa: Epidemiology and Prevention*. IARC Scientific Publication 153. IARC, Lyons.

Parkin, D.M., Bray, F., Ferlay, J. & Pisani, P. (2005) Global cancer statistics, 2002. *CA Cancer J Clin*, 55, 74–108.

Parkin, D.M., Whelan S.L. *et al.* (2002) *Cancer Incidence in Five* Continents. Vol. VIII. IARC Scientific Publications 155. IARC, Lyons.

Pavia, M., Pileggi, C., Nobile, C.G. & Angelillo, I.F. (2006) Association between fruit and vegetable consumption and oral cancer: a meta-analysis of observational studies. *Am J Clin Nutr*, 83(5), 1126–34.

Peek, R.M. Jr. & Blaser, M.J. (2002) *Helicobacter pylori* and gastrointestinal tract adenocarcinomas. *Nat Rev Cancer*, 2(1), 28–37.

Platz, E.A., Rimm, E.B. *et al.* (2000) Racial variation in prostate cancer incidence and in hormonal system markers among male health professionals. *J Natl Cancer Inst*, 20, 92(24), 2009–17.

Popkin, B.M. (2004) The nutrition transition: an overview of world patterns of change. *Nutr Rev*, 62, S140–3.

Popkin, B.M. (2007) Understanding global nutrition dynamics as a step towards controlling cancer incidence. *Nature Reviews. Cancer*, 7(1), 61–7.

Prentice, R.L. & Sheppard, L. (1990) Dietary fat and cancer: consistency of the epidemiologic data, and disease prevention that may follow from a practical reduction in fat consumption. *Cancer Causes Control*, 1, 81–7.

Qureshi, M., Thacker, H.L., Litaker, D.G. & Kippes, C. (2000) Differences in breast cancer screening rates: an issue of ethnicity or socioeconomics? *Journal of Women's Health & Gender-Based Medicine*, 9(9), 1025–31.

Rahman, M., Sakamoto, J. & Fukui, T. (2003) Bidi smoking and oral cancer: a meta-analysis. *Int J Cancer*, 106(4), 600–4.

Robb, K.A., Solarin, I. *et al.* (2008) Attitudes to colorectal cancer screening among ethnic minority groups in the UK. *BMC Public Health*, 8, 34.

Sewram V, De Stefani E, Brennan P, & Boffetta P., 2003. Maté consumption and the risk of squamous cell esophageal cancer in Uruguay. *Cancer Epidemiol Biomarkers Prev*, 12(6), 508–13.

Shibata A, & Whittemore A., 1997. Genetic predisposition to prostate cancer: possible explanations for ethnic differences in risk. *Prostate*, 32, 65–72.

Shikata, K., Kiyohara, Y. *et al.* (2006) A prospective study of dietary salt intake and gastric cancer incidence in a defined Japanese population: the Hisayama study. *Int J Cancer*, 1, 119(1), July, 196–201.

Sitas, F., Yarnell, J. & Forman, D. (1992) *Helicobacter pylori* infection rates in relation to age and social class in a population of Welsh men. *Gut*, 33, 1582.

Skinner, H.G. & Schwartz, G.G. (2009) The relation of serum parathyroid hormone and serum calcium to serum levels of prostate-specific antigen: a population-based study. *Cancer Epidemiol Biomarkers Prev.* 18(11), 2869–73.

Smigal, C., Jemal, A. *et al.* (2006) Trends in breast cancer by race and ethnicity: update 2006. *CA: a Cancer Journal for Clinicians*, 56(3), 168–83.

Szczepura, A., Price, C. & Gumber, A. (2008) Breast and bowel cancer screening uptake patterns over 15 for UK south Asian ethnic minority populations, corrected for differences in socio-demographic characteristics. *BMC Public Health*, 8, 346.

Van Cleave, T.T., Moore, J.H. *et al.* (2010) Interaction among variant vascular endothelial growth factor (VEGF) and its receptor in relation to prostate cancer risk. *Prostate*, 1, 70(4), March, 341–52.

Vyse, A.J., Gay, N.J. *et al.* (2002) The burden of *Helicobacter pylori* infection in England and Wales. *Epidemiol Infect*, 128(3), June, 411–17.

Ward, E., Jemal, A. *et al.* (2004) Cancer disparities by race/ethnicity and socioeconomic status. *CA: a Cancer Journal for Clinicians*, 54(2), March–April, 78–93.

Weikert, C., Dietrich, T. *et al.* (2009) Lifetime and baseline alcohol intake and risk of cancer of the upper aerodigestive tract in the European Prospective Investigation into Cancer and Nutrition (EPIC) study. *Int J Cancer*, 125(2), 406–12.

Wild, C.P. & Hardie, L.J. (2003) Reflux, Barrett's oesophagus and adenocarcinoma: burning questions. *Nat Rev Cancer*, 3(9), 676–84.

Wong, B.C., Lam, S.K. *et al.* (China Gastric Cancer Study Group) (2004) *Helicobacter pylori* eradication to prevent gastric cancer in a high-risk region of China: a randomized controlled trial. *JAMA*, 14, 291(2), 18794.

World Cancer Research Fund/American Institute for Cancer Research (2007) *Food, Nutrition, Physical Activity, and the Prevention of Cancer: A Global Perspective.* AICR, Washington, DC.

Zambon, P., Talamini, R. *et al.* (2000) Smoking, type of alcoholic beverage and squamous-cell oesophageal cancer in northern Italy. *Int Cancer*, 86(1), 1 April, 144–9.

Zeka, A.. Gore, R. & Kriebel. D. (2003)) Effects of alcohol and tobacco on aerodigestive cancer risks: a meta-regression analysis. *Cancer Causes Control*, 14(9), 897–906.

Zheng, X.Z., Yang, A.Q. *et al.* (2008) Ethnicity determines association of p53Arg72Pro alleles with cervical cancer in China. *European Journal of Cancer Prevention*, 17(5), 460–6.

Metabolic Syndrome and Polycystic Ovary Syndrome (PCOS) in Black and Minority Ethnic Groups

Abate, N., Carulli, L. *et al.* (2003) Genetic polymorphism PC-1 K121Q and ethnic susceptibility to insulin resistance. *Journal of Clinical Endocrinology & Metabolism*, 88.

American Association of Clinical Endocrinologists (2005). Position statement on metabolic syndrome and cardiovascular consequences of polycystic ovary syndrome. *Endocrine Practice*, 11(2), 125.

Azziz, R. (2006) How prevalent is metabolic syndrome in women with polycystic ovary syndrome? *Nat Clin Pract Endocrinol Metab*, 2(3), 132–3.

Barclay, A., Petocz, P. *et al.* (2008) Glycemic index, glycemic load, and chronic disease risk – a meta-analysis of observational studies. *American Journal of Clinical Nutrition*, 87(3), 627–37.

Barr, S., Hart, K., Reeves, S. & Jeanes, Y. (2007) Dietary composition of UK women with polycystic ovary syndrome. *Annals of Nutrition and Metabolism*, 51(Suppl. 1), 345.

Chang, R.J., Nakamura, R.M., Judd, H.L. & Kaplan, S.A. (1983) Insulin resistance in non-obese patients with polycystic ovarian disease. *J Clin Endocrinol Metab*, 57, 356–9.

Diamanti-Kandarakis, E. (2008) Polycystic ovarian syndrome: pathophysiology, molecular aspects and clinical implications. *Expert Reviews in Molecular Medicine*, 10(2), E3.

Dokras, A. (2008) Cardiovascular disease risk factors in polycystic ovary syndrome. *Seminars in Reproductive Endocrinology*, 26(1), 39–44.

Dokras, A., Bochner, M., *et al.* (2005) Screening women with polycystic ovary syndrome for metabolic syndrome. *Obstetrics and Gynaecology*, 106(1), 131–7.

Douglas, C., Gower, B.E. *et al.* (2006) Role of diet in the treatment of polycystic ovary syndrome. *Fertility and Sterility*, 85, 679–88.

Dunaif, A., Futterweit, W., Segal, K.R. & Dobrjansky, A. (1989) Profound peripheral insulin resistance, independent of obesity, in the polycystic ovary syndrome. *Diabetes*, 38, 1165–74.

Ehrmann, D., Barnes, R. *et al.* (1999) Prevalence of impaired glucose tolerance and diabetes in women with polycystic ovary syndrome. *Diabetes Care*, 22, 141–6.

Ehrmann, D., Kasza, K. *et al.* (PCOS/Troglitazone Study Group) (2005) Effects of race and family history of type 2 diabetes on metabolic status of women with polycystic ovary syndrome. *Journal of Clinical Endocrinology and Metabolism*, 90(1), 66–71.

Ehrmann, D., Liljenquist, D.R. *et al.* (PCOS/Troglitazone Study Group) (2006) Prevalence and predictors of the metabolic syndrome in women with PCOS. *Journal of Clinical Endocrinology and Metabolism*, 91, 48–53.

Escorbar-Morreale, H. & San Millan, J.L. (2007) Abdominal adiposity and the polycystic ovary syndrome. *Trends in Endocrinology and Metabolism*, 18(7), 266–72.

Essah, P. (2007) The metabolic syndrome in polycystic ovary syndrome. *Clinical Obstetrics and Gynaecology*, 50(1), 205–25.

European Society for Human Reproduction & Embryology (ESHRE) (2004) Revised 2003 consensus on diagnostic criteria and long term health risks related to polycystic ovary syndrome. *Fertility and Sterility*, 81(1), 19–25.

Farshchi, H., Rane, A., Love, A. & Kennedy, R.L. (2007) Diet and nutrition in polycystic ovary syndrome (PCOS): pointers for nutritional management. *Journal of Obstetrics and Gynaecology*, 27(8), 762–73.

Forouhi, N.G. (2000) The relationship between body fat distribution, insulin sensitivity, and postprandial lipids in Europeans and South Asians: a cross-sectional study. PhD thesis, London University.

Franks, S., McCarthy, M. & Hardy, K. (2006) Development of polycystic ovary syndrome: involvement of genetic and environmental factors. *International Journal of Embryology*, 29, 278–85.

Galgani, J., R. Uuauy, Aguirre, C., & Diaz, E. (2008) Effect of the dietary fat quality on insulin sensitivity. *British Journal of Nutrition* 100, 471–9.

Gamberini, A., Pelusi, C., *et al.* (2004) Glucose intolerance in a large cohort of Mediterranean women with polycystic ovary syndrome. *Diabetes*, 53, 2353–8.

Glueck, C. J. P., R. Wang, P. Goldenberg, N. & Sieve-Smith, L. (2003) Incidence and treatment of metabolic syndrome in newly referred women with confirmed polycystic ovarian syndrome. *Metabolism*, 52, 908–15.

Hayes, C. & Kriska, A. (2008) Role of physical activity in diabetes management and prevention. *Journal of American Dietetic Association*, 108, S19–S23.

Herriot, A.M., Whitcroft, S. & Jeanes, Y. (2008) A retrospective audit of patients with polycystic ovary syndrome: the effects of a reduced glycaemic load diet. *Journal of Human Nutrition and Dietetics*, 21, 337–45.

Holte, J., Bergh, T. *et al.* (1995) Restored insulin sensitivity but persistently increased early insulin secretion after weight loss in obese women with polycystic ovary syndrome. *Journal of Clinical Endocrinology and Metabolism*, 80(9), 2586–93.

Jeanes, Y.M., Barr, S., Smith, K. & Hart, K.H. (2009) Dietary management of women with polycystic ovary syndrome in the United Kingdom: the role of dietitians. *Journal of Human Nutrition and Dietetics*, 22, 551–8.

Kasim-Karakas, S., Almario, R.U. *et al.* (2004) Metabolic and endocrine effects of a polyunsaturated fatty acid-rich diet in polycystic ovary syndrome. *Journal of Clinical Endocrinology and Metabolism* 89(2), 615–20.

Kiddy, D., Hamilton-Fairley, D. *et al.* (1992) Improvement in endocrine and ovarian function during dietary treatment of obese women with polycystic ovary syndrome. *Clinical Endocrinology*, 36(1), 105–11.

Liepa, G., Sengupta A. & Karsies, D. (2008) Polycystic ovary syndrome (PCOS) and other androgen excess-related conditions: can changes in dietary intake make a difference? *Nutrition in Clinical Practice*, 23(1), 63–71.

Lindholm, A., Andersson, L. *et al.* (2008). Prevalence of symptoms associated with polycystic ovary syndrome. *International Journal of Gynecology and Obstetrics*, 102, 39–43.

Lo, J.C., Feigenbaum, S.L. *et al.* (2006) Epidemiology and adverse cardiovascular risk profile of diagnosed polycystic ovary syndrome. *J Clin Endocrinol Metab*, 91, 1357–63.

Lindström J, Ilanne-Parikka P, Peltonen M, Aunola S, Eriksson JG, Hemiö K, Hämäläinen H, Härkönen P, Keinänen-Kiukaanniemi S, Laakso M, Louheranta A, Mannelin M, Paturi M, Sundvall J, Valle TT, Uusitupa , M, Tuomilehto, J; Finnish Diabetes Prevention Study Group. (2003) Sustained reduction in the incidence of type 2 diabetes by lifestyle intervention: follow-up of the Finnish Diabetes Prevention Study. *Lancet*, 368(9548):1673–9.

Marsh, K. & Brand-Miller, J. (2005) The optimal diet for women with polycystic ovary syndrome? *British Journal of Nutrition*, 94, 154–65.

Mathur, R., Alexander, C.J. *et al.* (2008) Use of metformin in polycystic ovary syndrome. *American Journal of Obstetrics and Gynecology*, 199(6), 596–609.

McKeigue, P.M., Mermot, M.G. *et al.* (1988) Diabetes, hyperinsulinaemia and coronary risk factors in Bangladeshis in east London. *British Heart Journal*, 60, 390–6.

McKeigue, P.M., Shah, B. & Marmot, M.G. (1991) Relation of central obesity and insulin resistance with high diabetes prevalence and cardiovascular risk in South Asians. *Lancet*, 337(8738), 382–6.

McKeown, N.M., Meigs, J.B. *et al.* (2004) Carbohydrate nutrition, insulin resistance, and the prevalence of the metabolic syndrome in the Framingham Offspring Cohort. *Diabetes Care*, 27, 538–46.

McMillan-Price, J., Petocz, J.P. *et al.* (2006) Comparison of 4 diets of varying glycemic load on weight loss and cardiovascular risk reduction in overweight and obese young adults. *Archives of Internal Medicine*, 166, 1466–75.

Moran, L., Noakes P.M. *et al.* (2003) Dietary composition in restoring reproductive and metabolic physiology in overweight women with polycystic ovary syndrome.

Journal of Clinical Endocrinology and Metabolism, 88(2), 812–19.

Moran, L. & Norman, R.J. (2004) Understanding and managing disturbances in insulin metabolism and body weight in women with polycystic ovarian syndrome. *Best Practice and Research Clinical Obstetrics and Gynaecology*, 18(5), 719–36.

Qublan, H.S., Yannakoula, E.K., Al-Qudah, M.A. & El-Uri, F.I. (2007) Dietary intervention versus metformin to improve the reproductive outcome in women with polycystic ovary syndrome: a prospective comparative study. *Saudi Medical Journal*, 28(11), 1694–9.

Raji, A., Seely, E.W., Arky, R.A. & Simonson, D.C. (2001) Body fat distribution and insulin resistance in healthy Asian Indians and Caucasians. *Journal of Clinical Endocrinology and Metabolism*, 86, 5366–71.

Riccardi, G. & Rivellese, A.A. (2000) Dietary treatment of the metabolic syndrome – the optimal diet. *The British Journal of Nutrition*, 83(Suppl. 1), S143–8.

Rodin, D.A., Bano, G. et al. (1998) Polycystic ovaries and associated metabolic abnormalities in Indian subcontinent Asian women. *Clinical Endocrinology*, 49, 91–9.

Russo, G.L. (2009) Dietary n-6 and n-3 polyunsaturated fatty acids: from biochemistry to clinical implications in cardiovascular prevention, *Biochem Pharmacol*, 77, 937–46.

Sanders, T.A. (2009) Fat and fatty acid intake and metabolic effects in the human body. *Annuls of Nutrition and Metabolism*, 55(1–3), 162–72.

Sheehan, M. (2004) Polycystic ovarian syndrome: diagnosis and management. *Clinical Medicine and Research*, 2(1), 13–27.

Stamets, K., Taylor, D.S. et al. (2004) A randomized trial of the effects of two types of short-term hypocaloric diets on weight loss in women with polycystic ovary syndrome. *Fertility and Sterility*, 81(3), 630–7.

Tillen, T., Forouhi, N. et al. (2005) Metabolic syndrome and coronary heart disease in South Asians, African Caribbeans and White Europeans: a UK population-based cross-sectional study. *Diabetologia*, 48, 649–56.

Tonkin, A. (2004) The metabolic syndrome – a growing problem. *European Heart Journal Supplements*, 6(Suppl. A), A37–A42.

Weerakiet, S., Srisombut, C. et al. (2001) Prevalence of IGT and type 2 DM in Asian women with PCOS. *International Journal of Gynecology and Obstetrics*, 75, 177–84.

Westerveld, H., Hoogendoorn, M. et al. (2008) Cardiometabolic abnormalities in the polycystic ovary syndrome: pharmacotherapeutic insights. *Pharmacology and Therapeutics*, 119(3), 223–41.

Wijeyaratne, C., Balen, A.H., Barth, J.H. & Belchetz, P.E. (2002) Clinical manifestations and insulin resistance (IR) in polycystic ovary syndrome (PCOS) among South Asians and Caucasians: is there a difference? *Clinical Endocrinology*, 57, 343–50.

World Health Organization (1999) *Definition, Diagnosis and Classification of Diabetes Mellitus and its Complications*. Report of a WHO consultation. WHO, Geneva.

Vitamin D Deficiency in BME Groups

Allgrove, J. (2004) Is nutritional rickets returning? *Archives of Diseases in Childhood*, 89, 699–701.

Awumey, E.M.K., Mitra, D.A. et al. (1998) Vitamin D metabolism is altered in Asian Indians in the southern United States: a clinical research center study. *Journal of Clinical Endocrinology and Metabolism*, 83, 169–73.

Callaghan, A., Moy, R. et al. (2006) Incidence of symptomatic vitamin D deficiency. *Archives of Diseases in Childhood*, 91, 606–7.

Clemens, M.R. (1989) The problem of rickets in UK Asians. *Journal of Human Nutrition and Dietetics*, 2, 105–16.

COMA (Committee on Medical Aspects of Food Policy) (1980) *Working Party on Fortification of Food with Vitamin D*. HMSO, London.

Compston, J.E. (1998) Vitamin D deficiency: time for action. Evidence supports routine supplementation for elderly people and others at risk. *British Medical Journal*, 317, 1466–7.

Department of Health (1998) Nutrition and Bone Health: with particular reference to calcium and vitamin D no. 49. London: The Stationary Office.

El-Sonbaty, M.R. & Abdul-Ghaffar, N.U.A.M.A. (1996) Vitamin D deficiency in veiled Kuwaiti women. *European Journal of Clinical Nutrition*, 32, 338–9.

Falch, J.A. & Steihaug, S. (2000) Vitamin D deficiency in Pakistani premenopausal women living in Norway is not associated with evidence of reduced skeletal strength. *Scandinavian Journal of Clinical Laboratory Investment*, 60, 103–9.

Goswani, R., Gupta, N. et al. (2000) Prevalence and significance of low 25-hydroxyvitamin D concentrations in healthy subjects in Delhi. *American Journal of Clinical Nutrition*, 72. 472–5.

Harris, S.S. & Dawson-Hughes, B. (1998) Seasonal changes in plasma 25-hydroxyvitamin D concentrations of young American black and white women. *American Journal of Clinical Nutrition*, 67, 1232–6.

Hampson, G., Martin, F.C. et al. (2003) Effects of dietary improvement on bone metabolism in elderly underweight women with osteoporosis: a randomised controlled trial. *Osteoporosis International*, 14, 750–6.

Hamson, C., Goh, L. et al. (2003) Comparative study of bone mineral density, calcium and vitamin D status in the Gujarati and White populations of Leicester. *Postgraduate Medical Journal*, 79, 279–83.

Hanley, D. & Davison, K. (2005) Vitamin D insufficiency in North America. *J Nutr*, 135, 332–7.

Henderson, J.B., Dunnigan, M.G. *et al.* (1990) Asian osteomalacia is determined by dietary factors. *British Journal of Nutrition*, 4, 18–24.

Heaney, R.P. (2003) Long-latency deficiency disease: insights from calcium and vitamin D. *American Journal of Clinical Nutrition*, 78(5), 912–19.

Hirani, V. & Primatesta, P. (2005) Vitamin D concentrations among people aged 65 years and over living in private households and institutions in England: population survey. *Age and Ageing*, 10, 1–6.

Holick, M.F. (1995). Environmental factors that influence the cutaneous production of vitamin D. *American Journal of Clinical Nutrition*, 61, 38S–64S.

Iqbal, S.J., Featherstone, S. *et al.* (2001) Family screening is effective in picking up undiagnosed Asian vitamin D deficient subjects. *Journal of Human Nutrition and Dietetics*, 14, 371–6.

Ladhani, S., Srinivasan, L. *et al.* (2004) Presentation of vitamin D deficiency. *Archives of Diseases in Childhood*, 89, 781–4.

Lawson, M., Thomas, M. & Hardiman, A. (1999) Dietary and lifestyle factors affecting plasma vitamin D levels in Asian children living in England. *European Journal of Clinical Nutrition*, 53, 268–72.

McKinlay, A. (2006) Workshop round-up session. Rapporteur's report. *Progress in Biophysics and Molecular Biology*, 92, 179–84.

Norman A.W. (1998). Receptors for 1 (alpha), 25(OH) 2D3: past, present and future. *Journal of Bone and Mineral Research*, 13, 1360–9.

O'Hare, A.E., Uttley, W.S. *et al.* (1984) Persisting vitamin D deficiency in the Asian adolescent. *Archives of Disease in Childhood*, 59, 766–70.

Pal, B.R., Marshall, T. & James, C. (2003) Distribution analysis of vitamin D highlights differences in population subgroups: preliminary observations from a pilot study in UK adults. *Journal of Endocrinology*, 179, 119–29.

Pietrek, J., Window, J., Preece, M.A. & O'Riordan, J.L.H. (1976) Prevention of vitamin D deficiency in Asians. *Lancet*, 1, 1145–8.

Roy, D.K., Berry, J.L. *et al.* (2007) Vitamin D status and bone mass in UK South Asian women. *Bone*, 40(1), 200–4.

Shaw, N.J. & Pal, B.R. (2002) Vitamin D deficiency in Asian families: activating a new concern. *Archives of Diseases in Childhood*, 86, 147–9.

Shenoy, S., Swift, P. *et al.* (2005) Maternal vitamin D deficiency, refractory neonatal hypocalcaemia and nutritional rickets. *Archives of Diseases in Childhood*, 90(4), 437–8.

Solanki, T., Hyatt, R.H. *et al.* (1995). Are elderly Asians in Britain at a high risk of vitamin D deficiency and osteomalacia? *Age and Ageing*, 24, 103–7.

Stephens, W.P., Klimiuk, P.S., Berry, J.L. & Mawer, E.B. (1981) Annual high dose vitamin D prophylaxis in Asian immigrants. *Lancet*, 2, 1199–201.

Update on Vitamin D (2007) *Position Statement by the Scientific Advisory Committee on Nutrition*. The Stationary Office, London. www.sacn.gov.uk/pdfs/sacnpositionvitamind20070507.pdf.

Wharton, B. & Bishop, N. (2003) Rickets. *Lancet*, 362, 1389–400.

Willett, A.M. (2004) Factors affecting vitamin D status in older adolescents and their relevance to bone health. PhD Thesis, University of Cambridge.

Working Party on Fortification of Food with Vitamin D, COMA (Committee on Medical Aspects of Food Policy) (1980). HMSO, London.

Index

Multicultural Handbook of Food, Nutrition and Dietetics, First Edition. Edited by Aruna Thaker, Arlene Barton.
© 2012 Blackwell Publishing Ltd. Published 2012 by Blackwell Publishing Ltd.

for bottle feeds 331–7
for breastfeeding 327–31
for children 326
for pre-term infants 345–6
for preconception 317–19
for pregnancy 319–26
for weaning infants 337–45
heart disease *see* coronary heart disease and
    stroke
herbal remedies
    for coronary heart disease and stroke 128
    for diabetes 27–8, 56–7, 94, 230–1
herbs and spices
    East Asian 144–5, 174, 185–6
    Jewish traditions 206
    Mediterranean diets 217
    South Asian Sub-continent 13, 33, 76–7
    West Africa 260–1, 272–3
    West Indies 115–17
Hindu religion
    celebrations and festivals 5–6, 75–6
    demographic data and key features 4
    dietary implications 4–5, 86
HIV-positive mothers 330–1
Hoisin sauce 148
Holi festival 5–6
Homowo festival 269
hookah 220–1
hoppers 88
hospitality 4
'hot / cold' foods 14, 33, 90–1
    and pregnancy 69
Hunnan cuisine 141
hypercholesterolaemia 234
hypertension 58
    classifications 232
    dietary modifications 128–31, 152, 208, 232
    treatments 127–8
    see also coronary heart disease and stroke

Indian restaurants 74
infections, food-acquired 323–5
insulin 228
iodine deficiencies 97
iron
    deficiencies 20, 69, 97, 236
    sources 21
Islam
    demographic data and key features 42, 251,
      308

dietary influences and restrictions 43, 75, 86,
    237–8, 308–9
festivals and obligations 42–3, 75, 309
Israel 197–8
    see also Jewish diet

Jainism 5
Janmashtmi festival 6
Japanese diets 178–90
    common (traditional) foods 180–6
    cooking methods and food preservation 186–7
    cultural and religious influences 180
    demographic information 178–9
      UK migration 180
    further reading 190–1
    health and life expectancy 190
    meal patterns 188–90
    second-generation migrants 188–9
    use of alcohol and cigarettes 187–8
Jewish diets 197–211
    cultural and religious influences 199–205
      fasting 204–5
      festivals 203–5
      Hebrew calendar 201–3
      religious observances 201–5
    diet-related disorders 207–10
      cancer 209
      diabetes 208–9
      obesity 207–8
      stroke 208
    ethnographic information 197–9
      UK migration 199
    food production and preparation 201–6
      healthy eating alternatives 202, 205–7
      specific restrictions 200
    health practices 205
    nutritional support 209–10
    websites and resources 211
joint pain, therapeutic remedies 14

kadhi 8
karela (bitter melon gourd) 27–8, 56, 128, 147
Kashrut 200
kebabs 141–2, 302, 312
kenkey 271
Kill the Five Thieves 30
Kirat Karni 30
kosher foods 200
kulfi 49
Kuwait 219–20

lacto-vegetarian diets
  benefits 21
  South Asian populations 4
lactose intolerance 185, 272
lard 150, 283, 292
Lebanon 219
lentils *see* dal; pulses
lilva seeds 8
lime juice 10
linoleic acid 323, 324
listeriosis 324–5
locuma 311
low-fat dairy foods 130
lung cancer 356–7
lycopene 306

Macmillan Cancer support 362
mah ke dal 31
Maha Shivratri festival 5
maize and maize meal 270–1
Makar Sankranti (Kite Flying festival) 5
malawa pancake 240
malnutrition 95–6
masala 13
maternal and infant health 68–9, 96–7,
    317–51
  preconception 317–19
  pregnancy and lactation 319–26
  breastfeeding 326–31
  bottle feeding 331–7
  weaning 337–46
  food intolerances and allergies 346–7
  oral health problems 347–9
  websites and further reading 349–51
meat eating
  disease risk associations 66
  kosher preparations 200
  raw dishes 310
  religious observances 4, 43, 200–1
'Mediterranean' diets 117, 302–6, 314
metabolic syndrome 156, 363–6
  dietary modifications 365–6
  information sources 372–3
  prevalence 364
  treatments 364–5
  see also diabetes; hypertension; obesity
methionine 8
meze 312
milk and dairy products
  in East Asian diets 150, 173

in East and South–East European cuisines 282,
    299
in Eastern Mediterranean diets 239, 255
in Jewish traditions 201
in South Asian Sub–continent 9–10, 19, 37–8,
    76, 83
in West African diets 251, 272
in West Indian diets 116, 125
unpasteurized 334–5
use for infant feeds 334
miso 186
Mongolian dishes 140
monosodium glutamate (MSG) 151, 162, 174
Moon festival 144
Muharrem 309
mukhvas 14
mung flour 9
mushrooms 282

Naam Japna 30
naan bread 44
nasopharyngeal cancer 162, 361
nausea and vomiting, nutrition support 166
Navratri festival 6
New Year celebrations 6, 298
Nigerian diets 248–66
  common (traditional) foods 252–61
    healthy eating recommendations 254–8
    regional variations 250–1
  cultural and religious influences 250–3
    food taboos 253, 257, 258
  demographic information 248–50
    UK migration 250
  diet-related disorders 261–4
    coronary heart disease 263–4
    obesity 263–4
  eating patterns and meal preparations 251–2,
    253
  nutritional support 264–6
nitrosamines 66, 162
noodles 142, 148, 149, 171, 181
nutrition support 95–6, 117, 164–7, 209–10
  see also formula feeds; fortified foods
nutritional supplements 167, 368
nuts 9, 25
  sweet dishes 313

obesity
  cultural influences 53–4, 92–3, 122–3, 207
  definitions 51, 222–4